W0107498

IMMUNOPHARMACOLOGY
REVIEWS   VOLUME 1

A Continuation Order Plan is available for this series. A continuation order will bring delivery of each new volume immediately upon publication. Volumes are billed only upon actual shipment. For further information please contact the publisher.

IMMUNOPHARMACOLOGY REVIEWS
VOLUME 1

Edited by
John W. Hadden
and
Andor Szentivanyi

University of South Florida College of Medicine
Tampa, Florida

PLENUM PRESS • NEW YORK AND LONDON

ISBN 978-1-4615-7254-1   ISBN 978-1-4615-7252-7 (eBook)
DOI 10.1007/978-1-4615-7252-7

© 1990 Plenum Press, New York
Softcover reprint of the hardcover 1st edition 1990
A Division of Plenum Publishing Corporation
233 Spring Street, New York, N.Y. 10013

All rights reserved

No part of this book may be reproduced, stored in a retrieval system, or transmitted
in any form or by any means, electronic, mechanical, photocopying, microfilming,
recording, or otherwise, without written permission from the Publisher

CONTRIBUTORS

CHRISTINE M. ABARCA • Departments of Internal Medicine and Pharmacology, University of South Florida College of Medicine, Tampa, Florida 33612

MICHAEL CHIRIGOS • United States Army Medical Research Institute of Infectious Diseases, Frederick, Maryland 20701

RONALD G. COFFEY • Program of Immunopharmacology, Departments of Medicine, Pharmacology, and Medical Microbiology and Immunology, University of South Florida College of Medicine, Tampa, Florida 33612

JOEL B. CORNACOFF • Sterling Research Group, Rensselaer, New York 12144

JACK H. DEAN • Sterling Research Group, Rensselaer, New York 12144

JOHN W. HADDEN • Program of Immunopharmacology, Departments of Medicine, Pharmacology, and Medical Microbiology and Immunology, University of South Florida College of Medicine, Tampa, Florida 33612

EVAN M. HERSH • Section of Hematology and Oncology, Department of Internal Medicine, Arizona Cancer Center, University of Arizona, Tucson, Arizona 85724

JOSEPH J. KRZANOWSKI, JR. • Department of Pharmacology and Therapeutics, University of South Florida College of Medicine, Tampa, Florida 33612

MICHAEL I. LUSTER • National Toxicology Programs, National Institute of Environmental Health Science, Research Triangle Park, North Carolina 27709

JAMES B. POLSON • Department of Pharmacology and Therapeutics, University of South Florida College of Medicine, Tampa, Florida 33612

GERARD RENOUX • Faculty of Medicine, University of Tours, 37032 Tours Cedex, France

ANDOR SZENTIVANYI • Departments of Internal Medicine and Pharmacology, University of South Florida College of Medicine, Tampa, Florida 33612

CHARLES W. TAYLOR • Section of Hematology and Oncology, Department of Internal Medicine, Arizona Cancer Center, University of Arizona, Tucson, Arizona 85724

JOSEPH F. WILLIAMS • Department of Pharmacology and Therapeutics, University of South Florida College of Medicine, Tampa, Florida 33612

PREFACE

Immunopharmacology as a field of scientific endeavor had its origins more than thirty years ago in the application of antibody-based techniques to assays of hormones and drugs in tissues and body fluids. More recently, the field has been redefined to include a primary focus on the immune system as a target of xenobiotic action. Advances in the field of immunology have made it apparent that the immune system, like other organ systems, declines in its function as a result of aging, viral infections like AIDS, and other immunotoxic influences, giving rise to secondary immunodeficiency. Deficiency of the immune system in turn leads to infections, autoimmune diseases, and an increased incidence of certain cancers. The notion of treating the failing immune system is relatively new; however, more than a decade of research on cancer and AIDS has created the burgeoning new clinical field of immunotherapy.

Immunopharmacology then stands as the preclinical and clinical science of immune manipulation. As such, like its parent field of pharmacology, it includes within its scope basic studies of immune mechanisms as they relate to the pathogenesis of inflammation and immunologic disturbances. As with pharmacology, the perspective is always a therapeutic one. Studies of immune and inflammatory processes emphasize the use of pharmacologic probes and drugs to elucidate the underlying biochemical pharmacology. The development of drugs and biologicals for therapy is a central focus, and studies involving immunopharmacologic characterization of immunotherapeutic agents—in addition to the more conventional pharmacologic approaches to drug development—are thus a mainstream affair. Intrinsically linked to efforts to restore or stimulate the immune system are those to understand how immunosuppressive and immunotoxic influences operate. Thus immunotoxicology is an integral part of immunopharmacology.

With these pursuits at its core, immunopharmacology finds additional overlaps with other fields. Nutrition, for example, affects immune function, since specific defects, in zinc for example, can preferentially impair the immune system. The central nervous and endocrine systems play inordinately important roles in determining how the immune system functions; thus the fields of neuroendocrine immunology and chronobiology are intimately related. The biochemical pursuits of the mechanisms of transmembrane signaling and of the regulation of mediator release and action are central mechanistic concerns. Immunopharmacology therefore derives a distinctive "hybrid vigor" from its two parent fields, immunology and pharmacology, and from interdisciplinary interactions with many other fields.

As this definition of immunopharmacology has increasingly come into focus in the journals of the field and in the many published conference proceedings which reflect its development, it has become increasingly apparent to us that the field needs a primary reference series offering authoritative reviews.

This is the first volume of a new series of immunopharmacology reviews. We have intended these reviews to be "the best by the best." The compendium will over the years provide a strong reference background for use by research specialists and by the teachers and students of the field of immunopharmacology.

In this first volume we have selected reviews which discuss the immunopharmacologic and pharmacokinetic analyses of immunotherapeutic agents and the current status of their application to cancer; which reflect in depth on the molecular communications among the immune and central nervous systems and on transmembrane signaling processes involved in lymphocyte activation; and finally which cover the emerging field of immunotoxicology. Future volumes will expand on these reflections to examine the full range of cellular and molecular components and the disease processes intrinsic to our definitions of immunopharmacology.

John W. Hadden
Andor Szentivanyi

Tampa, Florida

CONTENTS

CHAPTER 2

PHARMACOKINETICS OF IMMUNOMODULATORS

JOSEPH F. WILLIAMS

CHAPTER 3

IMMUNOTHERAPY AND BIOLOGICAL THERAPY OF CANCER:
CURRENT CLINICAL STATUS AND FUTURE PROSPECTS

CHARLES W. TAYLOR AND EVAN M. HERSH

CHAPTER 4
THE PHARMACOLOGY OF MICROBIAL MODULATION IN THE
INDUCTION AND EXPRESSION OF IMMUNE REACTIVITIES: THE
PHARMACOLOGICALLY ACTIVE EFFECTOR MOLECULES OF
IMMUNOLOGIC INFLAMMATION, IMMUNITY, AND
HYPERSENSITIVITY

ANDOR SZENTIVANYI, JOSEPH J. KRZANOWSKI, JR., JAMES B. POLSON,
AND CHRISTINE M. ABARCA

CHAPTER 5

EARLY BIOCHEMICAL EVENTS IN T-LYMPHOCYTE ACTIVATION BY
MITOGENS

JOHN W. HADDEN AND RONALD G. COFFEY

CHAPTER 6

TOXICITY TO THE IMMUNE SYSTEM: A REVIEW

JACK H. DEAN, JOEL B. CORNACOFF, AND MICHAEL I. LUSTER

CHAPTER 1

THE CHARACTERIZATION OF IMMUNOTHERAPEUTIC AGENTS

JOHN W. HADDEN, GERARD RENOUX, and MICHAEL CHIRIGOS

1. INTRODUCTION

Two relatively recent scientific evolutions have raised therapeutic immunophar-macology to its present position of interest. The first concerns the progressive elucidation of primary and secondary immunodeficiency diseases over the last 25 years, and the second is the attempt to mobilize host resistance mechanism in the treatment of cancer over the last 15 years. Twenty-five years ago, immunodefi-ciencies were considered to be relatively rare clinical problems involving mainly patients who lacked the capacity to make antibody (Bruton agammaglobulinemia and acquired agammaglobulinemia) and patients with ataxia telangiectasia, Wiskott–Aldrich syndrome, or humoral immunodeficiency secondary to lym-phoid malignancy. With the development of the current concepts of the role of the thymus-dependent system of immunity and the cooperative roles of mac-rophages and natural killer cells with T lymphocytes in the expression of cellular immune response, there ensued an extensive analysis of the prevalence of cel-lular immune deficiencies in various human populations. Somewhat unexpected-ly, it was found that cellular immune deficiencies are not rare and that they occur to a degree in large percentages of the world's populations. In addition to a number of rare congenital deficiencies (such as the DiGeorge and Nezeloff syndromes), transient deficiencies were observed in neonates and in children

JOHN W. HADDEN • Program of Immunopharmacology, Departments of Medicine, Pharmacolo-gy, and Medical Microbiology and Immunology, University of South Florida College of Medicine, Tampa, Florida 33612.   GERARD RENOUX • Faculty of Medicine, University of Tours, 37032 Tours Cedex, France.   MICHAEL CHIRIGOS • United States Army Medical Research Institute of Infectious Diseases, Frederick, Maryland 20701.

1

with viral infections. As expected, cellular immune deficiency was found to be common in cancer patients and increased in severity with more widespread disease. It was compounded by intensive cytoreductive therapy with chemotherapy and irradiation. Similar deficiencies were seen following immunosuppressive drug therapy and exposure to immunotoxic chemicals. Impressive in terms of the numbers of people involved was the discovery of pronounced immune deficiencies associated with parasitosis, malnutrition, and aging. The general impression that was derived from these observations is that cellular immune deficiencies are a common precursor to a large variety of clinical diseases ranging from infection to cancer and autoimmunity. The degree of association is such as to indicate that the treatment of cellular immune deficiency is a clinical goal in itself to prevent these disease sequelae. Such an immunoprophylactic approach seems reasonable in the same context as we now treat coronary artery disease to prevent acute myocardial infarction or hypertension to prevent cerebral vascular accidents.

Estimations concerning the practicality and ultimate efficacy of such an approach rest on the progress in immunotherapy achieved over the last 20 years. Prior to 1968, when the first bone marrow transplant was performed for combined immunodeficiency syndrome, agammaglobulinemic patients had received γ-globulin, and a few with other diseases had received dialyzed leukocyte extracts called "transfer factor." With the opening of the clinical doors to cellular engineering in the form of bone marrow transplantation, much larger doors were opened to molecular engineering in a variety of diseases, most importantly cancer. After 15 years of experimental clinical immunotherapy in which thousands of human patients with cancer have been treated with a variety of drugs and biologicals, the need for a specific base, an immunopharmacology of immunotherapy, has never been more apparent.

It is our collected impression that the progress is sufficiently encouraging in cancer and even more so in viral infections and rheumatoid arthritis to warrant continued growth and development of immunotherapy. It is the intention of this chapter to describe what we consider to be some of the basic principles involved in how immunotherapeutic agents work. The process of characterizing immunotherapeutic agents has, heretofore, been an art; however, a sufficient number of basic principles have emerged to allow one to say that a science is in evolution. It is our intent to try to summarize some of its basics. Our attempt is to be totally comprehensive but, we hope, sufficiently liberal in its use of anecdotal examples to provide a solid grasp of the basic concepts. We apologize at the onset for biases that inherently derive from more experience with one drug or biological than another. The reader is referred to other texts for more comprehensive reviews of the immunopharmacologies of the agents involved (Chirigos, 1977a,b; Hadden et al., 1977a, 1981a,b, 1983a,b; Serrou and Rosenfeld, 1980; Hadden et al., 1980; Hersh et al., 1981; Serrou et al., 1982; Mihich, 1982; Hadden et al., 1983b; Fenichel and Chirigos, 1984; Fudenberg et al., 1984; Hadden and Spreafico, 1985, 1986). The discussion is restricted to the preclinical immunopharmacological analyses of chemically defined drugs and biologicals. Discussion of complex mixtures such as Bacille Calmette Guerin (BCG), *Corynebacterium parvum*, Krestin, picibanil (OK 432), and lentinan is largely avoided since these agents are chemically undefined in structure and have been covered extensively in several of the reviews mentioned above.

2. IMMUNOTHERAPEUTIC AGENTS

The agents to be included for discussion are listed in Table I, and a short discussion defining them has been included.

2.1. Immune System-Derived Biologicals

The advent of genetic engineering has created an explosion of development in this area that will continue unabated into the foreseeable future. The prospect of abundant quantities of inexpensive, pure, homogeneous molecules for prospective treatment carries with it an intense and exciting competition. The potential lack of toxicity, high degree of specificity, and lack of allergenic potential of

TABLE I
Substances That Affect the Immune System

Biologicals	Chemically defined drugs
Immune system	Sulfur-containing
Interferon α, β, γ	Levamisole
Thymic hormones	Immuthiol
Thymosin	NPT 16416
Thymostimulin (TP1)	Thiabendazole
Thymopoietin (TP5)	Benzimidazoles
Thymulin	Cimetidine
Thymic humoral factor	Purine/pyrimidine
Interleukin-2 (T-cell growth factor)	Isoprinosine
Interleukin-1 (lymphocyte-activating factor)	NPT 15392
Colony-stimulating factors	Pyrimidinoles
Tumor necrosis factor	Polynucleotides
Lymphotoxin	Poly A:U
Macrophage-activating factors	Poly I:C
Tuftsin	Miscellaneous
Bacteria/fungi	MVE-2
Glycans (e.g., krestin,	Azimexon
lentinan, glucan)	Bestatin
Muramyl dipeptides	LF 1695
Endotoxin	Indomethacin

the use of human regulatory molecules in human patients further support the appropriateness of the competitive development.

2.1.1. Interferons

The interferons are currently defined as α (leukocyte derived), β (fibroblast derived), and γ (lymphocyte derived) (Stewart, 1981). Representatives of each have been sequenced and genetically engineered in bacteria. All share the properties of inhibiting viral replication and cell growth and modulating immune function, particularly to activate macrophage and natural killer cell cytocidal functions. Activity in clinical cancer and in certain viral infections has been demonstrated.

2.1.2. Thymic Hormones

Thymopoietin, thymulin, and thymosin α_1 have been sequenced and either synthesized chemically or genetically engineered (Goldstein, 1984). Their structures differ, and evidence has been presented to indicate that they all derive from thymic epithelial cells and circulate in the blood. All three induce the differentiation of thymic cell precursors and modulate the function of mature T cells. They apparently do not induce intrathymic maturation. The purified hormones as well as partially purified thymic extracts [thymosin fraction V, thymostimulin (TP1), and thymic humoral factor] have shown activity clinically in primary immunodeficiency, cancer, and rheumatoid arthritis.

2.1.3. Interleukins

Soluble mediators produced by immune cells have often been termed lymphokines if produced by lymphocytes, monokines if produced by monocytes/macrophages, or cytokines if produced by any cells including lymphocytes or monocytes/macrophages (Hadden and Stewart, 1981). Thus far, interleukin-1 and II, tumor necrosis factor, lymphotoxin, and colony-stimulating factor have been sequenced and cloned. The cloning of other lymphokines regulating production, movement, and functions of various cell populations will soon follow.

Interleukin-1 or lymphocyte-activating factor is a monokine that induces T lymphocytes to make T-cell growth factor and B cells to differentiate and make immunoglobulin. It also functions as the fever regulator, endogenous pyrogen. Its therapeutic potential has not been fully explored.

Interleukin-2 (IL-2) or T-cell growth factor is a lymphokine that induces immature T-cell differentiation and operates as a second signal to complete the induction of proliferation of T lymphocytes from a G_1–S boundary restriction point. It therefore functions in both maturation and cloning of T cells. Deficiencies of IL-2 have been described in aging, autoimmunity, and acquired immunodeficiency syndrome (AIDS). Initial clinical trials in AIDS and cancer are currently in progress.

Tumor necrosis factor (TNF), a product mainly of macrophages, and lymphotoxin, a lymphokine, are structurally similar peptides that act directly to kill tumor cells of various types. Very recent data indicate that cloned human TNF has broad-spectrum antitumor activity in murine tumor systems.

Colony-stimulating factors (CSFs) govern the growth and maturation of granulocytes and macrophages. Several have been described as selective for either series or active on both series of cells. CSF_1, active on monocytes and macrophages, has been purified and is thought also to act as a macrophage-activating factor. Recently several CSFs have been reported to be cloned. Their therapeutic potential remains to be tested.

Other biologicals of therapeutic interest include lymphocyte chalones, transfer factor, dialyzable leukocyte factor, and suppressor factors. Purification and cloning efforts are awaited.

2.1.4. Tuftsin (Thr-Lys-Pro-Arg)

Tuftsin (Najjar and Bump, 1984), a tetrapeptide, represents the amino acids 289–292 of the immunoglobulin heavy chain and is thought to be selectively cleaved and liberated as an active fragment. It has been synthesized and shown to bind selectively to granulocytes, macrophages, and natural killer cells. It induces a modification of the functions of motility, secretion, and most importantly microbicidal and tumoricidal activity.

2.2. Bacteria and Fungi

The microbes represent rich sources of immunomodulator molecules, and considerable preclinical and clinical efforts support the biological activity of preparations of intact bacteria (including mixed bacterial vaccines), homogenized organisms, and extracts rich in peptidoglycans, lipopolysaccharides, or high-molecular-weight glycans. Selective chemical analysis in recent years has led to several relatively pure homogeneous preparations.

2.2.1. Glycans

A number of glycans have been described, including lentinan, krestin, levan, schizophyllan, and glucan (Aoki, 1984; DiLuzio, 1985; DiLuzio and Jacques, 1986). All share β_{1-3} glycosidic linkages, which appear to be essential for immunopharmacological activity. Particulate glycans persist in the body and induce granulomas; however, soluble forms are also active, and, for glucan itself, activity is seen in molecules as small as 10,000 daltons. The central action of glycans, exemplified by glucan, is the capacity to expand the reticuloendothelial system and to activate macrophages for enhanced microbicidal and tumoricidal activity. Many of the secondary features of their immunopharmacological action can be explained by the production of monokines such as interleukin 1 and colony-stimulating factor. Glucan itself has just entered clinical trials; however, extensive clinical testing of krestin and lentinan in Japan supports antitumor activity (when used in conjunction with cytoreductive therapy) and antiinfectious activity.

Muramyl dipeptide [N-acetylmuramyl-L-alanyl-D-isoglutamine (MDP)] (Chedid et al., 1978; Lederer and Chedid, 1982) represents the smallest component of the mycobacterial cell wall having adjuvant activity comparable to complete Freund's adjuvant and protective activity against pathogen challenge. More than 600 derivatives of MDP have been synthesized, and a spectrum of immunopharmacologies reported. All apparently have the capacity to activate macrophages and induce monokine production. Muramyl dipeptide itself is pyrogenic; however, several derivatives are not. Collectively the MDPs show antiinfectious and antitumor activity as well as adjuvancy with vaccines. Initial clinical trials have begun in several countries.

2.2.2. Endotoxins

Lipopolysaccharides (LPS) (Nowotny, 1983; Szentivanyi et al., 1986) have been extensively studied for action on the immune system, and many effects on macrophages and lymphocytes have been documented. Perhaps the most studied actions are those as polyclonal B-cell mitogens, activators of macrophages, and inducers of T-cell differentiation. The attendant toxicities including fever, cardiovascular collapse, RES blockade, and death have precluded serious thought about the clinical administration of LPS. Intensive efforts to define chemically the active components of various LPSs have been made, and evidence supports activity of both the polysaccharides and lipid A components. Recent reports of detoxification (Ribi, 1984) without loss of immunopharmacological activity suggest that LPSs or their components may yet become useful in clinical therapeutics.

2.3. Drugs

2.3.1. Sulfur-Containing Compounds

Levamisole [2,3,5,6-tetrahydro-6-phenylimidazo(2,1-b)thiazole] (Amery et al., 1977; Symoens and Rosenthal, 1977; Renoux, 1978; Amery and Hörig, 1984) is an immunopotentiating compound with mild effects to augment lymphocyte, macrophage, and neutrophil functions including proliferation, secretion, and motility. The action is evident with continued use (2–6 months) of intermittent doses (every week or every other week) in most but not all individuals tested. The action has been explained by effects on the GMP system similar to that of imidazole (Hadden *et al.*, 1975) and on the CNS–hepatic axis to produce a thymic-hormone-like substance, an action shared by other sulfur-containing compounds (Renoux and Renoux, 1977a,b; Renoux *et al.*, 1979a). The immunopharmacological actions have translated into mild clinical activity in a variety of neoplastic and infectious diseases and in rheumatoid arthritis.

Imuthiol (sodium diethyldithiocarbamate) (Renoux and Renoux, 1979, 1980, 1984) as an immunopotentiating compound shows some of the immunopharmacological features of levamisole, particularly those related to thymic-hormone-like activity; however, it is less toxic and in some systems more active. Clinical testing has been started in several diseases including AIDS.

Others—NPT 16416, thiabendazole, benzimidazoles, and cimetidine—all represent sulfur-containing compounds having immunopharmacological activity similar to levamisole (Hadden, 1985). The purine structure of NPT 16416 [7,8-dihydrothiazole(3,2-e)hypoxanthine] is thought to confer other immunopharmacological features to the levamisolelike structure (Hadden *et al.*, 1982). The thiabenzimidazoles [e.g., WY 18251, 3-*p*-chlorophenylthiazole(3,2-a)benzimidazole, 6-2 acetic acid (Fenichel *et al.*, 1980; Gregory *et al.*, 1980)] have additional antiinflammatory action. Cimetidine {N-cyano-N-methyl-N-[2'(5-methyl imidazole 4-ylmethylthio)ethyl]guanidine} (Friedman, 1981) also has an H_2-blocking capacity relevant to the inhibition of T suppressor activity.

2.3.2. Purines and Pyrimidines

Isoprinosine (N,N-dimethylaminoisopropanol plus *para*-aminobenzoic acid salt of inosine, 3 : 1 molar ratio) (Hadden and Giner-Sorolla, 1981; Tsang *et al.*, 1984; O'Neill *et al.*, 1984) has activity to induce T-lymphocyte differentiation comparable to thymic hormones and to potentiate the activity of antigens and lymphokines on lymphocytes and macrophages. It is nontoxic *in vivo* and stimulates cell-mediated immunity and human natural killer cell activity. It has seen extensive clinical use in viral infections and is licensed in 80 countries. It is currently being evaluated as an immunorestorative agent in AIDS and related diseases.

NPT 15392 (9-erythro-2-hydroxy-3-nonylhypoxanthine) (Hadden and Giner-Sorolla, 1981; Simon *et al.*, 1983) is a hypoxanthine derivative with an immunopharmacology very similar to that of isoprinosine; however, it is active at 1/101–1/1000 the concentration and has a longer duration of action *in vivo*. Its action as a thymomimetic compound has produced immunorestoration in a variety of immunodepressed conditions in animals including several cancer models. It is undergoing initial clinical testing in cancer patients.

Pyrimidinoles [2-amino-5-bromo- or 5-iodo-6-phenyl-4-pyrimidinoles (ABPP or AIPP)] (Stringfellow, 1981) activate macrophages and natural killer cells; apparently ABPP but not AIPP induces appreciable interferon levels. Both are active in murine viral and tumor models, and clinical tests have begun with ABPP.

Polynucleotides (Levy et al., 1981; Levy and Chirigos, 1984)—polyadenylate–uridylate (poly A : U), polyinosinate and cytidylate (poly I : C), and a complex of poly I : C with poly-e-lysine (poly lC : LC)—are polymers that to a greater or lesser degree induce interferon and activate macrophages and natural killer cells. Poly A : U induces T lymphocyte differentiation, perhaps mediated by cAMP. These polymers are antileukemic, particularly in high dose, and therefore potentially immunotoxic. Poly lC : LC has been under clinical evaluation in other cancers.

2.3.3. Other Compounds

MVE-2 (maleic anhydride divinyl ether) copolymers of molecular weight approximately 15,000 (Bartocci et al., 1980; Chirigos and Stylos, 1980; Carrano et al., 1984) are members of the pyran copolymer family. These compounds activate macrophages and natural killer cells, presumably through an interferon-mediated mechanism. MVE-2 also causes RES expansion associated with hepatosplenomegaly and drug retention. MVE-2 has shown activity in murine viral and tumor challenges and is undergoing initial clinical testing for toxicity and activity in cancer.

Azimexon [(2,2-cyanaziridinyl)-(1)-1-(2-carbamoylaziridinyl)-(1)-propane] (Chirigos and Mastrangelo, 1982; Bicker, 1984). This compound and its analogue ciamexon act to promote both lymphocyte and macrophage function in a potentiator mode of action. In addition to promotion of cellular immune response in vivo, azimexon expands the RES, perhaps through mediation of macrophage-derived colony-stimulating factor. It has shown activity in murine infections and tumor models using immunorestorative and adjuvant protocols. Initial clinical testing is under way in cancer and AIDS.

Bestatin [(2S, 3R)-3-amino-2-hydroxy-4-phenyl butyryl-1-leucine] (Umezawa, 1981), a dipeptide derivative of Streptomyces olivoreticuli, acts on macrophages, natural killer cells, promyelocytes, and perhaps T lymphocytes in a potentiator type of action. It reportedly enhances humoral and cellular immunity and partially protects mice against pathogen and tumor challenge. Clinical trials have been initiated in cancer.

Indomethacin   [1-(p-chlorobenzoyl)-5-methoxy-2-methylindole-3-acetic acid] is a nonsteroidal antiinflammatory drug used to treat inflammatory diseases (e.g., rheumatoid arthritis), presumably through its ability to inhibit the cyclooxygenase pathway of arachidonate metabolism and to prevent prostaglandin synthesis. This and related compounds have been considered for use in human cancer because, increasingly, prostaglandin-producing suppressor cells have been detected in cancer and are thought to contribute to tumor-induced immune suppression. Work in murine cancer models supports the possible future use of prostaglandin synthesis inhibitors in human cancer.

LF   1695   [(4-methyl-1-pyperidinyl)5-aminophenyl(4-chlorophenyl)methane] (Othmane *et al.*, 1984), a new immunostimulating compound probably can be classified as a thymomimetic drug since it induces T-cell differentiation and promotes various T-cell functions *in vitro* and *in vivo*. It is in a preclinical development phase and appears to be nontoxic in animals.

3. GENERAL FEATURES OF THE MODE OF ACTION OF IMMUNOTHERAPEUTIC BIOLOGICALS AND DRUGS

3.1. Classification

No simple nomenclature exists to conveniently describe the immunopharmacological actions of the various substances under study. Several are in popular use and are employed here because, although they do not serve to classify the agents, they do bring out nuances of their actions that are important to thinking about how best to analyze and to use them.

Most agents are classified as immunostimulants; however, the contexts in which stimulation occurs may differ widely. The most common setting to elicit stimulation is in combination with antigen, generally referred to as adjuvant action. Here it is useful to dissociate cellular immune responses from T-cell-dependent B-lymphocyte antibody responses, as they differ in their modulation. B-cell responses generally require a 24-hr inductive phase dependent on T helper cell and macrophage function prior to B-cell activation. Adjuvants of T-cell-dependent B-cell responses include almost all of the agents listed on Table I. Among the most active are the MDPs, endotoxins, and the polynucleotides. Of these the MDPs and polynucleotides are most active during the 24-hr inductive phase, whereas endotoxins are more active during B-cell activation. Polynucleotides actually inhibit the B-cell activation phase. A number of agents will act as adjuvants in preadministration protocols. In some cases the mechanisms are not clear; however, agents that act to induce RES expansion, e.g., MDP, glycans, azimexon, and MVE-2, are generally active in this regard. The chemically defined low-molecular-weight drugs such as levamisole and isoprinosine act best when given with or following antigen. Interferons have been reported to stimulate at low dose but inhibit at high dose. In general, the biologicals have not been extensively explored on T-cell-independent antibody responses.

Although it is well known that T-cell responses differ from B-cell responses in the triggering processes involved, the immunotherapeutic agents have not been carefully analyzed in this respect, and T-cell adjuvant is only recently recognized as a classification. A number of drugs including levamisole, imuthiol, isoprinosine, NPT 15392, and MDP stimulate cell-mediated immunity (CMI), and the biologicals, particularly the thymic hormones, do also.

As mentioned, one feature of some immunostimulating compounds is the capacity to augment not only the function but the number of cells of the re-

TABLE II

In Vivo Effects of Levamisole, Isoprinosine, and Thymic Hormones on Immune
Function of Experimental Animals[a] and Man

Immune function	Levamisole	Isoprinosine	Thymic hormones[b]
Experimental animals			
T-cell marker induction in athymic or thymectomized mice	+	+	+
T-cell mitogen response	+	+	+
Lymphokine production	+	+	+
Cytotoxicity of T cells	+	+	+
Immune function			
Cell-mediated immunity: DTH or graft rejection	+	+	+
T-dependent antibody production	+(variable)	+	+
Natural killer cell activity	?	+	?
Macrophage function	+	+	+
Resistance to pathogen challenge	+	+	+
Resistance to tumor recurrence			
Following cytoreductive therapy	+	NT[a]	+
Without cytoreductive therapy	0	0	0
Reduction of autoimmunity	+	+	+
Reversal of effects of aging on immune response	+	+	+
Man			
Active rosettes of T cells	+	+	+
T-cell mitogen response	±	+	+
Lymphocyte counts	±	±	±
DNCB or skin tests	+	+	+
Resistance to cancer	+ after chemo Rx	NT	+
Resistance to virus infection	+	+	+
Decreased autoimmunity	+	+	+

[a]Particularly in immunosuppressed mice.
[b]Particularly in thymectomized mice.
[c]NT, not tested.

ticuloendothelial (RES) system (e.g., glycans, MVE-2, and azimexon). This
action predicts increased clearance of intravascular particles and pathogens and
increased resistance to pathogens, particularly those infecting the RES.

Another useful grouping, in the context of immunostimulation and particularly immunorestoration, includes the thymic hormones and the thymomimetic

drugs. The thymic hormones have, as general features, the capacity to augment a variety of cellular immune functions, particularly in the thymus-deprived mouse or following suppression of the T-cell system as in cancer, aging, etc. See Table II for some of these features (Hadden, 1985).

There are two classes of agents that mimic thymic hormone action. One class includes levamisole, which on the basis of its sulfur moiety induces a thymic-hormone-like substance *in vivo* (Renoux and Renoux, 1977a,b). This action is shared by imuthiol and thiabendazole and probably the other sulfur-containing compounds listed in Table I. Notably these compounds do not induce T-cell differentiation *in vitro*. The second class is represented by isoprinosine, which on the basis of its 9-substituted hypoxanthine moiety induces T-cell differentiation, increases interleukin-2 production, and modulates T-cell functions. These actions are shared by NPT 15392 and other 9-substituted hypoxanthines (Hadden *et al.*, 1983).

Interferon induction is another common feature of the action of immunotherapeutic agents. The interferons are implicated in immunoregulatory phenomena leading to the activation of natural killer (NK) cells and macrophages for tumor cell killing. Agents such as the glycans, polynucleotides (poly A : U and poly IC : LC), polymers like MVE-2, and the pyrimidinoles induce interferon in association with the activation of macrophages and natural killer cells. In the case of NK cells, no direct relationship between level of interferon induced and degree of NK activation exists (Herberman *et al.*, 1979). It must be noted that other agents may activate one or the other of these tumoricidal populations in the absence of overt interferon induction (e.g., MDP activates macrophages, and isoprinosine, NPT 15392, and cyclomunine activate natural killer cells). Nevertheless, the interferon inducers share many immunopharmacological actions with each other and with the actions of exogenous administered interferons.

Another frequently observed feature of immunologically active compounds is the capacity to be immunomodulatory, that is, to stimulate at one dose and inhibit at another, usually at a higher dose. Virtually any substance at high enough dose can be observed to be inhibitory (Toman's law); therefore, it is important to distinguish whether the inhibitory effects represent physiological activation of suppressor mechanisms, antiproliferative effects on lymphocytes, specific immunotoxic effects, or nonspecific toxicity. The interferons are the most immunomodulatory of the immune-derived biological substances listed in Table I. Immunosuppressive effects of higher doses of interferons have been well documented and derive in part from their capacity to inhibit cellular proliferation. The bacterial and fungal agents have frequently been implicated in immune suppression, and the mechanism, where probed, generally involves macrophage-mediated prostaglandin production. The polymers MVE-2 and polynucleotides at higher doses have a particular propensity to be suppressive for T-cell responses and to be toxic for T cells. It is important not to ignore selective immunotoxicity at higher doses, since it may translate into antileukemic potential as with poly I : C and the interferons. A number of biologicals, e.g., thymic hormones, in-

terleukins, and tuftsin, and the drugs imuthiol, isoprinosine, NPT 15392, azimexon, and bestatin are relatively free of immunosuppressive influences at higher doses.

With these as well as the other agents listed in Table I, another common
feature of the action is immunologic activity at one dose and lack of effect at a
higher dose.

Another useful way of grouping agents has to do with their capacity to
activate one or the other of the two cyclic nucleotide systems, cyclic 3'-5'-
adenosine monophosphate (cAMP) or cyclic 3'-5'-guanosine monophosphate
(cGMP). A large body of evidence (see Hadden et al., 1977a; Hadden, 1977,
1983a, for review) indicates that agents that increase cGMP promote the functions of lymphocytes, macrophages, and granulocytes including proliferation,
secretion, and motility, and agents that increase cAMP generally inhibit these
functions but promote others such as T-cell differentiation. Table III reclassifies
the agents listed in Table I as to cyclic-nuceotide-related actions. This represents
a partial listing as only some of the agents have been analyzed. Several (e.g.,
cimetidine and indomethacin) can be predicted to be indirectly active by blocking
the production of substances known to act via the cAMP system.

3.2. Pharmacokinetics

The pharmacokinetics of immunotherapeutic agents have been generally
presumed to be basically similar to those of conventional drugs and, therefore,
have received relatively little interest. Unfortunately, as we have learned more
about the fundamental parameters of xenobiotic action as they apply to immunotherapeutics, we have been dealt surprises. The work of Stewart and co-
workers (Hanley et al., 1979) with interferons represents the first serious kinetic
study of biologicals derived from the immune system (Dianzini, 1985). These
works showed that following intramuscular administration, α-interferon distributed to blood and cerebrospinal fluid with a half-life of approximately 4 hr.

TABLE III
Cyclic Nucleotides Mediating the Actions of Various Agents

T lymphocyte		B lymphocyte	Macrophage
cGMP	cAMP	cGMP	cGMP
Thymosin V	Thymic humoral factor	Endotoxin	Tuftsin
Thymopoietin	Poly A:U		MDP
Interleukin I	Endotoxin		Levamisole
Interleukin II			Macrophage-activating factor
Levamisole			Interferons
Cimetidine			

The removal of the interferon was attributed to kidney catabolism and excretion. In contrast, β-interferon injected intramuscularly showed only a small fraction in the circulation; the remainder was lost as a result of local degradation. When given intravenously β-interferon showed a shorter half-life than α-interferon. Consider the implications of these observations. If β-interferon could only be given effectively intravenously and even then would be less active than α-interferon, what might the clinical results be. One might seriously question whether the clinical development of β-interferon was a worthy commercial effort. At the time these observations were made a number of pharmaceutical firms had already invested several million dollars in the production of β-interferon and a number of patients had been treated. It was notable that the only clinical responses seen were those following intravenous administration.

We are not aware of published data on the pharmacokinetics on the thymic hormones. Administration of thymosin fraction V intravenously leads to detectable serum levels of one of its constituents, thymosin α_1, which clear by 24 hr (A. Goldstein, personal communication). The serum half-life of thymopoietin pentapeptide given intravenously is apparently very short (<1 min) (G. Goldstein, personal communication). Similarly, the oligopeptide thymulin is thought to have a short half-life and needs stabilization with carboxymethylcellulose for effective administration.

Of the interleukins only IL-2 has been extensively reported on; its half-life following intravenous administration is <10 min (Cheever et al., 1985; Lotze et al., 1985). It is important, however, not to conclude that a relatively short half-life defines a lack of activity or a need to use higher doses or infusions to obtain sustained serum levels. The loss of a biological from the circulation may not represent biotransformation or excretion. In the case of interferons, thymic hormones, and interleukins, the target cells are thought to or have been shown to bear specific receptors. The loss from circulation may represent, in large part, specific absorption on target cell surfaces. More work is needed in this area to determine pharmacokinetics for the various biologicals using bioassay as well as radioimmunoassay in order to detect the true molecular turnover in relation to biological effect. Tissue distribution, biotransformation, and excretion are also essential features to explore.

Like the intact bacteria, the glycans and other polymers offer complexities in terms of pharmacokinetics. The particulate glycans induce granuloma formation and persist within the reticuloendothelial system for considerable time (DiLuzio, 1985). MVE-2 persists in the RES for up to 28 days (Chirigos and Mastrangelo, 1982; Carrano et al., 1981, 1984). The problem of persistence is a real one. It is a general impression that the persistence of inert materials in the body may have carcinogenic potential (e.g., cancers at sites of depot injections or tuberculosis scars). Although not documented as to mechanism, the prevalent impression of this association suggests that regulatory agencies will prefer readily metabolizable pharmaceuticals, and poorly biodegradable agents will be tolerated and approved only if therapeutic activity can only be gained in this manner.

In general, the chemically defined agents behave as drugs. The kinetics of clearance (half-life) have been published for such agents as MDP (Parant et al., 1979), levamisole (Schneiden, 1980), imuthiol (Brazier and Coquet, 1985; Guillaumin et al., 1986), and isoprinosine (T. Ginsberg, personal communication); the half-lives range from minutes to hours, but in general clearance is complete by 24 hr. The situation with levamisole is of interest. Levamisole is metabolized to the open-ring structure 2-oxo-3-(2-mercaptoethyl)-5-phenylimidazolidine (OMPI), whose metabolism and clearance from the circulation are considerably slower than those of levamisole itself (Schneiden, 1980). Both in vitro and in vivo OMPI has shown four to ten times the potency of levamisole (Symoens and Rosenthal, 1977). The appearance of intermediates with immunopharmacological activity is an important pharmacological issue that may have considerable implications in terms of patent security. Muramyl dipeptide offers some interesting nuances in terms of active metabolites. Chedid et al., (1984) have found that monoclonal antibodies to MDP will neutralize interleukin-1 activity, suggesting that MDP may be incorporated by macrophages into the molecular structure of interleukin-1. The persistence, then, of MDP in the circulation of the body may be that of interleukin-1.

As mentioned previously, the sulfur-containing compounds have been reported to induce a serum factor termed hepatosin (see Renoux et al., 1984). This factor has been observed in serum 12 hr after a single dose of imuthiol or levamisole, a time when no detectable drug exists in the serum. A similar factor having the capacity to induce T-cell differentiation in the Komuro–Boyse assay was reported 24 hr after a single dose of isoprinosine (Renoux et al., 1979b). The inference that immunostimulants induce hormonelike or lymphokine mediators that circulate and act in a cascade fashion over a prolonged period of time represents a distinct possibility.

3.3. Immunopharmacodynamics

It has been rather generally assumed that if an immunotherapeutic agent can no longer be found in the circulation, its biological activity has been completed, and, as with other pharmaceuticals, another dose is needed to sustain action. This concept appears to be completely erroneous as it applies to immunopharmacology. A number of examples support this statement with respect to compounds which are otherwise reasonably rapidly cleared from the circulation.

If a single dose of interferon is given, macrophage cytocidal activity increases to peak at 3 days and then declines slowly to near control levels (Saito et al., 1985). Natural killer cell activity also increases to peak at 3 days and declines by 5 days. When two or more doses of interferon are given consecutively, the macrophage increase occurs but not the NK cell increase. On this basis the strategy for augmenting NK cell activity with interferon would call for spaced interferon dosing, perhaps on a weekly basis.

The interferon inducer AIPP, as well as other interferon inducers, produces a refractory state for interferon induction following a single administration (Stringfellow, 1981). Despite clearance of the drug itself and the induced interferon after 24 hr, the protective effect to challenge with virus or tumor lasts up to 7 days. It was found that weekly administration of the drug gives persistent protection.

Levamisole when administered on a triple dose basis (i.e., three consecutive days a week) produced changes in immune parameters for up to 1 week (Sunshine et al., 1976) and when given as a single dose of 50 mg/week it still retained activity in rheumatoid arthritis. When it was administered more frequently on a daily basis, either no increase in positive effects occurred or an increase in negative effects resulted (Veys and Symoens, 1981). Imuthiol given as a single dose also modified immune parameters for up to 1 week; however, repeated administration was not inhibitory in man (Renoux and Renoux, 1984). Isoprinosine given as a single dose modified immune parameters for up to 1 week (Vecchi et al., 1978; Tsang et al., 1984); its analogue NPT 15392 has demonstrated effects up to 14 days following a single injection (Florentin et al., 1982). Cyclomunine, a fungus-derived oligopeptide similar to cyclosporin A, was shown, following a single dose of 250 μg/kg, to increase thymulin serum levels up to 240 days (Dardenne et al., 1980).

Such persistent effects on the immune system are unheard of in terms of pharmacodynamics associated with conventional pharmaceutical agents. Unfortunately, the extent to which other agents described in Table I have similar prolonged effects have not been tested. The possibility that they too have persistent activity over several days is real. It is disturbing that we may have learned, after years of clinical testing, a fundamental principle of immunopharmacology that redefines how that clinical testing might best be performed. It seems essential to examine in detail the optimal frequency of administration of each of the agents described in order to determine the best regimen to produce a response and to sustain it or to increase it cumulatively. We consider dose finding an important issue for defining the optimal efficacy of immunotherapy.

3.4. Toxicology

It is not possible within the scope of this review to develop the realm of general toxicology and immunotoxicology of the immunotherapeutic agents under discussion, as this will be dealt with in a later review in this series. It is, however, important to emphasize that most immunologically active agents are immunomodulatory; i.e., they can suppress immune responses at high dose. It is also important to determine the relationship of dose–response characteristics of an agent to augment and to suppress in order to predict effectively the margin of safety and the benefit-to-risk ratio. Given the considerable variability on a dose basis of individual response to immunotherapeutic agents, a wider margin of safety is needed than seems to be the case with other drugs. Also doses active of a particular agent for one disease may be quite different from those for another disease. Immunotoxicology is not often monitored carefully, as it is considered an undesirable effect to be avoided; however, the nature and character of any immunotoxic effects must be defined with the same care as the positive actions of the agent. Screening of body weight (as an index of general health), lymphoid organ weight and cellularity, and white blood cell counts and differential counts are important routine issues to consider in the course of an immunopharmacological evaluation in addition to the conventional tests for toxicity and immunotoxicity routinely performed to assess acute, subacute, and chronic toxicity. It is important to note frequency of infection and nature of death, as the toxicologist may not tend to relate the presence of infection, cancer, or inflammatory or wasting diseases to immunotoxic effects.

3.5. Side Effects

It is not possible here to catalogue the various side effects associated with any specific agent but only to emphasize those generally associated with immunologically active agents (see Werner et al., 1977; Georgiev, 1983a,b; Descotes, 1986; Mihich and Kantor, 1987). The first is that immunostimulating agents have a theoretical potential for augmenting allergic and inflammatory processes and perhaps to predispose to lymphoid malignancy. In fact, there are few if any examples of this happening. As an example, rheumatoid arthritis is improved by several thymic hormone preparations, levamisole, and isoprinosine. Incidence of spontaneous lymphoid malignancy has been reduced by pretreatment with isoprinosine (Sergiescu et al., 1981), levamisole, bestatin, and tuftsin (Bruley-Rosset et al., 1981, 1985). Nevertheless, these possibilities must be kept in mind.

In general, the agents listed in Table I are relatively nontoxic for systems other than the immune system. Alterations of the immune system leading to side effects are frequent. With the biologicals the first consideration is whether the proteins derive from heterologous species. For example, thymosin fraction V derived from bovine thymus contains proteins antigenic for the human, and clinical therapy is associated with local and systemic allergic problems. For the biologicals cloned from human genes in bacteria or yeast, the degree to which microbial substituents are added to the gene product will define their potential for allergy. Also requirements exist to purify the products from allergenic microbial constituents and from immunologically active endotoxin before a particular biological can be considered safe. Theoretically, the pure gene product will be remarkably safe except insofar as its action does not by definition induce symptoms; e.g., cloned interferon induces symptoms of fever, malaise, and myalgias, i.e., a "flulike syndrome," which can be considered an intrinsic part of the immunopharmacological action of interferon.

Other effects not generally considered may be produced by drugs and biologicals derived from the immune system or the endocrine and central nervous systems. For example, thymosin α_1 decreases luteinizing hormone release from the pituitary and increases serum corticosteroids, presumably through induction of ACTH; thymosin B_4 has the opposite effect (Hall et al., 1984). Lymphokines have been reported to increase serum corticosteroid levels (Besedovsky et al., 1983). Muramyl dipeptide is associated with fever and sleep regulation (Chedid, 1983) and imuthiol and isoprinosine are associated with CNS stimulation (Renoux et al., 1984; A. Glasky, personal communication). These endocrine and CNS interactions may be more than fortuitous and may reflect the coordinated integration of the immune, endocrine, and nervous systems (see Fabris et al., 1972; Cooper, 1984; Renoux and Biziere, 1985, for reviews).

3.6. Dose and Route of Administration

Bliznakov and Adler (1972), in studies with a variety of agents, were likely the first investigators to show that animal responses to bacterial, protozoal, or viral challenges were dose dependent and usually had two peaks of maximal action. It has become increasingly evident that most immunotherapeutic agents, such as BCG (Mitchell et al., 1973; Florentin et al., 1976; Piessen et al., 1977; Turcotte et al., 1978), LPS (Neter, 1969; Personn, 1977; Behling and Nowotny, 1977), Brucella extracts (Renoux et al., 1970), C. parvum (Kirchner et al., 1975; Nagoya et al., 1977), poly A : U (Morris and Johnson, 1978), MDP (Leclerc et al., 1979), tilorone (Megel and Gibson, 1984), lentinan (Hamuro and Chihara, 1984), levamisole (Renoux, 1978; Mantovani and Spreafico, 1975), isoprinosine (Hadden and Wybran, 1981), NPT 15392 (Floretin et al., 1982), Wy 18,251 or Wy 40,453, two thiazolobenzimidazole compounds (Fenichel et al., 1980; Gregory et al., 1980), and thymic hormones (Primus et al., 1978; Talmadge et al., 1984a) can have time-and dose-dependent regulatory characteristics causing either enhancement or inhibition of various immune responses as well as of tumor development. It should be pointed out that microorganisms are also immunomodulators. Small amounts of many bacterial products, as well as viral components, may serve as potent stimulators of specific and nonspecific host defense, whereas relatively large amounts of the same component are immunosuppressive and block various host defenses (Friedman et al., 1983).

As with other drugs, each immunotherapeutic agent will have its optimal dose. What may be unique features of their action include the following. (1) An action may be observed at extremely low doses otherwise considered homeopathic. For example, 2 mg/kg of levamisole once a week has been reported to be active in rheumatoid arthritis (Veys and Symoens, 1981), and 0.1 mg/kg of NPT 15392 as one dose is active for more than 1 week. (2) An extraordinary range of concentrations may be active; e.g., MDPs, NPT 15392, imuthiol, and endotoxin show activity over a range of several orders of magnitude of concentration. (3) Dose–response curves with two peaks of activity are seen with levamisole and isoprinosine on lymphocyte function. (4) Biphasic dose–response curves exist where activity is seen at one concentration and is lost or converted to suppression at higher concentrations.

A final point deserves special emphasis. The rules of conventional pharmacology generally dictate that increasing dose is associated with increased response, and the optimal dose is that which is most active given the limitation of side effects. It is almost axiomatic in immunopharmacology that increasing an active dose leads not to more effect but to less.

Most drugs and biological agents are administered to mice by the parenteral route (intravenous, intraperitoneal, and subcutaneous route). In man, similarly, these routes seem to be appropriate, since these sizable proteins are not expected to be orally active. For the drugs, a need exists to emphasize the oral route in the evaluation of an agent once it can be determined that this route is effective. Chemically defined agents that are orally active include the muramyl dipeptides, the sulfur-containing drugs, isoprinosine, NPT 15392, azimexon, and indomethacin. The glycans, endotoxin, polynucleotides, and pyran copolymers are only active parenterally.

The routes by which an agent is active are important to consider in relation to developmental perspectives. Because of cost and convenience factors, parenterally administered agents will ultimately have restricted application. If relatively devoid of side effects (e.g., thymosin and TP1), they may be administered like vitamin B_{12} in the doctor's office; however, if they are more complicated in their action, like the interferons and interleukin 2, their use may be restricted to the hospital setting. To justify the expense and inconvenient method of administration, their efficacy will need to be measurably greater. On a cost and convenience basis, the orally active drugs, given comparable efficacy, have been and will probably continue to be more desirable to the patient, clinician, and the pharmaceutical industry.

The frequency of administration is another issue that apparently dissociates immunotherapeutic agents from conventional drugs. Many appear to be active on an intermittent basis, and this phenomenon is discussed in greater detail in the next section.

3.7. General Clinical Pharmacology Principles Relating to Drug Development

Except for the situations mentioned above, the evaluation of immunotherapeutic biologicals and drugs is generally comparable to that for other drugs. Following discovery and initial testing, usually patent considerations pertain. In the case of biologicals, some unusual situations have arisen relevant to genetically engineered materials and monoclonal antibodies, which are in the process of being legally resolved (see Crespo, 1982). In the case of biologicals, it is important to analyze subunit structures in the search for patentable synthetic molecules constituting the active site; similarly, derivatives may yield more stable or active molecules. In the case of drugs these relationships are more easily understood as a result of past experience (see Hammer, 1982). Issues of basic chemistry formulation are not reviewed here, and the reader is referred to the extensive compendiums of Georgiev (1983a,b).

Because the waters of preclinical and clinical therapeutic immunopharmacology are only now being charted, the selection of a strategy of development for any particular substance is a complicated one often involving more intuition than science. Based on historical perspective the selection of an optimal compound of a series is generally better done in retrospect. Thus, on a prospective basis, a knowledge of the class of compound, its general characteristics, and the cellular targets of its action is very useful in the development of structure–function relationships. A general rule is that if the primary cellular target can be defined and the compounds are generally nontoxic, one or more simple and reliable *in vitro* assays can be selected to screen analogues. With demonstration of *in vivo* activity, one or the other of the two primary screening assays discussed in the next section (Jerne plaque assay or mitogen assay with spleen cells) can be used to comparatively test active analogues. It pays to remain simple at this stage. Once a prototype compound is selected, and with the establishment of molecular identity, purity, and an acceptable form or vehicle for *in vitro* and *in vivo* use, the preclinical evaluation may proceed.

The decision to proceed with the cost and effort involved in the general approach to development and licensing (see Table IV) cannot be reasonably made without an analysis of acute toxicity and, in particular, immunotoxicity. The definition of toxic potential in relation to therapeutic efficacy is an issue only recently defined for agents of this type. The biologicals, particularly if they are

TABLE IV

Flow Chart for Characterization of Potential Immunotherapeutic Agents: Toxicopharmacology

1. Chemistry: formula, identification procedures
2. Acute and chronic toxicities (two animal species); route of administration
3. Pyrogenicity; inflammatory reactions
4. General pharmacology: hematology, biochemistry, pathology; influences of the agent on heart, brain, liver, kidney, etc.; compatabilities with other drugs
5. Pharmacokinetics and biodisposition
6. Carcinogenesis, tumor-promoting influence, mutagenesis
7. Teratology

derived from the human and are to be administered to humans, can be generally considered remarkably safe with probably indeterminate or at least very high maximum tolerated and lethal doses. Their toxicity testing in a heterologous species capable of sensitization and, therefore, of irrelevant immunotoxicology is to be avoided. The immunotherapeutic drugs offer more complexity and are similar to other drugs in the sense that toxicities may be limiting (e.g., azimexon, MVE-2, poly IC : LC). The nature of the immunotoxicity of a particular compound (see Table IV) can be very important in understanding its mechanisms of action and should receive a careful analysis. The more important consideration is efficacy. The criteria of efficacy in relation to immunorestoration in secondary immunodeficiency or to the treatment of any of the diseases that result (i.e., cancer, autoimmunity, infection) remain to be firmly established.

The selection of preclinical end points and the rate and direction the development will take will depend to a considerable extent on a series of factors many of them unrelated to the agent itself (see Hammer, 1982). These features include management disposition and education, corporate marketing targets and expertise, funds available, experience with similar products, trained personnel able to perform the requisite testing, and/or an aggressive development psychology. Many pharmaceutical companies unaware of the requirements for specific training in therapeutic immunopharmacology have rechanneled inflammation-oriented pharmacologists into the area. The lack of a reasonably sophisticated background in immunology and in the relation of the immune system to disease predisposition and pathogenesis can be major impediments to a speedy and successful development strategy. We consider both on-site and consultative immunopharmacological expertise to be a necessity.

With a decision to proceed with development, the selection of preclinical end points is important in defining the timing of further toxicity, mutagenicity, and carcinogenicity testing and the setting of preclinical and clinical disease-related goals. From an immunopharmacological standpoint, the ability to establish targets of action is the first essential. Once a determination can be made that the prototype substance is a T-cell adjuvant or potentiator, a macrophage activator, an NK-cell stimulant, an interferon inducer, etc., a series of abstract as well as experimental comparisons can be made with existing compounds. Knowledge of some of the nuances and ambivalences of agents in a class may be very useful in considering the potential of the agent, e.g., whether a T-cell regulator promotes suppressor T-cells or a macrophage activator induces endogenous pyrogen production (i.e., fever) or prostaglandin production. Often carefully comparing *in vitro* and *in vivo* effects will reveal whether or not expectations have been consistently met. Any inconsistencies are important in indicating unique features of an agent, both positive and negative.

It is important to stress bottom-line interpretations. If a drug is active on T cells and/or macrophages, it should stimulate delayed hypersensitivity to sheep

TABLE V
Flow Chart for Characterization of Potential Immunotherapeutic Agents:
Immunopharmacology–Immunotoxicology

1. *In vitro* immunopharmacology: cellular targets, dose–response relationships, threshold of toxicity, biochemical mechanisms
2A. *In vivo* administration and tests: influences of doses and schedule of administration
   a. Lymphoproliferation: spleen, lymph node, thymus, liver weights; induction of lymphomas in a model such as NZB mice
   b. Immediate and delayed hypersensitivities induced by the agent
 B. *In vivo* administration, *ex vivo* tests
   a. Toxic effects on the hematopoietic system: blood cell counts, bone marrow colony-forming unit (CFU) counts, modifications in number or percentage of immunocytes
   b. Cellular immune response against the agent
   c. Immunoglobulin levels
   d. Induction of antibodies against the agent
   e. Induction of autoantibodies by the agent
   f. Increase in IgE specific for an allergen (e.g., ovalbumin)
3. Preclinical characterization of agents

erythrocytes or oxazolone. If it is active on B cells and/or macrophages, it should stimulate antibody levels following antigen challenge. If the agent is an activator of macrophages, it should increase macrophage number and/or function to kill facultative intracellular pathogens or tumor cells. If the agent stimulates natural killer cells, resistance to virus and tumor challenge should be affected. If any of these basic predictions do not pertain, a potentially serious immunopharmacological side effect or shortcoming may exist.

Once the principal immunobiological and/or immunorestorative effects can be established, appropriate disease models can be selected. The possibilities are many, and the scientific and commercial positioning of related products will factor into the decision. In general, large potential markets like cancer and rheumatoid arthritis tend to attract the most interest; however, chronic and recurrent infections and secondary immunodeficiency (e.g., the AID-related complex) are increasingly being seen as more facile therapeutic proving grounds. With the demonstration of a primary immunopharmacological action of a compound that is consistent with a potential to reverse the immunodeficiency or immunopathology of a particular disease state, the next step is the selection of the appropriate animal models for preclinical testing and the decision to proceed further with toxicopharmacology (Table V). The decision to go ahead, the pace, and the degree of investment of time and effort will depend on a constellation of features both tangible and intangible. This chapter is oriented toward maximizing the understanding of the tangible features of the process.

4. PRECLINICAL CHARACTERIZATION OF AGENTS

4.1. In Vitro Immunopharmacology

The *in vitro* approach offers several important advantages in the analyses of these agents (see Hadden, 1983b). It allows a dissection of cell populations so that principal cellular targets of an agent's action can be delineated, the dose–response relationships characterized, and the molecular mechanisms probed. It is only with primary cellular targets identified that the complexities of *in vivo* action can be deciphered. It is important to emphasize that the immune system is composed of an elaborate network of molecular intercommunications among the cells involved with both positive and negative feedback loops and that a predicted response can only be achieved with manipulations that are carefully constructed and timed.

4.1.1. Precursor Differentiation

Relatively little is known about therapeutic regulation of hematopoietic and myeloid cell growth and development. Colony-stimulating factors (CSFs) acting selectively on granulocytes (G) or macrophages (M) and on GM precursors have been described using bone marrow or spleen colony formation in soft agar assay. Similarly, growth inhibitors (chalones) have been described. Recent investigations have identified several immunotherapeutic agents that can stimulate the induction and secretion of CSF. Both azimexon and imuthiol stimulate the production of CSF (Mossalayi *et al.*, 1986; Schlick *et al.*, 1985). The MDPs induce production of a macrophage growth factor that is also a CSF (Schindler *et al.*, 1986), and it seems likely that other macrophage activators, e.g., glycans will show similar effects. Therapeutic regulation of myeloid growth can be envisioned to be beneficial in overcoming the suppressive effects of chemotherapy or radiotherapy by using chalones to suppress growth and thereby protect the population during the therapy or by using growth factors to restore proliferation following therapy.

Lymphocyte growth is thought to be regulated at the mature T-cell level by interleukin-2, and recent evidence indicates that the replication of T-cell precursors is also controlled by IL-2 (Hadden *et al.*, 1986). The regulation of B-lymphocyte growth at the precursor level remains to be clarified. Simple cloning assays are not generally available for assessment of the growth of lymphocyte precursors.

Perhaps best developed is our understanding of the regulation of T-lymphocyte differentiation and function. A variety of chemically defined thymic hormone preparations are available (e.g., thymosin α_1, thymopoietin, and thymulin; see Hadden *et al.*, 1986, for review). The *sine qua non* of the actions of these hormones *in vitro* is that they induce prothymocyte differentiation in the Komuro and Boyse assay or the Bach azathioprine-sensitive rosette assay. A number of chemically defined drugs will mimic these actions. Included are agents that are thought to act by increasing cAMP, such as poly A : U and endotoxin (LPS). Other agents such as isoprinosine and NPT 15392 also induce; however, their mechanisms are unknown. Agents containing sulfur such as levamisole and imuthiol are not directly active; however, *in vivo* they induce a serum factor that in turn is active *in vitro*.

B-cell differentiation is less well studied. Both bursapoietin and a splenin have been described, and nonspecific induction of maturation markers *in vitro* has been shown with endotoxin, poly A : U, and isoprinosine (Scheid *et al.*, 1975; Hadden and Giner-Sorolla, 1981; Audhya *et al.*, 1983).

T-cell markers such as T-cell rosettes with sheep erythrocytes (SRBC), particularly when depressed, have been useful in demonstrating the action of thymic hormone preparations, and drugs acting in a similar manner include isoprinosine, levamisole, NPT 15392, and lynestrenol (Hadden and Wybran, 1981). Restoration of trypsinized SRBC receptors has not in our hands proved to be a reliable assay for the action of these agents. Relatively little has come of efforts to modify the surface markers of T-helper or T-suppressor cells. The maturation of intrathymic lymphocytes has been poorly responsive to thymic hormone preparations; however, interleukin-2 and endotoxin are very active in inducing maturation in terms of surface markers as well as proliferative responses (Hadden *et al.*, 1986). Levamisole has also been described to be active (Otterness *et al.*, 1979).

4.1.2. T-Cell Functions

The most commonly used assays are those utilizing lectin mitogens such as phytohemagglutinin (PHA) or concanavalin A (Con A) or alloantigens in mixed leukocyte culture. Drugs such as isoprinosine, NPT 15392, lynestrenol, levamisole, imuthiol, and azimexon are active. The thymic hormones have been relatively inactive in these assays. T-cell functions such as lymphokine production and cytolytic, helper, and suppressor activity have also been studied. In the case in which thymic hormone preparations or the drugs have been shown to be active on proliferation, positive actions have also been seen in the other T-cell functions.

4.1.3. B-Cell Functions

The production of plasma cells with cytoplasmic immunoglobulin has been shown to be promoted by pokeweed mitogen or endotoxin. The effect of pokeweed mitogen has been reported to be stimulated and potentiated by NPT 15392 (Pompidou *et al.*, 1985). Isoprinosine is also active in this assay (A. Pompidou, personal communication). Antibody responses of murine plaque-forming cells to SRBC have been shown to be increased by levamisole and isoprinosine. A potent effect of levamisole to reverse the suppressive effect of soluble immune response suppressor factor (SIRS) and interferon has been reported (Aune and Pierce, 1983).

4.1.4. Macrophage Functions

The macrophage offers responsive assays for the action of agents; however, the significance of effects are often in doubt because this cell is so sensitive to manipulation. Responses such as chemotaxis, phagocytosis, pinocytosis, and chemiluminescence have been reported to be altered by a number of agents. The knowledge that the responses of macrophages to inflammatory stimuli (the ''inflammatory'' macrophage) are distinct from the responses to immunologic stimuli (the ''activated'' macrophage) indicates that tests involving bactericidal and tumoricidal activity or proliferation are the most germane to predicting whether macrophage-mediated resistance will be enhanced (see Hadden et al., 1981a). Lymphokines, interferons, and endotoxin are all potent inducers of macrophage activation for killing, and their interactions are potentiative. Muramyl dipeptide (MDP) and derivatives are potently active in this regard (Taniyama and Holden, 1979) and will potentiate the action of low concentrations of lymphokines (Fidler et al., 1981), particularly when encased in liposomes.

A number of agents do not directly activate macrophages; however, they do potentiate lymphokine effects to do so. Examples are the effects of levamisole, isoprinosine, azimexon, and NPT 15392 to potentiate lymphokine-induced macrophage microbicidal capacity or proliferation (Hadden et al., 1979). Muramyl dipeptide both modulates lymphokine-induced macrophage proliferation and acts itself to induce proliferation (Schindler et al., 1986). The production of soluble mediators having both positive [e.g., interleukin-1 (LAF), endogenous pyrogen, and collagenase] and negative effects [prostaglandins (PG)] has been reported with MDP (Wahl et al., 1979), and these observations deserve further study with analogues and other agents to know what the therapeutic significance may be. Certainly, the production of PG and endogenous pyrogen can be predicted to be limiting features of the action of agents, as both fever and suppressed proliferative and cytolytic responses of lymphocytes and macrophages result.

4.1.5. Interferon Induction

Interferon and interferon inducers can be assayed by inhibition of viral replication in a number of systems. Many inducers (e.g., poly I: poly C, poly IC : LC, poly A : U, and tilorone) are suppressive to lymphocytes (particularly of the T lineage), as are high concentrations of interferon itself. 6-Phenylpyrimidinone (ABPP) has been shown to induce interferon and is receiving attention as a less toxic therapeutic agent in this class (Stringfellow, 1981).

The foregoing represents only a sampling of the assays in use and some of the agents shown to be active.

4.2. In Vivo Characterization of Immunotherapeutic Agents

A general review of these agents has led to a conceptualization of the specifications of candidates for clinical trials. Before such trials, the agent should be well defined in its influences on sets or subsets of immunocompetent cells. As demonstrated by *in vivo* assays, the ideal agent should have no immunosuppressive effects with prolonged administration. The absence of carcinogenicity, of tumor-promoting influence, and of antigenicity or sensitizing effect is an important prerequisite. Known toxic levels and levels yielding pharmacological effects will help in delineating the range of doses and in predicting most adverse effects. Knowledge of cell targets defined *in vitro* will be essential for interpreting the *in vivo* effects as to direct versus indirect actions and, therefore, provides valuable information on the mechanisms of action of these agents.

Obviously, a principal aim of immunopharmacological investigation is the use of animal models for the exploration of human problems. The nature of the knowledge sought involves a treatment that for ethical reasons cannot be carried out in man until a detailed appraisal of the toxicopharmacological and immunologic properties of the agent has been performed.

4.2.1. Laboratory Mouse

Before discussing immunopharmacological studies in mice some general comments about the use of mice are important. The laboratory mouse is the animal of choice for characterization of immunotherapeutic agents, mainly because mouse immune cells and their gene products have activities similar, if not identical, to their human counterparts. In general, the results gained from mouse immune studies can be reasonably extended to human clinical testing.

Information on the characteristics of inbred and genetically defined strains of mice may be found in Altman and Dittmer Katz (1979), Festing (1979), Staats (1980), Greene (1981), and *Mouse News Letter* (Jackson Labs). The use of inbred animals (see Cohen, 1979) permits both testing of a specific treatment on the response of the animal with the potential for the repetition of the experiment at another time or in another laboratory and the exploitation of the unique properties of particular strains. The concept of uniqueness also includes the introduction of specific alleles into an inbred background to provide a line specifically created for particular studies (e.g., athymic nude, beige mice). Use of the F_1 hybrid from two inbred strains is sometimes preferred for bioassay; these animals retain the advantage of genetic uniformity while adding superior development and physiological homeostasis. The cost of the hybrid also is somewhat lower than that of pure strains.

We know from the studies of the mouse immunogeneticists that histocompatibility (H-2)-defined responsiveness bears a close relationship to resistance to engraftment of foreign tissues and to response to a number of selected antigens; however, resistance to complex infections such as herpes simplex (Lopez, 1975) or *Listeria monocytogenes* (Cheers and McKenzie, 1978) or to some spontaneous or induced cancers (Williams *et al.*, 1975) involve genetic loci outside of the H-2 complex.

Resistance to both infection (herpes viruses or *Listeria monocytogenes*) and tumor development is generally considered to be principally within the domain of cellular immune response (i.e., T lymphocyte and macrophage mediated). Although certain aspects of cellular immunity such as graft rejection, graft-versus-host reactions, and mixed leukocyte reactions are dictated by genes of the H-2 complex, it is perhaps not surprising that resistance characteristics might involve multiple genes outside the H-2 locus including those determining nonimmunologic resistance characteristics.

An examination of mouse strains relatively susceptible or resistant to herpes virus infection (Lopez, 1975), *Listeria monocytogenes* infection (Cheers and McKenzie, 1978), or mammary tumor development (Cotzias and Tang, 1977) reveals an interesting pattern. For each of these diseases the C57BL/6 strain of mice has been shown to be highly resistant. In contrast, the DBA/2 strain is highly susceptible. Other relatively susceptible strains include the C3H and the Balb/c. It is of note that these three strains all find common ancestry in DBA stock (Staats, 1980). A similar pattern of resistance and susceptibility emerges for H-2-linked susceptibility to leukemogenesis (Lilly and Pincus, 1973) and resistance to allogeneic engraftment following irradiation (Cudkowicz and Bennett, 1971).

Based on limited studies of comparative immune responses, it is not clear why one strain should be more resistant than the other. For example, the response of spleen cells to T-cell mitogens or to sheep erythrocytes does not show the C57BL/5 mouse to have greater intrinsic responsiveness than any of the other three strains (Williams and Benacerraf, 1972; Singhal *et al.*, 1978), nor are these strains markedly different in predisposition to autoimmune disease.

Of interest to the immunopharmacologist is that, insofar as it has been analyzed, responsiveness to immunopotentiator therapy appears to correlate directly with susceptibility and inversely with resistance. As demonstrated by the work of Renoux *et al.*, (1979a), the sheep erythrocyte plaque response of C57BL/6 mice is relatively resistant to modification by *in vivo* treatment with the immunopotentiator levamisole, whereas the responses of C3H and Balb/c mice are sensitive, and those of DBA/2 intermediate in sensitivity. Similarly, the spleen cell proliferative responses of C57BL/6 mice are much more resistant to stimulation by muramyl dipeptide than are those of DBA/2 mice (Damais *et al.*, 1978). Also, spleen cell mitogen responses of C57BL/6 mice are resistant to *in vivo* stimulation by isoprinosine, whereas those of C3H and Balb/c are quite responsive (L. Simon, personal communication). It appears then that for every comparison made here the C57BL/6 mouse emerges as resistant, and the C3H, Balb/c, and DBA/2 as susceptible.

The finding that C57BL/6 mice are resistant and DBA/2, Balb/c, and C3H are susceptible to three diseases involving cellular immunity and also to three immunopotentiators acting on cellular immune responses may be fortuitous; however, it seems likely that the observations may be linked in that the immunopotentiator sensitivity involves a dysfunction of those cells responsible for disease susceptibility. Although much of the cellular immune response is attributable to genes within the H-2 complex, the lack of a strict relationship of the above responses to the H-2 complex implies that the cells responsible for this type of resistance may not be lymphocytes. In this regard, it is notable that susceptibility to herpes infection and to allogeneic engraftment may be subverted by prior transplantation of bone marrow from resistant but compatible donors (C. Lopez, personal communication; Cudkowicz and Bennett, 1971), suggesting that if not lymphocytes, perhaps other marrow-derived cells such as natural killer cells may be involved.

As the work of Renoux et al. (1979a) points out, in addition to strain, age and sex are important determinants of responsiveness to immunopotentiators. Similarly, stress, nutrition, and concurrent disease would also be factors. Given the multiplicity of host variables, both genetic and epigenetic, it is perhaps not surprising that immunopotentiator studies in different mouse strains have yielded conflicting results. In light of these observations, it would seem wise in the future to select mouse strains for immunopotentiator studies based on some knowledge of their demonstrated responsiveness.

The value of mouse research results may be largely dependent on the care as well as the selection of the experimental animal. It is essential, therefore, that the investigator be deliberate in his choice of mice and be cognizant of the reputation of the supplier. A number of features are critical for mice used for % in vivo testing or as cell donors for in vitro assays. The major factors seem to be chronic stress, bacterial and parasitic load, virus infection, diet, and general maintenance procedures. Most laboratories have to buy mice from commercial sources. Travel and repeated handling are obvious sources of stress leading to transient thymic involution and possible contamination. It is, therefore, mandatory to quarantine animals for at least 10 days. Hair cleanliness and weight are two easy ways to evaluate mouse health. A reduced growth rate suggests either internal infection or ectodermic parasitism, and a spontaneous death among a new mouse lot indicates that the entire lot could be infected. An indirect indication of latent bacterial or viral infection may be the finding of an increased basal number of spontaneous plaque-forming cells (PFC) to sheep red blood cells (SRBC). The immune perturbations contributed by such infection with attendant actions of interferon, lymphokines, and endotoxin may greatly mask or modify the analysis of an immunotherapeutic agent.

4.2.2. Technical Details of Importance

We do not detail the techniques to be employed; however, the desirability of standardizing, as far as possible, all technical aspects is, nevertheless, to be emphasized, since all in vivo immunologic responses may be affected by nuances in the experimental procedures. We must also stress the role of contaminating endotoxin in immunopharmacological research. Bacterial endotoxin (LPS) is long known to possess multiple potent effects on the immunologic apparatus (Morrison and Ryan, 1979). It can modify results and lead to misinterpretation of experimental findings. Endotoxin has been the cause of variability in studies performed with mitogens, fetal calf serum, culture medium, reagents, transfer factor, interferon, and thymus extract preparations (Fumarola, 1981; Watson and Epstein, 1973; Shiigi and Mishell, 1975). The role of endotoxin as a widespread and potent contaminating agent in immunopharmacological research cannot be underestimated, and all possible precautions should be taken to avoid the danger of its inadvertent involvement in the results. All reagents and media should, therefore, be endotoxin-free, and syringes and glassware of the pyrogen-free grade for administration to animals and for immunologic tests. Producers should be able to certify, and investigators to test, the endotoxin content of their materials. For this, the *Limulus* endotoxin assay represents a valid tool to reduce the risk of incorrect interpretation and false results.

Finally, the appropriate appraisal of data by statistical tests if necessary; however, as pointed out by Hoffman (1976), the use of an incorrect test, such as a chi-square analysis when the total number of observations is less than 30, can lead to erroneous conclusions. Crude statistical analysis of the data, especially on long-term assays involving evaluation of survival rate, may also invite excessive conclusions (Casagrande and Pike, 1975). The help of a statistician on the design as well as the interpretation of trials is advised.

4.2.3. How to Characterize Immunotherapeutic Agents

In the framework of this chapter, we present a series of sequential and progressively more demanding assays through which immunotherapeutic agents can be screened for therapeutic potential (Tables VI and VII). The proposed sequence of progressive assays is (1) to show whether a new compound demonstrates a broad spectrum of activity, so that it could be tested in a more discriminating and specific manner; (2) to establish the parameters of dose, schedule, route, duration, and maintenance of activity on defined immune responses through *in vivo* activation and both *in vivo* and *in vitro* testing; such an approach to the screening of these agents is designed to define its effects on T-cell, B-cell, NK-cell, macrophage, and polymorphonuclear cell function; (3) immunotoxicology and toxicopharmacology of the agent should be evaluated at the earliest point of positive data, so as not to waste time and money on a toxic compound; (4) agents that have passed step 3 will then be tested for effects on models of immunodeficiencies, autoimmune and infectious diseases, and cancers; and (5) a comparison between *in vivo* and *in vitro* assays will give indications of how to initiate studies on the mode of action of the agent.

For some immunotherapeutic agents, the development of specific testing

TABLE VI

Flow Chart for Characterization of Potential Immunotherapeutic Agents:
First Step, Influences on Cell Populations and Immunomodulating Effects

Cell	Effect
T cell	Evaluation of T-cell subsets in spleen
	Mixed-lymphocyte culture (MLC) to alloantigens
	Plaque forming cells (PFC) to sheep erythrocytes (SRBC) (IgG class) and to trinitrophenyl-hemocyanin (TNP-KLH) conjugate
B cell	Evaluation of B cells in spleen
	Blastogenesis to pokeweed mitogen (PWM) and dextran sulfate
	PFC to TNP carrier conjugates with Ficoll or lipolysaccharide (LPS)
	Levels of circulating antibodies to the above antigens, including SRBC
Lymphokine induction	Evaluation of interferon or CSF levels in serum
NK cell	Cytotoxic assay on YAC-1 myeloma cells
Macrophages	Yeast and bacteria phagocytosis and killing
	Chemotaxis
	Lysosomal enzyme evaluation
	Antibody-dependent cellular cytotoxicity (ADCC) to SRBC
	Tumor cell cytotoxicity
Granulocytes	Phagocytosis and killing
	Chemotaxis
	Glucose metabolism [nitroblue tetrazolium test (NBT)]
	Oxygen radical formation (chemiluminescence)
Macrophage/ granulocyte precursor	Colony-forming units (CFUs)

might be required. For example, the activity of a monoclonal antibody against a tumor antigen can be assessed in a specific system of antibody-mediated cytotoxicity.

To determine whether a new drug is active on the immune system, testing ought to be both reliable and inexpensive. Random-bred mice can be satisfactorily employed at this stage. The most convenient assays are to evaluate the impact of the agent on the magnitude of the response to immunization and on lymphoproliferation induced by T- and B-cell mitogens (see Table VI).

The influence of immunization is easily evaluated by specific spleen cell responses to SRBC. Quantitation of the clear zones of lysis (plaques) in agar impregnated with erythrocytes by one or the other modification of the Jerne plaque assay (Jerne and Nordin, 1963) allows an estimation of the IgM-antibody plaque-forming cells (PFC) to SRBC. Other classes of antibodies can also be revealed with a second "developing" antibody reagent able to bind to the primary antibodies on the SRBC and to the added complement. The PFC response to SRBC is a macrophage- and T-cell-dependent response expressed through B

TABLE VII
Flow Chart for Characterization of Potential Immunotherapeutic Agents:
Second Step, Influences on Cell Populations and Immunomodulating Effects

Cell	In vivo activation, in vivo testing
T cells and macrophages	Delayed-type hypersensitivity to SRBC or oxazolone Skin graft rejection
T cells, B cells, and macrophages	Immediate and intermediate hypersensitivities to a carrier-hapten system, such as dinitrophenyl (DNP)–bovine γ-globulin (BGG)
	In vivo activation, in vitro testing
T cells	Detection assays for T-cell phenotypes (Komuro–Boyse) Mixed lymphocyte response (MLC) to allogeneic cells Suppressor cells
B cells	Jerne plaque assay to SRBC and TNP-KLH or TNP-Ficoll
Macrophages	Phagocytosis Chemotaxis Intracellular enzyme levels
Granulocytes	Phagocytosis Chemotaxis NBT test

cells, and the erythrocyte antigens are made up of a variety of T-dependent and T-independent epitopes. Activity in this test thus implies a follow-up delineating which is the precise cell target. A pilot study should involve at least four doses administered to at least five mice of the same age and sex concomitantly with (1) immunized untreated mice, (2) nonimmunized treated mice, and (3) diluent-treated mice as control groups. Evaluation of direct (IgM) and indirect (IgG) PFCs on days 2 to 4 post-immunization and -treatment, will show if the compound influences immune responsiveness. So far no agent active in vivo or in other specific immunologic tests has failed to show activity in this test.

The effect of treatment with the agent on lymphoproliferation can be assessed on responses of splenocytes to phytohemagglutinin (PHA) and concanavalin A (Con A) as T-cell mitogens and to LPS and dextran sulfate as B-cell mitogens. Stimulation or depression in this assay does not correlate with overall effect on cellular or humoral response (see Florentin et al., 1983); however, the test is useful to show immunopharmacological activity. With activity in the initial PFC and mitogen screen, in-depth analysis can proceed. The tests enumerated in Tables VI and VII represent the most frequently employed assays, as detailed in books (Hadden et al., 1977b; Chirigos, 1977a,b; Serrou and Rosenfeld, 1980; Hersh et al., 1981; Sirois and Rola-Pleszczynski, 1982; Yamamura et al., 1982; Klein et al., 1983; Fenichel and Chirigos, 1984; Talmadge et al.,

1985a) and journals such as the *International Journal of Immunopharmacology*, the *Journal of Immunopharmacology, Immunopharmacology*, and the *Journal of Biological Response Modifiers*.

A substantial literature indicates that the tests proposed to evaluate the influences of an agent on T cells, B cells, NK cells, macrophages, and granulocytes (Tables VI and VII) are presently sufficiently reliable to determine the activity of a drug. The technical details are not discussed here. The assays should be performed with a wide range of doses, including repeated administration, and given to mice from at least two inbred strains to show whether or not the agent displays an immunomodulatory influence that is controlled by the mouse MHC genome. For example, lentinan augments NK activity when administered to NK high-responder C3H/HEJ mice but not when administered to low-responder Balb/c mice (Hamuro and Chihara, 1984). Kinetic studies are also valuable, as changes in responsiveness may depend on the interval between treatment and test, and the action may persist for long periods. Isoprinosine augments the response to Con A of mouse splenocytes at days 1 and 3 after the last injection, and this effect is lost by day 5 (Vecchi *et al.*, 1978), whereas isoprinosine and imuthiol increased PCFs to SRBC for the 7 days of observation (Renoux *et al.*, 1979b; Renoux and Renoux, 1984). NPT 15392 modifies immune responses up to 14 days after a single injection (Florentin *et al.*, 1982), and pyrimidinones have effects for up to 1 week (Stringfellow, 1981).

To exemplify the usefulness of such screens, results from preliminary studies performed by the Biological Response Modifier Program of the National Cancer Institute (see Talmadge and Chirigos, 1985) and from published studies in the literature (see Hadden, 1981, 1983; Florentin *et al.*, 1981, 1983) are summarized in Table VIII. Presented are qualitative descriptions of actions of various biologicals and drugs on important functions of T cells, macrophages, and natural killer cells both *in vitro* and *in vivo*. From such a summary several fundamental points are evident. The interferons inhibit T-cell replication while promoting NK and macrophage killer function. These actions are generally shared by the interferon inducers. Somewhat paradoxically, both the interferons and their inducers have a degree of T-cell adjuvanticity *in vivo*, evident at low doses and dependent on the timing of the administration. Thymosin fraction V, a representative thymic hormone preparation known to contain thymopoietin, thymosin α_1, and thymulin, is fairly selective in its action to stimulate T-cell functions both *in vitro* and *in vivo*. These effects are reproduced both *in vitro* and *in vivo* by the purine thymomimetic drugs. The sulfur-containing thymomimetic drugs are inactive *in vitro* but active *in vivo*, presumably through the induction of a thymic-hormone-like substance. Azimexon shows a weak thymic-hormone-like profile and may also be classified as a thymomimetic drug, although the mechanism of its action is not clear. In general, the thymomimetic drugs augment NK-cell activity *in vivo* but not *in vitro*. This effect may be mediated in part by IL-2, as they all promote its production. Interleukin-2 itself shows a broad

TABLE VIII
Comparison of Immunomodulatory Properties

	Biologicals					Interferon inducers			Thymomimetic drugs				Others		
	rHuIFN-α	rHuIFN-γ	rHuIL-2	Thymosin fraction V	Tuftsin	MVE-2	Poly IC:LC	Poly A:U	Isoprinosine	NPT 15392	Levamisole	Imuthiol	MDP	Bestatin	Azimexon
In vitro															
T-cell function	−	−	+	+	+	0	0	0	+	+	±	+	0	+	±
Mitogen	−	−	+	+	+	0	+	+	+	+	±	0	+	+	±
MLR															
NK-cell activity	+	+	0	0	0	−	+	+	0	0	0	0	0	0	ND
Macrophage cytotoxicity	+	+	+	0	+	+	+	+	0	0	0	0	+	+	0
In vivo															
T-cell adjuvant	+	+	+	+	+	+	+	+	+	+	+	+	+	+	+
NK-cell activity	+	+	+	0	0	+	+	+	+	+	+	+	±	0	0
Macrophage cytotoxicity	+	+	+	0	+	+	+	+	0	0	0	0	+	+	0
IFN induction	0	0	+	0	0	+	+	+	0	0	0	0	0	0	0

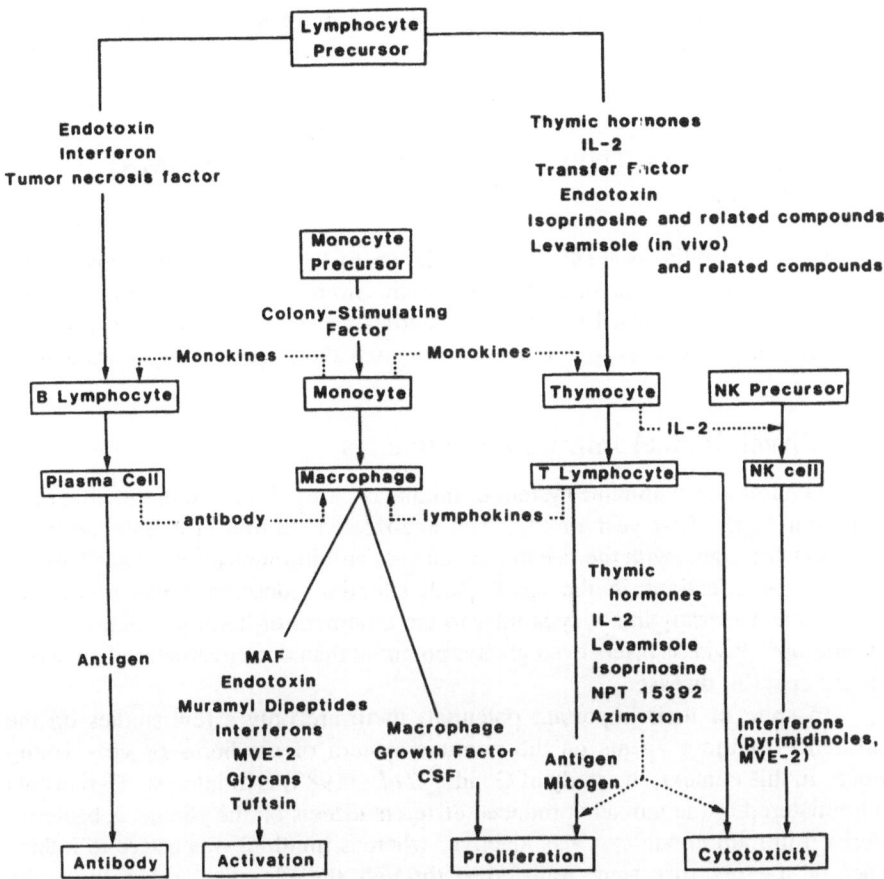

FIGURE 1. Immunorestorative and immunomodulation therapies.

spectrum of immunopharmacological effects in addition to known actions on T cells. Its effects on macrophage activation *in vitro* and *in vivo* may be mediated by γ-interferon induction. Tuftsin, MDP, and bestatin are primarily active on macrophages but show some T-cell-related effects, presumably mediated in part by induction of interleukin-1 (IL-1). It is apparent that the systematic preclinical evaluation of these immunotherapeutic agents will be able to delineate various classes and profiles of agents based on effector cell activity.

4.2.4. Summary of Cellular Mechanisms of Action

Based on the extensive literature of both *in vitro* and *in vivo* studies, beyond the scope of this review, we present a simplified combined schema (Figure 1) depicting the proposed mechanisms of action of a number of agents under discussion in this chapter.

5. PRECLINICAL THERAPEUTIC STUDIES IN ANIMAL MODELS

Once a candidate agent has been shown to be immunopharmacologically active and relatively free of undesirable toxic, immunotoxic, and pharmacological effects, it can then be entered in studies on animal models of immunologically based diseases to evaluate its potential therapeutic effectiveness.

5.1. Physiological Immunodeficiencies

The immature immune system of infants is partly the cause of the infections common to the first year of life. The age-related decline in cellular immune function correlates with the rise in incidence of autoimmune diseases and cancers as well as infections in the aged. Both situations deserve consideration for replacement therapy in a way similar to the treatment of hormonal deficiencies. Immunoprophylaxis offers even greater potential than does treatment of an established specific disease.

In spite of their important potential, there are only a few studies on the influence of those agents on the immune system of newborns or very young mice. In this context, the study of Gendre et al. (1983) is of interest. Two agents administered to the mothers produced different effects on the young. A bacteria-derived immunomodulator was inactive, whereas imuthiol was active to induce specific factors that were transferred through the placenta and milk to the offspring.

Correction of immunologic senescence is an attractive area of research as a model to evaluate the interrelationships among the decline in thymic hormone levels; T-cell number and function, IL-2 production, thymus atrophy, and growth and other hormone production. Impressive in this regard is the observation that the life span of dwarf mice, which are short-lived, hypopituitary, and growth hormone deficient, could be extended three- to fourfold and their immunity augmented by growth hormone and thyroxine treatment (Fabris et al., 1972). Studies on the effectiveness of these agents to modify age-induced changes in immunologic activities may predict their potential to prevent and treat autoimmune diseases, infections, and cancer in the elderly. Makinodan and Kay (1980) have summarized most of the available data up to 1980. Thymus grafts and thymic extracts have been employed with limited and transient effects; double-stranded polynucleotides and levamisole were used successfully to restore the declining immune functions of aging mice. More recently, bestatin, tuftsin (Bruley-Russet et al., 1981), and NPT 15392 (Florentin et al., 1983) were found to restore some of the T-cell and macrophage responses. Imuthiol restores T-cell-associated events in aged mice, thymus-hormone-like serum activity, and IL-1 and IL-2 production to the levels of young controls (Bruley-Russet et al., 1985; Chung et al., 1985). Isoprinosine increases T-cell activities and natural killer cell and monocyte function in old hamsters (Tsang and Fudenberg, 1984).

5.2. Iatrogenic Immunodeficiencies

Unwanted immunodeficiency occurs with therapies such as cytotoxic anti-cancer drugs, ionizing radiation, antibiotics, surgery, and anesthesia. There is a strong need for detailed studies on the effects of immunotherapeutic agents in conjunction with immunosuppressive or toxic drugs to reverse the development of iatrogenic immunodeficiencies.

5.3. Autoimmune Disease Models

The genetically determined and spontaneous autoantibody responses of the NZB mouse strain has long provided the most accepted model of autoimmunity (See Talal and Hadden, 1984, for review). Other mouse models of congenital autoimmunity are known, such as the F_1 hybrids between NZB and New Zealand white mice (NZB/W), MLF/1 pr mice, BXSB mice, or genetically manipulated NZB/W mice to which the X-linked immunodeficiency gene has been added. A comprehensive review of experimental models for acquired thyroiditis and allergic encephalomyelitis has been made by Weigle (1980). These models have increased our understanding of autoimmunity and of the relationships between immunodeficiency and autoimmunity; however, only a few reports have dealt with the influences of immunotherapeutic agents.

A temporary remission of symptoms and decrease in autoantibody titers can be induced in NZB mice injected with thymosin (Talal et al., 1975), ubiquitin (Gershwin et al., 1979), or thymulin (FTS) (Bach et al., 1980). Levamisole is inactive by itself but maintains a cyclophosphamide-induced remission (Zulman et al., 1978). Imuthiol delays symptoms, including lymphomas and proteinuria, and retards autoantibody production (Renoux, 1982). Isoprinosine restores depressed suppressor cells and prolongs life somewhat in Swan mice (Touraine et al., 1982). NPT 15392 retards the development of antierythrocyte antibody in young and/or old NZB mice (Jones et al., 1983). Thiazolobenzothiazole compounds do not modify the autoantibody response in NZB/W F_1 or MRL/1 pr mice (Gregory et al., 1980). Tilorone prevents experimental allergic encephalomyelitis if repeatedly administered for several weeks prior to encephalitogen challenge (Megel and Gibson, 1984). In contrast, C. parvum provokes an early autoimmune anemia in young NZB mice (Halpern and Fray, 1969), CBA mice (McCracken et al., 1971), and various other mouse strains (Cox and Keast, 1974). Finally, transfer factor may induce autoimmune hemolytic anemia in certain patients (Ballow et al., 1973).

Autoimmune recognition and low levels of autoantibodies are normal but can predispose to autoimmune disease if immune balance is altered. Immunomodulating agents may modify the balance among immunocyte populations, particularly after long-term administration. Studies on the influence of these agents on autoimmune processes are consequently needed. It will be important to determine whether or not the agent induces or augments the levels of autoantibodies in susceptible animals. Data thus gained may be able to avert the potential danger of an increased incidence of autoimmune disease in patients treated chronically.

5.4. Infections

The importance of the host in the natural history of infectious disease has been somewhat neglected during the flourishing years of antibiotic therapy. It has become apparent, however, that not all infections are cured by antibiotics. The role of host defense mechanisms has again been increasingly taken into consideration.

Disease or health, death or cure, is the outcome of a conflict between the pathogens and the invaded body. The latter mounts all possible defenses against the attacker, which has already taken advantage of a failure in the defense system for its primary invasion and has developed mechanisms to escape the immune system for its maintenance. In this context, the development of preventive and therapeutic immunotherapy will obviously be beneficial.

Vaccination, which relies on a well-functioning immune system to be effective, is out of the scope of this discussion on nonspecific immunotherapy; however, the use of well-chosen adjuvants, such as MDP, may increase the protection afforded by existing vaccines by specifically enhancing cellular immunity (Chedid et al., 1982).

5.4.1. Viral Infections

Specific antiviral responses are, in the main, T cell dependent (see Werner, 1979; Hadden, 1987). If T-cell-mediated immunity can be expanded or rescued during cytotoxic chemotherapy without altering the efficacy of the cytolytic agent, one might expect greater toxicity against tumor to be achieved together with less compromise of protection against viral diseases. In addition, agents increasing cytotoxic T-cell (CTL) number and activity are likely to be useful in the treatment of and protection against T-cell-dependent viral pathogens in populations at risk.

Isoprinosine has been shown to have antiviral activities in vivo against several virus infections in mice (Gordon et al., 1974; Muldoon et al., 1972; Hadden et al., 1977c; Simon and Glasky, 1978; Ohnishi et al., 1983). Interferons also possess antiviral effects, most frequently shown by in vivo prophylactic assays (Stewart, 1981). Lentinan has been shown to induce in mice a degree of protection against a variety of viruses, particularly when administered prophylactically (Hamuro and Chihara, 1984). A prophylactic influence of MVE-2 has also been reported (Chirigos *et al.*, 1983).

Questions concerning the efficacy of immunotherapeutic agents against viral diseases must be addressed in conveniently chosen experimental models, including drug-induced immunologic deficiencies.

5.4.2. Bacterial and Fungal Infections

The host response to intracellular microorganisms results in increased nonspecific resistance to antigenically unrelated viruses, rickettsia, bacteria, or fungi (see Hadden and Englard, 1977; Hibbs *et al.*, 1980). Nonspecific resistance mediated by activated macrophages is also the mechanism of the prophylactic influence of agents of bacterial or fungal origin against infections.

Although a number of clinical studies report beneficial influences of immunotherapeutic agents against infections, there are still a very limited number of experimental studies. Levamisole can prevent bacterial infection in suckling or adult mice (see Renoux, 1978). Lentinan also potentiates host resistance and prolongs survival time of mice infected with *Listeria, Klebsiella,* or *Streptococcus* (Chihara, 1983). Thymosin fraction V corrects the susceptibility to infection with *C. albicans* of mice from some inbred strains but lowers the resistance of otherwise resistant mice (Salvin and Neta, 1983). Thymosin α_1 given concurrently with 5-FU partially protects mice from lethal infections by opportunistic pathogens to which normal mice were highly resistant (Ishitsuka *et al.*, 1984). Other agents, such as tuftsin (Nishioka *et al.*, 1981) or imuthiol (Renoux, 1982; Corke *et al.*, 1984), enhance colloidal clearance and macrophage bactericidal activity. It remains to be seen if these agents prevent and cure infections in experimental models of immunodepression.

5.5. Cancer

Efforts to establish an immunopharmacology for cancer immunotherapy have been frustrated by the lack of animal tumor models that directly relate to human cancer (see Talmadge *et al.*, 1985a; Hadden and Spreafico, 1985). Prior emphasis on transplantable tumors that were often inadvertently immunogenic and the easily demonstrated effectiveness of BCG, *C. parvum*, and high-molecular-weight polysaccharide preparations led to the erroneous conclusion that such therapy in man would be equally effective. A considerable number of clinical trials have not generally supported this conclusion. The relative failure of these agents in the human can be attributed to a number of factors including the inadequacy of the models and the complexity and ambiguity of the actions of the agents in humans. The evolution of immunotherapy in human cancer has increasingly moved away from the complex bacterial preparations toward the use of biologicals and chemically defined agents. The apparent rule that has emerged from both murine tumor systems and human cancer trials is that these agents act to increase the number of individuals remaining in remission following effective cytoreductive therapy with chemotherapy, surgery, or irradiation. They have not been particularly active in treating progressive disease. Levamisole offers a case in point. In 34 animal tumor models in which it was used as a monotherapy, no effect was observed; however, following cytoreductive therapy it was active in 13 of 21 systems (Symoens and Rosenthal, 1977). The experience in human cancer generally parallels these results. If one accepts the contention that levamisole, although a weak agent, is the only agent in which studies with mice correlate with the human, then, logically, the models in which it has been effective are the most appropriate for testing related agents. One of the difficulties with this consideration is that very little is known about the mechanism by which levamisole exerts its antitumor action in either the animal models or human cancer.

Animal tumors like human tumors involve immunosuppressed hosts, and since cytoreductive therapy may contribute further to the immunosuppression, it is essential to know something about the immune status of the host prior to intervening with an immunotherapy. The first goal of immunotherapy should be to determine if immunologic reconstitution is effective. Secondary goals should include not only whether decreased growth of the primary tumor or of metastases and increased survival result but also whether increased resistance to secondary infection occurs. Finally, if survival is increased, it is important to determine whether resistance to rechallenge with the tumor indicates that specific antitumor mechanisms are involved. In designing combined therapy in these animal models, it is important to determine the degree of antigenicity of the tumor and to ensure that the tumor is syngeneic to the host and uninfected with antigenic pathogens so that only tumor antigenicity will determine specific host resistance.

We present a brief summary of the model approaches currently employed by the Biological Response Modifier (BRM) Program of the National Cancer Institute in order to allow the reader to assess the progress in the area and to evaluate the prospects for new strategies in the future. The reader is referred to other sources for technical details (Talmadge et al., 1985a).

5.5.1. Animal Models

A number of animal species have been useful in these investigations. With rare exceptions, such as osteogenic sarcoma in the beagle dog and some tumor models in the rat, species other than the mouse do not provide tumor models that are significantly better. Larger animals require more care and larger numbers to make evaluation significant, and experimentation with them takes longer and is more expensive. For all of these reasons, the bulk of the experimental animal work required for the development of immunotherapy has been done in the mouse. There are many obvious advantages to using the mouse as an experimental animal, including the existence in this species of an athymic mutant, the nude mouse, in which human tumors can be transplanted as well as the existence of many different mouse tumor types (leukemias, lymphomas, carcinomas, melanomas, osteogenic sarcomas, lymphosarcomas, mammary adenocarcinomas, etc.). Despite their limitations, the mouse tumor models have been useful in the past in predicting the efficacy of chemotherapeutic drugs in man.

5.5.2. Studies of Direct and/or Host-Mediated Antitumor Effects

Tumor cell lines capable of growing both *in vitro* and *in vivo* are essential. With the use of *in vitro* and *in vivo* techniques one can dissect the mechanisms by which various agents exert their antitumor effects. Several tumor lines fulfill these criteria. (1) Meth A sarcoma cells are derived from Balb/c mice that have been treated with the carcinogen 3-methylcholathrene; these cells can grow in suspension cultures in the ascites form as well as inoculated subcutaneously in syngeneic mice. In the ascites form they can be recovered from the peritoneal cavity of mice as a >95% viable cell suspension. Inoculation of 10 to 100 cells can cause a tumor in intraperitoneal and subcutaneous locations. (2) Lymphoid leukemia L1210 is derived from DBA mice that have been treated with 7,12-dimethylbenzanthracene; their growth characteristics are similar to the Meth A cells. (3) MBL-2 Moloney leukemia virus-induced tumor grows in C57BL/6 mice; its growth characteristics are similar to the Meth A and L1210 cell lines. These and similar tumor cell lines lend themselves to studying the *in vitro* as well as the *in vivo* antitumor effects of a therapeutic agent.

In vitro evaluation can be made by assessing the effects of various concentrations of the agent when incubated directly with tumor cells (direct antitumor effects) or incubated with host cells, particularly macrophages or lymphocytes, in the presence of tumor cells (tumor cell killing mediated by enhancement of host cells). Of the immunotherapeutic agents under discussion, only the interferons show significant direct antitumor action *in vitro*. This action is mediated by growth inhibition rather than cell killing. The recent development of cloned tumor necrosis factor and lymphotoxin as well as antitumor monoclonal antibodies will lead to rapid development in this area in the future. A number of agents, as discussed, will activate host cells to kill tumor cells (see Table IX).

In vivo evaluation of the agents can be done by treating normal or tumor-bearing mice with different concentrations via different routes (oral, i.p., i.v., i.m., s.c.), and at set time intervals following treatment, host cells can be harvested, particularly macrophages, lymphocytes, and NK cells. The separated

TABLE IX
Antitumor Properties[a]

	Biologicals					IFN Inducers				Others	
	rHu IFNα	rHu IFNγ	rHu IL-2	Thymosin fraction V	Tuftsin	MVE-2	Poly IC:LC	Poly A:U	MDP N or MLV	Bestatin	Azimexon
Nonspecific prophylaxis	+	+	+	0	0	+	+	+	0	0	0
Specific prophylaxis	+	+	+	+	+	+	+	+	+	+	0
Experimental metastases	+	+	+	+	+	0	+	+	+	+	0
Spontaneous metastases	+	+	+	+	+	±	+	+	+	+	+
Autochthonous tumors	NT	NT	NT	0	NT	NT	+	NT	0	NT	NT

[a] Symbols used: +, active; 0, inactive; NT, not tested.

cells are then incubated with tumor cells to assess host-cell-mediated tumor cell killing.

A compartmentalized system can be employed in which tumor cells (Meth A, L1210, or MBL-2) are inoculated i.p. and treatment is by the i.p. route. Macrophages can be harvested from the peritoneal cavity and separated by adherence for *in vitro* testing of tumor cell killing. Similarly, splenic lymphocytes can also be tested *in vitro*. Employing the MBL-2 compartmentalized system, Chirigos and Stylos (1980) demonstrated that interferon and maleic anhydride divinyl ether exerted antitumor activity by stimulating peritoneal macrophages to exert tumoricidal activity both *in vitro* and *in vivo*. Similar compartmentalized immune responses have been stimulated by MVE-2 treatment against a mouse mammary adenocarcinoma (Khato *et al.*, 1983). Augmentation of natural killer cells by immunotherapeutic agents in the lung and liver leads to a significant decrease in the number of B16 melanoma metastases in these organs (Wiltrout *et al.*, 1985).

Examples of tumor cell lines that can be maintained *in vitro* and also cause local growth subcutaneously leading to metastases include (1) osteosarcoma cells, transplantable mouse osteosarcoma cells derived from radionuclide-induced osteosarcomas of the mouse; (2) Madison 109 alveolar carcinoma, a spontaneous lung tumor that arose in a Balb/c mouse; and (3) B16 melanoma. Several lines of this latter tumor have been developed, particularly ones with a high metastic characteristic in C57BL/6 mice. These cell lines allow one to specifically address questions related to resistance to metastasis formation (Wiltrout *et al.*, 1985; Talmadge *et al.*, 1985b).

5.5.3. Nonspecific and Specific Prophylaxis Models

The BRM program has employed the ultraviolet light (UV 23–37) model to examine nonspecific prophylaxis. The resistance mechanisms in this model are probably primary ones dependent on natural killer cells and macrophages, predicting that interferon and its inducers and reticuloendothelial system expanders will be active.

In this model (see Table IX) the interferons, IL-2, and the interferon inducers have been confirmed to be active; MDP in multilamellar vesicles (MLV) but not free MDP is active. Thymosin, tuftsin, bestatin, and azimexon are inactive.

The model of specific prophylaxis employed by the BRM program involves the preadministration of the immunotherapeutic agent in conjunction with a tumor cell vaccine (UV 23–37) followed by tumor challenge. In this model immune mechanisms are involved as well as primary resistance mechanisms. It is important to note that suppressor cell phenomena and induction of progression rather than regression have been observed in such models with immunotherapy (Vecchi *et al.*, 1978), and simple interpretations without mechanistic studies may be hazardous. In any case, the BRM program has found all of the agents studied except azimexon active in this model (see Table IX). These models of prophylaxis are effective in delineating the action of various agents, particularly when combined with cellular mechanism studies, but bear no predictive relationships to human cancer since therapy with the human is invariably initiated not before but well after the onset of the cancer.

5.5.4. Metastasis Models: Spontaneous and Experimental

Metastatic potential is an all-important parameter of neoplasia. Several tumors lend themselves to studying the effect of these agents on *in vivo* metastases:

1. The Lewis lung carcinoma of C57BL/6 mice grows rapidly subcutaneously and develops macroscopic pulmonary metastases that can be counted within 3 weeks after tumor cell inoculation.
2. The B16 melanoma grows rapidly *in vivo*. Measured numbers of cells can be inoculated locally into the footpad or ears of C57BL/6 mice, and primary tumors can be removed easily after specific intervals. The primary tumors give rise to metastases that can be counted in the lung without prior fixation or staining.
3. Madison 109 alveolar carcinoma grows well *in vivo* and can be used similarly to the B16 melanoma (Papamatheakis *et al.*, 1978).

Sarcoma T241 (a malignant fibrosarcoma originally induced by dibenzanthracene in C57BL/6 mice, CD8F, and breast tumors are other examples of tumors possessing metastatic characteristics.

With these murine tumors, two models of immunotherapy have been employed. The first, a model of experimental metastasis, involves intravenous injection of the tumor into the mouse with subsequent enumeration of liver and/or lung metastases. In this model the primary resistance mechanisms lie within the target organs themselves (i.e., lung and liver) and initially depend on macrophages, Kuppfer cells, NK cells, and nonimmune barriers to implantation. All three tumors have been employed by the BRM program for this use, and a number of agents have been found to be active (see Table IX), including the interferons, IL-2, thymosin, tuftsin, poly IC:LC, poly A:U, MDP, and bestatin; only azimexon was not active (see Chirigos *et al.*, 1985; Wiltrout *et al.*, 1985). The second, a model of spontaneous metastasis, involves the implantation and subsequent removal of the primary tumor at a time when micrometastases are forming. In this manner, the behavior of the metastases independent of the primary can be examined. Resistance in this case is more complex because of the latency period between implantation and analysis in which immune mechanisms are observed. Based on the Lewis lung model, resistance relies on the activities of suppressor cells and cytolytic effector cells at the level of regional lymph nodes and spleen as well as on the primary resistance mechanisms in organs to which metastases seed (see Hadden and Spreafico, 1983). The BRM program has generally used the B16 melanoma system for its studies (see Talmadge and Chirigos, 1985), and other investigators have generally used the Lewis lung model (see Hadden and Spreafico, 1985). The BRM studies (see Table IX) have found all the immunotherapeutic agents studied active to a greater or lesser degree in this model. Other reports (see Hadden and Spreafico, 1985) have found levamisole to be variably active, and WY18251, NPT 15392, and cimetidine have been more consistently active. Another spontaneous metastasis model of note is the T241 fibrosarcoma in the B6 mouse, in which both levamisole and NPT 15392 have been shown to be active (Simon et al., 1983).

5.5.5. Autochthonous Tumor Models

Models of spontaneous or induced tumor development offer special problems and challenges in the study of the immunotherapy of cancer. As models of human cancer they are most relevant because of their low antigenicity, a probable background of yet uncharacterized secondary immunodeficiency, and sufficient latency to allow tumor growth and tumor-host interactions to become established. The problems include the time and cost requirement to carry the animals well into maturity before tumorigenesis occurs and low incidence of spontaneous tumor development, depending on the model. The BRM program has utilized two metastatic autochthonous tumor models in its studies (see Talmadge and Chirigos, 1985; Talmadge et al., 1985a). The first employs ultraviolet (UV) light-induced skin tumors (squamous cell carcinomas, fibrosarcomas, and others, which develop in mice 20–50 weeks after UV exposure. The second model utilizes the induction of mammary tumors in rats by N-nitrosomethylurea (NMU) 90–120 days after injection. In both models therapy is not initiated until palpable tumors develop. Response is measured by growth kinetics of the primary tumor, time of survival, and the development of metastases. The intrinsic variability of the tumorigenic response presents unique problems, as does the human counterpart. The resistance mechanisms are predictably complex in these systems, yet immunodeficiency with active suppressor cells has been documented in the UV model, a situation similar to a number of human cancers.

The BRM program has found positive effects with an MDP derivative MTP-PE incorporated into liposomes, OK 432, and poly IC:LC in the UV-induced model (Table IX). Thymosin fraction V is inactive. The positive effects observed with the active agents involve retardation of tumor progression, reduction of spontaneous metastasis, and prolongation of survival but no cures. Another model of this type successfully employed by Stolfi and Martin (1978) involves the development of spontaneous breast tumors in CD8F mice, in which MVE-2 has been shown to increase survival time. The limitation of these models is that cures are being sought during active progressive disease when it is only realistic to expect them following cytoreductive therapy. Logically, these models should be reconstructed to employ surgery and/or cytoreductive therapy prior to immunotherapy in order to achieve cures.

5.5.6. Transplanted Tumor Models: Adjunctive Therapy

For the reasons pointed out, we do not discuss the myriad of attempts to treat active progressive transplanted cancer in mice but focus on models in which immunotherapy has been introduced following cytoreductive treatment of the cancer using surgery, chemotherapy, or irradiation. These models are the most complex but are most comparable to the situation faced in man. In addition to involving an established host–tumor interaction (including such maladaptations as suppressor cells and antigen–antibody complexes), these models also introduce the additional immunosuppressive effects of anesthesia and surgery, irradiation, and/or chemotherapy. Such models make it mandatory to conduct mechanistic studies in order to interpret results. Unfortunately, we have relatively little information about the effects of anesthesia and surgery, irradiation, and chemotherapy on the immune response of normal mice (Davis and Shires, 1986). In immunodeficient tumor-bearing mice, the situation becomes more complex. At best, chemotherapy can be immunorestorative by reversing tumor-inducing immunosuppression, and at worst it can aggravate the immunosuppression (see Faanes et al., 1980; Spreafico et al., 1982; Berd et al., 1984; Ehrke and Mihich, 1985). The effects of subsequent immunotherapy can only be guessed at. Clearly, this area, as do many involving experimental immunotherapy, requires intense investigation to clarify the interactions involved.

As indicated, levamisole has shown activity in 13 of 21 adjunctive therapy studies in murine tumor models (Symoens and Rosenthal, 1977); however, the degree of activity was generally small, suggesting that the more potent agents currently under study would be more active than levamisole in similar systems. Thymosin fraction V and α_1 have yielded long-term cures and increased mean survival times in mice bearing MOPC 315 tumors and treated first with cyclophosphamide (Zatz et al., 1981). These thymic hormones have also reduced the susceptibility to tumor and pathogen challenge in chemotherapy-treated mice (Ishitsuka et al., 1983a,b; Ohta et al., 1985). More studies of this nature are warranted. Considering the extensive background of published experience with chemotherapy in various transplanted mouse tumor models, it is more feasible to exploit these models at the present time than it is to wait for the development of the same information in the autochthonous models.

5.5.7. Immunopharmacological Correlates of Antitumor Immunotherapy

All of the models discussed lend themselves to the analysis of the mechanisms involved. The selection of effector cells following treatment may vary depending on the type of tumor and inoculation route employed (ascites versus solid) and the route of treatment. The most accessible are spleen, peritoneal exudate cells, peripheral blood, bone marrow, lung, lymph nodes, and the primary tumor itself.

It is difficult in most cases to correlate directly the tumor cell killing achieved with specific effector cell population elicited by the immunotherapeutic agent. Table X (adapted from Talmadge and Chirigos, 1985) presents a correlation of effector cell augmentation by several immunotherapeutic agents in normal mice with immunoprophylaxis and immunotherapeutic results in mice bearing various tumors. From these studies Talmadge and Chirigos (1985) concluded that the nonspecific immunoprophylaxis model gave more positive results than the therapeutic models and probably reflected NK-cell-augmenting action on the part of the agent tested and that therapeutic effects could be correlated to an extent with macrophage activation and T-cell adjuvancy but not with systemic NK-augmenting effects. Such a conclusion supports the general interpretation that natural killer cells form a primary resistance barrier to spontaneous or transplanted tumor development and to metastasis formation; however, they constitute a weak barrier relatively easily overcome. Once overcome by progressive tumor growth, specific tumor resistance mechanisms involving sensitized T cells and activated macrophages (see Alexander, 1975) intervene and define whether tumor rejection can occur.

More explicit insights can be obtained by analyzing correlations of effector cell augmentation in the tumor-bearing mouse under treatment with tumor reduction. Depending on the tumor model employed, several correlations have been made. In a compartmentalized system, e.g., the ascites MBL-2, tumoricidal macrophages elicited in the peritoneal cavity by MVE-2, tumoricidal macrophages elicited in the peritoneal cavity by MVE-2 can be correlated with the reduction of MBL-2 tumor cells (Chirigos and Stylos, 1980). In this system, one can separate the macrophage population by adherence and test their tumoricidal activity *in vitro* against the same target tumor cell. Attempts to correlate the contribution of the NK cell to tumor cell killing is technically more difficult because of the inability to separate adequately the lymphocyte population containing NK cells from the tumor cell population. Monoclonal antibodies specific for tumor cells may be useful for allowing such a fractionation. Similarly, a case for the alveolar macrophages in containing or eradicating the growth of lung metastases can be made if the macrophages tested *in vitro* against the syngeneic tumor were to confirm such a role. The NK cells contained in lavages obtained from lungs bearing tumor lesions have been examined (Fidler *et al.*, 1981).

TABLE X

Correlation of Effector Cell Augmentation and Therapeutic Activity[a]

Agent	NK activation (spleen)	Macrophage activation	T-cell stimulator in vitro	T-cell adjuvant activity	Nonspecific immunoprophylaxis	Therapeutic activity
MVE-2	+	±	0	+	+	0
Poly IC:LC	++	++	0	++	+	++
rHu IFN-α	+	+	−	+	+	+
OK-432	++	+	+	+	+	+
Lentinan	+	0	0	+	+	0
Nor-MDP	0	+	+	+	0	+
MTP-PE in MLV	0[b]	++	+	++	+	++
Thymosin fraction V	0	0	++	++	0	+
NED-137	0	0	0	+	0	0
rHu IL-2	+	+	++	++ or [c]	+	++

[a]Symbols used: +, stimulated effector cell function; ±, slight stimulation of effector cell function; 0, no effect on effector cell function; −, depressed effector cell function.

[b]NK-cell activity noted in the lungs and liver but not in the spleen, blood, or peritoneal cavity.

[c]High IL-2 levels depressed cytotoxicity T-cell (CTL) activity, whereas low doses stimulated CTL activity.

Agents capable of blocking macrophage and/or NK-cell activity have been useful in determining the antitumor role of these effector cells. Carrageenan, silica, and methyl palmitate have been shown to suppress macrophage cytolytic activity, whereas antiasialo-G_{M1} serum selectively suppresses NK cells. Monoclonal antibodies selective for macrophages or NK cells may prove useful in delineating the specific effector cells elicited by immunotherapeutic substances that are directly responsible for tumor cell cytolysis. Generally, the administration of an active immunotherapeutic substance results in an increase in macrophage and/or NK-cell numbers and a decrease in tumor growth. In contrast, the administration of such blocking agents leads to a selective suppression of macrophages and/or NK cells that is associated with enhanced tumor growth. Several immunotherapeutic agents have been shown to nullify the suppressive effects of these blocking agents. DiLuzio (1985) demonstrated the importance of macrophage cytolytic function to growth and development of a murine mammary adenocarcinoma (BW 10232). Administration of glucan resulted in a decrease in tumor growth and enhanced the population of tumor macrophages. In contrast, macrophage suppression by methyl palmitate was associated with enhanced tumor growth and a decrease in the number of tumor macrophages, indicating that macrophages were essential effector cells.

The role of NK cells in retarding the establishment of lung and liver tumors has been demonstrated by the use of the NK-cell suppressive antiasialo-G_{M1} serum (Wiltrout et al., 1985). Mice treated with antiasialo-G_{M1} serum exhibited increased formation of experimental metastases in lung and liver after intravenous challenge with B16 melanoma or Lewis lung carcinoma. This increased metastasis formation coincided with decreased splenic NK activity and increased survival of intravenously injected radiolabeled tumor cells. In contrast, the injection of mice with maleic anhydride divinyl ether (MVE-2), a potent augmentor of NK-cell tumoricidal activity (Bartocci et al., 1980), augmented NK activity in the spleen and significantly depressed the formation of experimental metastases in the lungs and liver. These two examples demonstrate an association of macrophages and/or NK cells in inhibiting tumor cell growth and/or metastasis formation. The two experimental model systems described represent examples of how correlations can be made of specific effector-cell-mediated tumor cell killing with the use of effector-cell-blocking agents. The development of monoclonal antibodies specific for tumor target cells as well as specific effector cells would markedly improve the quantitative aspects of effector-to-target-cell kinetic studies.

5.5.8. Regimen of Treatment

For potential clinical usefulness in human cancer, the route by which the immunotherapeutic agent is administered and by which it elicits a regulatory role on effector cells is of critical importance. In clinical studies the oral, intravenous, and intramuscular routes are most often used. The bulk of information developed in preclinical studies of these agents, however, has been by administering the agents by the intraperitoneal (i.p.) route. The route by which the agent is administered may have an impact on its ability to regulate an effector cell response at a specific site. For example, Picibanil (OK 432), when administered by the i.p. route, augments NK-cell activity of spleen and peritoneal exudate cells (PEC) but not peripheral blood; in contrast, i.v. inoculation leads to significant augmentation in spleen and peripheral blood but not of PEC (Chirigos *et al.*, 1984). Similarly, NPT 15392 given i.p. augments PEC NK activity but not spleen NK but given i.v. augmented both (Florentin *et al.*, 1982). Results also show that augmentation of poly IC : LC depends on the route of treatment (Chirigos *et al.*, 1985). Responses were equivalent when it was administered by the i.v., i.m., and i.p. routes, less effective by the intradermal (i.d.) route, and completely ineffective by the oral route. In addition, augmented NK activity persisted longer when poly IC : LC was given by the i.v. route.

Selection of the route of treatment would depend, in part, on the site of the tumor and the ability of the immunotherapeutic agent to enhance effector cell responses at that site; e.g., if the site of the tumor is in the lung, selection of a treatment would be based on whether the agent selected would be more efficacious when administered by the i.v. route. To aid in making such evaluations, studies are needed in which the more potentially useful agents are administered by various routes (oral, i.v., i.m., i.p.) to determine whether effector cell responses are increased in the most critical organs and tissues (i.e., peripheral blood, spleen, lung, liver). Wiltrout *et al.* (1985) reported that i.v. injection of MVE-2 led to significant increases in NK cell activity in peripheral blood, spleen, lung, and liver. This increased NK activity correlated with a decrease in the number of B16 melanoma lung and liver metastases.

The dose is also of primary importance. In addition to the determination of maximum tolerated dose, it is important to determine an optimal immunomodulatory dose and an optimal therapeutic dose. Previous studies indicate that most of the immunotherapeutic agents under study are down-regulating and/or toxic when given frequently at high dose and that immunomodulating and therapeutic effects are greatest at low doses. For example, therapy studies of MBL-2 (a Moloney virus-induced lymphoma) tumor ascites using recombinant human IL-2 showed a dose-dependent prolongation of survival (Talmadge and Chirigos, 1985). The optimal therapeutic activity with rHu IL-2 observed at 100 units/animal, (either three times per week or daily i.p.). Less activity was observed with higher doses of the IL-2. The animals that had no apparent tumor burden on day 55 rejected a second tumor challenge, whereas control animals were not protected against tumor challenge. The schedule and dosage dependency of the therapeutic activity of IL-2 were also observed for the treatment of experimental M109 metastases and B16-BL6 experimental and spontaneous metastases. In this study, the optimal prolongation of survival was observed following the triweekly or daily administration of 100 units of rHu IL-2. In contrast, lower or higher doses of rHu IL-2 had less therapeutic activity. In parallel to these observations, it was found that a high dose of rHu IL-2 inhibits T-cell adjuvancy effects, indicating a probable close relationship between optimal immunomodulatory dose and therapeutic dose. These observations also underscore the need to analyze a broad range of doses in order to probe for the most effective.

Another more recently discovered variable in the optimum immunomodulatory dose is the frequency of administration. A number of agents have been reported to boost macrophage and NK activity; however, few studies have been reported describing the response of macrophages and NK cells to multiple treatments in various treatment protocols with these agents. Maintaining augmented levels of effector cells by repeated therapy is obviously desirable; however, recent results indicate that multiple treatments may be counterproductive in maintaining a sustained boosting of NK-cell activity. Piccoli et al., (1984) and Saito et al., (1985) reported on the lack of a sustained or cyclic augmentation of NK activity by repeated injections with MVE-2. Similarly, Saito et al., (1985) reported on the development of hyporesponsiveness of natural killer cells to augmentation of activity after multiple treatments with MVE-2, Corynebacterium parvum, poly IC:LC, and α-interferon. In these studies, in contrast to a significant increase in splenic NK activity obtained with a single treatment with each of these agents, multiple treatments led to a progressive decrease in the degree of augmentation of NK activity. In contrast, multiple injections with these agents resulted in sustained augmentation of macrophage-mediated reactivity. Recent results from mouse experiments show that multiple injections of interferon do not augment NK cytotoxicity but reduce this activity compared to the effect obtained with a single treatment (Saito et al., 1985).

The current results and those reported by others emphasize the necessity to determine the immunopharmacodynamics of these agents to establish the most effective treatment protocol to sustain the immunopharmacological response. Only such a protocol would be expected to be the most effective for the treatment of cancer.

The study of immunotherapeutic agents in vivo with various tumors and mouse strains, including the nude mouse inoculated with human tumors, will produce a wealth of new information of both fundamental and practical importance. It is essential to emphasize that although the understanding of targets and mechanisms of action of the various immunotherapeutic agents has progressed well, our knowledge about the use of such agents in the immunosuppressed, tumor-bearing individual, particularly following the use of other therapies, is grossly wanting. To conserve time, money, and manpower, it would seem prudent to emphasize tumor models directly analogous to the situation in man, i.e., the adjuvant use of immunotherapy in mice treated with conventional cytoreductive therapy with the goal of monitoring the premorbid status of the immune system, evaluating the impact of the immunotherapy on parameters related to resistance, establishing correlates of therapeutic response, and finally, determining whether cure is associated with resistance to rechallenge. The clear-cut demonstration of immune eradication of cancer remains a primary, yet generally unconfirmed, rationale for the use of immunotherapy.

Conceptually, such research will clarify the effects that immunotherapeutic agents have on the humoral as well as the cellular arm of the immune system and clarify their respective roles in antitumor action. The relative importance of the specific immune mechanisms and of the nonimmune recognition mechanisms operative needs to be determined in order to assess the ultimate usefulness of cancer vaccines as part of the immunotherapy protocol. These studies will have an important impact on present-day thinking concerning the etiology, pathogenesis, and therapy of not only cancer but other diseases such as the infectious complications that are so frequently attendant to cancer. At the pragmatic level, animal experimentation should provide useful guidelines for a more effective approach to the treatment with immunotherapy alone or, more likely, for combination therapies leading to new and more effective strategies of treatment for human cancer.

5.5.9. Future Directions: Synergistic Strategies

We have seen some benefit of immunorestorative therapy in situations where primary cytoreductive therapy has had a fair chance of cure. These responses have occurred almost totally as a result of the increasing numbers of animals that remain in remission. From a chemotherapeutic standpoint, these results constitute an effect on a small portion of the cancer population. The principle underlying this effect is that the immune system can only be expected to eradicate minimal residual tumor if the amount of tumor is small enough and the immune system sufficiently spared by the chemotherapy or other cytoreductive therapy to enable it to respond. No single agent in our immunotherapeutic repertoire can be seen to cure regularly spontaneous or syngeneic, poorly immunogenic cancers without concomitant cytoreductive therapy. We can say that in the repertoire we have many active biologicals and drugs and that we have learned a good deal about their immunopharmacologies. The specificity of the action of various agents is often unique, and this has allowed the prediction that ultimately these agents may be selectively applied in therapeutic settings where a specific deficit exists and that they may be used in combination to achieve a more complete reconstitution and therapeutic effect. By way of speculation, we think it is time to draw from our knowledge of the basic immunopharmacology of the agents discussed and from the existing examples of synergistic combinations of immunotherapeutic agents to make up, by prediction, new strategies for combination use.

In discussing these prospective strategies, we would like to highlight the possibilities of using the many immunotherapeutic agents in combined protocols. It should be noted that early antitumor synergism was seen by Mathé with BCG and *Pseudomonas* vaccine and by Old and co-workers with BCG and endotoxin in tumor necrosis serum (TNS) production (Carswell *et al.*, 1975).

Natural and cloned interferons have shown the capacity to modulate host resistance, particularly macrophage- and killer cell-mediated immunity, and to inhibit progression of human tumors. Synergistic interactions of α,-, β-, and γ-interferons have been described, and synergistic anticancer effects have been noted in laboratory animals using interferon in combination with such agents as isoprinosine (Cerutti *et al.*, 1978), cyclomunine, *Staph.* lysate, cimetidine (C. Chany, personal communication), and tumor necrosis factor (Sugarman *et al.*, 1985). Recent reports indicate that γ-interferon represents a major macrophage-activating factor (MAF) for tumoricidal macrophages. There are considerable data supporting synergistic interactions of liposomes, endotoxin, and muramyl dipeptides with MAF (see Fidler *et al.*, 1981). These agents now may logically be employed in combination with γ-interferon. It appears important to determine how the interferons interact with chemotherapy and radiation to ascertain if they should be used in combination or sequence. We need to decide whether to integrate interferon in combination with other immunotherapeutics following cytoreduction therapy. As well as the examples mentioned, the combination of interferon with mixed lymphokines, tumor necrosis factor, and lymphotoxin appears logical to enhance antitumor mechanisms, with thymic hormones, interleukin 1 and 2, thymomimetic drugs, and macrophage activators to enhance both specific and nonspecific host resistance.

The thymic hormones have shown the capacity, both individually and collectively, to modulate the number and, more importantly, the function of T-cell precursors and mature thymus-dependent lymphocytes. They have also been shown to improve cellular immune function. The effects of thymic hormones to reconstitute the T-cell system are somewhat limited, and recent evidence suggests that other factors, such as interleukin 2, may also be necessary in regulating the ontogeny of T lymphocytes (see Hadden *et al.*, 1986). Other recent evidence indicates that thymic hormones and IL-2 may be complementary in their effects to reconstitute the T-cell system (Trevers and Goldstein, 1980; Hadden *et al.*, 1986). The combination of thymic hormones with thymomimetic drugs and other lymphokines seems logical in terms of efforts to reconstitute T-cell immunity. Their eventual combination with macrophage-based approaches, antitumor therapy, and antisuppressor cell therapy also seems warranted.

Lymphokines offer many possibilities for multimodality therapy. Mixtures of lymphokines (free of interferon) have shown interferonlike effects to induce tumor regression in tumors of both mice and humans. Synergistic interactions on macrophages of lymphokines with endotoxin, muramyl dipeptides, and thymomimetic drugs such as isoprinosine, NPT 15392, and levamisole are well documented. Their use in combination therapy with thymic hormones suggests that it would be appropriate to test the capacity of detoxified endotoxin to synergize with lymphokines; this needs to be tested. It appears that the muramyl dipeptides now offer the potential of replacing mycobacterial therapy with defined macrophage-activating molecules that confer protection against pathogen challenge, are adjuvant active, and prime for TNF production. It also appears that endotoxin has been successfully detoxified as monophosphoryl lipid A by Ribi and shown to elicit TNF following MDP or BCG priming (Bloksma et al., 1985). We now have the prospect of harnessing the TNF phenomenon using detoxified forms of both MDP and endotoxin in humans. These advances represent important steps in anticancer immunopharmacology and should translate into more effective human protocols that can be employed in parallel with existing strategies.

Cloned lymphotoxin and TNF offer the prospect of introducing two new cytotoxic agents into anticancer protocols both alone and in combination with other cytotoxins (e.g., chemotherapy, radiotherapy, interferon) and other immunorestorative agents.

In addition to the previously mentioned chemically defined immunotherapeutic agents, thymomimetic drugs (isoprinosine, NPT 15392, levamisole, and imuthiol) and macrophage-active agents (e.g., glycans and muramyl dipeptides) have shown potent immunopharmacological activity, particularly as immunorestoratives. It now seems logical to examine their use in combination with other immunotherapeutic agents since their immunopharmacologies have been elucidated.

Recent technological developments with hybridomas offer exciting new prospects. A number of monoclonals (MoAbs) have been raised to human tumorassociated antigens and appear to be selective enough to use for diagnostics and therapy. A variety of animal and human tumors have been successfully localized and imaged using isotopically labeled antitumor MoAbs, particularly when double isotopes are used to allow computer-based techniques for subtracting vascular background. Unarmed mouse MoAbs have shown activity to regress both animal and human tumors. A variety of immunotoxins are being developed including, as arming agents, toxins, anticancer drugs, and isotopes. Despite difficulties relating to the use of heterologous proteins, circulating antigen–antibody complexes, only partial localization in the tumor, etc., the potential of this "silver bullet" approach is evident. The combining of MoAbs with other cytotoxins seems natural in the same way we now employ multidrug combined chemotherapy in cytoreduction protocols.

The capacity of monoclonals to improve our efforts to produce anticancer vaccines is of obvious importance. Batch preparation of tumor antigens using affinity chromatography with immobilized antitumor MoAbs will yield volumes of antigen in a highly pure state. This will allow them to be used directly as antigens for vaccine, or, more importantly, in the future it will allow purified antigens to create genes for recombinant engineering of large quantities of tumor-related antigens for synthetic vaccine formation. The development of modern technology in this area makes it clear that by preparation of the proper vaccine, cell-mediated immunity can be specifically invoked. The prospect of employing this technology in the development of more effective antitumor responses is feasible.

Finally, it is apparent that human antitumor responses are limited by immunosuppressive influences deriving from the tumor and from the immune system. The use of selective chemotherapy to reduce tumor-induced immunosuppression can have important beneficial effects. Obviation of the immunosuppression deriving from the host by use of such agents as cylophosphamide and cimetidine, which act to inhibit T-cell-induced suppression, or indomethacin to inhibit macrophage-induced suppression via prostaglandins has been shown experimentally to be of benefit to survival and longevity in animals with cancer.

The appropriate use of both nutritional support and growth factors to restore immune cell populations decimated by toxic cytoreductive therapy figures into a comprehensive ''prohost'' approach to cancer.

Combined immunotherapy of cancer in light of the many recent developments is an idea whose time has come (see Figure 2). It is currently impossible to imagine its placement in any setting other than following the cytoreductive methods currently available. It appears that chemotherapy, radiotherapy, and surgery can only be improved when conjoined with interferons, antitumor MoAbs, immunotoxins, lymphotoxin, and tumor necrosis factor. The toxicities of the latter agents would allow their use collectively. The complementary strategies of reversing immunosuppression and of augmenting both specific and nonspecific resistance mechanisms directed toward the tumor by using the various approaches described can only enhance the cleanup of minimal residual tumor and prevent metastasis formation. Additionally, the restoration of natural

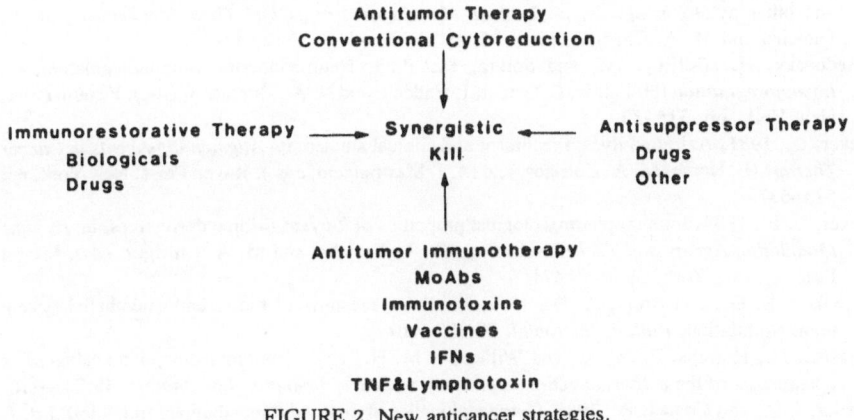

FIGURE 2. New anticancer strategies.

and specific resistance will inevitably improve cancer management by reducing the incidence and severity of opportunistic infections, which complicate cancer and its treatment.

REFERENCES

Alexander, P. 1975, The role of macrophages in the host defense against cancer, in: *Host Defense against Cancer and Its Potentiation* (D. Mizuno, G. Chihara, F. Fukjoka, T. Yamamoto, and Y. Yamamura, eds.), University of Tokyo Press, Tokyo, pp. 113–130.

Altman, P. L., and Dittmer Katz, D. (eds.), 1979, *Inbred and Genetically Defined Strains of Laboratory Animals*, Federation of American Societies for Experimental Biology, Bethesda.

Amery, W. K., and Hörig, C., 1984, Levamisole, in: *Immune Modulation Agents and Their Mechanisms* (R. L. Fenichel and M. A. Chirigos, eds.), Marcel Dekker, New York, pp. 383–408.

Amery, W. K., Spreafico, F., Rojas, A. F., Denissen, E., and Chirigos, M. A., 1977, Adjuvant treatment with levamisole in cancer: A review of experimental and clinical data, *Cancer Treat. Rev.* **4**:167–194.

Aoki, T., 1984, Lentinan, in: *Immune Modulation Agents and Their Mechanisms* (R. L. Fenichel and M. A. Chirigos, eds.), Marcel Dekker, New York, pp. 63–77.

Audhya, T., Scheid, M. P., and Goldstein, G., 1983, Contrasting biological activities of thymopoietin and splenin, two closely related polypeptide products of thymus and spleen, *Proc. Natl. Acad. Sci. U.S.A.* **81**:2847–2849.

Aune, T. M., and Pierce, C. M., 1983, Inhibition of interferon or soluble immune response suppressor (SIRS) mediated suppression by levamisole, *Int. J. Immunopharmacol.* **5**:91–98.

Bach, M., Droz, D., Noel, L., Blanchard, D., Dardenne, M., and Peking, A., 1980, Effects of long-term treatment with circulating thymic factor on murine lupus, *Arthritis Rheum.* **23**:1351–1358.

Ballow, M., Dupont, B., and Good, R. A., 1973, Autoimmune hemolytic anemia in Wiskott-Aldrich syndrome during treatment with transfer factor, *J. Pediatr.* **83**:771–780.

Bartocci, A., Papademitriou, V., and Chirigos, M. A., 1980, Enhanced macrophage and natural killer cell antitumor activity by various molecular weight maleic anhydride divinyl ethers, *J. Immunopharmacol.* **2**:149–158.

Behling, U., and Nowotny, A., 1977, Immune adjuvancy of lipopolysaccharide and a non toxic hydrolytic product demonstrating oscillating effects with time, *J. Immunol.* **118**:1905–1907.

Berd, D., Maguire, H. C., and Mastrangelo, M. J., 1984, Immunopotentiation by cyclophosphamide and other cytotoxic agents, in: *Immune Modulation Agents and Their Mechanisms* (R. L. Fenichel and M. A. Chirigos, eds.), Marcel Dekker, New York, 39–61.

Besedovsky, H., DelRey, A., and Sorkin, E., 1983, Neuroendocrine immunoregulation, in: *Immunoregulation* (N. Fabris, E. Garaci, J. Hadden, and N. A. Mitchison, eds.), Plenum Press, New York, pp. 315–339.

Bicker, U., 1981, Aziridine dyes: Preclinical and clinical studies, in: *Augmenting Agents in Cancer Therapy* (E. Hersh, M. A. Chirigos, and M. J. Mastrangelo, eds.), Raven Press, New York, pp. 523–537.

Bicker, U. F., 1984, Immunopharmacological properties of 2-cyanaziridine derivatives, in: *Immune Modulation Agents and Their Mechanisms* (R. L. Fenichel and M. A. Chirigos, eds), Marcel Dekker, New York, pp. 447–474.

Bliznakov, E. G., and Adler, A. D., 1972, Nonlinear response of the reticuloendothelial system upon stimulation, *Pathol. Microbiol.* **38**:393–410.

Bloksma, N., Hofhuis, F. M. A., and Willers, J. M. N., 1985, Muramyl dipeptide analogues as potentiators of the antitumor action of endotoxin, *Cancer Immunol. Immunother.* **19**:205–210.

Brazier, J. L., and Coquet, B., 1985, Pharmacokinetics of diethyldithiocarbamate (imuthiol), *Int. J. Immunopharmacol.* **7**:336–341.

Bruley-Rosset, M., Hercend, T., Martinez, J., Rappaport, H., and Mathé, G., 1981, Prevention of spontaneous tumors of aged mice by immunopharmacological manipulations: Study of immune antitumor mechanisms, *J. Natl. Cancer Inst.* **66**:1113–1119.

Bruley-Rosset, M., Vergnon, I., and Renoux, G., 1985, Influences of sodium diethyldithiocarbamate, DTC (imuthiol), on T-cell defective responses of aged Balb/c mice, *Int. J. Immunopharmacol.* **8**:287–297.

Carrano, R. A., Kinashita, K., Imondi, A. R., and Duliucci, J. D., 1981, MVE-2: Preclinical pharmacology and toxicology, in: *Augmenting Agents in Cancer Therapy*, Volume 16 (E. Hersh, M. A. Chirigos, and M. J. Mastrangelo, eds.), Raven Press, New York, pp. 345–349.

Carrano, R. A., Iuliucci, J. D., Luce, J. K., Page, J. A., and Irriondi, A. R., 1984, MVE-2: Development of an immunoadjuvant for cancer treatment, in: *Immune Modulation Agents and Their Mechanisms* (R. L. Fenichel and M. A. Chirigos, eds.), Marcel Dekker, New York, pp. 243–260.

Carswell, E. A., Old, J., Kassel, R. L., Green, S., Flor, N., and Williamson, B., An endotoxin-induced serum factor that causes necrosis of tumors, *Proc. Natl. Acad. Sci. U.S.A.* **72**:3666–3670, 1975.

Casagrande, J., and Pike, M. D., 1975, Reduced incidence of spontaneous tumors: Another statistical analysis, *Science* **190**:808–809.

Cerutti, I., Chany, C., and Schlumberger, J., 1979, Isoprinosine increases the antitumor action of interferon, *Int. J. Immunopharmacol.* **1**:59–63.

Chedid, L., 1983, Muramyl peptides as possible endogenous immunopharmacologic mediators, *Microbiol. Immunol.* **27**:723–732.

Chedid, L., Audibert, F., and Johnson, A. G., 1978, Biological activities of muramyl dipeptides, a synthetic glycopeptide analogous to bacterial immunoregulating agents, *Prog. Allergy* **25**:63–68.

Chedid, L., Parant, F. J., Lederer, C., Choay, J. P., and Lefrancier, P. L., 1982, Biological activity of a new muramyl peptide adjuvant devoid of pyrogenicity, *Infect. Immun.* **35**:417–424.

Chedid, L., Bahr, G., Riveau, G., and Kreuger, J., 1984, Specific absorption with monoclonal antibody to muramyl dipeptide of the pyrogenic and somnogenic activities of rabbit monokines, *Proc. Natl. Acad. Sci. U.S.A.* **81**:5888–5891.

Cheers, C., and McKenzie, I. F. C., 1978, Resistance and susceptibility of mice to bacterial infections: Genetics of listeriosis, *Infect. Immun.* **19**:755–770.

Cheever, M. A., Thompson, J. A., Kern, D. E., and Greenberg, P. D., 1985, Interleukin 2 (IL-2) administered *in vivo:* Influence of IL-2 route and timing on T cell growth, *J. Immunol.* **134**:3895–3900.

Chihara, G., 1983, Preclinical evaluation of lentinan in animal models, in: *Biological Response Modifiers in Human Oncology and Immunology* (T. Klein, S. Specter, H. Friedman, and A. Szentivanyi, eds.), Plenum Press, New York, pp. 189–197.

Chirigos, M. A. (ed.), 1977a, *Modulation of Host Immune Resistance in the Prevention or Treatment of Induced Neoplasia, Fogarty International Center Proceedings* 28, U.S. Government Printing Office, Washington.

Chirigos, M. A. (ed.), 1977b, *Control of Neoplasia by Modulation of the Immune System*, Raven Press, New York.

Chirigos, M. A., 1981, Enhanced antitumor response to combined treatment with maleic vinyl ether, *Exp. Pathol.* **19**:19–23.

Chirigos, M. A., and Mastrangelo, M. J., 1982, Immunorestoration by chemicals, in: *Immunological Approaches to Cancer Therapeutics* (E. Mihich, ed.), John Wiley & Sons, New York, pp. 191–240.

Chirigos, M. A., and Stylos, W. A., 1980, Immunomodulatory effect of various molecular weight maleic anhydride vinyl ethers and other agents *in vivo, Cancer Res.* **40**:1967–1972.

Chirigos, M. A., Schlick, E., Piccoli, M., Read, E., Hartung, K., and Bartocci, A., 1983, Characterization of agents, in: *Advances in Immunopharmacology* (J. W. Hadden, ed.), Pergamon Press, Oxford, pp. 669–677.

Chirigos, M. A., Saito, T., and Talmadge, J. E., 1984, *Immunomodulatory Activity of Picibinal (OK432), Excerpta Medica, Amsterdam,* pp. 20–31.

Chirigos, M. A., Schlick, E., Ruffman, R., Budzynski, W., Sinibaldi, P., and Gruys, E., 1985, Pharmacokinetics and therapeutic activity of poly ICLC, *J. Biol. Resp. Mod.* **4:**721–627.

Chung, V., Florentin, I., and Renoux, G., 1985, Increased production of interleukins 1 and 2 after imuthiol administration to young immunocompetent and aged immunodepressed mice, *Int. J. Immunopharmacol.* **7:**335–340.

Cohen, C., 1979, Inbred animals, history, use and classification, in: *Inbred and Genetically Defined Strains of Laboratory Animals* (P. L. Altman and D. Dittmer Katz, eds.), Federation of American Societies for Experimental Biology, Bethesda.

Cooper, E. (ed), 1984, *Stress, Immunity, and Aging,* Marcel Dekker, New York.

Corke, C. F., Sedgwick, A. D., MacKay, A. R., Bates, M. B., and Willoughby, D., 1984, Enhancement of colloidal clearance in normal rats by sodium diethyldithiocarbamate (DTC), *Int. J. Immunopharmacol.* **6:**535–537.

Cotzias, G. C., and Tang, L. C., 1977, An adenylate cyclase of brain reflects propensity for breast cancer in mice, *Science* **197:**1094–1096.

Cox, K. O., and Keast, D., 1974, Studies of the *Corynebacterium parvum-associated anemia in mice, Clin. Exp. Immunol.* **17:**199–207.

Crespo, R. S. (ed.), 1982, *Potentiating in the Biological Sciences,* Wiley Interscience, New York.

Cudkowicz, G., and Bennett, M., 1971, Peculiar immunobiology of bone marrow allografts, *J. Exp. Med.* **134:**83–102.

Damais, C., Parant, M., Chedid, L., Lefrancier, P., and Choay, J., 1978, *In vitro* spleen cell responsiveness to various analogs of MDP (N-acetylmuramyl-L-alanyl-D-isoglutamine), a synthetic immunoadjuvant in MDP high responder mice, *Cell. Immunol.* **35:**173–179.

Dardenne, M., Niaudet, P., Simon-Lavoine, N., and Bach, J.-F., 1980, Stimulation of thymic humoral functions by cyclomunine, a cyclic peptide in mice, *Int. J. Immunopharmacol.* **2:**154.

Davis, J., and Shires, C. (eds.), 1986, *Host Defenses in Trauma and Surgery,* Raven Press, New York.

Descotes, J. (ed.), 1986, *Immunotoxicology of Drugs and Chemicals,* Elsevier, Oxford.

Dianzani, F., 1985, The biology of the interferon system, ES, **5:**59–63. DiLuzio, N. R., 1985, Update on the immunomodulating activities of glucans, *Springer Semin. Immunopathol.* **8:**387–400.

DiLuzio, N. R., and Jacques, P., 1986, Glucans as immunodulators, in: *Advances in Immunopharmacology 3* (L. Chedid, J. Hadden, F. Spreafico, P. Dukor, and D. Willoughby, eds.), Pergamon Press, London, pp. 369–375.

Ehrke, M. J., and Mihich, E., 1985, Immunoregulation by cancer chemotherapeutic agents, in: *The Reticuloendothelial System,* Volume 8 (J. W. Hadden and A. Szentivanyi, eds.), Plenum Press, New York, pp. 309–347.

Faanes, R. B., Merluzzi, V. J., Ralph, P., Williams, N., and Tarnowski, G. S., 1980, Restoration of tumor and drug-induced immune dysfunction, in: *International Symposium on New Trends in Human Immunology and Cancer Immunotherapy* (B. Serrou and C. Rosenfeld, eds.), Doin Editeurs, Paris, pp. 953–964.

Fabris, N., Pierpaoli, W., and Sorkin, E., 1972, Lymphocytes, hormones and aging, *Nature* **240:** 557–559.

Fenichel, R. L., and Chirigos, M. A. (eds.), 1984, *Immune Modulation Agents and Their Mechanisms,* Marcel Dekker, New York.

Fenichel, R. L., Alburn, H. E., Schreck, P. A., Bloom, R., and Gregory, F. J., 1980, Immunomodulating and antimetastatic activity of 3-(*p*-chlorophenyl)thiazolo(3,2-a)benzimidazole-2-acetic acid (Wy-18,251, NSC 310633), *J. Immunopharmacol.* **2:**491–508.

Festing, M. R. W. (ed.), 1979, *Inbred Strains in Biomedical Research,* Macmillan, London.

Fidler, I. J., Sone, S., Fogler, W. E., and Barnes, Z. L., 1981, Eradication of spontaneous metastases and activation of alveolar macrophages by intravenous injections of liposomes containing muramyl dipeptide, *Proc. Natl. Acad. Sci. U.S.A.* **78:**1680–1685.

Florentin, I., Huchet, R., Bruley-Rosset, M., and Halle-Pannenko, O., 1976, Studies on the mode of action of BCG, *Cancer Immun. Immunother.* **1:**31–39.

Florentin, I., Bruley-Rosset, M., Schulz, J., Davigny, M., Kiger, N., and Mathé, G., 1981, Attempt at functional classification of chemically-defined immunomodulators, in: *Advances in Immunopharmacology* (J. W. Hadden, L. Chedid, P. Mullen, and F. Spreafico, eds.), Pergamon Press, Oxford, pp. 311–325.

Florentin, I., Taylor, E., Davigny, M., Mathé, G., and Hadden, J. W., 1982, Kinetic studies of the immunopharmacologic effects of NPT 15392 in mice, *Int. J. Immunopharmacol.* **4:**225–234.

Florentin, I., Kraus, L., Bruley-Rosset, M., and Mathé, G., 1983, *In vivo* functional characterization of immunomodulators, in: *Advances in Immunopharmacology 2* (J. W. Hadden, L. Chedid, P. Dukor, F. Spreafico, and D. Willoughby, eds.), Pergamon Press, New York, pp. 661–668.

Friedman, H., 1981, Immunomodulating effects of cimetidine, in: *Augmenting Agents in Cancer Therapy* (E. M. Hersh, M. A. Chirigos, and M. J. Mastrangelo, eds.), Raven Press, New York, pp. 417–425.

Friedman, H., Klein, T. W., and Specter, S., 1983, Infection and immunosuppression, in: *Advances in Immunopharmacology 2* (J. W. Hadden, L. Chedid, P. Dukor, F. Spreafico, and D. Willoughby, eds.), Pergamon Press, New York, pp. 773–783.

Fudenberg, H. H., Whitten, H. D., and Ambrogi, F. (eds.), 1984, *Immunomodulation: New Frontiers and Advances*, Plenum Press, New York.

Fumarola, D., 1981, Contaminating endotoxin: A serious problem in immunological research, *Cell. Immunol.* **58:**216–217.

Georgiev, V. (ed.), 1983a, *Survey of Drug Research in Immunologic Disease*, Volume 1, *Aliphatic Derivatives*, S. Karger, Basel.

Georgiev, V. (ed.), 1983b, *Survey of Drug Research in Immunologic Disease*, Volume 2, *Noncondensed Aromatic Derivatives*, S. Karger, Basel.

Gershwin, M. E., Kruse, W., and Goldstein, G. 1979, The effect of thymopietin and ubiquitin on spontaneous immunopathology of New Zealand mice, *J. Rheum.* **6:**610–620.

Goldstein, A. L. (ed.), 1984, *Thymic Hormones and Lymphokines*, Plenum Press, New York.

Gordon, P., Rosen, B., and Brown, E. R., 1974, Anti-herpes virus action of isoprinosine, *Antimicrob. Agents Chemother.* **5:**153–156.

Greene, M. C. (ed.), 1981, *Genetic Variants and Strains of the Laboratory Mouse*, Gustav Fischer Verlag, Stuggart, New York.

Gregory, F. J., Alburn, H. E., Carlson, R. P., and Lewis, A. J., 1980, Wy-40,453: A mesoionic thiabenzothiazole with novel immunomodulator activity, *Int. J. Immunopharmacol.* **2:**166–167.

Guillaumin, J. M., Lepape, A., and Renoux, G., 1986, Fate and distribution of radioactive sodium diethyldithiocarbamate (imuthiol) in the mouse, *Int. J. Immunopharmacol.* **8:**859–865.

Hadden, J. W., 1977, Cyclic nucleotides in lymphocyte proliferation and differentiation, in: *Immunopharmacology* (J. W. Hadden, R. G. Coffey, and F. Spreafico, eds.), Plenum Press, New York, pp. 1–28.

Hadden, J. W., 1980, The immunopharmacology of immunotherapy: An update, in: *Advances in Immunopharmacology* (J. Hadden, L. Chedid, F. Spreafico, and P. Mullen, eds.), Pergamon Press, Oxford, pp. 327–342.

Hadden, J. W., 1983a, Cyclic nucleotides and related mechanisms in immune regulation: A mini review, in: *Immunoregulation* (N. Fabris, E. Gonaci, J. Hadden, and A. Mitchison, eds.), Plenum Press, New York, pp. 201–230.

Hadden, J. W., 1983b, Characterization of immunotherapeutic agents: An overview, in: *Advances in Immunopharmacology 2* (J. Hadden, L. Chedid, P. Dukor, F. Spreafico, and D. Willoughby, eds.), Pergamon Press, New York, pp. 691–702.

Hadden, J. W., 1985, Thymomimetic drugs, in: *Symposium on Immunopharmacology*, Volume 3 (P.A. Meischer, L. Bolis, and M. Ghione, eds.), Serona Symposia, Raven Press, New York, pp. 183–192.

Hadden, J. W., 1987, Immunotherapy in the treatment of infectious diseases, in: *Proceedings of the International Symposium on Immunological Adjuvants* (J. A. Majde, ed.), Alan R. Liss, New York, pp. 337–349.

Hadden, J. W., and Delmonte, L., 1978, Cyclic nucleotides in immunopotentiators action, in: *Handbook of Cancer Immunology*, Volume 5 (H. Waters, ed.), Garland Publishing, New York, pp. 109–134.

Hadden, J. W., and England, A., 1977, Molecular aspects of macrophage activation, in: *Immunopharmacology* (J. W. Hadden, R. G. Coffey, and F. Spreafico, eds.), Plenum Press, New York, pp. 87–100.

Hadden, J. W., and Giner-Sorolla, A., 1981, Isoprinosine and NPT 15392: Modulators of lymphocyte and macrophage development and function, in: *Augmenting Agents in Cancer Therapy* (E. Hersh, M. A. Chirigos, and M. J. Mastrangelo, eds.), Raven Press, New York, pp. 497–522.

Hadden, J. W., and Spreafico, F., Animal tumor models for evaluating chemically defined immunomodulators, in: Biological response modifiers in human oncology and immunology (T. Klein, S. Specter, H. Friedman, and A. Szentivanyi, eds.), Plenum Press, New York, pp. 309–315.

Hadden, J. W., and Spreafico, F. (guest eds.), 1985, New strategies of immunotherapy, in: *Springer Seminars in Immunopathology*, Volume 8 (P. A. Miescher and H. J. Muller-Eberhard, eds.), Springer-Verlag, Heidelberg.

Hadden, J. W., and Spreafico, F. (guest eds.), 1986, *Springer Seminars in Immunopathology: New Perspectives in Immunotherapy (II)*, Volume 9 (P. A. Miescher and H. J. Muller-Eberhard, eds.), Springer-Verlag, Heidelberg.

Hadden, J. W., and Stewart, W. E. II (eds.), 1981, *The Lymphokines: Biochemistry and Biological Activity*, Humana Press, New York.

Hadden, J. W., and Wybran, J., 1981, Isoprinosine, NPT 15392, and azimexon: Modulators of lymphocyte and macrophage development and function, in: *Advances in Immunopharmacology* (J. Hadden, L. Chedid, P. Muller, and F. Spreafico, eds.), Pergamon Press, Oxford, pp. 457–468.

Hadden, J. W., Coffey, R. C., Hadden, E. M., Lopez-Corrales, E., and Sunshine, G. H., 1975, Effects of levamisole and imidazole on lymphocyte proliferation and cyclic nucleotide levels, *Cell. Immunol.* **20:**98–103.

Hadden, J. W., Delmonte, L., and Oettgen, H., 1977a, Mechanisms of immunopotentiation, in: *Immunopharmacology* (J. W. Hadden, R. G. Coffey, and F. Spreafico, eds.), Plenum Press, New York, pp. 279–313.

Hadden, J. W., Coffey, R. G., and Spreafico, F. (eds.), 1977b, *Immunopharmacology*, Plenum Press, New York.

Hadden, J. W., Lopez, C., O'Reilly, A. J., and Hadden, E. M., 1977c, Levamisole and inosiplex: Antiviral agents with immunopotentiating action, *Ann. N.Y. Acad. Sci.* **284:**139–152.

Hadden, J. W., England, A., Sadlik, J. R., and Hadden, E. M., 1979, The comparative effects of isoprinosine, levamisole, muramyl dipeptide, and SM 1213 on lymphocyte and macrophage proliferation and activation *in vitro*, *Int. J. Immunopharmacol.* **1:**17–27.

Hadden, J. W., England, A., Sadlik, J., and Hadden, E. M., 1981a, Lymphokine-induced macrophage proliferation and activation, in: *Lymphokines and Thymic Hormones: Their Potential Utilization in Cancer* (A. Goldstein and M. Chirigos, eds.), Raven Press, New York, pp. 159–172.

Hadden, J. W., Chedid, L., Mullen, P., and Spreafico, F. (eds.), 1981b, *Advances in Immunopharmacology*, Pergamon Press, Oxford.

Hadden, J. W., Hadden, E. M., Spira, T., Settineri, R., Simon, L., and Giner-Sorolla, A., 1982, Effects of NPT 15392 *in vitro* on human leukocyte functions, *Int. J. Immunopharmacol.* **4:**225–234.

Hadden, J. W., Chedid, L., Dukor, P., Spreafico, F., and Willoughby, D. (eds.), 1983a, *Advances in Immunopharmacology 2*, Pergamon Press, New York.

Hadden, J. W., Cornaglia-Ferraris, P., and Coffey, R. G., 1983b, Purine analogs as immunomodulators, in: *Progress in Immunology IV* (Y. Yamamura and T. Kishimoto, eds.), Academic Press, Tokyo, pp. 1393–1408.

Hadden, J. W., Specter, S., and Hadden, E. M., 1986, Effects of T cell growth factor/interleukin II on prothymocytes, *Lymphokine Res.* 5:s49–s54.

Hall, N. R. S., McGillis, J. P., and Goldstein, A. L., 1984, Activation of neuroendocrine pathways by thymosin peptides, in: *Stress, Immunity and Aging*, Volume 24 (E. Cooper, ed.), Marcel Dekker, New York, pp. 209–223.

Halpern, B., and Fray, A., 1969, Declanchement de l'anemie hemolytique autoimmune chez de jeunes souriceaux NZB par l'administration de *C. parvum*, *Ann. Inst. Pasteur* 117:778–781.

Hammer, C. (ed.), 1982, *Drug Development*, CRC Press, Boca Raton, FL.

Hamuro, J., and Chihara, G., 1984, Lentinan, a T-cell oriented immunopotentiator: Its experimental and clinical applications and possible mechanisms of immune modulation, in: *Immune Modulation Agents and Their Mechanisms* (R. L. Fenichel and M. A. Chirigos, eds.), Marcel Dekker, New York, pp. 409–436.

Hanley, D. F., Wiranowska-Stewart, M., and Stewart, W. E. II, 1979, Pharmacology of interferons, I. Pharmacologic distinctions between human leukocyte and fibroblast interferons, *Int. J. Immunopharmacol.* 1:219–226.

Herberman, R. B., Djeu, J. Y., Kay, H. D., Ortaldo, J. R., Riccardi, C., Bonnard, G. D., Holden, H. T., Fagnani, R., Santoni, A., and Pucetti, P., 1979, Natural killer cells: Characteristics and regulation of activity, *Immunol. Rev.* 44:43–70.

Herberman, R. B., Brunda, M. J., Cannon, G. B., Djeu, J. Y., Nunn-Hargrove, M., Jett, J. R., Ortaldo, J. R., Reynolds, C., Riccardi, C., and Santoni, A., 1981, Augmentation of natural killer (NK) cell activity by interferon and interferon inducers, in: *Augmenting Agents in Cancer Therapy* (E. M. Hersh, M. A. Chirigos, and M. J. Mastrangelo, eds.), Raven Press, New York, pp. 253–265.

Hersh, E., Chirigos, M. A., and Mastrangelo, M. J. (eds.), 1981, *Augmenting Agents in Cancer Therapy*, Raven Press, New York.

Hibbs, J. B., Remington, J. S., and Stewart, C. C., 1980, Modulation of immunity and host resistance by micro-organisms, *Pharmacol. Ther.* 8:37–69.

Hoffman, J. I. E., 1976, The incorrect use of chi-square analysis for paired data, *Clin. Exp. Immunol.* 24:227–229.

Ishitsuka, H., Umeda, Y., Sakamoto, A., and Yagi, Y., 1983a, Protective activity of thymosin α_1 against tumor progression in immunosuppressed mice, in: *Biological Response Modifiers in Human Oncology and Immunology*, Volume 166 (T. Klein, S. Specter, H. Friedman, and A. Szentivanyi, Plenum Press, New York, pp. 87–100.

Ishitsuka, H., Umeda, Y., Nakamura, J., and Yagi, Y., 1983b, Protective activity of thymosin against opportunistic infections in animal models, *Cancer Immunol. Immunother.* 14:145–150.

Ishitsuka, H., Umeda, Y., Tzuka, E., Ohta, Y., and Yagi, Y., 1984, Efficacy of thymosin α_1 in animal models, in: *Thymic Hormones and Lymphokines* (A. L. Goldstein, ed.), Plenum Press, New York, pp. 425–438.

Jerne, N. R., and Nordin, A. A., 1963, Plaque formation in agar by single antibody producing cells, *Science* 140:405–408.

Jones, C., Lee, C., Hoehler, F., Koyama, P., Skinner, W., and Lamott, J. A., 1983, Observations on the immunomodulator NPT 15392 in New Zealand black mice, *Int. J. Immunopharmacol.* 5:85–90.

Khato, J., Chirigos, M. A., and Sieber, M., 1983, Antimetastatic effects of maleic anhydride divinyl ether in rats and mammary adenocarcinoma, *J. Immunopharmacol.* 5:65–75.

Kirchner, H., Glaser, M., and Herberman, R. B., 1975, Suppression of cell-mediated tumor immunity by *Corynebacterium parvum*, *Nature* 257:396–399.

Klein, T., Specter, S., Friedman, H., and Szentivanyi, A. (eds.), 1983, *Biological Response Modifiers in Human Oncology and Immunology*, Plenum Press, New York.

Leclerc, C., Judy, D., and Chedid, L., 1979, Inhibitory and stimulatory effects of a synthetic glycopeptide (MDP) on the *in vitro* PFC response: Factors affecting the response, *Cell. Immunol.* **42**:336–343.

Lederer, E., and Chedid, L., 1982, Immunomodulation by synthetic muramyl peptides and trehalose diesters, in: *Immunological Approaches to Cancer Therapeutics* (E. Mihich, ed.), John Wiley & Sons, New York, pp. 107–136.

Levy, H. B., and Chirigos, M. A., 1984, Studies with the interferon inducer and immune modulator, poly ICLC, in: *Clinical Applications of the Interferon System* (I. Lascostiz, ed.), *Contrib. Oncol.* **20**:358–375.

Levy, H. B., Stephen, E. S., Harrington, D., Engel, K., Riley, F., and Lvovsky, E., 1981, Polynucleotides in the treatment of disease, in: *Augmenting Agents in Cancer Therapy*, Volume 16 (E. Hersh, M. Chirigos, and M. Mastrangelo, eds.), Raven Press, New York, pp. 135–150.

Lilly, F., and Pincus, J., 1973, Genetic control of viral leukemogenesis, *Adv. Cancer Res.* **17**:231–277.

Lopez, C., 1975, Genetics of natural resistance to herpes virus infections in mice, *Nature* **258**:152–153.

Lotze, M. T., Frana, L. W., Sharrow, S. O., Robb, R. J., and Rosenberg, S. A., 1985, *In vivo* administration of purified human interleukin 2. I. Half-life and immunologic effects of the Jurkat cell line-derived interleukin 2, *J. Immunol.* **135**:2865–2875.

Makinodan, T., and Kay, M. M. B., 1980, Age influence on the immune system, *Adv. Immunol.* **29**:287–330.

Mantovani, A., and Spreafico, F., 1975, Allogeneic tumor enhancement by levamisole, a new immunostimulatory compound: Studies on cell-mediated immunity and humoral antibody response, *Eur. J. Cancer* **11**:537–544.

McCracken, A., McBride, W. H., and Weir, D. M., 1971, Adjuvant-induced anti red blood cell activity in CBA mice, *Clin. Exp. Immunol.* **8**:949–955.

Megel, H., and Gibson, J. P., 1984, Tilorone and related analogs, in: *Immune Modulation Agents and Their Mechanisms of Action* (R. L. Fenichel and M. A. Chirigos, eds.), Marcel Dekker, New York, pp. 97–119.

Mihich, E. (ed.), 1982, *Immunological Approaches to Cancer Therapeutics*, John Wiley & Sons, New York.

Mihich, E., and Kanter, P. M., 1987, The toxicology of biological response modifiers, in: *Immunotoxicology* (A. Berlin, J. Dean, M. H. Draper, E. M. B. Smith, and F. Spreafico, eds.), Martinus Nijhoff, Boston, pp. 208–218.

Mitchell, M., Kirkpatrick, D., Hoky, W., and Gery, I., 1973, On the mode of action of BCG, *Nature* **243**:216–218.

Morris, C. K., and Johnson, A. C., 1978, Regulation of immune system by synthetic polynucleotides, VII. Suppression induced by pretreatment with poly A : U, *Cell. Immunol.* **39**:345–354.

Morrisson, D. C., and Ryan, J. L., 1979, Bacterial endotoxins and host immune responses, *Adv. Immunol.* **28**:293–450.

Mossalayi, M. D., Descombe, J. J., Musset, M., Tanzer, J., and Goube deLaforet, P., 1986, *In vitro* effects of sodium diethyldithiocarbamate (imuthiol) on human T lymphocytes, *Int. J. Immunopharmacol.* **8**:841–844.

Muldoon, R. L., Menzy, L., and Jackson, G. G., 1972, Effects of isoprinosine against influenza and some other viruses causing respiratory diseases, *Antimicrob. Agents Chemother.* **2**:224–228.

Nagoya, T., Kobayashi, F., and Nomota, K., 1977, Immunological properties of *Propionobacter acnes:* Potentiation and suppression of antibody response to sheep and hamster erythrocytes in mice, *Microbiol. Immunol.* **21**:33–44.

Najjar, V. A., and Bump, N. J., 1984, Tuftsin (Thr-Lys-Pro-Arg): A stimulator of all known functions of macrophage, in: *Immune Modulation Agents and Their Mechanisms* (R. L. Fenichel and M. A. Chirigos, eds.), Marcel Dekker, New York, pp. 229–242.

Najjar, V. A., Chaudhuri, M. K., Konopinska, D., Beck, B. D., Layne, P. P., and Linehan, L., 1981, Tuftsin (Thr-Lys-Pro-Arg), a physiological activator of phagocytic cells: A possible role in cancer suppression and therapy, in: *Augmenting Agents in Cancer Therapy* (E. Hersh, M. A. Chirigos, and M. J. Mastrangelo, eds.), Raven Press, New York, pp. 459–478.

Neter, E., 1969, Endotoxin and the immune response, *Curr. Top. Microbiol. Immunol.* **47**:82–124.

Nishioka, K., Amoscato, A. A., and Babcock, G. F., 1981, Tuftsin: A hormone-like tetrapeptide with antimicrobial and antitumor activities, *Life Sci.* **28**:1081–1090.

Nowotny, A. (ed.), 1983, *Beneficial Effects of Endotoxin*, Plenum Press, New York.

Ohnishi, H., Kosuzume, H., Iraba, H., Ohkusa, M., Shimada, S., and Suzuki, Y., 1983, The immunomodulatory action of inosiplex in relation to its effects in experimental viral infection, *Int. J. Immunopharmacol.* **5**:181–196.

Ohta, Y., Tizuka, E., Tamara, S., and Yagi, Y., 1985, Thymosin α_1 exerts protective effect against the 5-FU induced bone marrow toxicity, *Int. J. Immunopharmacol.* **7**:761–768.

O'Neill, G., Ginsberg, T., and Hadden, J. W., 1984, Immunopharmacology of the hypoxanthine containing compounds isoprinosine and NPT 15392, in: *USFDA Conference on Immunomodulation in Veterinary Medicine* (M. Kende, J. Gainer, and M. Chirigos, eds.), Alan R. Liss, New York, pp. 525–542.

Papamatheakis, J. D., Chirigos, M. A., and Schultz, R. M., 1978, Effect of dose, route, and timing of pyrancopolymer therapy against the Madison lung carcinoma, in: *Immune Modulation and Control of Neoplasia by Adjuvant Therapy* (M. A. Chirigos, ed.), Raven Press, New York, pp. 427–443.

Parant, M., Parant, F., Chedid, L., Yapo, A., Petit, J. F., and Lederer, E., 1979, Fate of the synthetic immunoadjuvant, muramyl dipeptide (^{14}C-labelled) in the mouse, *Int. J. Immunopharmacol.* **1**:35–41.

Personn, U., 1977, Lipopolysaccharide-induced suppression of the primary immune response to a thymus-independent antigen, *J. Immunol.* **118**:787–789.

Picolli, M., Saito, T., and Chirigos, M. A., 1984, Bimodal effects of MVE-2 on cytotoxic activity of natural killer cells and macrophage tumoricidal activities, *Int. J. Immunopharmacol.* **6**:597–676.

Piessen, W. F., Campbell, M., and Churchill, W. H., 1977, Inhibition or enhancement of rat tumor dependent on the dose of BCG, *J. Natl. Cancer Inst.* **59**:207–211.

Primus, P. J., de Martino, C., MacDonald, R., and Hansen, J. H., 1978, Immunological reconstitution of T-cell deprived mice. I. Inability of thymosin to restore spleen cell mitogen and tumor allograf response, *Cell. Immunol.* **35**:25–31.

Renoux, G., 1978, Modulation of immunity by levamisole, *Pharmacol. Ther. A* **2**:397–423.

Renoux, G., 1982, Immunopharmacologie et pharmacologie du diethyldithiocarbamate de sodium (DTC), *J. Pharmacol.* **13**:95–134.

Renoux, G., and Biziere, K., 1985, Brain neocortex lateralized control of immune recognition, *Integr. Psychiatry* **4**:32–40.

Renoux, G., and Renoux, M., 1977a, Thymus-like activities of sulphur derivatives on T-cell differentiation, *J. Exp. Med.* **145**:466–471.

Renoux, G., and Renoux, M., 1977b, Roles of the imidazole or thiol moiety in the immunostimulant action of levamisole, in: *Control of Neoplasia by Modulation of the Immune System* (M. A. Chirigos, ed.), Rovers Press, New York, pp. 67–80.

Renoux, G., and Renoux, M., 1979, Immunopotentiation and anabolism induced by sodium diethyldithiocartamate, *J. Immunopharmcol.* **1**:247–267.

Renoux, G., and Renoux, M., 1980, The effects of sodium diethyldithiocarbamate, azathioprine, cyclophosphamide or hydrocortisone acetate administered alone or in association for 4 weeks on the immune response of balb/c mice, *Clin. Immunol. Immunopathol.* **15**:23–32.

Renoux, G., and Renoux, M., 1984, Diethyldithiocarbamate (DTC). A biological agent specific for T cells, in: *Immune Modulation Agents and Their Mechanisms* (R. L. Fenichel and M. A. Chirigos, eds.), Marcel Dekker, New York, pp. 6–20.

Renoux, G., Renoux, M., and Tinelli, R., 1970, Influence of *Brucella* endotoxins on the initiation of antibody-forming spleen cells in mice immunized with sheep red blood cells, *Infect. Immun.* **2**: 1–6.

Renoux, G., Renoux, M., and Guillaumin, J. M., 1979a, Genetic and epigenetic control of levamisole-induced immunostimulation, *Int. J. Immunopharmacol.* **1**:43–48.

Renoux, G., Renoux, M., and Guillaumin, J. M., 1979b, Isoprinosine as an immunopotentiator, *J. Immunopharmacol.* **1**:337–356.

Renoux, G., Renoux, M., Guillaumin, J. M., and Gouzien, C., 1979c, Differentiation and regulation of lymphocyte populations: Evidence for immunopotentiator-induced T cell recruitment, *J. Immunopharmacol.* **1**:415–422.

Renoux, G., Bardos, P., Degenne, D., and Musset, M., 1982, Sodium diethyldithiocarbamate (DTC)-induced modifications of NK activity in the mouse, in: *Natural Cell-Mediated Immunity* (R. B. Herberman, ed.), Academic Press, New York, pp. 443–448.

Renoux, G., Renoux, M., Biziere, K., Guillaumin, J. M., Bardos, P., and Degenne, D., 1984, Involvement of brain neocortex and liver in the regulation of T cells: The mode of action of sodium diethyldithiocarbamate (imuthiol), *Immunopharmacology* **7**:89–100.

Ribi, E., 1984, Beneficial modification of endotoxin molecule, *J. Biol. Resp. Mod.* **3**:1–9.

Saito, T., Ruffman, R., Welher, R. D., Herbermann, R. B., and Chirigos, M. A., 1985, Development of hyporesponsiveness of natural killer cells to augmentation of activity after multiple treatments with histological response modifiers, *Cancer Immunol. Immunother.* **19**:130–135.

Salvin, S. B., and Neta, R., 1983, Resistance and susceptibility to infection in inbred murine strains, I. Variation in the response to thymic hormones in mice infected with *Candida albicans, Cell. Immunol.* **75**:160–172.

Scheid, M., Goldstein, G., and Boyse, E. A., 1975, Differentiation of T cells in nude mice, *Science* **190**:1211–1213.

Schindler, T., Coffey, R. G., and Hadden, J. W., 1986, Stimulatory effects of muramyl dipeptide and its butyl ester derivative on the proliferation and activation of macrophages *in vitro*, *Int. J. Immunopharmacol.* **8**:487–498.

Schlick, E., Hartung, K., and Chirigos, M. A., 1984, Comparison of *in vitro* and *in vivo* modulation of myelopoiesis by biological response modifiers, *Cancer Immunol. Immunother.* **8**:226–232.

Schlick, E., Ruffman, R., Hartung, K., and Chirigos, M. A., 1985, Modulation of myelopoiesis by CSF or CSF-inducing biological response modifiers, *J. Immunopharmacol.* **7**:141–166.

Schnieden, H., 1980, Levamisole—a general pharmacological prespective, *Int. J. Immunopharmacol.* **3**:9–13.

Sergiescu, D., Cerutti, I., Kahan, A., Piatier, D., and Efihymiou, E., 1981, Isoprinosine delays the early appearance of autoimmunity in NZB/NZWF mice, *Clin Exp. Immunol.* **43**:36–45.

Serrou, B., and Rosenfeld, C. (eds.), 1980, *New Trends in Human Immunology and Cancer Immunotherapy*, Doin, Paris,

Serrou, B., Rosenfeld, C., Daniels, J. C., and Saunders, J. P. (eds.), 1982, *Current Concepts in Human Immunology and Cancer Immunomodulation*, Volume 17, Elsevier Biomedical Press, Amsterdam.

Shiigi, S. M., and Mishell, R. I., 1975, Sera and the *in vitro* induction of immune responses, I. Bacterial contamination and the generation of good fetal bovine sera, *J. Immunol.* **115**:741–749.

Simon, L., and Glasky, A. J., 1978, Isoprinosine: An overview, *Cancer Treat. Rep.* **62**:1963–1969.

Simon, L. N., Hoehler, F. K., McKensie, D. T., and Hadden J. W., 1983, Isoprinosine and NPT

15392: Immunomodulation and cancer, in: *Biological Response Modifiers in Human Oncology and Immunology* (T. Klein, S. Spector, H. Friedman, and A. Szentivanyi, eds.), Plenum Press, New York, pp. 241–259.

Singhal, S. K., Roder, J. C., and Duwe, A. K., 1978, Suppressor cells in immunosenescence, *Fed. Proc.* **37**:1245–1252.

Sirois, P., and Rola-Pleszczynski, M. (eds.), 1982, *Immunopharmacology*, Elsevier, Amsterdam.

Spreafico, F., Tagliabue, A., and Vecchi, A., 1982, Chemical immunodepressants, in: *Immunopharmacology* (P. Sirois and M. Rola-Pleszczynski, eds.), Elsevier, Amsterdam, pp. 315–348.

Staats, J., 1980, Standardized nomenclature for inbred strains of mice, seventh listing, *Cancer Res.* **40**:2083–2128.

Stewart, W. E. II (ed.), 1981, *The Interferon System*, Springer Verlag, New York.

Stolfi, R. L., and Martin, D. S., 1978, Therapeutic activity of maleic anhydride–vinyl ether copolymers against spontaneous, autochthonous murine mammary tumors, *Cancer Treat. Rep.* **62**:1791–1796.

Stringfellow, D., 1981, 6-Arylpyrimidinoles: Interferon inducers-immunomodulators-antiviral and antineoplasic agents, in: *Augmenting Agents in Cancer Therapy* (E. M. Hersh, M. A. Chirigos, and M. J. Mastrangelo, eds.), Raven Press, New York, pp. 215–228.

Sugarman, B. J., Aggarival, B. B., Hass, P. E., Figari, I. S., Palladino, M. A., and Shepard, H., 1985, Recombinant human tumor necrosis factor-α: Effects on proliferation of normal and transformed cells *in vitro*, *Science* **230**:943–945.

Sunshine, G., Lopez-Corrales, E., Hadden, E. M., Coffey, R. G., Wanebo, H., and Hadden, J. W., 1976, Levamisole and imidazole: *In vitro* effects in mouse and man and their possible mediation by cyclic nucleotides, in: *Modulation of Host Immune Resistance* (M. Chirigos, ed.) Fogarty International Center Proceedings 28, DHEW (NIH# 77-893), Washington, pp. 31–38.

Symoens, J., and Rosenthal, M., 1977, A review: Levamisole in the modulation of the immune response. The current experimental and clinical state, *J. Reticuloendothel. Soc.* **21**:175–221.

Szentivanyi, A., Friedman, H., and Nowotny, A. (eds.), 1986, *Immunobiology and Immunopharmacology of Bacterial Endotoxins*, Plenum Press, New York.

Talal, N., and Hadden, J. W., 1984, Hormones, immunomodulating drugs and autoimmunity, in: *Handbook of Inflammation*, Volume 5 (L. Glynn, J. Houck, and G. Weissman, eds.), Elsevier/North Holland, Amsterdam, pp. 355–369.

Talal, N., Dauphinee, M., Pillarsetty, R., and Goldblum, R., 1975, Effect on thymosin on thymocyte differentiation and autoimmunity in NZB mice, *Ann. N.Y. Acad. Sci.* **249**:438–450.

Talmadge, J. E., and Chirigos, M. A., 1985, Comparison of immunomodulatory and immunotherapeutic properties of biological response modifiers, *Springer Semin. Immunopathol.* **8**: 429–443.

Talmadge, J. E., Benedict, K. L., Uithoven, K. A., and Lenz, B. F., 1984a, The effect of experimental conditions on the assessment of T cell immunomodulation by biological response modifiers (thymosin fraction five), *Immunopharmacology*. **7**:17–26.

Talmadge, J. E., Oldham, R. K., and Fidler, I. J., 1984b, Practical considerations for the establishment of a screen procedure for the assessment of biological response modifiers, *J. Biol. Resp. Mod.* **3**:88–109.

Talmadge, J. E., Fidler, I. J., and Oldham, R. K. (eds.), 1985a, *Screening for Biological Response Modifiers: Methods and Rationale*, Martinus Nijhoff, Boston.

Talmadge, J. E., Adams, J., Phillips, H., Collins, M., Levy, H., Schneider, M., and Chirigos, M. A., 1985b, Immunotherapeutic potential in murine tumor models of polyinosinic-polyeytidylic acid and poly-L-lysine solubilized by carboxymethylecellulose, *Cancer Res.* **45**:1066–1072.

Taniyama, T., and Holden, H. T., 1979, Direct augmentation of cytotoxic activity of tumor-derived macrophages and macrophage cell lines by muramyl dipeptide, *Cell. Immunol.* **48**:369–374.

Touraine, J.-L., Gay-Ferret, G., Sanadji, K., Othmane, O., Tournie, G. J., and Touraine, F., 1982,

Isoprinosine: Synergistic effects with NPT 15392 *in vitro* and activity on suppressor T lymphocytes in autoimmune mice *in vivo*, in: *Current Concepts in Human Immunology and Cancer*, Volume 17 (B. Serrou, C. Rosenfeld, J. C. Daniels, and J. P. Saunders, eds.), Elsevier Biomedical, Amsterdam, pp. 491–499.

Tsang, K.Y., and Fedenberg, H. H., 1984, Restoration of immune response in aging animal models, in: *Stress, Immunity, and Aging* (E. L. Cooper, ed.), Marcel Dekker, New York, pp. 257–269.

Tsang, K.-Y., Fudenberg, H. H., Hoehler, F. K., and Hadden, J. W., 1984, Immunostimulant compounds, isoprinosine and NPT 15392, in: *Immune Modulation Agents and Their Mechanisms* (R. L. Fenichel and M. A. Chirigos, eds.), Marcel Dekker, New York, pp. 79–95.

Turcotte, R., Lafleur, L., and Labreche, M., 1978, Opposite effects of BCG on spleen and lymph node cells: Lymphocyte proliferation and immunoglobulin synthesis, *Infect. Immun.* **21:**696–704.

Umezawa, H. (ed.), 1981, *Small Molecular Immunomodifiers of Microbial Origin*, Pergamon Press, Oxford.

Vecchi, A., Sironi, M., and Spreafico, F., 1978, Preliminary characterization of mice of the effect of isoprinosine on the immune system, *Cancer Treat. Rep.* **62:**1975–1979.

Veys, E. M., and Symoens, J., 1981, Immunopharmacologic therapy of connective tissue diseases, in: *Advances in Immunopharmacology* (J. Hadden, L. Chedid, P. Mullen, and F. Spreaticos, eds.), Pergamon Press, Oxford, pp. 139–147.

Wahl, L. M., Wahl, M., McCarty, J. B., Chedid, L., and Mergenhagen, S. E., 1979, Macrophage activation by mycobacterial water soluble compounds and synthetic muramly dipeptide, *J. Immunol.* **122:**2226–2231.

Watson, J., and Epstein, R., 1973, The role of humoral factors in the initiation of *in vitro* primary immune responses. I. Effects of deficient fetal bovine serum, *J. Immunol.* **110:**31–42.

Weigle, W. O., 1980, Analysis of autoimmunity through experimental models of thyroiditis and allergic encephalomyelitis, Adv. Immunol. **30:**159–273.

Werner, G. H., 1979, Immunopotentiating substances with antiviral activity, *Pharmacol. Ther.* **6:** 235–240.

Werner, G. H., Maral, R., Floc'h, F., and Jouanne, M., 1977, Toxicological aspects of immunopotentiation by adjuvants and immunostimulating substances, *Bull. Inst. Pasteur* **75:**5–84.

Williams, R. M., and Benacerraf, B., 1972, Genetic control of thymus cell function, *J. Exp. Med.* **135:**1279–1292.

Williams, R. M., Dorf, M. E., and Benacerraf, B., 1975, H-2 linked genetic control of resistance to histocompatible tumors, *Cancer Res.* **35:**1481–1590.

Wiltrout, R. H., Mathieson, B. J., Talmadge, J. E., Reynolds, C. W., Zhang, S.-R., Herberman, R. B., and Ortaldo, J. R., 1984, Augmentation of organ-associated natural killer activity by biological response modifiers, *J. Exp. Med.* **160:**1431–1449.

Wiltrout, R. H., Herberman, R. B., Zhang, S., Chirigos, M. A., Ortaldo, J. R., Green, K. M., and Talmadge, J. E., 1985, Role of organ associated NK cells in decreased formation of experimental metastasis in lung and liver, *J. Immunol.* **134:**4267–4275.

Yamamura, Y., Kotani, S., Azuma, I., Koda, A., and Shiba, T. (eds.), 1982, *Immunomodulation by Microbial Products and Related Synthetic Compounds*, Excerpta Medica, Amsterdam.

Zatz, M. M., Glaser, M., Seals, C. M., and Goldstein, A., 1981, Effects of combined cyclophosphamide and thymosin treatment on tumor growth and host survival in mice bearing a synergistic tumor, in: *Lymphokine and Thymic Hormones: Their Potential Utilization in Cancer Therapeutics* (A. Goldstein, and M. A. Chirigos, eds.), Raven Press, New York, pp. 249–256.

Zulman, J., Michalski, J., McCoombs, C., Greenspan, J., and Talal, N., 1978, Levamisole maintains cyclophosphamide-induced remission in murine lupus erythematosus, *Clin. Exp. Immunol.* **31:**321–329.

CHAPTER 2

PHARMACOKINETICS OF IMMUNOMODULATORS

JOSEPH F. WILLIAMS

1. INTRODUCTION: PHARMACOKINETICS

Immunopharmacology is a relatively new but rapidly developing discipline devoted to unraveling the pharmacological basis of agents whose primary target is
the immune system. Presently, considerable attention is being directed to the
therapeutic application of these agents for their activity to augment or suppress
the responsiveness of various cellular constituents of the immune network. Such
immunotherapeutic approaches to modulate immunologic mechanisms can be
considered analogous to the well-established therapeutic application of diverse
pharmacological agents to treat pathophysiological states resulting from dysfunction of the cardiovascular, renal, nervous, or other systems. Thus, the goal of
immunopharmacology is to regulate chemically the activity of the immune system for biological and therapeutic benefit.

The list of immunologically active agents currently being investigated is
quite extensive and constantly enlarging. The term *biological response modifiers*
(BRMs) has been proposed to encompass this group of agents of widely divergent nature (Oldham, 1983). Biological response modifiers include chemically
defined agents, extracts and preparations from microbial products, and preparations of natural or synthetic biological substances produced by recombinant DNA
procedure. Functionally these agents may be divided into those whose cellular
targets may be the T cell, B cell, NK cell, or macrophage and those agents that
are more nonspecific in their interaction. Some of the agents may act on a given
cell type directly or indirectly because of the marked interdependence of the

JOSEPH F. WILLIAMS • Department of Pharmacology and Therapeutics, University of South
Florida College of Medicine, Tampa, Florida 33612.

65

immune cells as modulated by their communication and regulation via lympho-kine and monokine secretion.

Although extensive information has accumulated on the immunophar-macological activity of the BRMs, only recently have data become available on their pharmacokinetic characterization, and for some agents this information is still lacking. In many cases, the unavailability of sufficient quantities of various BRMs or the lack of available sensitive assay procedures to monitor their pres-ence in biological tissues at low concentrations has significantly hampered such pharmacokinetic studies. However, because of the critical interplay of pharma-cokinetic considerations with the onset, intensity, and duration of phar-macodynamics, immunotherapeutics is at a critical threshold of development where the pharmacokinetics of BRMs must be assessed by formalized and sys-tematic approaches. From such studies may come information that may allow the establishment of a more rational, effective, and safe protocol for therapeutic dosage regimens.

This chapter briefly considers some of the salient aspects of pharmacokinet-ic studies and reviews the current information available on selected BRMs. More extensive coverage of pharmacokinetics can be found in textbooks devoted to that subject (Gibaldi and Perrier, 1982). The present review is simply to high-light those features that currently appear critical to the immunotherapeutic ap-plication of the BRMs and possibly to call attention to important considerations that at the present time may have been inadequately addressed.

Pharmacokinetics in a strict sense implies the mathematical assessment of the relationship between the administered dose of an agent and the temporal changes in the systemic concentration of the agent that occur following its administration. In general, drug concentration is determined in the blood or plasma, and the measured drug concentration–time curve is a function of the major pharmacokinetics determinants, i.e., those factors that affect absorption, distribution, metabolism, and excretion. Although for some drugs no clear rela-tionship has been found between the drug concentration in the systemic circula-tion and the pharmacological effect, for many agents serum or plasma concentra-tions have been established that serve as indices for proper institution and maintenance of therapeutic effect. In such cases, the systemic concentration presumably is correlated with the effective concentration of the agent at the site of action and serves to link pharmacokinetics and pharmacodynamics. Applica-tion of information gleaned from pharmacokinetic studies can thus be utilized to establish appropriate dosage and dose interval and to predict and manage the onset, intensity, and duration of drug effect. In other cases, the relationship between serum drug concentration and therapeutic effect may be indirect, and indices of dose activity may be the more appropriate guide for therapeutic man-agement. For example, peak serum levels of the anticoagulant warfarin occur at approximately 6 hr after a single dose, but the maximum effect on prothrombin times does not occur until 2 days. Warfarin inhibits the synthesis of various blood coagulation factors, but the manifestation of reduced synthesis is not seen until circulating levels of the various factors decline through their degradation. Therefore, measurement of prothrombin time rather than serum warfarin concentration is a better estimate for drug management. Finally, there are instances where no correlation between pharmacokinetics and pharmacodynamics has been established.

At the present time there are insufficient pharmacokinetic and pharmacodynamic data to predict the most relevant approach to immunotherapy with the BRMs. In some instances there appears to be a temporal dissociation between serum concentration and biological effect. This may represent, as indicated above in the case of warfarin, an initial effect that either requires a lag time before its expression is observed or one that initiates a cascade of events leading ultimately to the desired biological effect. Despite the possible discrepancies between serum concentration and therapeutic effect, adequate knowledge of the pharmacokinetics of the BRMs is important for a complete understanding of those processes involved in the absorption, distribution, metabolism, and excretion of these agents.

For the following discussion, we assume that there exists a pharmacologically definable relationship among the doses of the BRM administered, the serum concentration achieved, and the desired immunopharmacological effect. The particular relationship among these three modalities is yet to be deciphered and understood.

1.1. Absorption

With the exception of instances, such as intravenous administration, where a drug is introduced directly into the systemic circulation, plasma drug concentration is achieved only after the drug traverses membranes from its site of application, i.e., the route of administration. The plasma concentration–time curve may differ markedly for the same drug depending on the route of administration. The transfer of drug across membranes is influenced by many factors including the physiochemical properties of the drug, the particular drug delivery system employed, as well as physiological variables such as the presence of metabolizing enzyme systems and the level of blood supply to the area of drug administration.

The main pharmacokinetic parameters generally associated with the absorption processes are the estimate of bioavailability and the rate of drug absorption. Bioavailability is defined as the fraction of the dose that appears in the systemic circulation in the unchanged form. Generally, the fractional absorption (F) is determined by comparing the total area under the plasma drug concentration–time curve (AUC) of a single dose given by one route (e.g., oral, I.M.) relative to the AUC obtained after a single intravenous administration of the drug. Thus,

$$F = (dose)_{i.v.} (AUC)_x / (dose)_x (AUC)_{i.v.}$$

where $dose_x$ and AUC_x are the dose and the area under the curve for the drug administered by a particular route of administration, and $dose_{i.v.}$ and $AUC_{i.v.}$ are the corresponding values for the drug given intravenously. Other approaches, such as determining the total quantity of drug excreted in the urine, can also be used to assess fractional absorption.

Failure of F to be equal to unity may indicate either incomplete absorption or metabolic destruction of the drug at the site of administration prior to or during the absorption transfer across membranes. For oral dosage forms, incomplete availability may result from a number of factors including instability of the compounds in the fluids of the gastrointestinal tract, destruction by the gastrointestinal enzymes, or metabolism of part of the dose during its "first pass" through the liver. Bioavailability may also be influenced by the pharmaceutical preparations, and different formulations may not have equivalent bioavailability. Although bioavailability of oral dosage forms has received the greatest attention, bioavailability by other routes of administration is equally worthy of concern and evaluation and may be of considerable importance with respect to several of the biological BRM products.

In addition to bioavailability, the rate of drug absorption is also of pharmacokinetic importance. The rate of drug absorption mainly influences the initial part of the serum drug concentration–time curve following a single dosage. Rapid absorption leads to high peak plasma concentrations occurring shortly after drug administration, whereas slow absorption is characterized by lower and later peak concentrations. Rapid absorption is desirable where clinically effective serum concentrations and/or rapid onset of clinical effect is desired soon after dose administration. Slow absorption may delay or even present the achievement of effective serum concentrations. On the other hand, a slow, sustained absorption rate may allow a great duration of clinical effect by maintaining effective serum concentrations for a longer period of time. It should be emphasized that the time to peak serum concentrations is not necessarily of major concern for the onset of drug effect. Once the plasma concentration exceeds the minimal effective concentration, the effect will ensue. Thus, the pharmacodynamic aspects of drug action may occur at serum concentrations considerably less than those maximally achieved following administration of a given dose. The most appropriate dose–response relationship may be ascertained only after exhaustive exploration of various dosage schedules and monitoring for clinical effectiveness. In contrast, for agents administered on a chronic basis the absorption rate may be of less importance than the completeness of absorption. The steady-state plasma concentration of an agent given chronically is influenced more by the extent than by the rate of absorption. Thus, barring the development of tolerance or significant toxic effects from chronic drug exposure, the appropriate dosage schedule may be accurately determined only following repeated drug administration.

An important exception to the consideration discussed previously is where the biological activity results in part or completely from the metabolic activation of the parent compound. At the extreme, where the administered compound is inactive and only the metabolite is active, the best correlation between effect and serum drug concentration would be with the active metabolite and not the parent drug. In such cases more complex pharmacokinetic evaluations are required to assess the relative bioavailability of the drug and the rate of formation and elimination of the metabolite. Although beyond the scope of the present overview, it should be readily apparent that the route of drug administration is an important consideration in such circumstances. Thus, the formation of active metabolite may differ quantitatively as well as temporally depending on the route of administration.

In summary, initial pharmacokinetic consideration relative to the absorption of BRMs needs to focus on bioavailability after different routes of administration and the consideration of different dosage formulations of the same preparations relative to both the completeness of absorption and the rate of absorption.

1.2. Distribution

Distribution refers to the reversible transfer of a drug from one site to another in the body. In most instances pharmacokinetic analysis considers the body as consisting of "compartments." The simplest model is the one-compartment model in which the body is considered as a single homogeneous compartment. Although applicable for some agents, most drug distributions have been shown to be best described by a two-compartment model where there is a central compartment and a second peripheral compartment into which the drug distributes.

The fundamental pharmacokinetic parameter used to describe drug distribution is the apparent volume of drug distribution, which relates the amount of drug in the body to the concentration of drug in the blood, plasma, or serum, depending on the measured fluid. This volume is not necessarily correlated with any identifiable physiological volume or space but simply is the volume required to account for the measured serum drug concentration:

$$V = \text{amount of drug in body/concentration in plasma, etc.}$$

There are several methods used to determine the volume of distribution depending on the pharmacokinetic model and other factors, but all relate the amount of drug in the body to plasma concentration for those particular circumstances.

Volume of drug distribution in influenced by many factors. It can vary as a function of patient's age, sex, or body composition. In addition, the pK_a of the drug, the degree of plasma protein binding, the partition coefficient of the drug, and differences in regional blood flow may also modify the volume of drug distribution. Finally, various disease processess may also cause significant changes in the distribution volume. Thus, although the volume of distribution may be considered a constant relating the plasma concentration and the amount of drug in the body, it is only appropriate for a particular circumstance and may vary manyfold under various conditions.

1.3. Elimination

The elimination of an agent from the body may be considered as resulting from two pharmacokinetic factors—metabolism and excretion. Two pharmaco-kinetic parameters most frequently used to characterize elimination are plasma half-life ($T_{1/2}$) and clearance. Drug half-life is the time it takes for the plasma drug concentration to be reduced by 50% and is usually determined from the terminal or elimination phase of the plasma concentration–time curve:

$$T_{1/2} = 0.693/B$$

where B is the apparent rate constant for elimination determined from the slope of the elimination phase. Although $T_{1/2}$ is a good indicator of the time to reach steady-state concentrations (approximately 90% of a new steady state will be achieved in four half-lives), the time required for drug to be removed from the body, or a means to estimate the appropriate dosage interval, $T_{1/2}$ is not as good an indicator of the body's ability to eliminate a drug as is clearance (CL):

$$CL = B \cdot V$$

Clearance is the volume of drug distribution from which drug is removed by the eliminating organs per unit time. Clearance is additive in character and reflects the contribution of all systems responsible for drug elimination, e.g., liver, kidney, lungs, bile, sweat. Clearance is thus dependent on both the ability of the organs to eliminate the drug and the volume in which the drug is distributed. For a constant clearance, these two parameters are reciprocally related. For example, a decrease in drug elimination rate and an increase in the volume of distribution may offset one another and may result in no change in the clearance, but an increase in $T_{1/2}$ would be determined.

The two major sites of drug elimination are the liver and kidney. For the majority of chemical agents the liver is the site of major drug biotransformation reactions resulting in the administered agent being converted to one or more metabolites. The ability of the liver to eliminate an agent via biotransformation is dependent on two variables, the rate of delivery of the agent to the elimination organ and the intrinsic activity of the liver processes of biotransformation. For some agents the intrinsic activity may be so high that the rate of elimination is dependent on the rate of drug delivery, i.e., blood flow. In other instances, elimination may be determined by the intrinsic activity and the unbound fraction of drug in the blood. Thus, drugs may be spoken of as high-extraction-ratio drugs whose elimination via the liver is blood-flow dependent and low-extraction-ratio agents whose elimination is blood-flow independent. In other cases, clearance may be dependent on blood flow as well as intrinsic clearance and plasma protein binding. Similar considerations apply to renal clearance of an agent, but consideration must also be given to the particular contributions made by glomerular filtration, active secretion, and reabsorption. The rate of filtration depends on the unbound concentration of drug in the plasma and the volume of fluid filtered, usually estimated by inulin or creatinine clearance. Secretion by the kidney will depend on the intrinsic activity of the active transport systems to handle the agent and the rate of delivery of the drug to the secretory site, i.e., renal blood flow and the unbound fraction of the drug. Reabsorption depends on the urine pH, the pK_a of the chemical agent, and the rate of urine flow.

Hepatic intrinsic activity can be markedly altered by either induction or inhibition of the enzyme systems involved in drug biotransformation as a result of exposure to various agents or hepatic disease. In addition, genetic differences within the population may result in significantly different rate of biotransformations. Likewise, hepatic blood flow may be affected by numerous physiological, pathological, and pharmacological factors. Similarly, renal drug clearance may be altered by various factors that affect either intrinsic activity or blood flow. Consequently, much of the consideration needed in establishing an appropriate dosage and dose schedule is dependent on understanding the concepts involved in drug clearance and the factors that may modify these processes.

The liver and kidney also appear to play major roles in the metabolic disposition of circulating proteins (Strober and Waldmann, 1974; Schwartz, 1984). Although the mechanisms involved are presently less well understood than those involved in the oxidative and conjugation enzyme systems, it is appreciated that receptors exist for proteins on the cell surface in these organs. Specific binding of glycosylated proteins can be demonstrated and is followed by internalization and subsequent proteolysis, presumably in the lysosome. Such clearance mechanisms may be of considerable relevance with respect to the pharmacokinetics of the BRMs that are protein in nature, in particular the natural and recombinant interferons, interleukins, and tumor necrosis factor, to name but a few. Current information indicates that clearance of biological immunoactive substances may differ significantly from related material produced by recombinant procedures. Thus, further investigation and understanding of these clearance mechanisms is imperative.

2. PHARMACOKINETICS OF IMMUNOMODULATORS

In this section a brief review of the currently available information concerning the pharmacokinetic behavior of selected immunomodulators is presented. Although I attempted to conduct an extensive and comprehensive search of the literature, because of the large number of disciplines engaged in immunomodulator research and the rapid state of development of research in this area, I fear that important observations may have been unintentionally overlooked. What is presented is hoped to bring into focus, perhaps as a candid snapshot, those features of immunomodulator pharmacokinetics currently recognized and perhaps to provide a perspective for future studies. There has been only a minimal attempt in this review to extend the available pharmacokinetic data to explain or predict how this information might interface with pharmacodynamic considerations. However, it is assumed that, given sufficient understanding of each of these independently, a more appropriate meshing can and will be achieved.

2.1. Biologically Derived Immunomodulators and Related Derivatives

2.1.1. Interferon

Of all the biologically derived immunomodulators, interferon is the one for which the most information is available regarding its pharmacokinetic behavior. However, the situation is far from being completely resolved because of the multiplicity of interferons. In addition to the well-recognized three classes (α, β, and γ) of naturally occurring interferon, current techniques of molecular biology using recombinant DNA procedures are providing additional material that has to be independently investigated. Admittedly, the recent availability of purified recombinant interferon preparations has greatly augmented investigations of the pharmacokinetic parameters, but it perhaps has overshadowed the equally important studies of the pharmacokinetic profile of naturally occurring interferon. However, if interferon inducers are to be developed as important therapeutic tools, information must be available not only on the pharmacokinetics of the inducers but also on the biological substances that they elicit.

A number of reviews have been previously published on the pharmacokinetics of interferon (Ho, 1973; Bocci, 1981, 1984; Scott, 1982; Billiau, 1983; Mannering and Deloria, 1986). The reader is referred to these articles for a more thorough discussion of various topics concerning interferon not addressed in the present chapter. Suffice it to say that many factors, including the type of interferon (α, β, γ), the source of the interferon (natural versus recombinant), and the species of animals used in the study (rat, rabbit, monkey, human, etc.) (Gomi et al., 1984) add to the complexity of the subject.

Despite the numerous complexities alluded to above, a general impression regarding the pharmacokinetic behavior of interferon is emerging.

2.1.1a. Absorption of Interferon. Interferon preparations, both natural and recombinant, of various types have been administered via a number of routes, including oral, intramuscular, subcutaneous, and intranasal, to estimate their systemic availability (Davies *et al.*, 1983; Yoshikawa *et al.*, 1983; Shah *et al.*, 1984; Wills *et al.*, 1984a,b; Gibson *et al.*, 1985). In some but not all studies, the intravenous administration of the same interferon preparation has also been studied, allowing for the determination of bioavailability. Unfortunately, there are also instances where although both intravenous and other routes have been used in the same study for a single interferon preparation, more attention has been given to the plasma concentration achieved relative to another interferon preparation than to the estimation of the bioavailability of a given preparation.

In general, it appears relatively conclusive that interferon is not bioavailable after the oral route of administration (Wills *et al.*, 1984b). This is not too surprising considering the protein nature of interferon and the presence of various proteases, etc., within the gastrointestinal tract. Intranasal administration of interferon preparations also does not appear to yield significant systemic concentrations (Davies *et al.*, 1983), a possible desirable feature with respect to limiting the effect of interferon to a local area.

The systemic availability of interferon after intramuscular or subcutaneous administration appears to depend on the particular type and source of the interferon preparations as well as on the species of animal used in the investigation (Hanley *et al.*, 1979; Gutterman *et al.*, 1982; Sarkar, 1982; Gomi *et al.*, 1984; Satoh *et al.*, 1984). For most preparations, both the intramuscular and the subcutaneous routes of administration result in more sustained blood concentrations and a longer half-life than is observed after intravenous administration (Gutterman *et al.*, 1982; Gomi *et al.*, 1984; Shah *et al.*, 1984; Kurzrock *et al.*, 1985). The bioavailability of the interferon from these sites, particularly the intramuscular route, differs depending on whether the interferon is glycosylated (Hanley *et al.*, 1979; Satoh *et al.*, 1984). Natural β-interferon, which is glycosylated, is apparently less bioavailable via intramuscular administration than is either naturally occurring α-interferon or recombinant β-interferon, neither of which is glycolysated (Cantell *et al.*, 1983). One observation that may modify this impression is that recombinant β-interferon has been shown to display flip-flop kinetics in which the rate of absorption is significantly slower than the rate of distribution or elimination (Satoh *et al.*, 1984). Another possibility that may complicate current approaches to pharmacokinetic evaluation is that absorption and distribution may be occurring through other systems, e.g., lymphatic drainage (Yoshikawa *et al.*, 1983), than the cardiovascular system. In such instances monitoring plasma concentrations is not valid, and alternative approaches must be utilized for pharmacokinetic evaluation. Thus, with present techniques it may be difficult to conclude whether the absolute bioavailability of β-interferon is less after intramuscular administration or whether lower area under plasma concentration curve reflects more rapid and extensive tissue uptake and/or elimination or unique physiological handling.

2.1.1b. Distribution of Interferon. Few studies have extensively examined the tissue distribution of various interferon preparations to determine whether a preferential difference might exist for the particular classes of interferon. A total apparent volume of distribution of 2.5 liters has been reported for human IFN-α, suggesting extensive binding to cellular receptors (Bocci *et al.*, 1985a). Although in many studies significant concentrations of interferon have not been found in the CNS following systemic administration (Habif *et al.*, 1975; Abreu, 1983; Smith *et al.*, 1985), side effects referable to the CNS frequently accompany interferon administration. The presence of the blood–brain barrier for interferon seems appropriate and has led to the intrathecal route of interferon administration being investigated (Billiau *et al.*, 1981). However, whether such a blood–brain barrier precludes an important clinical consideration is presently not completely established (Abreu, 1983). For example, it is well known that penicillin does not normally gain access to the CNS because of the blood–brain barrier, but in cases of inflamed meninges penicillin can cross into the brain and is therapeutically effective. Whether clinical instances may exist that modify interferon distribution into the CNS remains unknown.

2.1.1c. Elimination of Interferon. A major consideration in the pharmacokinetics of interferon has been its rapid disappearance from the systemic circulation. Following intravenous administration, the plasma half-life is 1 hr or less (Abreu, 1983). This could reflect a rapid and extensive distribution and/or elimination. Extensive rapid and prolonged tissue uptake of interferon may argue against the application of pharmacokinetic principles in establishing appropriate dose and dose-interval parameters. On the other hand, if plasma half-life actually reflects the elimination phase, then such data may be of more heuristic value. In other words, it needs to be established whether plasma levels of interferon do or do not reflect levels of interferon at critical target sites.

Several experimental studies have established that the kidney appears to be the major organ involved in the metabolic elimination of interferon (Bino *et al.*, 1982; Bocci, 1982; Bocci *et al.*, 1981, 1982b, 1983a,b). Urinary levels of interferon are negligible, but renal ligation or bilateral nephrectomy (Bocci *et al.*, 1981; Tokazewski-Chen *et al.*, 1983) results in a prolonged half-life. Thus, ligation of renal blood vessels resulted in a large increase in the detectable plasma interferon activity following administration of human leukocyte-derived α-interferon to rat (Rosenberg *et al.*, 1985). There was no increase in the interferon degradation products in other organs. This and other studies have suggested that at least for nonglycosylated interferons, the kidney plays the predominant role in the metabolic clearance of interferon. It has been proposed that interferon is filtered at the glomerulus, reabsorbed in the renal tubule, and metabolically destroyed within the renal cells (Bino *et al.*, 1982; Bocci *et al.*, 1984), similar to the handling of other low-molecular-weight proteins such as the Bence Jones proteins.

The liver has also been implicated as a possible organ of elimination or metabolism for certain interferon preparations. This appears to be particularly true for glycosylated preparations such as naturally elicited β-interferons (Bocci *et al.*, 1982a). An auxiliary role of the liver in the catabolism or elimination of nonglycosylated interferon preparations has also been reported (Bocci *et al.*, 1985b). With respect to the latter observation, it is as yet unknown whether in the face of altered states of renal function the liver may adaptively increase its capacity to clear interferon.

Somewhat relevant to the preceding is the question of species difference in the pharmacokinetic handling of interferon. From the extant studies there do appear to be differences between species in various pharmacokinetic parameters, which may have major importance when considering the therapeutic implications with respect to man. Thus, the most relevant species to study with respect to absorption may not be the most relevant with respect to distribution and/or elimination. Such species considerations with regard to pharmacokinetics coupled with reported species variation in pharmacodynamic effects magnify the complexity of the resolution of the dilemma. Given the relatively well-established species-dependent nature of interferon pharmacodynamics, the question is pertinent to the possible species-dependent nature of the pharmacokinetic parameters (Billiau *et al.*, 1981).

2.1.2. Interleukins

Limited information is available on the pharmacokinetic behavior of the interleukins because of the only very recent availability of sufficient quantities. From the available studies, the pharmacokinetics of IL-2 mirrors that of interferon (Cheever *et al.*, 1985): IL-2 administered intravenously to mice has a mean $T_{1/2}$ of 3.7 min (Donohue and Rosenberg, 1983), whereas a $T_{1/2}$ of 22.5 min has been reported for humans (Bindon *et al.*, 1983). As with IFN, intraperitoneal or subcutaneous injection of IL-2 results in a more prolonged $T_{1/2}$ and lower serum concentration, probably influenced by a slow but continued absorption from the site of administration (Chang *et al.*, 1984; Cheever *et al.*, 1985). Thus, the reported values may not be an accurate reflection of independent pharmacokinetic disposition but a composite of two or more factors. The liver and kidney are the major sites of IL-2 concentration (Koths and Halenbeck, 1985). Also, similar to interferon, renal clearance of IL-2 appears to be the major mechanism for elimination. No IL-2 is excreted in the urine, and renal vascular pedicle ligation, but not ligation of the ureters, increases the serum IL-2 half-life (Donohue and Rosenberg, 1983). These results suggest that renal filtration and intrarenal catabolism play a significant role in IL-2 elimination. In addition, other results suggest that hepatic parenchymal or Kupffer cells probably do not contribute significantly to IL-2 elimination. Examination of studies attempting to correlate plasma levels and the effect of IL-2 to induce growth of T cells shows that the intraperitoneal or subcutaneous administration of IL-2 was more effective than the transient high serum titers produced by intravenous administration.

The fate of interleukin 1 (IL-1) has not been extensively studied. Interleukin 1 is rapidly cleared from the circulation, but, contrary to IL-2, the kidney does not appear to represent the major route of IL-1 elimination (Kampschmidt and Jones, 1985).

2.1.3. Muramyl Dipeptide and Analogues

N-Acetylmuramyl-L-alanyl-D-isoglutamine, more commonly referred to as muramyl dipeptide (MDP), is the smallest subunit of the bacterial peptidoglycan component of the cell wall that retains biological activity as an immunoadjuvant. In addition, this molecule has also been shown to elicit other immunostimulating activities.

Although no definitive pharmacokinetic studies on MDP and/or its analogues have been published, a number of studies (Parent et al., 1979; Ambler and Hudson, 1984) have examined to a limited degree some of the pharmacokinetic aspects. After intravenous administration circulating MDP rapidly decline with a initial half-life of 4–5 min. A logarithmic plot of circulating amounts of MDP versus times shows the presence of multiphasic clearance from the circulation. After intraperitoneal or subcutaneous injection, peak blood levels are attained at about 10 min, being about 6% of the dose, and then steadily decline, reaching low levels by 2 hr. Between 75% and 95% of the original dose of MDP was recovered intact in the urine, indicating minimal metabolism. The MDP is extensively distributed to all tissues, but liver and kidney showed the highest percentage of the injected material (Ambler and Hudson, 1984). Liver was the tissue in which the most extensive metabolism of MDP was observed (Ambler and Hudson, 1984). Surprisingly, the tissue distribution of MDP 3 hr after oral administration was similar to that seen 30 min after intravenous injection, suggesting that the liver did not preferentially remove MDP from the portal circulation.

It has been known for some time that when a protein antigen is administered to an animal as an oil–water emulsion, e.g., Freund's complete adjuvant, a greatly augmented immunostimulant activity occurs, presumably because of the mineral oil component serving to establish a depot form at the site of injection. Parent et al. (1979) and Hudson (1984) have shown that MDP or nor-MDP was retained for a longer time at the site of injection when given as an water-in-oil emulsion. Of interest is that Hudson (1984) showed that the retention of the MDP emulsion in the foot did not necessarily reflect a reduced efficacy in eliciting delayed-type hypersensitivity reaction.

Since the macrophage appears to be the primary cellular target for MDP, targeted drug delivery approaches may circumvent some of the problems of the rapid elimination of MDP. Incorporation of MDP in liposomes may direct its uptake in organs with high RES activity, such as the liver, spleen, and lymph nodes. Indeed, Schroit et al. (1983) showed that liposome-encapsulated MDP and MTP were retained in the lungs and that alveolar macrophages isolated 24 hr later displayed greater tumoricidal activity than if free MDP or MTP had been injected. Such targeted delivery of MDP and other immunostimulants deserves further study.

I am not aware of significant published information on the pharmacokinetics of other biologically derived immunostimulants. Thymopentin, the active moiety of thymopoietin, is being developed as an immunoregulatory agent. Audhya and Goldstein (1985) reported this pentapeptide to be rapidly degraded ($T_{1/2} = 30$ sec) in human plasma. The biological potency varied greatly according to the route and rate of administration, with intravenous infusion providing the greatest efficacy. Tumor necrosis factor has been reported in mice to have a serum half-life of 10.5 min and a volume of distribution consistent with that of the extra-cellular space (Flick and Gifford, 1986). It might be anticipated that when more extensive studies are conducted, aspects similar to those discussed above for interferon, IL-2, and MDP will be encountered.

2.2. Chemically Synthesized Immunomodulators

Agents that fall into this category are numerous, and only selected ones will be discussed. In many cases, unlike the biologicals discussed above, the pharma-cokinetics of the chemically synthesized modulators have been extensively ex-amined. In part this is because of the ready availability of sufficient quantities of the pure chemical and of radiolabeled material as well as the existence of sen-sitive and specific procedures to detect the small amounts of chemical agent present in plasma and/or tissues. Despite the knowledge of the pharmacokinetics of these compounds, a chasm still exists in utilizing this information and linking it to appropriate therapy for achieving the desired immunotherapeutic response. Although perhaps not directly applicable, understanding the interplay of the pharmacokinetics and -dynamics of these chemically synthesized immu-nomodulators may provide insights into comparable interrelationships for the biologically derived agents.

Many of the chemically synthesized agents appear to act either directly or indirectly by eliciting various endogenous factors, some of which have been discussed. Discussion of the pharmacokinetics of chemically synthesized agent must be viewed from these perspectives. Thus, although understanding the phar-macokinetics may provide information for the biological handling of these agents, their immunopharmacodynamic and immunotherapeutic effects may re-quire additional integrative approaches.

2.2.1. Levamisole

Levamisole is a readily aqueous-soluble compound. It is the *levo*-isomer of tetramisole, a synthetic anthelmintic used against nematodes of animals and man. Levamisole is rapidly absorbed from all routes of administration (Galtier *et al.*, 1983a,b). It is extensively metabolized in the liver and excreted in bile (Galtier *et al.*, 1983b), undoubtedly accounting for its better bioavailability after intramuscular or subcutaneous injection than after oral administration. The biological half-life of levamisole has been reported to vary from 30 min in rats to about 4 hr in man (Kouassi *et al.*, 1986), possibly reflecting species differences in hepatic metabolic activity. *Para*-hydroxylation of the phenyl ring of levamisole occurs but represents only a small percentage of the urinary metabolite (Graziani and DeMartin, 1977; Galtier *et al.*, 1983a,b), most occurring as the glucuronide conjugate (Kouassi *et al.*, 1986). Symoens *et al.* (1979) reported that 2-oxo-3(2-mercaptoethyl)-5-phenylimidazolidine, produced by the opening of the thiazole ring of levamisole, is a major metabolite *in vivo*. Levamisole appears to be widely distributed throughout the body, the highest concentrations being found in lungs, liver, and kidneys (Benard *et al.*, 1980; Galtier *et al.*, 1983b). The distribution to the latter two tissues probably reflects their role in the elimination of levamisole, since mainly products other than levamisole are found in these organs (Galtier *et al.*, 1982). The biological half-life of the metabolites of levamisole appears to be much longer (16 hr) than that of the parent compound (Symoens *et al.*, 1979), suggesting the possibility that the immunobiological effect may be more closely correlated with an active metabolite than with levamisole itself. Further studies are certainly necessary to explore this point as well as the levamisole-induced production of an active serum factor, as discussed by Renoux (1980).

2.2.2. Isoprinosine

Isoprinosine (Isosiplex) is composed of inosine and the *p*-acetamidobenzoate (PAcBA) salt of N,N-dimethylaminoisopropanol (DIP) in a 1 : 3 molar ratio. Very little data is apparently available on the pharmacokinetics of this agent.

There have been two studies on the metabolism and excretion of PAcBA and DIP (Nielsen and Beckett, 1981; Streeter and Pfadenhauer, 1984). In man, Nielsen and Beckett (1981) showed that orally administered PAcBA was rapidly eliminated ($T_{1/2}$ 50 min), primarily as PAcBA glucuronide (55%) and as unchanged PAcBA (30%). The elimination half-life of DIP was 3.5 hr; DIP-N-oxide (65%) and unchanged DIP (30%) represented the urinary metabolites. In rhesus monkeys (Streeter and Pfadenhauer, 1984) a similar pattern of metabolism and elimination was seen after oral administration of PAcBA, but the glucuronide metabolite accounted for only 31% of the administered intravenous dosage. In addition, a minor metabolite was identified as the hippuric acid conjugate of PAcBA. DIP-N-oxide was the only metabolite of DIP identified after either intravenous or oral dosage and accounted for only 17–18% of the administered dose. The importance of understanding the pharmacokinetics of these components of isoprinosine is suggested by the observation that the biological activity of this compound is dependent on the administration of the complex rather than the individual components.

2.2.3. Maleic Anhydride Divinyl Ether (MVE-2)

Information on the pharmacokinetic behavior and pharmacology of MVE-2 has recently been summarized by Carrano et al. (1981) and Munson et al. (1981). After intravenous and intraperitoneal administration, a long half-life for MVE-2 is found, and the compound is concentrated in cells of the reticuloendothelial system. Twenty-eight days after administration, 8–9% of the administered dose was found in the liver. Approximately 19–20% of the total dose was eliminated in the urine and feces in the first 48 hr following administration. Detectable blood levels were observed for up to 2 weeks after administration. These data indicate the MVE-2 is rapidly cleared from the circulation following its administration, probably by rapid uptake into the RES. This cellular storage site may serve as a depot from which MVE-2 may be available for systemic release for extended periods of time, resulting in a sustained source for immunomodulatory activity. Carrano et al. (1981) showed that substantial levels of MVE-2 or its metabolites remained in rat liver 28 days after intravenous administration. Thus, weekly doses may be needed to maintain adequate tissue levels (Shopp and Munson, 1984). Further information on the integration of pharmacokinetic information to the use of MVE-2 may produce increased pharmacological effect and reduce toxicity, as suggested by Shopp and Munson (1984).

3. ALTERATION OF DRUG BIOTRANSFORMATION BY IMMUNOMODULATORS

As investigation of the immunomodulators has progressed, it has become apparent that these agents also possess the ability to interact with and affect cellular metabolism in non-immune-system tissues. With respect to pharmacokinetics, an effect common to many BRMs is to decrease the activity of the hepatic cytochrome P-450-dependent drug-oxidation system (Descotes, 1985; Kasai and Egawa, 1985; Williams and Szentivanyi, 1985). This enzyme system, located primarily in the endoplasmic reticulum of the liver but also found to lesser degree in other organelles and extrahepatic tissues, is responsible for the biotransformation of many drugs, other xenobiotics, and various endogenous substances including steroids, fatty acids, prostaglandins, and arachadonic acid. It is now recognized that the terminal oxidase of the system exists in a number of isozymic forms, collectively referred to as cytochromes P-450 but differing with respect to substrate specificity, catalytic activity, and gene regulation. Alteration in one or more of these cytochrome P-450 isozymes may lead to either increased or decreased duration of action and/or toxicity of compounds dependent on biotransformation for their inactivation or activation. Differences in specific iso-zymic forms of cytochrome P-450 have been shown to occur as a result of drug and other chemical exposures, genetic differences, sex differences, environmen-tal and nutritional effects, age, and species variation.

The inhibitory effect of the various immunomodulators on hepatic drug biotransformation reactions appears to result from a decrease in the level of cytochromes P-450. Generally, the effect of the immunomodulators can be seen within 24 hr after injection and persists for at least 72 hr. More prolonged depression of cytochrome P-450-dependent drug-metabolizing enzyme activity has been observed after *B. pertussis* and Freund's complete adjuvant (Williams and Szentivanyi, 1985). With these two agents the monooxygenase activity was depressed for 15 days and 30 days, respectively. It is presently unclear whether this decrease in hemoprotein level is a nonselective effect or if only specific isozymic forms are affected. Zerkle *et al.* (1980) reported that pretreatment of rats with tilorone, poly I–poly C, and Freund's adjuvant all caused a loss of cytochrome P-450, but these compounds differed with respect to which isozymic form was altered. A selective effect of endotoxin on the isozymes of cytochrome P-450 in untreated, phenobarbital-pretreated, and 3-methylcholanthrene-pretreated rats has also been suggested by Williams (1986).

The mechanism by which the immunomodulators cause the decrease in cytochromes P-450 is at present unknown. In many instances, an increase in heme oxygenase activity, the rate-limiting step in heme catabolism, occurs con-comitant with the loss of cytochrome P-450. In addition, an increased heme saturation of tryptophan oxygenase and a decrease in the activity of δ-ALA synthetase, the rate-limiting step in heme biosynthesis, is also observed. It has been suggested (Bissell and Hammaker, 1976a,b, 1977) that these results indi-cate either an increased dissociation or decreased association of heme with apo-cytochrome P-450. Whether an increased degradation or a decreased synthesis of apocytochromes P-450 occurs is not known.

Recently, Ghezzi *et al.* (1984, 1985, 1986) proposed a role for reactive oxygen intermediates in the loss of cytochromes P-450. These workers observed that the administration of poly I–poly C, endotoxin, or interferon caused a marked increase in xanthine oxidase activity in the liver and other organs. Xanthine oxidase is well known for its ability to generate reactive oxygen inter-mediates, particularly superoxides and hydrogen peroxide. It is also known that microsomal cytochrome P-450 is sensitive to peroxidative attack. Ghezzi *et al.* (1985) also demonstrated that concomitant oral administration of N-acetylcys-teine, a free radical scavenger, protected against the poly I–poly C and inter-feron-induced depression of cytochrome P-450 without altering the increased xanthine oxidase activity. In addition, the ability of different interferon species (i.e., IFLrA, IFLrD, and ILFrA/DLBglII) to induce xanthine oxidase correlated with their ability to depress liver cytochrome P-450-dependent drug metabolism (Ghezzi *et al.*, 1986). However, DeLoria *et al.* (1985) caution that the increased xanthine oxidase activity may be a consequence of the loss of cytochrome P-450 rather than the cause.

It is also unresolved whether the effect of various immunomodulators to cause a loss of cytochrome P-450 is the consequence of a direct effect on hepatic parenchymal cell metabolism or whether the effect may be indirectly mediated by endogenous substances released from cellular constituents of the immune network. Renton and Mannering (1976) have suggested that the effects of various agents on cytochrome P-450 resulted from their activity as interferon inducers. Indeed, injections of interferon have been shown to cause a decrease in hepatic microsomal cytochrome P-450 (Parkinson et al., 1982; Singh et al., 1982; Renton and Singh, 1984; Franklin and Finkle, 1985, 1986; Taylor et al., 1985; Roh et al., 1986). However, some of the agents that are the most effective in reducing cytochrome P-450 levels are not very effective inducers of interferon. Also, the incubation of either poly I–poly C or interferon with isolated hepatocytes caused an increase rather than a decrease in cytochrome P-450 (Renton et al., 1978).

Peterson and Renton (1984, 1986a) and Williams (1985) have shown that cellular products of macrophages other than interferon may be involved in eliciting the loss of cytochrome P-450. Peterson and Renton (1984) coincubated hepatocytes and Kupffer cells, the cells types beings separated by a semipermeable membrane. If dextran sulfate or latex particles were incubated with the hepatocytes, no loss of cytochrome P-450 was seen. However, if dextran or latex was incubated with the Kupffer cells, phagocytosis of the particles occurred, and a loss of cytochrome P-450 was observed in the parenchymal cells. No interferon was detectable in the culture medium. Williams (1985) incubated peritoneal macrophages with endotoxin and then injected an aliquot of the culture medium into endotoxin-tolerant rats and mice. No interferon was present in the culture medium, but injection of the medium caused a loss of cytochrome P-450. These results lend support to the suggestion of Soyka et al. (1979) that the macrophage was involved in the effect of Corynebacterium parvum on cytochrome P-450. These investigators showed that treatments such as UV irradiation and injection of silica that destroy macrophages ablated the loss of cytochrome P-450 caused by C. parvum. Recently, Peterson and Renton (1986b) have shown that antilymphocyte sera did not alter the effect of dextran to decrease cytochrome P-450 but that incubation of hepatocytes with interleukin 1, a macrophage mediator of immune function, did produce a loss of cytochrome P-450.

A possible T-cell-dependent activity in the effect of B. pertussis was suggested by Williams et al. (1981). The duration of the inhibition of drug-metabolizing activity caused by B. pertussis was attenuated in athymic mice compared to euthymic animals. On the other hand, Klinger et al. (1983) have shown that thymectomy or splenectomy per se did not alter microsomal cytochrome P-450 levels or the ability of the animals to respond to inducing agents such as phenobarbital or 3-methylcholanthrene. These observations may indicate the implicit involvement of the immune system in regulation of hepatic enzymatic activity only in response to immunologic challenge of various types. Other studies have implicated interleukin 1 as the effector of the increased hepatocyte production of acute-phase proteins and other hepatic metabolic alteration (Dinarello, 1984; Roh et al., 1986). Thus, it will be interesting to ascertain whether these two responses are related. In addition, it is not inconceivable that the effects of different immunomodulators on hepatic cytochrome P-450 may also be caused by a combination of the various immune effector substances acting independently, additively, or synergistically. The availability of adequate quantities of purified material should significantly facilitate research in this area. Further work is necessary to unravel this intriguing interrelationship between the immune system and hepatic parenchymal cell metabolism.

In summary, definitive information on the pharmacokinetics of the various immunomodulators is just beginning to be obtained. This has been greatly aided by the availability of recombinant molecules. However, it is apparent that the pharmacokinetics of the recombinant products may differ significantly not only from the endogenously produced substance but also among themselves. Thus, extrapolation of information about recombinant molecules may not be relevant for naturally occurring interferon, interleukins, or tumor necrosis factor, for example. Finally, the intimate and essential relationship between pharmacokinetics and pharmacodynamics needs to be elucidated. If only a minimal, transient level of BRM needs to be present for subsequent pharmacodynamic activation, then dose and dose interval will obviously differ from those for cases in which sustained levels are required.

The clinical relevance of the effect of BRMs on hepatic biotransformation is critical because of the drug–drug interactions that are possible where other agents are used either in conjunction with the BRMs for immunotherapy or to treat other disease processes. Continued effort is needed so that patients on medications for other disease processes are not compromised by the immunotherapy. In addition, information in this area may be important if BRMs are to be used in combination immunotherapy.

REFERENCES

Abreu, S. L., 1983, Pharmacokinetics of rat fibroblast interferon, *J. Pharmacol. Exp. Ther.* **226**: 197–200.

Ambler, L., and Hudson, A. M., 1984, Pharmacokinetics and metabolism of muramyl dipeptide and nor-muramyl dipeptide [^{3}H-labelled] in the mouse, *Int. J. Immunopharacol.* **6**:133–139.

Audhya, T. K., and Goldstein, G., 1985, Thymopentin: Stability considerations and potency by various routes of administration, *Surv. Immunol. Res.* **4** (Suppl. 1):17–23.

Benard, P., Brunet, C., Cazin, M., Braun, J. P., Burgat-Sacaze, V., and Rico, A. G., 1980, Whole body distribution of ^{3}H-levamisole in rats and mice, in: *Mechanisms of Toxicity and Hazard Evaluation* (B. Holmstedt, R. Lauwerys, M. Mercier, and M. Roberfroid, eds.), Elsevier/North-Holland Biomedical Press, New York, pp. 529–532.

Billiau, A., 1983, The pharmacokinetics and toxicology of interferon, *Soc. Gen. Microbiol.* **35**:255–276.

Billiau, A., Heremans, H., Ververken, D., Van Damme, J., Carton, H., and Desomer, P., 1981, Tissue distribution of human interferons after exogenous administration in rabbits, monkeys, and mice, *Arch. Virol.* **68**:19–25.

Bindon, C., Czerniecki, M., Ruell, P., Edwards, A., McCarthy, W. H., Harris, R., and Hersey, P., 1983, Clearance rates and systemic effects of intravenously administered interleukin 2 (IL-2) containing preparations in human subjects, *Br. J. Cancer* **47**:123–133.

Bino, J., Edery, H., Gertter, A., and Rosenberg, H., 1982, Involvement of the kidney in catabolism of human leukocyte interferon, *J. Gen. Virol.* **59**:39–45.

Bissell, D. M., and Hammaker, L. E., 1976a, Cytochrome P-450 heme and the regulation of hepatic heme oxygenase activity, *Arch. Biochem. Biophys.* **176**:91–102.

Bissell, D. M., and Hammaker, L. E., 1976b, Cytochrome P-450 heme and the regulation of δ-aminolevulinic acid synthetase in the liver, *Arch. Biochem. Biophys.* **176**:103–113.

Bissell, D. M., and Hammaker, L. E., 1977, Effect of endotoxin on tryptophan pyrrolase and delta-amino levulinate synthetase. Evidence for an endogenous regulatory heme fraction in rat liver, *Biochem. J.* **166**:301–304.

Bocci, V., 1981, Pharmacokinetic studies of interferons, *Pharmacol. Ther.* **13**:421–440.

Bocci, V., 1982, Catabolism of interferons, *Surv. Immunol. Rev.* **1**:137–143.

Bocci, V., 1984, Evaluation of routes of administration of interferon in cancer: A review and a proposal, *Cancer Drug Deliv.* **1**:337–351.

Bocci, V., Pacini, A., Muscettola, M., Paulesu, L., and Pessing, G. P., 1981, Renal metabolism of rabbit serum interferon, *J. Gen. Virol.* **55**:297–304.

Bocci, V., Pacini, A., Bandinelli, L., Pessina, G. P., Muscettola, M., and Paulesu, L., 1982a, The role of the liner in the catabolism of human δ-β-interferon, *J. Gen. Virol.* **60**:397–400.

Bocci, V., Pacini, A., Muscettola, M., Pessina, G. P., Paulesu, L., and Bandinelli, L., 1982b, The kidney is the main site of interferon catabolism, *J. Interferon Res.* **2**:309–314.

Bocci, V., Difrancesco, P., Pacini, A., Pessina, G. P., and Rossi, G. B., and Sorrentino, V., 1983a, Renal metabolism of homologous serum interferon, *Antiviral Res.* **3**:53–58.

Bocci, V., Mogensen, K. E., Muscettola, M., Pacini, A., Paulesu, L., Pessina, G. P., and Skiftas, S., 1983b, Degradation of human ^{125}I-interferon alpha by isolated perfused rabbit kidney and liver, *J. Lab. Clin. Med.* **101**:857–863.

Bocci, V., Maunsbach, A. B., and Mogensen, E. K., 1984, Autoradiographic demonstration of human ^{125}I-interferon alpha in lysosomes of rabbit proximal tubule cells, *J. Submicrosc. Cytol.* **16**:753–757.

Bocci, V., Pessina, G. P., Pacini, A., Paulesu, L., Muscettola, M., Naldini, A., and Lunghetti, G., 1985a, Pharmacokinetics of human lymphoblastoid interferon in rabbits, *Gen. Pharmacol.* **16** (3):277–279.

Bocci, V., Pacini, A., Pessina, G. P., Paulesu, L., Muscettola, M., and Lunghetti, G., 1985b, Catabolic sites of human interferon-γ, *J. Gen. Virol.* **66**:887–891.

Cantell, K., Hirvonen, S., Pyhala, L., DeReus, A., and Schellekens, H., 1983, Circulating interferon in rabbits and monkeys after administration of human gamma interferon by different routes, *J. Gen. Virol.* **64**:1823–1826.

Carrano, R. A., Kinoshita, F. K., Imondi, A. R., and Iuliucci, J. D., 1981, MVE-2: Preclinical pharmacology and toxicology, in: *Augmenting Agents in Cancer Therapy: Current Status and Future Prospects* (M. Chirigas and E. M. Hersh, eds.), Raven Press, New York, pp. 345–372.

Chang, A. E., Hyatt, C. L., and Rosenberg, S. A., 1984, Systemic administration of recombinant human interleukin-2 in mice, *J. Biol. Resp. Mod.* **3**:561–572.

Cheever, M. A., Thompson, J. A., Kern, D. E., and Greenberg, P. D., 1985, Interleukin 2 (IL 2) administered *in vivo*: Influence of IL 2 route and timing on T cell growth, *J. Immunol.* **134**: 3895–3900.

Davies, H. W., Scott, G. M., Robinson, J. A., Higgins, P. G., Wootton, R., and Tyrrell, D. A. J., 1983, Comparative intranasal pharmacokinetics of interferon using two spray systems, *J. Interferon Res.* **3**:443–449.

DeLoria, L., Abbott, V., Gooderham, N., and Mannering, G. J., 1985, Induction of xanthine oxidase and depression of cytochrome P-450 by interferon inducers: Genetic difference in the responses of mice, *Biochem. Biophys. Res. Commun.* **131**:109–114.

Descotes, J., 1985, Immunomodulating agents and hepatic drug-metabolizing enzymes, *Drug Metab. Rev.* **16**:175–184.

Dinarello, C. A., 1984, Interleukin-1 and the pathogenesis of the acute phase response, *N. Engl. J. Med.* **311**:1413–1418.

Donohue, J. H., and Rosenberg, S. A., 1983, The fate of interleukin-2 after *in vivo* administration, *J. Immunol.* **130**:2203–2208.

Flick, D. A., and Gifford, G. E., 1986, Pharmacokinetics of murine tumor necrosis factor, *J. Immunopharmacol.* **8**:89–97.

Franklin, M. R., and Finkle, B. S., 1985, Effect of murine gamma-interferon on the mouse liver and its drug-metabolizing enzymes: Comparison with human hybrid alpha-interferon, *J. Interferon Res.* **5**:265–272.

Franklin, M. R., and Finkle, B. S., 1986, The influence of recombinant DNA-derived human and murine gamma interferons on mouse hepatic drug metabolism, *Fund. Appl. Toxicol.* **7**:165–169.

Galtier, P., Coche, Y., and Camguilhem, R., 1982, Incidence of experimental cirrhosis on hepatic disposition of [^{3}H]levamisole in rats, *J. Pharm. Pharmacol.* **34**:310–313.

Galtier, P., Escoula, M. S., and Alvinerie, M. S., 1983a, Pharmacokinetics of [^{3}H]levamisole in pigs after oral and intramuscular administration, *Am. J. Rev.* **44**:583–587.

Galtier, P., Coche, Y., and Alvinerie, M., 1983b, Tissue distribution and elimination of [^{3}H]levamisole in the rat after oral and intramuscular administration, *Xenobiotica* **13**:407–413.

Ghezzi, P., Bianchi, M., Mantovani, A., Spreafico, F., and Salmona, M., 1984, Enhanced xanthine oxidase activity in mice treated with interferon and interferon inducers, *Biochem. Biophys. Res. Commun.* **119**:144–149.

Ghezzi, P., Bianchi, M., Gianera, L., Landolfo, S., and Salmona, M., 1985, Role of reactive oxygen intermediates in the interferon-mediated depression of hepatic drug metabolism and protective effect of N-acetylcysteine in mice, *Cancer Res.* **45**:3444–3447.

Ghezzi, P., Saccardo, B., and Bianchi, M., 1986, Induction of xanthine oxidase and heme oxygenase and depression of liver drug metabolism by interferon: A study with different recombinant interferons, *J. Interferon Res.* **6**:251–256.

Gibaldi, M., and Perrier, D., 1982, *Pharmacokinetics*, 2nd ed., Marcel Dekker, New York.

Gibson, D. M., Cotler, S., Spiegel, H. E., and Colburn, W. A., 1985, Pharmacokinetics of recombinant leukocyte A interferon following various routes and modes of administration to the dog, *J. Interferon Res.* **5**:403–408.

Gomi, K., Morimoto, M., Inone, A., Kobayachi, H., DeGuchi, T., Harg, T., and Nahansizo, N., 1984, Pharmacokinetics of human recombinant interferon-β in monkeys and rabbits, *Gann* **75**:292–300.

Graziani, G., and DeMartin, G. L., 1977, Pharmacokinetic studies on levamisole, *Drugs Exp. Clin. Res.* **2**:235–240.

Gutterman, J. U., Fine, S., Quesada, J., Horning, S. J., Levine, J. F., Alexanian, R., Bornhardt, L., Kramer, M., Spiegel, H., Colburn, W., Trown, P., Merigan, T., and Dziewanowski, Z., 1982, Recombinant leukocyte A interferon: Pharmacokinetic, single-dose tolerance, and biologic effects in cancer patients, *Ann. Intern. Med.* **96**:549–556.

Habif, D. V., Lipton, R., and Cantell, K., 1975, Interferon crosses blood–cerebrospinal fluid barrier in monkeys, *Proc. Soc. Exp. Biol. Med.* **149**:287–289.

Hanley, D. F., Wiranowska-Stewart, M., and Stewart, W. E. II, 1979, Pharmacology of interferons.

1. Pharmacologic distinctions between human leukocyte and fibroblast interferons, *Int. J. Immunopharmacol.* **1**:219–226.

Ho, M., 1973, Pharmacokinetics of interferons, in: *Interferons and Interferon Inducers* (N. Finter, ed.), Elsevier, Amsterdam, pp. 241–249.

Hudson, A. M., 1984, The fate of nor-muramyl dipeptide (^{3}H-labelled) after local administration in incomplete Freund's adjuvant in the guinea pig, *Int. J. Immunopharmacol.* **6**:119–124.

Kampschmidt, R. F., and Jones, T., 1985, Rate of clearance of interleukin-1 from the blood of normal and nephrectomized rats, *Proc. Soc. Exp. Biol. Med.* **180**:170–173.

Kasai, N., and Egawa, K., 1985, Effect of endotoxin on cytochrome P-450 activity, in: *Handbook of Endotoxin*, Volume 3: *Cellular Biology of Endotoxin* (L. J. Berry, ed.), Elsevier, New York, pp. 185–198.

Klinger, W., Muller, D., Danz, M., Kob, D., and Madry, M., 1983, Influence of impairment of the immune system on hepatic biotransformation reactions, their postnatal development and inducibility, *Exp. Pathol.* **24**:219–225.

Koths, K., and Halenbeck, R., 1985, Pharmacokinetic studies on ^{35}S-labeled recombinant interleukin-2 in mice, in: *Cellular and Molecular Biology of Lymphocytes:* Proceedings of the 4th International Lymphokine Workshop (C. Song and A. Schmipl, eds.), Academic Press, New York, pp. 779–783.

Kouassi, E., Caille, G., Lery, L., Lariviere, L., and Vezina, M., 1986, Novel assay and pharmacokinetics of levamisole and *p*-hydroxylevamisole in human plasma and urine, *Biopharm. Drug Disp.* **7**:71–89.

Kurzrock, R., Rosenblum, M. G., Sherwin, S. A., Rios, A., Talpaz, M., Quesada, J. R., and Gutterman, J. U., 1985, Pharmacokinetics, single-dose tolerance, and biological activity of recombinant δ-interferon in cancer patients, *Cancer Res.* **45**:2866–2872.

Mannering, G. J., and Deloria, L. B., 1986, The pharmacology and toxicology of the interferons: An overview, *Annu. Rev. Pharmacol. Toxicol.* **26**:455–515.

Munson, A. E., White, K. L., Jr., and Klykken, P. C., 1981, Pharmacology of MVE polymers, in: *Augumenting Agents in Cancer Therapy: Current Status and Future Prospects* (M. Chirigos and E. Hersh, eds.), Raven Press, New York, pp. 329–343.

Nielsen, P., and Beckett, A. H., 1981, The metabolism and excretion in man of N,N-dimethylamino-isopropanol and *p*-acetamido-benzoic acid after administration of isoprinosine, *J. Pharm. Pharmacol.* **33**:549–550.

Oldham, R. K., 1983, Biological response modifiers, *J. Natl. Cancer Inst.* **70**:789–796.

Parant, M., Parant, F., Chedid, L., Yapo, A., Petit, J. F., and Lederer, E., 1979, Fate of the synthetic immunoadjuvant, muramyl dipeptide (^{14}C-labelled) in the mouse, *Int. J. Immunopharmacol.* **1**:35–41.

Parkinson, A., Lasker, J., Kramer, M. J., Huang, M.-T., Thomas, P. E., Ryan, D. E., Reik, L. M., Norman, R. L., Levin, W., and Conney, A. H., 1982, Effects of three recombinant human leukocyte interferons on drug metabolism in mice, *Drug Metab. Disp.* **10**:579–585.

Peterson, T. C., and Renton, K. W., 1984, Depression of cytochrome P-450-dependent drug biotransformation in hepatocytes after the activation of the reticuloendothelial system by dextran sulfate, *J. Pharmacol. Exp. Ther.* **229**:299–304.

Peterson, T. C., and Renton, K. W., 1986a, The role of lymphocytes, macrophages and interferon in the depression of drug metabolism by dextran sulfate, *Immunopharmacology* **11**:21–28.

Peterson, T. C., and Renton, K. W., 1986b, Kupffer cell factor mediated depression of hepatic parenchymal cell cytochrome P-450, *Biochem. Pharmacol.* **35**:1491–1497.

Renoux, G., 1980, The general immunopharmacology of levamisole, *Drugs* **19**:89–99.

Renton, K., and Mannering, G. J., 1976, Depression of hepatic cytochrome P-450 dependent monooxygenase systems with administered interferon inducing agents, *Biochem. Biophys. Res. Commun.* **73**:343–348.

Renton, K. W., and Singh, G., 1984, Relationship between the antiviral effects of interferons and their abilities to depress cytochrome P-450, *Biochem. Pharmacol.* **33**:3899–3902.

Renton, K. W., Deloria, L. B., and Mannering, G. J., 1978, Effects of polyriboinosinic acid–polyribocytidylic acid and a mouse interferon preparation on cytochrome P-450-dependent monooxygenase systems in cultures of primary mouse hepatocytes, *Mol. Pharmacol.* **14:**672–681.

Roh, M. S., Moldawer, L. L., Ekman, L. G., Dinarello, C. A., Bistrian, B. R., Jeevanandam, M., and Brennan, M. F., 1986, Stimulating effect of interleukin-1 upon hepatic metabolism, *Metabolism* **35:**419–424.

Rosenberg, H., Madar, Z., Gertler, A., Rubinstein, M., and Bino, T., 1985, The fate of [^{125}I]-labeled human leukocyte-derived alpha interferon in the rat, *J. Interferon Res.* **5:**121–127.

Sarkar, F. H., 1982, Pharmacokinetic comparison of leukocyte and *Escherichia coli*-derived human interferon type alpha, *Antiviral Res.* **2:**103–106.

Satoh, Y., Kasama, K., Kajita, A., Shimizu, H., and Ida, J., 1984, Different pharmacokinetics between natural and recombinant human interferon beta in rabbits, *J. Interferon Res.* **4:**411–422.

Schroit, A. J., Galligioni, E., and Fidler, I. J., 1983, Factors influencing the *in situ* activation of macrophages by liposomes containing muramyl dipeptide, *Biol. Cell.* **47:**87–94.

Schwartz, A. L., 1984, The hepatic asialoglycoprotein receptor, *CRC Crit. Rev. Biochem.* **16:**207–233.

Scott, G. M., 1982, Interferon: Pharmacokinetics and toxicity, *Phil. Trans. R. Soc. Lond. [Biol.]* **299:**91–107.

Shah, I., Band, J., Samson, M., Young, J., Robinson, R., Bailey, B., Lerner, A. M., and Prasad, A. S., 1984, Pharmacokinetics and tolerance of intravenous and intramuscular recombinant alpha$_2$ interferon in patients with malignancies, *Am. J. Hematol.* **17:**363–371.

Shopp, G. M., and Munson, A. E., 1984, Modification of the pharmacokinetics of MVE-2 to enhance its effects on host resistance, *Prog. Clin. Biol. Res.* **161:**501–509.

Singh, G., Renton, K. W., and Stebbing, N., 1982, Homogeneous interferon from *E. coli* depresses hepatic cytochrome P-450 and drug biotransformation, *Biochem. Biophys. Res. Commun.* **106:**1256–1261.

Smith, R. A., Norris, F., Palmer, D., Bernhardt, L., and Wills, R. J., 1985, Distribution of alpha interferon in serum and cerebrospinal fluid after systemic administration, *Clin. Pharmacol. Ther.* **37:**85–88.

Soyka, L. F., Stephens, C. C., MacPearson, B. R., and Foster, R. S., Jr., 1979, Role of mononuclear phagocytes in decreased hepatic drug metabolism following administration of *Corynebacterium parvum*, *Int. J. Immunopharmacol.* **1:**101–112.

Streeter, D. G., and Pfadenhauer, E. H., 1984, Inosiplex: Metabolism and excretion of the dimethylaminoisopropanol and *p*-acetamidobenzoic acid components in rhesus monkeys, *Drug Metab. Disp.* **12:**199–203.

Strober, W., and Waldmann, T. A., 1974, The role of the kidney in the metabolism of plasma proteins, *Nephron* **13:**35–66.

Symoens, J., DeCree, J., Van Bever, W. F. M., and Janssen, P. A. J., 1979, Levamisole, in: *Pharmacological and Biochemical Properties of Drug Substances*, Volume 2 (M. E. Goldberg, ed.), American Pharmaceutical Association. Academy of Pharmaceutical Sciences, Washington, pp. 408–464.

Taylor, G., Marafino, B. J., Jr., Moore, J. A., Gurley, V., and Blaschke, T. F., 1985, Interferon reduces hepatic drug metabolism *in vivo* in mice, *Drug Metab. Disp.* **13**(4):459–463.

Tokazewski-Chen, S. A., Marafino, B. J., and Stebbing, N., 1983, Effects of nephrectomy on the pharmacokinetics of various cloned human interferons in the rat, *J. Pharmacol. Exp. Ther.* **227:**9–15.

Williams, J. F., 1985, Induction of tolerance in mice and rats to the effect of endotoxin to decrease the hepatic microsomal mixed-function oxidase system. Evidence for a possible macrophage-derived factor in the endotoxin effect, *Int. J. Immunopharmacol.* **7:**501–509.

Williams, J. F., 1986, Effect of endotoxin on cytochrome P-450 monooxygenase system of phenobarbital and 3-methylcholanthrene treated rats, *Pharmacologist* **28**:215.

Williams, J. F., and Szentivanyi, A., 1985, Pharmacokinetic and pharmacodynamic parameters affected by RE cell activators, in: *The Reticuloendothelial System*, Volume 8 (J. W. Hadden and A. Szentivanyi, eds.), Plenum Press, New York, pp. 1–25.

Williams, J. F., Winters, A. L., Lowitt, S., and Szentivanyi, A., 1981, Depression of hepatic mixed-function oxidase activity by *B. pertussis* in splenectomized and athymic nude mice, *Int. J. Immunopharmacol.* **3**:101–106.

Wills, R. J., Dennis, S., Spiegel, H. E., Gibson, D. M., and Nadler, P. I., 1984a, Interferon kinetics and adverse reactions after intravenous, intramuscular, and subcutaneous injection, *Clin. Pharmacol. Ther.* **35**:722–727.

Wills, R. J., Spiegel, H. E., and Soike, K. F., 1984b, Pharmacokinetics of recombinant alpha A interferon following IV infusion and bolus, IM, and PO administrations to African green monkeys, *J. Interferon Res.* **4**:399–409.

Yoshikawa, H., Takada, K., Muranishi, S., and Satoh, Y., 1983, Pharmacokinetic property of human interferon after administration by different routes: Promotion of intestinal absorption and specific transfer into lymphatics, *J. Pharm. Dyn.* **6**:s-91.

Zerkle, T. B., Wade, A. E., and Ragland, W. L., 1980, Selective depression of hepatic cytochrome P-450 hemoprotein by interferon inducers, *Biochem. Biophys. Res. Commun.* **96**:121–127.

CHAPTER 3

IMMUNOTHERAPY AND BIOLOGICAL THERAPY OF CANCER
Current Clinical Status and Future Prospects

CHARLES W. TAYLOR and EVAN M. HERSH

1. INTRODUCTION

The major modalities of modern cancer therapy are surgery, radiotherapy, chemotherapy, and hormonal therapy. A role in the cancer treatment armamentarium is being established for immunotherapy and biological therapy. Biological therapy of cancer can be defined as the modification and exploitation of the cellular and molecular mechanisms of host defense and of the regulation of tissue proliferation, tissue differentiation, and tissue survival for use in the treatment of cancer. Cancer immunotherapy was first conceived in 1900 by Paul Erlich (1906), who postulated that antibodies could be used for targeting drugs and toxins to tumor cells. As we shall discuss, the production of highly specific monoclonal antibodies (MoAbs) using the hybridoma methodology of Kohler and Milstein (1975) has led to a present-day reappraisal of Erlich's hypothesis.

Modern clinical immunotherapy of cancer began in the 1960s with Klein's (1967, 1968, 1969) studies of delayed hypersensitivity reactions as therapy for localized skin malignancies. The rationale behind these studies was that a locally applied immunogenic material would elicit a non-tumor-specific local immune response and that this response should lead to the regression of diversified tumor types. Indeed, it was found that immune stimulants such as Bacillus Calmette

CHARLES W. TAYLOR and EVAN M. HERSH • Section of Hematology and Oncology, Department of Internal Medicine, Arizona Cancer Center, University of Arizona, Tucson, Arizona 85724.

Guerin (BCG), the purified protein derivative of tuberculin (PPD), dinitrochlorobenzene (DNCB), and crude lymphokine preparations caused regression of a
variety of primary or metastatic skin malignancies including basal cell carcinoma, mycosis fungoides, lymphangiosarcoma, reticulum cell sarcoma, and
breast cancer (Klein *et al.*, 1976). Interestingly, this local cytotoxic response
appeared to be selective for tumor cells and relatively sparing of the adjacent
normal tissue (Klein *et al.*, 1976).

The immunologic and related host defense basis of cancer immunotherapy
includes the presence of tumor-associated antigens and tumor immunity, the
well-defined phenomenon of immunodeficiency in cancer patients prior to therapy (Bast, 1982), and the presence of immunosuppressive cellular components
and serum factors in cancer patients (Hersh *et al.*, 1980; Roth *et al.*, 1982). The
presence of immunologically specific and nonspecific cellular host defense
mechanisms gives further validity to the application of cancer immunotherapy.
Effector cells and cellular responses with the potential to contribute to the eradication of tumor cells include T cells, cytolytic T lymphocytes (CTL), B-cells,
antibody-dependent cell-mediated cytotoxicity (ADCC), natural killer (NK)
cells, lymphokine-activated killer (LAK) cells, and the monocyte/macrophage
system. In addition, cytokines secreted by these cells such as the interferons, the
interleukins, tumor necrosis factors (TNF), and certain cellular growth factors
may have direct antitumor activity or the ability to modulate cellular antitumor
activity.

Classic immunologic approaches to cancer therapy may be subdivided into
various categories (Table I). The goal of active cancer immunotherapy is to
stimulate *in vivo* a host immune response directed toward the tumor. This approach assumes an immunocompetent host. Active nonspecific immune stimulation has been attempted with the use of BCG as intact organisms (Bast *et al.*,
1974; Baldwin and Pimm, 1978), the methanol extraction residue (MER) of
BCG (Weiss, 1972; Weiss *et al.*, 1964), or purified BCG cell wall components
such as muramyl dipeptide (MDP) (Lederer and Chedid, 1982). For each of these
agents as well as those described below, extensive animal model work preceded
the clinical therapeutic studies (Baldwin and Pimm, 1973; Tokunaga *et al.*,
1974; McLaughlin *et al.*, 1980; Scott, 1974). Other crude microbial agents,
either as intact organisms or as extracted bacterial cell components, have also
been used. A partial list includes *Corynebacterium parvum* (Halpern, 1975),
Bordetella pertussis (Finger *et al.*, 1970), the penicillin-inactivated *Streptococcus* OK 432 (Oyama *et al.*, 1975), endotoxin (Carswell *et al.*, 1975), and the
fungal extracts zymosan (Martin *et al.*, 1964) and glucan (Mansell *et al.*, 1975).
These agents have the ability to enhance the immune response or nonspecific
host defense reactions to tumor antigens or tumor cells. However, with a few
notable exceptions (intralesional BCG for cutaneous melanoma, intravesical
BCG in the treatment of superficial bladder cancer), when introduced into the
clinic this approach has met with little reproducible success.

TABLE I
Classification of Immunotherapeutic Approaches

A. Active nonspecific immunotherapy
  1. Natural products
    a. Intact organisms (BCG, *C. parvum*)
    b. Crude extracts (MER BCG)
    c. Purified components (MDP, MTP)
  2. Synthetics
    a. Pyrans (MVE-2)
    b. Pyrimidinols (ABPP, AIPP)
B. Active specific immunotherapy
  1. Tumor cell vaccines
  2. Tumor antigen vaccines
C. Adoptive immunotherapy
  1. Cellular
    a. Leukocyte transfusions
    b. Bone marrow transplantation
    c. Transfer of interleukin-II-induced killer cells
  2. Subcellular
    a. Immune RNA
    b. Transfer factor
  3. Cytokine therapy
    a. Interferons
    b. Interleukins
    c. Tumor necrosis factor
    d. Lymphotoxin
    e. Colony-stimulating factors
    f. Macrophage-activating factors
D. Serotherapy
  1. Cytotoxic antitumor antibodies
  2. Antibody carriers of drugs, toxins, radioisotopes
E. Immunomodulation/immunorestoration
  1. Natural hormones
    a. Thymosin F5
    b. TP 1
    c. Thymosin α_1
    d. Thymic humoral factor
    e. Facteur thymique serique
  2. Synthetics
    a. Levamisole
F. Depletive therapy
  1. Plasma exchange
  2. Plasma immunoabsorption

Active specific immunotherapy is based on the premise that tumor antigens are immunogenic and that a host organism is capable of mounting an immune response to autologous tumor. This concept was controversial at one time but has become well established through the identification of tumor-associated antigens using murine and human monoclonal antibodies. In addition, a weak or suppressed host immune response may be overridden by active immunization. Vaccines composed of so-called autologous tumor extracts have been used to treat patients with malignant melanoma (Berd et al., 1986). Attempts to augment the antitumor response to tumor cell vaccines have been made by virus infection of tumor cells and the production of melanoma viral oncolysates (Wallack et al., 1986a,b). More recently vaccines composed of so-called purified melanoma tumor-associated antigens (e.g., gangliosides) have been shown to elicit antibody responses in melanoma patients (Livingston et al., 1987).

Another approach that has been studied combines specific immunization by tumor cells plus nonspecific immunostimulation with BCG (Reid et al., 1982). Although this should be an effective combination, there is experimental evidence that nonspecific immune stimulation may induce suppressor mechanisms for T-cell, B-cell, and NK activity (Lichtenstein et al., 1982).

Adoptive immunotherapy involves the transfer of components of the immune system in an attempt to confer on the recipient some properties of the donor's immune or host reactivity or immunocompetence. In past years adoptive immunotherapy was practiced using transfer factor (Spitler et al., 1972; Oettgen et al., 1974), or immune RNA (Pilch et al., 1974; Veltman et al., 1974). Today adoptive immunotherapy may be accomplished with the transfer of viable autologous cells that have been activated in vitro for antitumor activity (lymphokine-activated killer cells) or cellular products (e.g., cytokines). The in vitro incubation of peripheral blood mononuclear cells (PBMC) from cancer patients with interleukin-2 (IL-2) stimulates the development of an activated cell population termed lymphokine-activated killer (LAK) cells (Grimm et al., 1982). These IL-2-induced LAK cells have recently been shown to be capable of lysing autologous and allogeneic tumor cells in vitro as well as in vivo in animal models and patients with cancer (Mulé et al., 1984; Rosenberg et al., 1985a).

Cytokines may be considered derivatives of the classical adoptive immunotherapy approach. They are the polypeptide products of immune or host defense cell activation. Cytokines may effect the proliferation and differentiation of various cell types (T cell, B cell, macrophage/monocyte, myeloid, or other hematopoietic cells). Both paracrine (effects on cells in the immediate vicinity) and autocrine (effects on the cell type by which they are produced) functions of cytokines have been documented (Dinarello and Mier, 1987). The availability of large amounts of pure cytokines produced by recombinant DNA technology has revolutionized modern cancer immunotherapy research. The biological and clinical effects of these agents alone and in combination with classic chemotherapeutic agents is an expanding area of both basic and clinical investigation.

The prime approach to modern serotherapy involves the use of MoAbs for tumor targeting of other therapeutic or diagnostic agents. The most commonly available MoAbs are of murine origin and thus, when injected into humans, elicit a human-antimouse immune response (Shawler *et al.*, 1985; Jaffers *et al.*, 1983). The production of human MoAbs that are potentially less immunogenic has been accomplished by human somatic cell hybridization (Olsson and Kaplan, 1980) and by the use of Epstein–Barr virus (EBV)-immortalized human B-lymphocyte cell lines (Steinitz *et al.*, 1977). Other potential problems associated with the use of MoAbs in humans and their possible solutions are discussed below. Monoclonal antibodies have significant promise as diagnostic and therapeutic modalities. Current applications include use for tumor imaging when coupled to radioisotopes (Pimm, 1987) and use for cancer therapy either unmodified or coupled to toxins (Frankel *et al.*, 1986), drugs (Baldwin and Byers, 1987), or isotopes (Humm, 1986). All of these issues are discussed in detail below.

In a general sense, immunomodulation refers to the mechanisms for regulating the activity of the immune system. This includes both immunopotentiation and immunosuppression (up- and down-regulation of immune responses). Thymic hormones (as represented by various thymic extracts and factors that have been studied) are felt to be important in regulating cell-mediated immunity in general and T-cell functions specifically (Bach *et al.*, 1975; Hooper *et al.*, 1975). Immunorestorative therapy has been attempted in malignant diseases (Azizi *et al.*, 1984; Bedikian *et al.*, 1984) and the acquired immunodeficiency syndrome (Schulof *et al.*, 1986).

Immunodepletive therapy attempts to remove "blocking factors" that may be responsible for the inhibition of host humoral or cell-mediated immune responses against tumor cells. Clinically, this may be attempted by extracorporeal perfusion of patient plasma over *Staphylococcus aureus* protein A (SPA). Possible mechanisms for the antitumor activity of this approach include complement activation, binding of immune complexes, and removal of plasma IgG (Korec *et al.*, 1984; Bensinger *et al.*, 1984; Solal-Celigny *et al.*, 1986). However, minimal clinical antitumor activity and significant toxicity have been the results of most clinical studies in humans (Korec *et al.*, 1984; Bensinger *et al.*, 1984; Solal-Celigny *et al.*, 1986; Messerschmidt *et al.*, 1984). A multicenter trial in patients with diverse tumor types has recently been reported (Messerschmidt *et al.*, 1988). In this study, the therapy was relatively well tolerated. No complete remissions were seen, but 12 of 87 (14%) patients developed partial remissions. These responses were seen in patients with AIDS-related Kaposi sarcoma, breast cancer, and colon cancer.

With this brief introduction, the remainder of this chapter focuses on the current status and future prospects for immunotherapy of the following solid tumors: malignant melanoma, renal cancer, bladder cancer, gastrointestinal malignancies, gynecologic malignancies, lung cancer, breast cancer, head and neck cancers, central nervous system tumors, and Kaposi sarcoma. In addition, the following specific modalities are given special consideration: IL-2-induced LAK cell therapy, colony-stimulating factors, and monoclonal antibody therapy.

2. MALIGNANT MELANOMA

The incidence of malignant melanoma in the United States and in other countries appears to be increasing (Schreiber et al., 1981; Magnus, 1977). Patients with surgically resectable disease have the best chance for cure. Treatment of metastatic disease with standard cytotoxic chemotherapeutic agents results in an overall response rate of only 10–20% (Mastrangelo et al., 1985) and no survival benefit. The most single active agent is dimethyltriazenoimidazole carboxamide (DTIC). There is no convincing evidence that combination chemotherapy using DTIC and other cytotoxic agents results in an improved response rate for patients with malignant melanoma.

Immunologic agents that modulate the host response to tumor are being studied as treatment for malignant melanoma both as a means of preventing recurrence and dissemination after primary resection and for metastatic disease. Several aspects of the biology and natural history of malignant melanoma make the use of immune-modulating agents attractive. It is known that host immune factors play a role in regulating the growth of malignant melanoma (Bystryn, 1985). The primary lesion of cutaneous melanomas may be observed to undergo a partial spontaneous regression, resulting in depigmentation and the "halo phenomenon." A complete spontaneous regression of the primary lesion may also occur and result in metastatic lesions without a known primary site (Balch and Milton, 1985). The occasional prolonged interval between primary tumor excision and recurrence (10 years or longer) suggests that host factors are able to inhibit but not totally eradicate residual unresected disease and that with time, because of changes in tumor immunogenicity and/or host immune competence, the melanoma may recur (Clark et al., 1975).

Several antigens of relevance to immune therapy and biological therapy are known to be expressed on the surface membrane of malignant melanoma cells. These include HLA A,B (Pellegrino et al., 1982), HLA DR (Winchester et al., 1978), the cell surface glycoprotein, p97 (Plowman et al., 1983), the ganglioside GD_3 (Dippold et al., 1984), and a high-molecular-weight melanoma-associated antigen (Hellstrom et al., 1983). The last three are considered tumor-associated antigens and have very limited representation on normal cells. The human interferons α, β, and γ (IFN-α, IFN-β, IFN-γ) are known to modulate the expression and shedding of HLA and the other melanoma-associated antigens (Dolei et al., 1983; M. Herlyn et al., 1985; Giacomini et al., 1984). Up-regulation of the expression of both HLA and tumor-associated antigens has obvious immunotherapeutic implications. A human melanoma cell line selected for resistance to the antiproliferative results of IFN-γ has been shown to have an increased expression and shedding of HLA class II antigens after IFN-γ exposure when compared with the IFN-γ-sensitive parent cell line (Ziai et al., 1985).

The relevance of the expression of these antigens to host immune response and tumor lysis by immunologic agents is being actively studied. In the earlier years of clinical research on melanoma there was some evidence that it responded to immunotherapy. Intralesional BCG inoculation caused the regression of both injected and distant, noninjected nodules (Morton, 1971; Morton et al., 1970). This suggested activation of specific antitumor immunity. Bacillus Calmette Guerin administered repeatedly onto the skin after surgical extirpation of stage I and II disease was initially felt to be associated with prolonged remission and survival (Morton et al., 1974; Ikonopisou, 1975). These early studies employed historical control groups. However, when concurrent randomized control groups were used, the initially encouraging results could not be confirmed (Pinsky et al., 1976; Sterchi et al., 1985; Paterson et al., 1984), and this approach has not been pursued in recent years. Similarly, randomized studies have shown no benefit for melanoma patients who receive adjuvant Corynebacterium parvum alone or in combination with DTIC (Thatcher et al., 1986a,b).

The immunologic treatment modalities for primary or metastatic malignant melanoma that we discuss in this chapter include interferons as single agents or in combination with other cytokines or cytotoxic drugs, monoclonal antibodies for imaging and therapy, and melanoma vaccines.

The initial studies of human interferon in metastatic melanoma were begun in the early 1980s. The material used in these studies was leukocyte interferon, partially purified from the supernatants of preparations of activated leukocytes or lymphoblastoid cells. These studies were limited by the purity of the material and the quantity available. Three of these early studies are summarized in Table II. Although only minor activity was seen (overall response rate 2–9%), the occasional complete remission (two out of 94 patients treated) affirmed that further study of the interferons in melanoma was justified.

The availability of unlimited quantities of purified interferon by recombinant DNA technology has led to more in-depth clinical studies of the interferons. Currently, the most actively studied interferon is recombinant IFN-α (rIFN-α). Currently available commercial preparations of rIFN-α include rIFN-α2a or interferon αA (Hoffman-LaRoche, Inc.) and rIFN-α2b or interferon α2 (Schering-Plough Corp.). The mechanism by which the interferons act as anticancer agents has not been totally elucidated. In addition to the effects on cell surface antigens as mentioned above, the interferons are also known to induce the enzyme 2′,5′-oligoadenylate synthetase, which accelerates mRNA degradation and inhibits protein synthesis (Sen, 1984; Revel et al., 1980), down-regulate oncogenes that may be associated with inhibition of cellular proliferation (Clemens, 1985), and modulate host T-cell, B-cell, natural killer cell, and macrophage activity (Paulnock and Borden, 1985; Herberman and Ortaldo, 1981).

Published studies of rIFN-α2a are summarized in Table III. As with natural

TABLE II

Human Leukocyte or Lymphoblastoid Interferon as Therapy for Metastatic Malignant Melanoma

Reference	Dose	Schedule	Route	Duration	Number of patients	CR	PR	Percentage total responses
Retsas et al. (1983)	2.5×10^6 u/m^2	Daily	i.m.	30 days	17	0	1	6
Krown et al. (1984)	1, 3, or 9 $\times$ 10^6 u	Daily	i.m.	42 days	44	0	1	2
Goldberg et al. (1985)	0.5×10^6 u/m^2	Daily	i.m.	42 days	33	2	1	9
	5.0×10^6 u/m^2	Weekly	i.m.					
	15×10^6 u/m^2	Day 1, 3, 5, 8, 10, 12; q 3 weeks	i.m.					

TABLE III

rIFN-α_{2a} as Therapy for Metastatic Malignant Melanoma

Reference	Dose	Schedule	Route	Duration	Number of patients	CR	PR	Percentage total responses
Creagan et al. (1984a)	1.2×10^6 u/m²	TIW	i.m.	12 weeks	30	1	5	20
Creagan et al. (1984b)	50×10^6 u/m²	TIW	i.m.	12 weeks	31	3	4	23
Creagan et al. (1985)	50×10^6 u/m²	TIW	i.m.	12 weeks	35	0	8	23
	Cimetidine 300 mg	Qid	p.o.					
Hersey et al. (1985, 1986)	15–50×10^6 u/m²	TIW	i.m.	2–20 weeks	20	2	0	10
McLeod et al. (1987)	3×10^6 IU, then	D 1–3	s.c.	6 months	44	6	7	30
	9×10^6 IU, then	D 4 to week 10	s.c.					
	9×10^6 IU	TIW	s.c.					
	DTIC 200–800 mg/m²	q 21 day	i.v.					
Legha et al. (1987)	3–36×10^6 u/day	Daily	i.m.	2.5 months	35	0	3	9
	18×10^6 u/day	TIW	i.m.	2.5 months	31	0	2	6

or partially purified interferon, occasional complete remissions were seen (12 out of 226 patients treated). The overall response rate varied from 6% to 30%. Numerous doses, schedules, routes of administration, and durations of treatment have been studied. Generally, higher doses are associated with more toxicity but not higher response rates (Creagan et al., 1984a,b). The combination of cimetidine and rIFN-α2a was not found to be more effective than rIFN-α2a as a single agent. The addition of DTIC to rIFN-α2a resulted in a total response rate of 30% with six complete remissions out of 44 total patients treated. The utility of combination therapy with DTIC has not, however, been studied in a randomized trial, and thus the above-cited study must be considered unconfirmed.

Three published studies of rIFN-α2b are summarized in Table IV. In general, the complete remission and total response rates were similar to those seen with rIFN-α2a. When rIFN-α2b was administered intravenously in the study by Coates et al. (1986), no responses were seen. It was suggested that this interferon may be less effective when administered intravenously because of a rapid clearance and a decreased half-life. However, Kirkwood et al. (1985a) reported two complete responses using intravenous rIFN-α2b.

Interferon β shares many biological properties with IFN-α. Together they are referred to as type I interferons; IFN-γ is considered to be a type II interferon. The distinction between type I and type II was originally based on the acid stability of type I and acid lability of type II (Rubin and Gupta, 1980). Interferons α and β have similar antiviral and antiproliferative activities (Taylor-Papadimitrous, 1984). In distinction, IFN-γ is a relatively more potent immunostimulator (Vilcek et al., 1985). In addition, IFN-α and -β share a common surface membrane receptor, whereas IFN-γ is felt to have a distinct, unique receptor (Branca and Baglioni, 1981).

The initial studies of IFN-β used material that was produced from human fibroblast culture systems. These studies were limited by the difficulties associated with production of human fibroblast IFN-β, with the resultant expense and paucity of material. As has been previously discussed, recombinant DNA technology has allowed the relatively inexpensive production of unlimited amounts of IFN-β. The IFN-β used in clinical trials (IFN-β_{SER}) differs from natural human IFN-β by a substitution of serine for cysteine at amino acid position 17. This substitution was necessary for decrease disulfide bridging. Disulfide bridging in the unsubstituted recombinant molecule resulted in a tenfold less biological activity compared to naturally produced IFN-β (Mark et al., 1983, 1984).

A limited number of studies of IFN-β in cancer patients have been published. The majority of these studies are phase I trials in patients with varied types of cancer (Sarna et al., 1986; Abdi et al., 1986; Hawkins et al., 1985; Rosso et al., 1985). Only minor activity has been seen in patients with malignant melanoma. In the phase I study by Sarna et al. (1986), two of four melanoma patients had a minor response to doses of $0.006-500 \times 10^6$ u/m^2 administered

TABLE IV
rIFN-α_{2b} as Therapy for Metastatic Malignant Melanoma

Reference	Dose	Schedule	Route	Duration	Number of patients	CR	PR	Percentage total responses
Kirkwood et al. (1985a)	$3–100 \times 10^6$ u/day	Daily	i.m.	4 weeks	7	0	2	17
			i.v.		16	2	0	
Robinson et al. (1986)	10×10^6 IU/m^2	TIW	s.c.	52 weeks	51	4	6	20
Coates et al. (1986)	20×10^6 IU/m^2	Daily for 5 days each 14 days	i.v.	Variable	15	0	0	0

intravenously twice weekly. Interferon β has also been shown to be active when injected directly into melanoma tumor nodules. Rosso (1985) observed objective responses in five of six melanoma nodules (partial response in three, complete response in two) injected with 1×10^6 u/cm^3 of tumor tissue.

As was the case with IFN-β, few studies have been published using IFN-γ for melanoma patients, and most of these are, again, broad phase I studies. In four phase I studies (Brown et al., 1987; Foon et al., 1985; van der Burg et al., 1985; Vadhan-Raj et al., 1986) a total of nine melanoma patients received varied doses and routes of administration of recombinant IFN-γ with only one patient showing a true partial response.

The interferons continue to be an active area of investigation in malignant melanoma. Many studies with the interferons in combination with each other and other agents are under way. Preliminary results are available in abstract form. Combinations that have been studied in patients with malignant melanoma include IFN-β and IFN-γ (Schiller et al., 1987), IFN-β and interleukin-2 (Krigel et al., 1987), and IFN-γ and BCNU (Weiner et al., 1987).

In summary, IFN-α has been shown to have clinical activity in patients with metastatic malignant melanoma. However, at this time a definite impact of IFN-α on the overall outcome of patients with this disease remains to be proven. There is certainly reason for cautious optimism and further thoughtful investigation. Adjuvant studies using various interferons after surgical resection of primary disease have been initiated in an attempt to delay or prevent recurrence. This is theoretically attractive because patients in this setting should have minimal tumor burdens and may potentially have tumors that are more homogeneous with regard to IFN sensitivity and surface antigen expression. Further investigation is needed using in vitro and animal models to determine the mechanism of action of the interferons and to define potential clinically synergistic combinations of interferons with other cytokines, MoAbs, or cytotoxic drugs.

As was briefly discussed in Section 1, vaccines composed of autologous tumor cells have been used as therapy for malignant melanoma. The premise has been that antigens on tumor cells should elicit a host antitumor response. However, in practice these responses have been difficult to document (Livingston et al., 1985). Attempts to increase the immune response have been made by modifying the tumor cells or modifying the host immune system.

One approach to increase immunogenicity has been to use virally infected tumor cells for vaccination. In animal models potent antitumor responses have been documented after the administration of viral oncolysates (Sharpless et al., 1950). In a Southeastern Cancer Study Group phase I/II study (Wallack et al., 1986a), vaccinia melanoma oncolysates (VMO) were administered to 48 patients with high-risk stage I or pathological stage II malignant melanoma. Patients were vaccinated immediately after surgical resection or after a 6-week delay. Serological antimelanoma activity was seen in 13 of 23 (56%) patients who received immediate vaccination. This compares with serological responses in only two of 19 patients who received delayed vaccination. Side effects of this therapy were minimal. Twenty-eight of the 48 patients treated remained free of disease, whereas 20 have suffered recurrence.

It is known that host T lymphocytes are capable of suppressing the host immune response to tumor antigens (Fujimoto et al., 1976). It is known that cyclophosphamide causes a depletion of suppressor T lymphocytes (North, 1982). Berd et al. (1986) were able to demonstrate delayed-type hypersensitivity to autologous melanoma cells in seven of eight patients who received treatment with cyclophosphamide as compared with responses in only two of seven patients who did not receive cyclophosphamide pretreatment. Livingston et al. (1987) also found an enhanced antibody response in resected stage II melanoma patients who received pretreatment with cyclophosphamide in combination with a vaccination of the melanoma ganglioside GM_2 and BCG. The use of cyclophosphamide in combination with IL-2 for patients with metastatic melanoma is discussed in Section 12.

The use of MoAbs in the therapy of patients with malignant melanoma has potential both as a diagnostic and therapeutic modality. The technical aspects of MoAb therapy are discussed in detail in Section 14. Clinical aspects as they specifically relate to malignant melanoma are discussed here.

Radioisotopes that have been conjugated to MoAbs and used for tumor imaging include ^{131}I, ^{123}I, ^{111}In, ^{99m}Tc, and ^{67}Ga (Pimm, 1987). The ability to locate accurately metastatic tumor deposits is of obvious clinical importance for melanoma patients with early-stage disease. Whether or not to perform a regional lymph node dissection in these patients remains a controversial issue. The ability to select patients with positive lymph nodes preoperatively would be an important advance.

Lotze et al. (1986) at the National Cancer Institute have used ^{131}I- and ^{111}In-labeled Fab fragments of monoclonal antibodies to the high-molecular-weight and p97 melanoma-associated antigens in patients with metastatic and clinical stage II disease. Patients with metastatic disease received an intravenous injection of antibody, and 22 of 38 patients (58%) were found to have positive scans at sites of known metastatic disease. Patients with clinical stage II disease received local subcutaneous injections of antibody followed by lymph node resection. It was found that local lymph nodes could be imaged but that specificity was poor because of nonspecific tumor binding. Two other melanoma imaging studies have reported positive results with 68% and 88% of known metastatic nodules being imaged (Buraggi et al., 1984; Larson et al., 1983). Murray and his colleagues (1985, 1987a,b) have reported radioimmunoimaging studies in melanoma patients using the ^{111}In-labeled MoAbs 96.5 and ZME-018. These murine antibodies have specificity for the p97 and gp240 melanoma antigens, respectively. Fifty to sixty percent of previously documented metastatic tumor sites were successfully imaged in these studies. Although consistent nontumor uptake was seen (especially in the liver and spleen), no serious toxicity was observed.

Unconjugated monoclonal antibodies alone may have cytotoxic activity.

The processes by which this cytotoxic activity may occur include antibody-dependent cellular cytotoxicity (ADCC) and complement activation. Indeed, antitumor responses have been seen in melanoma patients treated with unconjugated MoAb. Thus, Houghton et al. (1985) have reported a phase I trial in which 12 patients were treated with R24, a mouse MoAb specific for the GD_3 ganglioside. Three partial responses were seen in patients with primarily skin and soft tissue metastases. Cheung et al. (1987) recently reported another phase I trial using an antibody directed to the GD_2 ganglioside. In this study, two of nine melanoma patients were found to have a partial response that lasted 22 and 56+ weeks. In pilot studies by Goodman et al. (1985) using the murine antimelanoma MoAbs 96.5 and 48.7 and by Oldham et al. (1984) using the murine anti-melanoma MoAb 9.2.27, localization of antibody to tumor was seen, but no objective tumor regressions were observed.

The use of monoclonal antibodies in patients with malignant melanoma is an area of very active research. Further studies are in progress using MoAb conjugated to toxins and drugs. The results of these studies are eagerly anticipated.

Another modality that has been shown to be of benefit to patients with malignant melanoma is the use of IL-2-induced LAK cells plus high-dose IL-2 or high-dose IL-2 alone (Rosenberg et al., 1985a, 1987). This is discussed in Section 12, devoted totally to IL-2-induced LAK cell therapy.

3. RENAL CANCER

The yearly incidence of and mortality from renal cancer in the United States are 20,000 and 9000, respectively (Silverberg and Lubera, 1987). The only proven effective therapy for this type of cancer is surgical removal (nephrectomy) prior to local or distant tumor dissemination.

Treatment of metastatic disease is largely ineffective. Standard treatment modalities include chemotherapy and hormonal therapy. Cytotoxic drugs with activity as single agents include hydroxyurea, vinblastine, and cyclohexylchloroethylnitrosourea (CCNU) (Hrushesky and Murphy, 1977; Harris, 1983). Response rates for these single agents are in the range of 9–15%. Combinations of cytotoxic drugs do not increase the response rate. Hormonal agents including antiestrogens and progesterones are associated with response rates of less than 10% (Hrushesky and Murphy, 1977; Harris, 1983; Prout, 1973).

An interesting phenomenon seen in renal cancer patients is spontaneous regression of distant, usually pulmonary, metastases (Everson and Cole, 1966; Garfield and Kennedy, 1972). Spontaneous regression may occur after nephrectomy as well as in patients who have not had their primary disease resected, but the overall incidence is less than 0.4% (Montie et al., 1977; Myers et al., 1968). One can speculate that host immune factors may play a role in these spontaneous regressions. There is evidence that host immune factors may be important in renal cancer (Holland, 1975).

Immunotherapeutic approaches to renal cancer that have shown some promise include the interferons, active specific immunotherapy with autologous tumor cells, and adoptive immunotherapy with IL-2-induced LAK cells. In this section we discuss the interferons and therapy with autologous tumor cells; LAK cell therapy is discussed in Section 12.

Prior to the availability of rINF-α, human leukocyte- and lymphoblastoid-derived IFN-α were used to treat patients with renal cancer. These studies are summarized by Table V.

The first report on the use of IFN-α in renal cancer was made by Quesada et al. (1983). The partially purified material used in this early study was prepared from human leukocytes. An update of the Quesada et al. (1985a) study has been reported. At the time of that report, 50 evaluable patients had been treated with a daily intramuscular (i.m.) dose of 3×10^6 units. Three complete remissions (CR) and ten partial remissions (PR) were seen for an overall response rate of 26%. In this study a correlation between tumor response and interferon-induced leukopenia (median leukocyte count) was reported. However, this correlation has not been seen in subsequent studies (Kirkwood et al., 1985; Buzaid et al., 1987).

Kirkwood et al. (1985b) performed a randomized study of low-dose (2×10^6 units per day) versus high-dose (10×10^6 units per day) human leukocyte IFN-α (HLE IFN-α). Although more responses were seen in patients who received the high-dose regimen, these patients also had significantly more toxicity. The question of the dose–response effect of IFN-α in renal cancer is discussed further below.

Figlin et al. (1985) have reported a combination study of HLE IFN-α and weekly vinblastine for renal cancer. The results of this study were disappointing in that the combination was associated with greater toxicity but not greater antitumor activity than that seen with IFN-α alone (Table V).

The human lymphoblastoid IFN-α (HLB IFN-α) studies summarized in Table V indicate an overall response rate of 16% (29 CR plus PR out of 184 patients treated). The study by Trump et al. (1987) is worthy of mention with regard to toxicity. An initial dose of 30×10^6 u/m^2 was found to be intolerable because of fever, fatigue, myelosuppression, and liver dysfunction.

More recently, recombinant IFN-α has been used to treat patients with renal cancer. These studies using rIFN-α2a and rIFN-α2b are summarized in Table VI. Numerous doses, schedules, and routes of administration have been employed in these investigations. Overall, 63 responses (six CR and 57 PR) have been documented in a total of 433 patients (15%). Diluted within this total is evidence for a significant dose–response relationship. This is best demonstrated in the study by Quesada (1985a). In this study patients were randomized to receive rIFN-α at 2×10^6 u/m^2 versus 20×10^6 u/m^2 on a daily schedule. No

TABLE V

Human Leukocyte and Lymphoblastoid IFN-α as Therapy for Renal Cancer

Reference	Interferon[a]	Dose	Schedule	Route	Number of patients	CR	PR	Percentage total responses
Quesada et al. (1985b)	HLE IFN-α	3×10^6 units	Daily	i.m.	50	3	10	26
Kirkwood et al. (1985b)	HLE IFN-α	1×10^6 units versus 10×10^6 units	Daily Daily	i.m. i.m.	16 14	0 1	0 2	0 21
Figlin et al. (1985)	HLE IFN-α	3×10^6 IU/day	5 days per week	i.m.	24	0	3	31
		Vinblastine 0.1– 0.5 mg/kg	Weekly	i.v.				
Neidhart et al. (1984)	HLB IFN-α	5×10^6 units/m^2	TIW	i.m.	33	0	5	15
Marumo et al. (1984)	HLB IFN-α	3×10^6 IU	Daily	i.m.	18	1	0	6
Vugrin et al. (1985)	HLB IFN-α	3×10^6 units/m^2	TIW	i.m.	21	0	1	5
Trump et al. (1987)	HLB IFN-α	$3–30 \times 10^6$ units/m^2	Daily for 10 days, q 3 weeks	i.m.	39	0	5	13
Umeda and Niijima (1986)	HLB IFN-α	5×10^6 IU	BIW, TIW, then daily	i.m.	73	1	16	23

[a]HLE IFN-α, human leukocyte IFN-α; HLB IFN-α, human lymphoblastoid IFN-α.

TABLE VI

rIFN-α as Therapy for Renal Cancer

Reference	Dose	Schedule	Route	Number of patients	CR	PR	Percentage total responses
Kempf et al. (1986)	2×10^6 IU/m^{2b}	TIW	s.c.	10	0	0	0
	3×10^7 IU/m^{2b}	Daily × 5, 2–3 weeks	i.v.	10	0	1	10
Quesada et al. (1985a)	2×10^6 units/m^{2a}	Daily	i.m.	15	0	0	0
	20×10^6 units/m^{2a}	Daily	i.m.	41	1	11	29
Umeda and Niijima (1988)	3–36×10^6 IU^a	Daily	i.m.	108	2	13	14
	6–10×10^6 IU^b	3–5 times weekly	i.m.	45	1	7	18
Muss et al. (1987)	2–10×10^6 IU/m^{2b}	TIW	s.c.	58	1	4	9
	30–50×10^6 IU/m^{2b}	Daily × 5, q 3 weeks	i.v.	54	1	2	6
Buzaid et al. (1987)	3–36×10^6 units^a	Daily	i.m.	22	0	5	23
Sarna et al. (1987)	3–36×10^6 units^a	5 days per week	i.m.	19	5		26
Fossa and de Garis (1987)	36×10^6 IU^a Vinblastine 0.1–0.5 mg/kg	TIW q 2–3 weeks	i.m. i.v.	18	0	6	33
	18–33×10^6 IU^a Vinblastine 0.1 mg/kg	TIW q 3 weeks	i.m. i.v.	13	0	3	23

[a]rIFN-α$_{2a}$ (Hoffman-La Roche, Inc.).
[b]rIFN-α$_{2b}$ (Schering-Plough Corporation).

responses were seen with the low-dose regimen, whereas the high-dose regimen was associated with a 29% response rate (one CR and 11 PR out of a total of 41 patients). Although the incidence of toxicity was similar in the two treatment groups, toxicity in the high-dose group was generally more severe and persisted longer.

Further evidence to support a dose–response effect for IFN-α in renal cancer patients is given in a review by Krown (1987). In this review of numerous studies a statistically significant improved response rate was found in patients who receive "intermediate" versus "low"-dose regiments. In the same review it was felt that the source of IFN-α and the schedule of administration were not important with regard to overall response rate.

The toxicities of IFN-α in renal cancer patients have been reviewed by Neidhart (1986). As has been previously mentioned, high-dose regimens are generally associated with greater toxicity. Commonly reported toxicities include fatigue, fever, chills, myalgias, myelosuppression, headache, diarrhea, nausea, anorexia, weight loss, hepatic dysfunction, and neurotoxicity (confusion, somnolence, decreased ability to concentrate, and psychomotor retardation).

Because of the small number of patients responding to single-agent IFN-α in any one study, it is difficult to strictly analyze response duration. In the present studies, response duration has been found to vary widely from a few months to greater than 2 years. Likewise, a beneficial effect on the survival of renal cancer patients who receive IFN-α has not been proven. Generally, responding patients survive longer than nonresponding patients. However, as has been suggested by Sarna et al. (1987), it is unclear whether the treatment has a direct effect on survival or whether it serves to select a group of patients with good prognostic factors such as lung-only metastases and good performance status. Interferon α should not be considered standard therapy for patients with renal cancer. Sufficient activity has been seen, however, to warrant preclinical investigations searching for synergistic combinations and future combination clinical trials.

Because of the modest but reproducible remission-inducing activity of IFN-α in patients with renal cancer, studies of IFN-α in combination with other modalities are of great interest. Fossa and de Garis (1987) have reported a combination study of rIFN-α and vinblastine. A 29% response rate (no CR and nine PR out of 31 patients treated) was reported. Although this is moderately encouraging, further confirmation of the efficacy of rIFN-α and vinblastine combination therapy awaits further study in randomized trials. Future prospects include combinations of IFN-α and other cytotoxic drugs, other interferons (IFN-β, IFN-γ), and other cytokines (IL-2, TNF).

A limited number of studies have been published using IFN-β and IFN-γ in patients with renal cancer. Three of these studies are presented in Table VII.

As has been previously discussed, rIFN-β_{SER} has been genetically altered to decrease disulfide bridging. Rinehart et al. (1986a) treated 15 patients with this material in a phase I/II trial and saw partial remissions in two patients.

TABLE VII

rIFN-β_{ser} and rIFN-γ as Therapy for Renal Cancer

Reference	Interferon	Dose	Schedule	Route	Number of patients	CR	PR	Percentage total responses
Rinehart et al. (1986a)	rIFN-β_{ser}	$0.01–600 \times 10^6$ units/m^2	Twice weekly	4-hour i.v. infusion	15	0	2	13
Rinehart et al. (1986b)	rIFN-γ	$0.01–600 \times 10^6$ units/m^2	Twice weekly	4-hour i.v. infusion	13	0	0	0
Quesada et al. (1987)	rIFN-γ	$5–20 \times 10^6$ units/m^2	Daily	i.m.	14	0	1	7
		$0.2–1.0 \times 10^6$ units/m^2	Daily	i.v. continuous infusion	16	0	1	6

Minimal activity has been seen with rIFN-γ in renal cancer patients. In the studies by Rinehart *et al.* (1986b) and Quesada *et al.* (1987), two partial remissions were seen in a total of 43 patients treated (5%) (Table VII).

The toxicities seen with IFN-β and IFN-γ in renal cancer patients are dose dependent and qualitatively similar to those seen with IFN-α. Reported toxicities include fever, chills, headaches, myalgias, fatigue, anorexia, nausea/vomiting, diarrhea, weight loss, and hypotension.

Active specific immunotherapy in the form of autologous or allogeneic tumor antigen with or without a nonspecific adjuvant has also been used as therapy for renal cancer patients. An early study by Tykka (1981) reported a 52% regression rate of pulmonary metastases in 21 patients. However, subsequent studies using more stringent response criteria have not been as encouraging. Fowler (1986) saw no objective responses in 23 patients treated with autologous or allogeneic tumor antigen plus *Candida albicans* antigen.

More recently attempts have been made to modulate T-suppressor lymphocyte function by administering cyclophosphamide prior to tumor cell immunization. Sahasrubudhe *et al.* (1986) treated 20 patients with weekly injections of irradiated autologous tumor cells plus *Corynebacterium parvum*. Intravenous cyclophosphamide was given prior to the initial week's injection of tumor cells. Five patients (26%) were found to have objective responses (one CR and four PR). The results of this pilot study are intriguing and indicate that further investigations using T-suppressor cell modulation in conjunction with this or other forms of immunotherapy should be undertaken. We subsequently discuss the use of cyclophosphamide plus IL-2 for patients with renal cancer.

One of the more exciting new modalities being investigated as therapy for renal cancer is the administration of IL-2-induced LAK cells plus high-dose IL-2 or IL-2 alone. This form of therapy is discussed in great detail in Section 12.

To summarize for now, the response of renal cancer to standard cytotoxic chemotherapeutic agents is dismal. A modest improvement in response rate has been made by the use of the interferons. However, the effect on long-term survival is unproven. Prospects for the future look brighter primarily because of advances in immunotherapy. It is likely that more effective therapies for renal cancer will be developed when knowledge is gained into the requirements for synergy among cytokines, cytotoxic drugs, and activated cellular systems with antitumor activity (LAK cells).

4. SUPERFICIAL BLADDER CANCER

In 1984 it was estimated there would be 38,700 new cases of bladder cancer and 10,700 deaths from bladder cancer (Silverberg, 1984). Histologically, 90% of cases are transitional cell carcinoma, 6–8% are squamous cell carcinoma, and 2% are adenocarcinoma (Richie *et al.*, 1985).

A brief discussion of the natural history and staging of bladder cancer is relevant to any therapeutic considerations. Bladder cancers arise from the superficial epithelial layer. The staging system is based on the depth of penetration of tumor into the underlying tissue layers. Superficial bladder tumors are confined to the epithelium and may be characterized as carcinoma *in situ* (CIS) or papillary carcinoma. In the staging system of Jewett, Marshall, and Strong (Marshall, 1952), superficial bladder cancers are stage 0. In the TNM classification they are referred to as TIS (CIS) or Ta (papillary).

After initial local therapy (transurethral resection), 40–85% of superficial bladder tumors will recur, usually within 6–12 months (Torti and Lum, 1984). Factors that are predictive of the tendency for bladder tumors to recur include stage (TIS or Ta versus higher stage), histological grade, degree of multicentricity, and presence of CIS with or without papillary tumors (Torti and Lum, 1987).

Because of the tendency for recurrence, patients with superficial bladder tumors must undergo repeated cystoscopies for surveillance. Recurrent tumors may be removed endoscopically, but the potential exists with each recurrence for deeper invasion and dissemination.

Since the early 1900s many agents have been infused into the bladders of patients with superficial bladder tumors either as primary therapy or as adjuvant therapy after surgical tumor removal. Agents demonstrated to have activity in this setting include thiotepa, ethoglucid (Epodyl[R]), mitomycin C, doxorubicin, VM-26 (Teniposide[R]), and BCG (Torti and Lum, 1984).

BCG is an attenuated form of *Mycobacterium bovis* originally isolated by Calmette and Guerin. In an early review of BCG and cancer, Bast *et al.* (1974) proposed five factors that existing data indicated were important for the success or failure of BCG as cancer therapy. These included (1) tumor size—studies in animals indicated that large tumor burdens were difficult to eradicate with BCG, (2) the ability of the host to develop an immune response to mycobacterial antigens, (3) a sufficient number of viable BCG organisms, (4) proximity of BCG to tumor cells, and (5) host ability to develop an immune response to tumor-associated antigens. These factors may serve as at least a partial explanation for the relative success of BCG when administered intralesionally for melanoma and intravesically for superficial bladder tumors and the relative lack of success of BCG when used for other diseases by other routes of administration.

The initial studies of BCG in superficial bladder cancer were reported by Morales (1980, 1984) and Morales *et al.* (1976). These studies showed that intracavitary BCG was effective as prophylaxis after primary tumor removal and for CIS as well as established early-stage tumors (Morales *et al.*, 1976; Morales, 1980). The 10-year experience of Morales (1984) in which more than 80 patients were treated was reported in 1984 (Table VIII). After prophylactic therapy, 48% of patients (20/42) remained disease-free with a mean follow-up of 61 months.

TABLE VIII

Phase II Studies of BCG for Superficial Bladder Tumors

Reference	BCG strain	Dose (number of organisms)	Cutaneous inoculation	Schedule	Prophylaxis[a]		CIS[a]		Therapy[a]	
					CR[b] (%)	Mean duration (mos)	CR (%)	Mean duration (mos)	CR (%)	Mean duration (mos)
Morales (1984)	Pasteur	1.2×10^9 CFU	Yes	Weekly × 6	20/42 (48)	61	10/17 (59)	51	14/23 (60)	47
Dekernion et al. (1985)	Tice	$2\text{–}8 \times 10^8$	No	Weekly × 6, then monthly until recurrence	15/22 (67)	15	13/19 (68)	14.5	8/22 (36)	13
Kelly et al. (1985)	Pasteur	6×10^6 to 1×10^{12} CFU[c]	No	Weekly × 6, repeat if residual tumor present	16/17 (94)	11	8/12 (67)	10.8	8/11 (73)	14.3
Schellhammer et al. (1986)	Pasteur	1×10^9	No	Weekly × 6	[d]		12/18 (67)	12.9	8/10 (80)	8.31

[a] Prophylaxis, no evidence of tumor after resection; CIS, carcinoma in situ. Therapy, documented residual superficial bladder tumor.
[b] CR indicates absence of recurrence of tumors treated prophylactically or complete response in CIS or therapy categories.
[c] Colony-forming units.
[d] Prophylaxis group not included in this study.

For CIS, 59% of patients (10/17) remained disease-free with a mean follow-up of 51 months. Finally, for residual tumors, 60% of patients (14/23) were disease-free with a mean follow-up of 47 months. These patients were treated with the Frappier strain of BCG (Institut Armand Frappier, Montreal, Quebec, Canada), which was given as 1.2×10^9 colony-forming units (CFU) intravesically and 5 $\times 10^7$ CFU intradermally weekly for 6 weeks.

Since the initial reports by Morales, a number of other phase II studies using BCG for various categories of superficial bladder tumors have been reported (Table VIII). Because of the short follow-up time, the mean duration of response in the studies by DeKernion et al. (1985), Kelley et al. (1985), and Schellhammer et al. (1986) was much less than that seen in the Morales study. The mean complete response rate of these four studies for patients treated in the therapy category was 62%. This compares favorably with the compiled complete response rates for other agents reported in the review by Torti and Lum (1984): thiotepa, 38%; epodyl, 45%; mitomycin-C, 49%; doxorubicin, 31%; VM-26, 33%.

A number of randomized studies have compared treatment of recurrent superficial bladder tumors by transurethral resection alone versus transurethral resection plus intravesical BCG (Lamm et al., 1982; Pinsky et al., 1985; Lamm, 1985; Herr et al., 1985, 1986). Pinsky et al. (1985) treated 43 patients with postresection BCG (120 mg intravesically; 5×10^7 viable units percutaneously) on a weekly schedule for 6 weeks and compared them with 43 randomized control patients who received resection alone. The BCG group was found to have fewer tumors on follow-up ($P < 0.001$) and a longer time to first recurrence ($P < 0.001$).

Lamm et al. (1982) randomized 57 patients with histologically documented transitional cell carcinoma of the bladder in whom all visible tumor had been resected to receive an every-3-month cytoscopy alone versus BCG (120 mg intravesically; 5 mg percutaneously) weekly for 6 weeks. With a minimum follow-up of 1 year or to time of tumor recurrence, 14 of 27 (52%) control patients recurred versus six of 30 (20%) BCG-treated patients.

In other studies patients have been randomized to receive BCG versus other active agents after transurethral resection of superficial bladder tumors. Brosman (1982) randomized patients to receive BCG (6×10^9 organisms) or thiotepa (60 mg) after resection. No recurrences were seen in the BCG group (39 patients) compared with a 40% recurrence rate in the thiotepa group (19 patients).

In a Southwest Oncology Group study, 169 patients were randomized to receive BCG (intravesically and percutaneously, weekly for 6 weeks, at 3 and 6 months, and every 6 months thereafter) or doxorubicin (intravesically, weekly for 4 weeks, then monthly for 1 year) (Mori et al., 1986). In the BCG group there was an 18% incidence of tumor recurrence (16/88 patients). This compares with a 54% incidence of recurrence in the doxorubicin group (45/83 patients). In addition, the complete response rates in 87 of these patients who were found to have CIS were 85% for BCG and 39% for doxorubicin.

Finally, Soloway and Perry (1987) treated 30 patients with persistent or recurrent superficial bladder tumors despite previous therapy with thiotepa and/or mitomycin-C. These patients received Tice strain BCG (intravesically, weekly for 6 weeks) and were found to have a 50% (15/30 patients) complete response rate with a mean follow-up of 16 months.

The studies discussed above indicate a significant advantage in decreasing recurrence and persistence of superificial bladder tumors in patients treated with intravesical BCG as compared with other agents intravesically or repeated transurethral surveillance and resection. However, most of these studies have not been specifically designed to answer the question of the ability of BCG to decrease the need for cystectomy or increase survival. Nevertheless, there is at least circumstantial evidence that by causing prolonged remissions BCG may delay the need for cystectomy (Pinsky et al., 1985; Herr et al., 1986).

The optimum duration of intravesical BCG therapy for patients treated prophylactically or for documented CIS or residual tumor deserves further discussion. It has been demonstrated that a significant number of patients who have recurrences or fail to respond after an initial course of therapy (weekly for 6 weeks) will have a favorable result after a second course of therapy (Kelley et al., 1985; Haaff et al., 1986b).

Catalona et al. (1987) performed a risk–benefit analysis of repeated courses of intravesical BCG (120 mg weekly for 6 weeks) in 100 patients. For patients who had failed one course of therapy, the risk-to-benefit ratio favored giving a second course. However, in patients who had failed two or more courses of therapy, the risk of local invasion (30%) or metastatic spread (50%) exceeded the chance of responding to further therapy (20%).

A recent randomized study by Badalament et al. (1987) investigated the efficacy of maintenance therapy with intravesical BCG for patients with superficial bladder cancer. Ninety-three patients with CIS or superficial papillary tumors underwent transurethral resection followed by BCG (120 mg intravesically, weekly for 6 weeks). Patients were then randomized to receive only follow-up cystoscopy or intravesical BCG monthly for 2 years. The two groups were found to have similar recurrence and progression rates even when correction was made for the presence or absence of tumor after the initial course of BCG. The major difference between the two groups was that the maintenance group had increased local toxicity.

The toxicities associated with BCG therapy in patients with bladder cancer have recently been reviewed by Lamm et al. (1986). The toxicities are reported for a total of 1278 patients compiled from the authors' personal experience, a literature review, and a questionnaire sent to other investigators. Over 95% of the patients treated had no serious complications. Toxicities that were seen using various BCG strains, doses, and schedules include fever $>103°F$ (3.9%), granulomatous prostatitis (1.9%), arthritis/arthralgia (0.5%), major hematuria (0.5%), skin rash (0.4%), skin abscess (0.4%), urethral obstruction (0.3%), orchitis/epididymitis (0.2%), contracted bladder (0.2%), renal abscess (0.1%), hypotension (0.1%), and cytopenia (0.1%).

The mechanism by which BCG leads to regression of superficial bladder tumors has not been fully elucidated. One suggestion is that intravesical BCG causes a nonspecific local inflammatory response, which results in local sloughing of normal as well as tumor tissue (Droller, 1987). However, other investigators have shown a correlation between response to intravesical BCG therapy and conversion of purified protein derivative (PPD) skin tests and the formation of a granulomatous response in the bladder (Lamm et al., 1982; Kelley et al., 1986). In addition, it is known that transitional cell carcinomas express ABO blood group antigens (Sadoughi et al., 1982) as well as other tumor-specific antigens (Bubenik et al., 1970). It is therefore possible that nonspecific immune stimulation with BCG results in a specific host immune response against these antigens and subsequent cytotoxicity. It has been speculated that intracavitary BCG may lead to increased NK-cell activity and/or to the release of cytokines such as IFN, IL-2, or tumor necrosis factor (TNF), which may then directly or indirectly lead to tumor regression (Torti and Lum, 1984; Droller, 1987). Haaff et al. (1986a) have demonstrated the presence of IL-2 in the urine of patients who received intravesical BCG.

Other biological response modifiers have been used to treat superificial bladder cancers. Responses have been seen with IFN-α administered intravesically, intralesionally via cystoscopy, and systemically (Ikic et al., 1981; Scorticatti et al., 1982; Torti et al., 1984). In a recent study by Torti et al. (1988), intravesical rIFN-α2b was given to 35 patients with recurrent superficial bladder cancer. Overall response rates of 58% (six CR and five PR out of 19 patients treated) and 25% (four CR and no PR out of 16 patients treated) were seen for patients with CIS or papillary transitional cell carcinoma, respectively. The optimum route, schedule, dose, and efficacy of IFN-α relative to BCG remain to be defined. Other biological agents with some activity but as yet an undefined role in bladder cancer include IL-2 (Pizza et al., 1984; Merguerian et al., 1987), levamisole (Romics et al., 1985), and the streptococcal preparation, OK-432 (Fujita, 1987).

5. GASTROINTESTINAL MALIGNANCIES

In the past, immunotherapy of gastrointestinal malignances has met with little success. In recent years encouraging results have been seen using immunotherapy as an adjuvant to surgical resection of colon cancer.

Cancer of the gastrointestinal tract is the second most common cause of cancer death in the United States. In 1986, it was estimated that there would be 98,000 new cases and 51,800 deaths from colon cancer (Silverberg and Lubera, 1986). In the last 40 years, little progress has been made in treating the remainder of patients with residual primary or metastatic disease. The 5-year survival rate of patients with colon cancer is directly related to the depth of tumor extension through the bowel wall and involvement of local lymph nodes (Astler and Coller, 1954). Patients with involvement of the mucosa and submucosa only have a >90% 5-year survival rate. In patients whose tumors do not involve local lymph nodes and do not penetrate the bowel wall (B_1) or those with bowel wall penetration but negative local lymph nodes (B_2), the 5-year survival rates vary from 65% to 43%. Patients with local lymph node involvement (C_1 or C_2) have a significantly decreased 5-year survival rate of less than 25% (Sinkovics, 1986).

In adjuvant colon cancer trials, standard cytotoxic drugs such as thiotepa, 5-fluorouracil (5-FU), floxuridine (FUDR), and 5-FU plus methyl-CCNU have not been shown to significantly prolong survival over untreated concurrent control groups. The addition of nonspecific immune-stimulating agents such as BCG or MER of BCG was again not associated with a survival benefit (Gastrointestinal Tumor Study Group, 1984; Panettiere and Chen, 1981). This trend of discouraging results in colon cancer adjuvant therapy may soon be broken.

The presence of tumor-associated antigens (TAA) for colon cancer has been suggested by the work of Hellstrom et al. (1970) and Hollinshead et al. (1970). Hollinshead et al. (1970) have isolated two colon cancer cell membrane antigens (72 kD and 88 kD) that are felt to be distinct from carcinoembryonic antigen (CEA). In a phase I study 22 colon cancer patients received varying doses of the 72-kD and 88-kD TAA after surgical resection of Dukes B_2, C, or D lesions (Hollinshead et al., 1985). The toxicity of this treatment consisted primarily of skin ulcers at the vaccination site and occasional fever and chills. A consistent immune response was seen when patients were tested by delayed hypersensitivity skin test to TAA and migration inhibition assays. Given the demonstrated safety and immune reactivity, a phase III randomized trial of adjuvant-active specific immunotherapy with TAA versus no further therapy after surgery has begun in colon cancer patients. Results are not yet available.

In 1985, Hoover et al. reported a randomized trial of adjuvant-active specific immunotherapy for colorectal cancer patients. In this study, patients with Dukes stage B_2 or C lesions were vaccinated postoperatively with a combination of 1×10^7 irradiated autologous tumor cells and 1×10^7 viable BCG organisms. The vaccinations were given weekly for 2 weeks approximately 4–5 weeks after surgery. A third injection of 1×10^7 irradiated tumor cells alone was given in the third week. Randomized control patients received no further therapy after surgery. At the time of this report 40 patients had been randomized and followed with a mean follow-up of 28 months. Three of 20 patients in the treatment group have recurred compared to nine of 20 control patients. Significant improvements in disease-free interval ($p = 0.035$) and overall survival ($p = 0.023$) were seen in the immunized patients. Toxicities associated with this regimen were minimal and consisted primarily of local injection site ulcers and mild fever. Further patient follow-up for this study continues.

Jessup *et al.* (1986) recently reported a comparison trial of vaccination with two doses of autologous tumor cells. Patients with Dukes B_2 or C colorectal carcinomas received vaccinations with 3×10^6 or 1×10^7 irradiated autologous tumor cells combined with 1×10^7 colony-forming units of BCG. Immune response, as measured by delayed-type hypersensitivity reactions to autologous tumor cells, was initially similar for high-dose and low-dose patients. However, on repeat testing at 3 months post-vaccination, none of seven low-dose patients as compared to three of four high-dose patients maintained positive cutaneous reactions. In a recent follow-up it has been suggested that autologous tumor cell–BCG vaccine may enhance cell-mediated immunity by inhibiting a CD8-positive suppressor cell mechanism (Jessup, 1987). Based on these results a randomized multicenter trial in the Eastern Cooperative Oncology Group (ECOG) is now in progress.

Levamisole is an antihelminthic agent that is felt to have immune-modulating activity (Terry and Rosenberg, 1982). Sertoli *et al.* (1987) have reported a randomized trial of chemotherapy (5-FU plus methyl-CCNU) versus chemotherapy plus levamisole. An untreated control group was not included. After 8 years no significant differences in disease-free interval or overall survival were seen between the two groups.

More encouraging results with levamisole can be found in a North Central Cancer Treatment Group and Mayo Clinic study (Laurie *et al.*, 1987). In this study 408 patients with resected B_2 or C colorectal carcinomas were randomized to receive levamisole or levamisole plus 5-FU or no further therapy. With a median follow-up of 56 months both levamisole groups have shown a significantly prolonged disease-free interval relative to control patients. In addition, patients with C lesions in the levamisole-alone group have shown a significant increase in survival. Confirmation of these results may be forthcoming from a large inter-cooperative-group study.

An effective therapy for metastatic colorectal cancer has not been found. Recently, biological agents have been used for patients with metastatic colorectal cancer in phase I and II trials. One of the most extensively studied biological agents is IFN-α. However, the results reported in a series of trials since 1984 have been disappointing (Krown *et al.*, 1987; Silgals *et al.*, 1984; Lundell *et al.*, 1984; Eggermont *et al.*, 1985, 1986). In these studies, more than 90 patients were treated with various high-dose recombinant or lymphoblastoid IFN-α regimens with significant toxicity. No complete responses were seen, and the partial response rate was only 5–10%. Although the possibility of enhanced response rates resulting from synergy between IFN-α and other standard cytotoxic or biological agents exists, the activity of IFN-α as a single agent in colorectal cancer patients must be considered minimal.

A new area of investigation that is under development for patients with colorectal cancer is the use of monoclonal antibodies for tumor detection and/or therapy. Colcher *et al.* (1987) have performed a radioimmunolocalization study in patients with metastatic colon cancer using ^{131}I-labeled murine IgG MoAb B 72.3. Tumor labeling was determined by γ scanning and by direct analysis of biopsy material obtained at the time of surgery. Of the surgical specimens, 99 of 142 (70%) tumor lesions showed significant antibody binding, whereas only 12 of 210 (6%) histologically confirmed normal tissues were found to have significant antibody binding.

Sears et al. (1985) and Douillard et al. (1986) have reported therapeutic trials of murine IgG MoAb 17-1A alone or in combination with autologous leukocytes for patients with metastatic colorectal carcinoma. This therapy was generally well tolerated, and occasional tumor stabilization or shrinkage was observed. However, in these studies 20 of 39 patients tested developed a human antimouse antibody (HAMA) response, and one patient had an anaphylactic reaction to a second dose of antibody.

Antiidiotype (anti-id) antibodies have been used in an attempt to initiate an antitumor immune response in cancer patients. The anti-id are antibodies that recognize an epitope associated with the combining site of an immunoglobulin molecule. It has been suggested that anti-id may have a beneficial effect in colon cancer patients who received the murine MoAb CO17-1A (D. Herlyn et al., 1985, 1986a,b). It was felt that the anti-id would contain an internal image of the tumor antigen and thereby selectively stimulate antigen-specific B and/or T cells. In a clinical study of 30 patients with advanced colorectal cancer, six partial remissions (defined as a >20% decrease in tumor for >4 weeks) were observed using alum-precipitated polyclonal goat anti-id antibodies to the MoAb CO17-1A (D. Herlyn et al., 1987). This remains an intriguing area of research. As we shall discuss later, anti-id antibodies that develop in vivo in response to tumor-specific MoAb therapy may potentially have detrimental effects by blocking the MoAb binding site and preventing tumor binding.

It is hoped that with the use of human MoAbs, host immune response against the antibody will be avoided. Smith et al. (1987) have reported in abstract form a radioimmunolocalization and pharmacokinetic study of the radiolabeled (^{131}I) human IgM MoAb 28A32. Although no antitumor responses were seen, metastatic tumor deposits were imaged, and the treatment was essentially nontoxic. Further studies of this and other human MoAbs with specificity for colon cancer using conjugates with drugs, toxins, or therapeutic radioisotopes are being planned or are underway.

Finally, two studies using human leukocyte IFN for gastrointestinal tumors other than colorectal cancer are worthy of mention. Oberg et al. (1986) treated 36 patients with malignant carcinoid tumors with daily intramuscular doses of 3–6 × 10^6 units of leukocyte IFN. Responses were defined as a >50% reduction of tumor size and/or principal marker (e.g., 5-HIAA). Objective responses were seen in 17 of 36 patients (47%) with a median duration of response of 34 months. Subjective responses of decreased symptoms of carcinoid syndrome (e.g., flushing, diarrhea) were seen in 23 of 36 patients (64%).

Eriksson et al. (1987) have evaluated the effects of human leukocyte IFN in

12 patients with malignant endocrine pancreatic tumors. Responses were defined as in the above study by Oberg. Ten of 12 patients were found to have a >50% reduction in tumor markers, and four of 12 had a >50% reduction in tumor size. The median duration of response was 11 months.

In summary, previous prospects for therapy of gastrointestinal malignancies were poor. However, there is cause for cautious optimism considering the possible leads to effective therapy discussed in this section (MoAb therapy, adjuvant autologous tumor cell vaccine–BCG combinations, and possibly adjuvant levamisole for colorectal cancer). Prospects for the future include further development of these and other modalities for colorectal cancer and new approaches for the notoriously resistant tumor types such as gastric and esophageal cancer.

6. GYNECOLOGIC MALIGNANCIES

Of the gynecologic malignancies, immunotherapy has been most actively studied in ovarian cancer. Ovarian cancer accounts for 4% of female cancers and 5% of female deaths from cancer (Silverberg and Lubera, 1988). The majority of patients with ovarian cancer present with advanced disease (57% stage III and IV) (Richardson et al., 1985). The 5-year survival rate of these patients is only 10%. Standard cytotoxic agents with activity in advanced ovarian cancer include cisplatin, doxorubicin, cyclophosphamide, chlorambucil, melphalan, and methotrexate. Nonspecific immunotherapy has been added to combination chemotherapy regimens with the hope of increasing response rates and survival. The rationale for using immunotherapy in ovarian cancer has been reviewed (Creasman and Clarke-Pearson, 1983; Bast and Knapp, 1984).

In 1979, Alberts et al. reported a Southwest Oncology Group randomized trial of chemotherapy (doxorubicin, cyclophosphamide) plus BCG versus chemotherapy alone in 154 patients with stage III or IV ovarian cancer. Patients who received immunotherapy were found to have significantly increased response rates (53% versus 36%, $P = 0.05$) and median survival (23.5 months versus 13.1 months, $P < 0.004$). A long-term follow-up of this trial has not been reported. However, a randomized study by the same group indicated no advantage for BCG in conjunction with combination chemotherapy including doxorubicin, cyclophosphamide, and cisplatin (Alberts et al., 1986). It seems possible that the addition of cisplatin might have overcome the contribution of BCG to the two-drug chemotherapy regimen.

In a Gynecologic Oncology Group (GOG) study, Creasman et al. (1979) reported an improved response rate and survival of stage III ovarian cancer patients who received melphalan plus levamisole as compared with a comparable group of patients who received levamisole alone. This study was not prospectively randomized. A randomized confirmation of these results has not been reported.

In 1981, a pilot study from the GOG indicated that a combination of mephalan and levamisole could be administered without serious toxicity to patients with ovarian cancer (Gudson *et al.*, 1981). However, when levamisole was studied in a randomized, placebo-controlled trial in conjunction with chemotherapy, no beneficial effect of the levamisole was found (Khoo *et al.*, 1984). In addition, in this setting, levamisole was associated was associated with significant toxicity.

In summary, nonspecific immunotherapy alone or combined with cytotoxic chemotherapy is of no proven long-term benefit to patients with ovarian cancer and should not be considered standard therapy.

Intraperitoneal administration of *Corynebacterium parvum* to patients with ovarian cancer has resulted in response rates (CR + PR) of 32–45% (Berek *et al.*, 1985c; Bast *et al.*, 1983). The responses were seen primarily in patients with minimal residual disease (<0.5 cm maximum tumor diameter). Increased activity of intraperitoneal natural killer cell activity and antibody-dependent cell-mediated cytotoxicity have been documented (Berek *et al.*, 1985c; Bast *et al.*, 1983; Lichtenstein *et al.*, 1984). However, this therapy was associated with significant toxicity (abdominal pain, fever, nausea/vomiting), which limits its clinical usefulness.

More recently, the activity of the IFNs in human ovarian cancer has been evaluated. Using human lymphoblastoid IFN administered intramuscularly (i.m.) to patients with chemotherapy- and radiotherapy-resistant disease, Abdulhay *et al.* (1985) observed responses in five of 28 (18%) patients (two CR and three PR). However, in a study using i.m. rIFN-α2a in a similar group of 15 patients, Niloff *et al.* (1985) noted no complete or partial responses.

Intraperitoneal (i.p.) IFN is probably more active in patients with ovarian cancer. Using IP rIFN-α2b, Berek *et al.* (1985a,b) reported a pathologically confirmed response rate of 45% in 11 patients (four CR and one PR). Patients with minimal residual disease were more likely to respond. Significant toxicity of this therapy was seen, including fever, nausea/vomiting, and abdominal pain. Welander (1987) recently reported a preliminary observation of the combination of rIFN-α2b and doxorubicin administered intravenously to 24 patients with relapsing ovarian cancer. A response rate of 29% (one CR and six PR) was seen. Finally, in a study by Rambaldi *et al.* (1985), i.p. IFN-β led to no tumor regressions in eight patients, but four of seven patients had a temporary resolution of ascites. In this study a modest increase in peritoneal natural killer cell activity was seen in response to IFN-β. Sufficient activity has been seen to warrant further studies of i.p. IFN in combination with other cytokines or chemotherapeutic agents. Available evidence indicates this form of therapy to be most effective in patients with low tumor burdens or minimal residual disease. However, the toxicity encountered with this approach may limit its overall usefulness.

Another approach to therapy of advanced ovarian cancer involves the use of MoAbs. Symonds *et al.* (1985) administered ^{131}I-labeled mouse MoAb (791 T/36) to patients with primary and recurrent ovarian cancer. Tumor was visualized in all 11 patients with ovarian malignancy, and the imaged sites of MoAb uptake were confirmed surgically in eight of eight patients.

Epenetos *et al.* (1987) used i.p. cocktails of ^{131}I-labeled murine MoAbs in a therapeutic trial of antibody-guided irradiation in 24 patients with ovarian cancer. Eight patients with tumor diameter >2 cm did not respond. However, nine of 16 (56%) patients with tumor diameter <2 cm did respond. Three of these patients were confirmed to have complete remissions at laparoscopy. This approach appears promising for patients with low tumor burdens. Further clinical applications could include patients with minimal residual disease after surgery. In this setting further studies should be undertaken using MoAbs conjugated to radioisotopes, drugs, or toxins.

Finally, a limited number of trials using immunotherapy in cervical cancer have been reported. In a GOG study patients with stages II B, III B and IV A cervix cancer were randomized to receive radiotherapy alone or radiotherapy plus *Corynebacterium parvum* (DiSaia *et al.*, 1987). The immunotherapy patients were found to have more hematological toxicity and fever and chills but no improvement in disease-free interval or overall survival. Interferon α has been found to have activity when injected perilesionally (six CR out of seven patients treated) or applied intravaginally in gel form (two CR and three PR out of seven patients treated) for cervical intraepithelial neoplasia (Choo *et al.*, 1985, 1986).

7. LUNG CANCER

Is is estimated that lung cancer caused 35% of the cancer deaths in males and 20% in females in 1988 (Silverberg and Lubera, 1988). The relative 5-year survival rate for patients with lung cancer during the period from 1979 to 1984 was approximately 12% (Silverberg and Lubera, 1988). Only patients with localized disease who are able to undergo complete surgical resection have a hope of cure. However, at the time of diagnosis spread to regional nodes or distant sites has occurred in 70% of patients (Cancer patient Survival Report Number 5, 1977). As the above 5-year survival rates indicate, a large number of patients who initially appear potentially curable with surgery have recurrences locally or distantly and die of this disease.

Patients with lung cancer have deficits in T-cell number and activity (Oldham *et al.*, 1976; Dellon *et al.*, 1975). Braun *et al.* (1983) have reported that recurrence after surgical resection of stage I and II disease may be associated with an increase in activity of a suppressor mononuclear cell population.

Adjuvant immunotherapy after surgical resection has been given in an attempt to increase disease-free interval and overall survival in non-small-cell lung cancer patients. The majority of randomized controlled studies indicate no benefit from adjuvant immunotherapy in this setting. Negative randomized adjuvant immunotherapy trials include levamisole in conjunction with postoperative radiotherapy (Herskovic *et al.*, 1988), intrapleural BCG and levamisole versus chemotherapy (cyclophosphamide, doxorubicin, cis-platinum) (Holmes *et al.*, 1985; Holmes and Gail, 1986), preoperative, intratumoral BCG (Matthay *et al.*, 1986), and intrapleural and intravenous *Corynebacterium parvum* (Ludwig Lung Cancer Study Group, 1985, 1986).

A randomized study from Japan using *Nocardia rubra* cell wall skeleton intrapleurally versus control for patients with small-cell and non-small-cell lung cancer indicated a trend toward prolonged survival in the treatment group (Yasumoto *et al.*, 1985). However, this difference did not reach statistical significance when only non-small-cell lung cancer patients were considered.

Takita *et al.* (1985) have reported a randomized trial of specific immunotherapy (allogeneic tumor-associated antigen vaccination plus complete Freund's adjuvant) versus nonspecific immunotherapy (complete Freund's adjuvant alone) versus control. This trial was done in patients with resectable squamous cell lung cancer. A significant improvement in survival was seen only in patients without hilar lymph node metastases who received nonspecific immunotherapy. However, this group accounted for only 19 patients out of the total of 86 randomized patients.

Finally, there is a report that adjuvant transfer factor causes a significant increase in survival in a group of primarily non-small-cell lung cancer patients with resected stage I and II disease (Fujisawa *et al.*, 1984). Kirsh *et al.* (1984) performed a randomized study of transfer factor versus control in 63 patients with resected non-small-cell lung cancer. A significant survival advantage was reported for the treatment group with a median follow-up of 25 months. At this time these reports should be considered preliminary and unconfirmed. Confirmation in large groups of patients with long-term follow-up is needed.

Immunotherapy in combination with chemotherapy and/or radiotherapy has been studied in patients with unresectable or metastatic non-small-cell lung cancer. A variety of immunotherapeutic agents including MER BCG, levamisole, and *Corynebacterium parvum* were found to be of no benefit (Robinson *et al.*, 1985; Krauss *et al.*, 1984; Thatcher *et al.*, 1984).

Corynebacterium parvum has been used as a sclerosing agent in patients with malignant pleural effusions caused by lung cancer (Millar *et al.*, 1980). McLeod *et al.* (1985) reported prevention of reaccumulation of effusion in 24 of 26 patients (92%). Toxicities included fever, mild chest pain, and nausea. A study by Rossi *et al.* (1987) indicates that response to intrapleural *Corynebacterium parvum* is not associated with an enhanced local cellular immunity. Rather, it is felt that this agent results in the development of pleural fibrosis. Another study using radiolabeled *Corynebacterium parvum* has shown that following intrapleural administration of this agent, radioactivity remains confined to the pleural cavity (Kaufmann *et al.*, 1986). More recently, intrapleural IL-2 has been shown to induce pleural LAK cells and result in the disappearance of malignant pleural effusions in nine of 11 patients with lung cancer (Yasumoto *et al.*, 1987).

Immunotherapy has also been used in combination with chemotherapy and radiotherapy in patients with small-cell lung cancer. Randomized trials of MER BCG (Maurer et al., 1985), *Propionibacterium granulosum* KP 45 (Roszkowski et al., 1985), and levamisole (Ainslie et al., 1983) have not resulted in prolongation of survival. A randomized trial of thymosin fraction V in conjunction with combination chemotherapy did not improve the complete response rate but did significantly prolong the survival of small-cell lung cancer patients (Cohen et al., 1979). A confirmation and long-term follow-up of this trial have not been reported.

Based on the above discussions, it is clear that immunotherapy does not significantly and reproducibly prolong the survival of lung cancer patients. However, further study of new immunotherapeutic agents including cytokines and monoclonal antibodies is warranted.

8. BREAST CANCER

Breast cancer has now been replaced by lung cancer as the most common cause of death from cancer in women (Silverberg and Lubera, 1988). However, breast cancer remains a significant problem. In 1988 it is estimated that 135,000 women will be newly diagnosed with breast cancer and that 42,000 women will die of breast cancer (Silverberg and Lubera, 1988). The prognosis and risk of recurrence of patients with resectable breast cancer depends on many factors, including size of primary tumor, number of axillary nodes involved, estrogen receptor status, menopausal state, and pathological factors such as presence of high nuclear grade or blood vessel or lymphatic invasion.

Adjuvant therapy has been successful in prolonging disease-free interval and overall survival in certain groups of patients at high risk for recurrence. The antiestrogen agent tamoxifen has been found to decrease mortality in postmenopausal patients with estrogen-receptor-positive tumors (National Institutes of Health Consensus Development Panel, 1986). A number of studies have documented a survival benefit for premenopausal patients with axillary node involvement who receive adjuvant combination chemotherapy (Bonadonna et al., 1986; Fisher et al., 1986).

Nonspecific immunostimulatory and immune-modulating agents such as BCG, MER BCG, *Corynebacterium parvum,* and levamisole have been used in conjunction with adjuvant chemotherapy and/or radiotherapy in patients with resectable breast cancer. With very few possible exceptions (to be discussed below), nonspecific immunotherapy has not been found to prolong significantly survival in randomized controlled studies (Treurniet-Donker et al., 1987; Schreml et al., 1983; Hubay et al., 1985).

In 1983 the Auckland Breast Cancer Study Group reported on 135 patients with positive axillary nodes who were randomized to receive *l*-phenylalanine mustard (L-PAM) plus levamisole or L-PAM plus placebo (Kay et al., 1983).

Patients less than 50 years old with one to three positive nodes who received levamisole had a shorter disease-free survival than those who received placebo ($p = 0.05$). In patients greater than 50 years old who received levamisole, there was a trend of prolonged disease-free survival. The effect of levamisole in overall survival was not discussed in this report.

A Finnish group has studied 72 patients with stage II breast cancer who were randomized to receive levamisole or placebo after postoperative radiotherapy (Klefstrom et al., 1985). Postmenopausal patients randomized to receive levamisole had significantly increased disease-free survival ($p = 0.003$) and overall survival ($p = 0.008$). The same Finnish group has recently reported a randomized study of stage III breast cancer patients (Klefstrom et al., 1987). In this study patients who received combined radiotherapy and chemotherapy (vincristine, doxorubicin, cyclophosphamide) plus levamisole had a prolonged disease-free interval compared with a combined therapy group that did not receive levamisole ($p = 0.035$). However, the ability of adjuvant levamisole in combination with radiotherapy and/or chemotherapy to prolong not only disease-free but overall survival of resected breast cancer patients has not been confirmed. Levamisole should not be considered standard therapy for breast cancer patients, and if used at all it should be only in the setting of randomized controlled clinical trials.

Many standard chemotherapy drugs have activity in patients with metastatic breast cancer. Attempts have been made to increase the response rate, response duration, or survival of metastatic breast cancer patients by the addition of immunotherapy to standard chemotherapy. However, immunotherapeutic agents such as levamisole (Carpenter et al., 1986), MER BCG (Aisner et al., 1987), and Corynebacterium parvum (Fritze et al., 1984) have generally not been effective.

As single agents, human lymphoblastoid IFN (Sarna and Figlin, 1985) and rIFN-α (Muss et al., 1984; Padmanabhan et al., 1985) have shown no activity in patients with metastatic breast cancer. There was also no evidence of increased therapeutic response when human lymphoblastoid IFN was added to chemotherapy (cyclophosphamide, vincristine, 5-FU, hydrocortisone) for metastatic breast cancer patients (Ashford et al., 1986).

In early murine studies, monoclonal antibodies to breast cancer antigens have led to successful tumor imaging (Estabrook et al., 1987) and tumor regressions (Ceriani et al., 1987). These studies have currently been reported only in abstract form. The latter study illustrates an attempt to overcome the problem of tumor antigenic heterogeneity. "Cocktails" of several MoAbs were more effective than single MoAbs when tested in this human breast tumor xenograft system. This and other potential difficulties of MoAb therapy are discussed in Section 14. Further studies using monoclonal antibodies in humans with breast cancer are anticipated.

9. HEAD AND NECK CANCER

In 1988, it is estimated there will be 42,400 new cases and 12,850 deaths from head and neck cancers (lip, tongue, mouth, pharynx, larynx) (Silverberg and Lubera, 1988). Five percent of cancers in the United States are squamous cell carcinomas of the head and neck (Kies *et al.*, 1985). Only one-third of these patients will have early-stage, localized disease at presentation such that they have a potential for cure using the standard modalities of surgery and radiotherapy (Hong and Bromer, 1983). Immunotherapy has been used in attempts to improve the disease-free survival, overall survival, and cure rate of these patients.

The rationale for using immunotherapy in head and neck cancer patients includes the well-documented occurrence of cellular and humoral immune deficits in these patients and the presence of tumor-associated antigens. These concepts have been reviewed previously (Newbill and Johns, 1983; Hollinshead, 1987; Scully, 1983; Naclerio, 1985). In spite of this rationale, current immunotherapy techniques have failed to have a major impact on the clinical outcome of patients with head and neck cancers.

In a retrospective review, Schantz *et al.* (1980) reported an improved survival for laryngeal cancer patients who developed postoperative wound infections. The implication was that the infection resulted in immune stimulation. In the early 1970s, Donaldson (1972) reported promising results for advanced head and neck cancer patients who received methotrexate plus BCG. In the later 1970s, other positive (Richman *et al.*, 1976) and negative (Suen *et al.*, 1977; Woods *et al.*, 1977) BCG studies for head and neck cancer were reported. More recently, Taylor *et al.* (1983) reported a randomized trial of 52 patients with advanced squamous cell carcinoma of the head and neck. After local therapy, patients who received BCG were reported to have significantly prolonged disease-free and overall survival. However, Medina (1983) has detailed the deficiencies in this study, including the use of other immunotherapies in addition to BCG (four patients in the BCG group received an autologous tumor cell vaccine), failure of eight patients to complete the immune therapy regimen, nonuniform follow-up, and poor compliance with the chemotherapy regimen.

Other immunotherapeutic modalities have been studied in this group of patients. Neifeld *et al.* (1985) found no benefit to presurgery intratumoral and postoperative subcutaneous *Corynebacterium parvum* in a randomized study of patients with squamous cell carcinomas of the oral cavity, pharynx, and larynx. Likewise, Goldenberg *et al.* (1985) found no benefit of transfer factor for patients with nasopharyngeal carcinoma. In a study from India, Padmanabhan *et al.* (1987) reported a trend towards enhanced disease-free survival in patients with early-stage cancer of the oral cavity who received levamisole following radiotherapy. However, this did not reach statistical significance.

In summary, there is no firm evidence that nonspecific immunotherapy as an adjuvant results in a significant improvement in disease-free or overall survival of patients with head and neck cancer.

Few studies using cytokines in the the therapy of head and neck cancers have been reported. Nasopharyngeal cancer is closely associated with Epstein–Barr virus infection. Because the IFNs have both antiviral and antiproliferative properties, they are of interest in this disease. Connors et al. (1985) treated 12 patients with recurrent nasopharyngeal carcinoma with human leukocyte IFN. Two objective partial responses were seen.

Juvenile laryngeal papillomatosis is a condition felt to be caused by papilloma viruses (Gissmann et al., 1983). These benign epithelial tumors occur during childhood, are typically recurrent, and may require frequent surgical removal to maintain a patent airway. Lundquist et al. (1984) treated 17 patients with this disease using intramuscular human leukocyte IFN. Some tumor control was seen in all patients, and nine were felt to be cured and no longer required therapy. Zenner et al. (1985) used rIFN-α to treat 20 patients with documented recurrent laryngotracheobronchial papillomatosis. Eleven of 20 patients were found to have complete responses. Further study of the IFNs in this disease is under way.

10. CENTRAL NERVOUS SYSTEM TUMORS

It is estimated that in 1988 there will be 14,700 new cases and 10,900 deaths from primary tumors of the brain and central nervous system (CNS) (Silverberg and Lubera, 1988). Approximately 50% of all intracranial neoplasms are metastases from primary tumors with origin outside the CNS (most commonly lung and breast cancer) (Walker et al., 1985). Of the primary CNS tumors, about 60% are malignant gliomas. The malignant gliomas are composed of a large group of histological types that have in common neuroectodermal origin. These tumors vary in grade, biology, and malignant potential. Included in this category are astrocytoma, oligodendroglioma, medulloblastoma, and ependymoma (Kornblith et al., 1985).

Standard treatment of primary CNS tumors includes surgical resection to the extent possible and radiation therapy with or without chemotherapy. The most active chemotherapeutic agents are the nitrosoureas (BCNU, CCNU, methyl-CCNU). The remainder of this discussion deals primarily with the results and potential of immunotherapy for malignant gliomas and to a lesser extent metastatic brain tumors.

Gliomas are known to express tumor-associated antigens (Carrel et al., 1982; Coakham, 1974; Coakham and Lakshmi, 1975) and to share antigens with malignant melanoma cells (M. Herlyn et al., 1983; Hersey, 1985). Patients with malignant gliomas have an altered immune status including depressed delayed hypersensitivity reactions to recall antigens, decreased numbers of total lymphocytes and T lymphocytes, and impaired lymphocyte blastogenic responses to mitogens (Bullard et al., 1986).

Nonspecific immune-stimulating and immune-modulating agents have been used as adjuvants to surgical resection and/or radiotherapy in patients with malignant gliomas. When evaluated in a randomized controlled manner, agents such as levamisole and the streptococcal component OK-432 did not produce a significant prolongation of survival (Fischer et al., 1985; Shibata et al., 1987). A similar randomized study using levamisole and CCNU as an adjuvant to radiotherapy also failed to demonstrate survival benefit in patients with multiple metastatic brain tumors (Robustelli della Cuna et al., 1984).

Preliminary investigations of the activity of the IFNs in patients with malignant gliomas and metastatic tumors have recently been reported. Obbens et al. (1985) saw a slight regression by CT scan in one of three patients with malignant astrocytoma who received intratumoral human leukocyte IFN. More dramatically, four of four patients with leptomeningeal metastatic disease (primary: small-cell lung, renal cell, breast, and large-cell lymphoma) had a transient (6–10 weeks) normalization of CSF after intrathecal human leukocyte IFN ($3–8 \times 10^6$ units, 3 times weekly) (Obbens et al., 1985). However, the neurological status of these patients generally did not improve.

Mahaley et al. (1985) treated 19 patients with recurrent gliomas using human lymphoblastoid IFN administered intravenously or intramuscularly. Tumor reductions of at least 25% by serial CT scans were seen in seven patients.

Early reports from Japan indicated that IFN-β was an active agent for patients with primary brain tumors (Nagai and Arai, 1984). Phase I and II studies of partially purified human IFN-β have also been reported in the United States (Bogdahn et al., 1985; Duff et al., 1986). Duff et al. (1986) treated 12 patients with recurrent, biopsy-proven glioblastoma multiforme using intravenous and intratumor IFN-β. No significant responses were seen.

Jacobs et al. (1986a) have demonstrated that IL-2-activated autologous lymphocytes from patients with gliomas have the ability to lyse autologous malignant glioma cells in vitro. In phase I studies this group demonstrated that it was feasible to administer IL-2 and autologous LAK cells alone or in combination by direct tumor injection in patients with malignant glioma (Jacobs et al., 1986b,c). This therapy was found to be relatively nontoxic. Further in vitro studies demonstrated the ability of IL-2-induced LAK cells from these patients to lyse autologous glioma cells but not normal peripheral blood lymphocytes. Further treatment and follow-up are necessary to define the efficacy of this form of treatment.

Finally, monoclonal antibodies are under active investigation in vitro and in vivo in patients with primary brain tumors. The potential of these agents as diagnostic and therapeutic modalities for primary brain tumor patients has recently been reviewed (Bullard and Bigner, 1985). Of the primary brain tumors, the malignant gliomas have been most actively studied with regard to MoAbs. One of their most striking characteristics is heterogeneity. This includes morphology, growth kinetics, expression of biochemical markers, ability to form tumors in nude mice, response to chemotherapy, as well as antigen expression (Bullard and Bigner, 1985). This heterogeneity will cause obvious difficulty with single-MoAb imaging and therapeutic studies. Another consideration is the ability of intravenously administered MoAbs conjugated to radioisotopes, drugs, or toxins to cross the blood–brain barrier. Possible solutions to these problems include the use of cocktails of MoAbs or MoAb conjugates injected directly into the CSF or intratumorally at the time of surgery. However, this remains a very complex problem, and much further investigation is needed.

11. KAPOSI SARCOMA

Kaposi sarcoma (KS) was originally described by Kaposi in 1872 (Hood *et al.*, 1982). In its classic form KS presents as reddish-brown nodules or plaques on the lower extremities of elderly men. The clinical course is usually one of slow local progression. The therapy is usually surgical excision or local radiotherapy, with systemic chemotherapy being reserved only for patients with advanced disease. A variant of classic KS that is much more common and aggressive is seen in Africa (Kaminer and Murray, 1950).

Since the initial descriptions of the acquired immune deficiency syndrome (AIDS) in the early 1980s, a marked increase in the incidence of KS has been seen. More than 30% of AIDS patients develop KS (Fauci *et al.*, 1984). In this setting, the clinical course may be one of multiple atypical skin lesions, multiorgan dissemination (commonly GI tract), and possible death (Friedman-Kien *et al.*, 1982). Standard chemotherapeutic agents found to have some degree of activity in the epidemic or AIDS-associated form of KS include vinblastine, doxorubicin, VP-16, and bleomycin. The reported response rate to these agents alone or in combination is in the range of 60–85% (Odajnyk and Franco, 1985). However, the majority of these remissions are partial, of short duration, and of questionable significance to survival. Despite a response to chemotherapy, most AIDS patients with KS continue to die of immunosuppression with widespread opportunistic infections. In fact, it is possible that chemotherapy in these patients leads to further immune suppression.

Because of its known antiviral, antiproliferative, and immunomodulatory effects, it was of great interest to study IFN-α in patients with AIDS-associated KS. One of the original reports of the usefulness of IFN-α in these patients was by Krown *et al.* (1983). In this phase I trial using rIFN-α2a, five of 12 evaluable patients with epidemic KS had objective responses (three CR and two PR). Immune function as measured by natural killer (NK) cell activity and lymphocyte proliferative response to PHA was found to increase in response to rIFN-α2a therapy. However, in this small group of patients, improvement in immune function was not significantly correlated with tumor response.

Rios *et al.* (1985a) treated 12 patients with epidemic KS using human lymphoblastoid IFN at a dose of 20×10^6 units/m^2 daily i.m. for 2 months. Two-thirds of the patients responded (four CR and four PR) with a median response duration of 28 weeks. Interestingly, immunologic parameters (T-cell levels, lymphocyte blastogenic response to PHA and CON-A, and ADCC) were found to decrease while on therapy.

In a study by Gelmann *et al.* (1985), 30 patients with AIDS-related KS received human lymphoblastoid IFN at a dose of $7.5-25 \times 10^6$ units/m^2 daily for 28 days. Three partial responses were seen. Responding patients were found to have significantly higher pretherapy total lymphocyte counts and CD4-positive lymphocytes and an absence of prior opportunistic infection (OI).

Most early studies of IFN in KS suffer from small numbers of patients treated with a wide range of doses resulting in variable response rates. The combined experiences of the Universities of California at San Francisco (UCSF) and Los Angeles (UCLA) have been reported recently (Volberding *et al.*, 1987; Abrams and Volberding, 1986). A total of 114 men with AIDS-related KS were treated with rIFN-α2b using low (1×10^6 IU/m^2), intermediate (30×10^6 IU/m^2), and high (50×10^6 IU/m^2) doses. The overall response rate was 35% (CR + PR). The three dosages were not randomly assigned, and the patients in these groups were not balanced for prognostic factors. However, patients who received the high-dose regimen had a higher response rate (45%) than the intermediate and low-dose regimens (28%, 33%). Important prognostic factors for response were low-stage disease and absence of "B" symptoms. The therapy was generally well tolerated, with only 6% of patients requiring treatment to be discontinued because of toxicity. Immunologic parameters did not improve with therapy or correlate with response.

The combined Memorial Sloan-Kettering Cancer Center experience with rIFN-α2b in AIDS-related KS has also been reported recently (Real *et al.*, 1986; Krown *et al.*,1986). In this combined experience in 75 patients, those who received high doses (36×10^6 units, 36 patients) as compared with low doses (3×10^6 units, 39 patients) had a significantly better response rate (38% versus 3%). The median duration of response in the high-dose patients was 18 months. The absence of prior OI correlated best with response to high-dose therapy. Large tumor burden and the presence of GI involvement did not correlate with response. The high-dose regimen was found to be more toxic, with 27% of patients requiring dose reduction as compared with none in the low-dose group. The most important pretherapy immune function parameters for predicting response were lymphocyte proliferative response to *E. coli* and presence of delayed-type hypersensitivity reactions to recall antigens (Krown *et al.*, 1986).

To summarize, current studies indicate IFN-α to be an active agent in AIDS-related KS. Although more toxic, higher doses are probably more effective, but this has not been proven in a randomized trial. In general, the best predictor of response to IFN-α is the pretherapy status of immune function as measured by any number of parameters including the presence of previous OI. Interferon therapy has not been shown to significantly improve immune function, and the antitumor activity that has been seen is probably more related to its antiproliferative effects.

Studies using IFN in combination with chemotherapeutic agents are currently under way (Lonberg et al., 1985; Rios et al., 1985b; Fischl et al., 1987). Other cytokines and combinations of cytokines are also being studied. To significantly alter the natural history of AIDS with KS will likely require improvement of immune function and/or the ability to control HIV replication. Agents with these potential properties are being actively sought and studied.

12. IL-2-INDUCED LAK CELL THERAPY

In 1981, Lotze (1981) and his co-workers at the National Cancer Institute (NCI) reported that the incubation of peripheral blood mononuclear cells (PBMC) from cancer patients in the presence of T-cell growth factor resulted in the generation of cells with lytic activity against fresh and cultured autologous tumor cells. T-cell growth factor has now been given the designation interleukin 2 (IL-2). The population of cells that result from the incubation of IL-2 with PBMC is referred to as lymphokine-activated killer or LAK cells. A somewhat later report from the group at the NCI indicated that LAK cells could be induced from the PBMC of both cancer patients and normal individuals and that these LAK cells were lytic in vitro against a broad range of both autologous and allogeneic tumor cells (Grimm et al., 1982). The LAK cells may be included in the group of cellular responses with potential antitumor activity as discussed in Section 1. The LAK cells are felt to be distinct from classical cytotoxic T lymphocytes (CTL) because they do not require prior immunization and there is no HLA restriction to their cytolytic activity. Several lines of evidence were initially reported to indicate that LAK effector cells are distinct from NK cells: (1) LAK cells will lyse NK-resistant targets (Daudi cell line); (2) the necessary and sufficient stimulus for LAK cell activation is IL-2 (Grimm et al., 1983a); (3) there is a dissociation of LAK from NK activity in strains of immunodeficient mice (Andriole et al., 1985); and (4) studies of the phenotypes of LAK precursors and effector cells, NK cells, and CTL have indicated a distinct functional nature of each system (Grimm et al., 1983b). The LAK effector cell was initially reported to be CD3 (pan T cell) and CD8 (suppressor/cytotoxic T cell) positive (Grimm et al., 1983b). This was not confirmed in further studies. A generally accepted marker for the LAK precursor cell in the human system has not been detected. It has recently been suggested that "LAK" is not a unique cell type but is a phenomenon or an activity that arises from IL-2-activated NK cells (Lotzova,

1987). Phillips and Lanier (1986) have suggested that this LAK phenomenon may be mediated by an IL-2-activated population of Leu-19-positive, CD-3-negative peripheral blood NK cells. Another report has suggested that LAK precursors arise from a population of CD16-positive NK cells (Itoh *et al.*, 1985).

In animal tumor models the combination of LAK cells and IL-2 has been found to be very effective at reducing pulmonary and liver metastases from immunogenic and nonimmunogenic murine tumors (Mulé *et al.*, 1984, 1985; Lafreniere and Rosenberg, 1985a,b; Rosenberg *et al.*, 1985b). In these animal studies high doses of IL-2 alone were found to be effective. However, the best activity was seen when IL-2 was given in combination with LAK cells.

In 1985, Rosenberg and his colleagues (1985a) at the NCI published the initial report of the use of autologous LAK cells and IL-2 in patients with disseminated malignancy. At the time of the most recent detailed update of this study a total of 157 patients with advanced cancer had been treated (Rosenberg *et al.*, 1987). The treatment procedure used for these patients included a 5-day period of high-dose IL-2 (1×10^5 units/kg q 8 hr). After a 2-day rest period, this was followed by five daily leukaphereses. The PBMC obtained by this procedure were incubated *in vitro* with IL-2 and then returned to the patient by an intravenous infusion in combination with further intravenous doses of IL-2 on the same dosage schedule. Of the 157 total patients treated, 108 received IL-2 plus LAK cells, and 49 received IL-2 alone. The overall response rate (CR + PR) in this broad group of patients with varied tumor types who received LAK cells plus IL-2 was 22%. The most frequent tumor types were renal cell cancer, melanoma, and colorectal cancer, for which the response rates were 33% (12/36), 23% (6/26), and 12% (3/26), respectively. Although the overall response rate is admittedly modest, it is very significant considering the refractory nature of metastatic disease in patients with these tumor types, as has been discussed previously. In addition, a number of complete responses were seen (four with renal cancer, two with melanoma, and one with colorectal cancer). Responses were also seen using high-dose IL-2 alone. However, with the exception of melanoma patients (no CR and five PR out of 16 total patients treated), high-dose IL-2 alone was not as active as the combination therapy. It has recently been reported that a total of 315 patients at the NCI have now received either LAK cells plus IL-2 or high-dose IL-2 alone (Rosenberg, 1988). Although specific details were not given, it was stated that the results have remained similar to that seen in the first 157 patients.

Shortly after the initial report of the effectiveness of clinical LAK/IL-2 therapy by Rosenberg *et al.*, in December, 1985, the Interleukin-2/Lymphokine-Activated Killer Cell Extramural Working Group was established. The initial objectives of these six extramural centers were to confirm the antitumor activity seen at the NCI and determine the feasibility of administering this complex treatment program in other institutions. The results of a phase II study using IL-2-induced LAK cell therapy for patients with renal cancer at the six extramural centers have recently been reported (Fisher *et al.*, 1988). The overall response rate in 32 patients with metastatic renal cancer was 16% (two CR, three PR). The two patients in CR remain so at 12 and 9 months. It was reported that this response rate was not significantly different from recently updated results from the NCI. Toxicity was commonly severe, and one patient had a myocardial infarction attributed to therapy. However, the toxicities were generally short-lived, and there were no treatment-related deaths. This report indicates that LAK/IL-2 therapy can be effectively administered outside of the NCI and that significant tumor responses will occur.

Although these results are exciting, they are obtained only at the expense of considerable toxicity. The majority of the side effects are related to the high-dose IL-2 therapy and are mediated via a diffuse capillary leak syndrome. This results in hypotension, weight gain, azotemia, oliguria, and respiratory distress associated with interstitial pulmonary edema. Four patients had documented myocardial infarctions, and there were four treatment-related deaths among the 157 patients treated at the NCI. Other less serious but nonetheless distressing side effects included malaise, fever, chills, nausea/vomiting, diarrhea, hyperbilirubinemia, and neuropsychiatric disorders. A final factor that must be considered in the evaluation of these results is the cost and lengthy hospital stay required to complete this complicated regimen of therapy.

In summary, these initial reports of IL-2-induced LAK cell therapy should be considered encouraging. The toxicity should not deter further study of this form of cancer treatment. This remains a very active area of investigation, and attempts are being made to decrease side effects and enhance effectiveness. Some new approaches have been suggested by Rosenberg (1988) and are summarized below.

From the early *in vitro* and *in vivo* animal studies it was evident that LAK cells are nonspecific in their recognition of tumor cells. It has subsequently been shown that sensitized mononuclear cells obtained from tumor-draining lymph nodes or from actual tumor tissue have a more effective antitumor activity (Shu *et al.*, 1987; Rosenberg *et al.*, 1986). Studies of these so-called tumor-infiltrating lymphocytes (TIL) have subsequently been initiated.

A recent report by Mitchell *et al.* (1988) has evaluated a regimen of low-dose cyclophosphamide in combination with lose-dose IL-2 for patients with disseminated melanoma. The premise behind this approach was that the low-dose cyclophosphamide would selectively deplete suppressor T lymphocytes and allow more effective induction of LAK cells. There is experimental evidence to support this hypothesis (Berd *et al.*, 1984a,b). In addition to the low-dose cyclophosphamide, a significantly lower IL-2 dose as compared with that in Rosenberg's original regimen was employed (3.6×10^6 units/m^2 daily versus 1×10^5 units/kg q 8 hr). Significant responses with this regimen were seen, including one complete remission and five partial remissions out of a total of 24 patients treated (overall response rate 25%). The mean duration of response was greater than 5 months. However, remissions of longer duration have been noted, and two patients remained on treatment for more than 1 year. Only moderate toxicity was seen, and this regimen was generally able to be given on an outpatient basis. All patients with a partial or complete remission after this form of therapy were found to have *in vitro* evidence of LAK-cell activation.

Rosenberg's group at the NCI have reported that LAK cell activity is enhanced *in vitro* and in animal models *in vivo* by prior exposure of tumor cells to tumor-specific antibody. This activates the mechanism of antibody-dependent cellular cytotoxicity (ADCC) (Shiloni *et al.*, 1987; Eisenthal *et al.*, 1987). An attractive clinical application of these results is the use of tumor-specific monoclonal antibodies prior to LAK cell therapy.

Finally, there is preliminary evidence that LAK cells or IL-2 may be synergistic with IFN-α (Brunda *et al.*, 1987), tumor necrosis factor (Winkelhake *et al.*, 1987), combination chemotherapy (Papa *et al.*, 1988), or interleukin-4 (Mulé *et al.*, 1987).

IL-2-induced LAK cell therapy cannot currently be considered standard therapy for any disease. However, enough activity has been demonstrated to warrant further study in patients with malignant melanoma, renal cancer, and colorectal cancer. There is every reason for optimism that in the future more effective and less toxic treatment strategies will be developed.

13. COLONY-STIMULATING FACTORS

Intensive treatment of patients with solid tumor malignancies using classical cytotoxic chemotherapy commonly results in bone marrow suppression with resultant granulocytopenia, anemia, or thrombocytopenia. In solid tumors that are relatively chemosensitive (e.g., large-cell lymphoma, testicular cancer, breast cancer), the ability to deliver full doses of chemotherapy may have important consequences with regard to response rates and patient survival.

A number of human hematopoietic colony-stimulating factors have recently been identified and reviewed (Clark and Kamen, 1987). These include erythropoietin, which is a regulator of erythropoiesis (Jacobs *et al.*, 1985), granulocyte colony-stimulating factor (G-CSF), which stimulates the formation of granulocytes (Nicola *et al.*, 1983), macrophage colony-stimulating factor (M-CSF), which stimulates macrophage colony formation (Clark and Kamen, 1987), granulocyte–macrophage colony-stimulating factor (GM-CSF), which acts on both granulocyte and macrophage progenitors (Metcalf, 1986), and interleukin-3 (multi-CSF), which supports proliferation of erythroid progenitors, granulocytes, macrophages, eosinophils, and megakaryocytes (Yang *et al.*, 1986). Other regulatory molecules that may be important in the process of hematopoiesis via synergism with other colony-stimulating factors or by acting as intermediaries include hematopoietin-1, interleukin-1 (IL-1), interleukin-4 (also known as B-cell stimulatory factor-1 or BSF-1), and interleukin-6 (also known as B-cell stimulatory factor-2) (Clark and Kamen, 1987; Paul and Ohara, 1987; Ikebuchi *et al.*, 1987).

Early clinical trials using colony-stimulating factors have recently been reported. Recombinant human GM-CSF has been shown to increase circulating leukocyte counts in neutropenic AIDS patients (Groopman *et al.*, 1987) and bone marrow transplant patients (Brandt *et al.*, 1988). In addition, the anemia of chronic renal failure has been effectively treated with human recombinant erythropoietin (Eschbach *et al.*, 1987).

This continues to be an area of exciting, active investigation. Studies are currently under way or will soon begin using erythropoietin or GM-CSF in solid-tumor patients who are undergoing chemotherapy as well as patients with a wide variety of bone marrow failure states including myelodysplastic syndromes, aplastic anemia, bone marrow failure caused by radiation therapy, and cyclic neutropenia. Finally, phase I clinical studies of recombinant human IL-3 and IL-4 are soon to be initiated.

14. MONOCLONAL ANTIBODY THERAPY

The use of monoclonal antibodies (MoAb) as a diagnostic and therapeutic tool in the treatment of cancer patients was briefly discussed in the introduction of this chapter. Clinical studies using MoAbs have been discussed under the heading of each specific solid tumor category. This section includes a general discussion of the practical and theoretical aspects of MoAbs and their diagnostic and therapeutic capabilities. In addition, potential problems that may alter the efficacy of MoAb therapy as well as their possible solutions are discussed.

As was mentioned in the introduction, it was Paul Erlich (1906) who first conceived of using antibodies to target drugs and toxins to tumor cells. Modern hybridoma methodology has led to the availability of relatively large amounts of highly specific monoclonal antibodies (MoAbs). Such MoAbs have been affectionately referred to as "magic bullets" or "guided missiles." Because of the potential problems with their clinical use, pessimists might be inclined to refer to them as "dull spears." The term "magic bullet" conjures up visions of an agent that has an innate ability to "seek out" and specifically bind to a tumor cell. Although the specificity of MoAbs in *in vitro* models is well documented, their use in intact organisms is much more complex.

In the ideal situation, for MoAbs to have specific tumor binding requires that tumor cells express unique antigens. As we shall see, in the practical situation of clinical cancer therapy this does not always occur. Tumor-associated antigens may be divided into two broad categories: oncofetal antigens and differentiation antigens. Oncofetal antigens are expressed during fetal development but are not present on normal adult cells. However, oncofetal antigens may be expressed on malignant cells (Sell, 1980). Examples of oncofetal antigens include carcinoembryonic antigens (CEA) (Shively and Todd, 1980) and alpha-fetoprotein (AFP) (Sell, 1982). The other broad category of tumor-associated antigens includes differentiation antigens. These have been defined as surface antigens that distinguish cells belonging to distinct differentiation lineages or distinguish cells at different phases in the same differentiation lineage (Houghton *et al.*, 1986). Examples with regard to human melanocytes and malignant melanoma include adenosine deaminase-binding protein (Houghton *et al.*, 1986) and the ganglioside GD_3 (Dippold *et al.*, 1984).

Unconjugated MoAbs may have antitumor effects by at least two mechanisms. Specific antibody binding to tumor cells may lead to fixation of complement and subsequent complement-mediated tumor cell lysis. Via an interaction with the Fc portion of tumor-cell-bound MoAbs, the process of antibody-dependent cellular cytotoxicity (ADCC) may also result in tumor cell lysis. As was previously discussed in Section 2, Houghton *et al.* have used the unconjugated R24 mouse MoAb in melanoma patients. This antibody has specificity for the GD_3 ganglioside, and tumor responses have been seen with its use (Houghton *et al.*, 1985).

Monoclonal antibodies may also be used as carriers for radioisotopes, drugs, or toxins. Much of the early work in this area has involved imaging studies wherein a radioisotope is conjugated to a MoAb. The utility of these studies lies in their ability to determine specificity of binding before a potentially more toxic drug or toxin conjugate is infused. The ideal radioisotope to use in imaging studies is one that is readily available, has a low cost, is easily conjugated to MoAbs, has a low-energy γ emission, which is best suited for γ imaging cameras, and has no associated emission of β particles. The most commonly used isotope is ^{131}I. Although ^{131}I is relatively cheap and readily available, it results in a high-energy γ emission associated with a β emission. Other, possibly more advantageous radioisotopes include ^{123}I, ^{111}In, ^{99m}Tc, and ^{67}Ga. A detailed discussion of the dosimetric aspects of radioisotopes with regard to MoAb tumor imaging is beyond the scope of this review. This subject has, however, recently been reviewed (Humm, 1986). ^{131}I and ^{123}I are readily conjugated to MoAbs by oxidative incorporation into tyrosine amino acids. However, for most other radioisotopes a more complex process involving chelating agents is required. The most frequently used chelating agent currently is diethylenetriaminepentaacetic acid (DTPA).

Conventional cytotoxic drugs may be conjugated to MoAbs in an attempt to specifically target their cytotoxic effects to tumor cells. The theoretical advantages of this approach would be to decrease systemic toxicity and perhaps increase antitumor efficacy. However, there are several potential problems with this approach. Nonspecific antibody binding could lead to significant toxicity in non-tumor-bearing tissues. Theoretical questions may also be raised regarding the intracellular transport of drugs that are conjugated to MoAbs. This may be accomplished by drug release after antibody–tumor binding and subsequent transcellular transport of unconjugated drug. Another possibility is the internalization of the intact drug–antibody conjugate with subsequent intracellular release of drug. In general, the details of these processes have not been specifically defined. One could argue that by conjugating a drug to an antibody, specificity may be increased, but that the drug may be limited in its ability to enter the cell, which thereby decreases its overall efficacy. A number of drugs have currently been conjugated to MoAbs. Examples include daunomycin, desacetylvinblastine, and methotrexate (Garnett and Baldwin, 1986; Rowland *et al.*, 1985).

Finally, MoAbs may be conjugated to immunotoxins and used therapeutically. The immunotoxins may be obtained from plant or bacterial sources and include ricin, diphtheria toxin, *Pseudomonas* exotoxin A, pokeweed antiviral protein, and gelonin. The immunotoxins have several advantages as MoAb-targeted cytotoxic agents. Ricin toxin (obtained from castor bean) illustrates two of these advantages. It is composed of two polypeptide chains designated the A chain and B chain. When internalized, the A chain leads to inactivation of cellular protein synthesis (Vitetta and Uhr, 1985). The potency of this toxin is such that it has been estimated that one molecule entering the cell is sufficient for cytotoxicity. The increased potency of toxins relative to drugs on a molecule-to-molecule basis provides an obvious advantage when one considers the problem of intracellular delivery. In addition, the A- and B-chain polypeptides of the ricin toxin may be separated enzymatically or by individual molecular cloning. The advantage afforded by the separation of the A and B chains is that the B chain is responsible for cellular binding of the intact toxin. When present, the B chain may lead to nonspecific binding and subsequent toxicity to normal tissues. A MoAb conjugated to a single A chain should theoretically have specific tumor binding afforded by the MoAb in the absence of the B chain. A detailed discussion of immunotoxin therapy in cancer patients is again beyond the scope of this chapter. However, this topic has recently been reviewed (Frankel *et al.*, 1986).

A major obstacle to effective therapy using MoAbs is that of tumor heterogeneity (Levy, 1987). All biological systems may be considered heterogeneous. Tumor cells have a characteristic genetic instability. Antigenic expression by tumor cells is also known to be variable. This is best illustrated by malignant melanoma patients, in whom different metastatic lesions from the same patient may have different antigenic phenotypes (Natali *et al.*, 1983). One approach to the problem of tumor cell antigenic heterogeneity is the use of "cocktails" of antibodies with varying antigenic specificity. In a human breast carcinoma xenograft system, a cocktail of antibodies was shown to be more effective than a single antibody (Ceriani *et al.*, 1987). Other related problems include the presence of free-circulating antigen, which may lead to nonspecific antibody binding and antigenic modulation. Antigenic modulation may result in the disappearance of an antigen from the cell surface.

In the early radioisotope-labeled MoAb imaging studies, a large degree of nonspecific binding was seen. This was particularly evident in the reticuloendothelial structures such as the liver and spleen. As was discussed above, antibody binding in an intact organism is a complex situation. Antibodies do not have a "homing mechanism" by which they are able to seek out the tumor cell. Their delivery to the tumor cells depends on a number of complex factors including pharmacokinetics (circulation half-life of antibody or antibody conjugate), blood flow to tumor tissue, and catabolism of antibody or antibody conjugate. In general, only a very small proportion of an antibody dose accumulates within the tumor (<0.05% of the dose per gram) (Larson et al., 1983; Armitage et al., 1985). A potential solution to these problems lies in the use of antibody fragments (Fab). In general, Fab fragments are more rapidly catabolized, penetrate more quickly and effectively into tumor tissue, and achieve higher tumor-to-blood ratios (Buraggi et al., 1984; Pimm et al., 1985).

The immunogenecity of murine MoAbs in humans has been previously discussed. The development of this human antimouse antibody (HAMA) response can, at the minimum, lead to decreased circulating half-lives of murine MoAbs. In addition, anaphylactic reactions have been reported with repeated antibody injections. The influence of HAMA on the overall efficacy of murine antibodies has not been fully determined. Two approaches to this problem are currently being studied. The first is the use of chimeric antibodies. A chimeric antibody contains the mouse antigen-binding region, but the remainder of the antibody has human origin and is potentially less immunogenic. These antibodies are produced through complex molecular cloning techniques. The second approach is through the use of human MoAbs (Larrick and Bouria, 1986). These may be produced by human somatic cell hybridization (Olsson and Kaplan, 1980) or by the use of Epstein–Barr virus-immortalized human B-lymphocyte cell lines (Steinitz et al., 1977). It is hoped that the human MoAbs will be less immunogenic. As discussed in Section 5 on colon cancer, clinical studies using a human IgM MoAb (28A32) with specificity for colon cancer have been initiated.

With the development of human MoAbs the prospects for future MoAb treatment programs appear bright. However, human MoAbs may not necessarily eliminate the problem of immunogenicity. The potential still exists for the development of antiidiotype antibodies. Antiidiotype antibodies are directed against the antigen-combining site of the immunoglobulin molecule and may effect antigen–antibody binding (Roitt et al., 1985). Potential approaches to prevent the development of antiidiotype antibodies include pretreatment with passive antiidiotype antibody to suppress subsequent active antiidiotype antibody development and the use of immunosuppressive drugs such as cyclophosphamide.

In spite of all of the obstacles, cautions, and considerations discussed above as well as others, MoAbs will likely become extremely useful agents in the clinical diagnosis and treatment of cancer. This continues to be a very promising area of research.

15. FINAL CONSIDERATIONS

In the past 10 to 20 years much has been learned regarding the immunotherapy and biological therapy of cancer. For the most part the nonspecific immune-stimulating agents such as BCG, levamisole, and *Corynebacterium parvum* have been found to be ineffective. Specific exceptions have been discussed. However, future prospects for the immunotherapy of solid tumors are very exciting. A number of cytokines including the interferons (α, β, and γ) as well as interleukin-2 have undergone clinical trials. Interferon α has been shown to have activity in malignant melanoma, renal cancer, and superificial bladder cancer. In the future, combinations of cytokines and classical cytotoxic chemotherapeutic agents will, we can hope, prove to be more active than either modality alone. These clinical studies should be guided by further *in vitro* and *in vivo* animal investigations, which demonstrate synergy between combinations of agents and should further delineate the mechanism of action of the various cytokines. Furthermore, the therapeutic use of activated cell populations (LAK, TIL) as well as MoAbs will provide many novel approaches to cancer treatment. It is likely that in the future the new approaches discussed in this chapter as well as those yet to be discovered will revolutionize clinical cancer therapy.

ACKNOWLEDGMENTS. The authors wish to acknowledge the patient and skilled assistance of Ann E. Barrett and B. Kathryn Monroe through the many revisions of this work.

REFERENCES

Abdi, E. A., Kamitomo, V. J., McPherson, T. A., Konrad, M. W., Inque, M., and Tan, Y. H., 1986, Extended phase I study of human β-interferon in human cancer, *Clin. Invest. Med.* 9:33–40.

Abdulhay, G., DiSaia, P. J., Blessing, J. A., and Creasman, W. T., 1985, Human lymphoblastoid interferon in the treatment of advanced epithelial ovarian malignancies: A Gynecologic Oncology Group study, *Am. J. Obstet. Gynecol.* 152:418–23.

Abrams, D. I., and Volberding, P. A., 1986, Alpha interferon therapy of AIDS-associated Kaposi's sarcoma, *Semin. Oncol.* 13 (Suppl. 2):43–47.

Ainslie, J., Burdon, J. G. W., Henderson, M. M., Ilbery, P. L. T., and Matthews, J. P., 1983, The use of levamisole as an adjunct to chemotherapy and radiotherapy in the treatment of small cell carcinoma of the lung, *Med. J. Aust.* 2:285–287.

Aisner, J., Weinberg, V., Perloff, M., Weiss, R., Perry, M., Korzun, A., Ginsberg, S., and Holland, J. F., 1987, Chemotherapy versus chemoimmunotherapy (CAF v CAFVP v CMF each ± MER) for metastatic carcinoma of the breast: A CALGB study, *J. Clin. Oncol.* 5:1523–1533.

Alberts, D. S., Moon, T. E., Stephens, R. A., Wilson, H., Oishi, N., Hilgers, R. D., O'Toole, R., and Thigpen, J. T., 1979, Randomized study of chemoimmunotherapy for advanced ovarian carcinoma: A preliminary report of a Southwest Oncology Group study, *Cancer Treat. Rep.* 63:325–331.

Alberts, D., Mason, N., O'Toole, R., Kronmal, R., Hilgers, R., Surwit, E., Eyre, H., Baker, L., Boutsellis, J., Rivkin, S., Green, B., and Hannigan, E., 1986, Randomized phase III trial of doxorubicin (D) + cyclophosphamide (C) + BCG vs DC + displatinum (P) vs DC + P + BCG in stages III and IV ovarian cancer, *Proc. ASCO* 5:119.

Andriole, G. L., Mule, J. J., Hansen, C. T., Linehan, W. M., and Rosenberg, S. A., 1985, Evidence that lymphokine-activated killer cells and natural killer cells are distinct based on an analysis of congenitally immunodeficient mice, *J. Immunol.* 135:2911–2913.

Armitage, N. C., Perkins, A. C., Pimm, M. V., Wastie, M. L., Baldwin, R. W., and Hardcastle, J. D., 1985, Imaging of primary and metastatic colorectal cancer using an ^{111}In-labelled antitumor monoclonal antibody (791T/36), *Nucl. Med. Commun.* 6:623–631.

Ashford, R., Priestman, T., Mott, T., and Bottomley, J. M., 1986, Combining interferon with cytotoxic chemotherapy in patients with advanced breast cancer, *Cancer Immunol. Immunother.* 23:217–219.

Astler, V. B., and Coller, F. A., 1954, The prognostic significance of direct extension of carcinoma of the colon and rectum, *Ann. Surg.* 139:846–852.

Azizi, E., Brenner, H. J., and Shoham, J., 1984, Postsurgical adjuvant treatment of malignant melanoma patients by the thymic factor thymostimulin, *Drug Res.* 34:1043–1046.

Bach, J. F., Dardenne, M., Pleau, J. M., and Bach, M. A., 1975. Isolation, biochemical characteristics and biological activity of a circulating thymic hormone in the mouse and in the human, *Ann. N.Y. Acad. Sci.* 249:186–210.

Badalament, R. A., Herr, H. W., Wong, G. Y., Gnecco, C., Pinsky, C. M., Whitmore, W. F., Jr., Fair, W. R., and Oettgen, H. F., 1987, A prospective randomized trial of maintenance versus nonmaintenance intravesical bacillus Calmette–Guerin therapy of superficial bladder cancer, *J. Clin. Oncol.* 5:441–449.

Balch, C. M., and Milton, G. W., 1985, Diagnosis of metastatic melanoma at distant sites, in: *Cutaneous Melanoma* (C. M. Balch and G. W. Milton, eds.), J. B. Lippincott, Philadelphia, pp. 221–250.

Baldwin, R. W., and Byers, V. S., 1987, Monoclonal antibody targeting of cytotoxic agents for cancer therapy, in: *Immunology of Malignant Diseases* (V. S. Byers and R. W. Baldwin, eds.), MTP Press, Lancaster, pp. 44–54.

Baldwin, R. W., and Pimm, R. V., 1973, BCG immunotherapy of rat tumors of defined immunogenicity, *Natl. Cancer Inst. Monogr.* 39:11–17.

Baldwin, R. W., and Pimm, M. V., 1978, BCG in tumor immunotherapy, *Adv. Cancer Res.* 28:91–147.

Bast, R. C., 1982, Effects of cancers and their treatment on host immunity, in: *Cancer Medicine* (J. F. Holland and E. Frei, eds.), Lea & Febiger, Philadelphia, pp. 1134–1173.

Bast, R. C., Jr., and Knapp, R. C., 1984, Immunologic approaches to the management of ovarian carcinoma, *Semin. Oncol.* 11:264–274.

Bast, R. C., Zbar, B., Borsos, T., and Rapp, H. J., 1974, BCG and cancer, *N. Engl. J. Med.* 290:1413–1420, 1458–1469.

Bast, R. C., Jr., Berek, J. S., Obrist, R., Griffiths, C. T., Berkowitz, R. S., Hacker, N. F., Parker, L., Lagasse, L. D., and Knapp, R. C., 1983, Intraperitoneal immunotherapy of human ovarian carcinoma with *Corynebacterium parvum, Cancer Res.* 43:1395–1401.

Bedikian, A. Y., Patt, Y. Z., Murphy, W. K., Umsawasadi, T., Carr, D. T., Hersh, E. M., Bodey, G. P., and Valdivieso, M., 1984, Prospective evaluation of thymosin fraction V immunotherapy in patients with non-small cell lung cancer receiving vindesine, doxorubicin, and cisplatin (VAP) chemotherapy, *Am. J. Clin. Oncol.* 7:399–404.

Bensinger, W. I., Buckner, C. D., Clift, R. A., and Thomas, E. D., 1984, Clinical trials with staphylococcal protein A, *J. Biol. Respir. Mod.* 3:347–351.

Berd, V., Maguire, H. C., Jr., and Mastrangelo, M. J., 1984a, Impairment of concanavalin A inducible suppressor activity following administration of cyclophosphamide to patients with advanced cancer, *Cancer Res.* 44:1275–1280.

Berd, V., Maguire, H. C., Jr., and Mastrangelo, M. J., 1984b, Potentiation of human cell-mediated and humoral immunity by low-dose cyclophosphomide, *Cancer Res.* **44**:5439–5443.

Berd, D., Maguire, H. C., Jr., and Mastrangelo, M. J., 1986, Induction of cell-mediated immunity to autologous melanoma cells and regression of metastases after treatment with a melanoma cell vaccine preceded by cyclophosphamide, *Cancer Res.* **46**:2572–2577.

Berek, J. S., Hacker, N. F., Lichtenstein, A., Jung, T., Spina, C., Know, R. M., Brady, J., Greene, T., Ettinger, L. M., Lagasse, L. D., Bonnem, E. M., Spiegel, R. J., and Zighelboim, J., 1985a, Intraperitoneal recombinant α-interferon for "salvage" immunotherapy in stage III epithelial ovarian cancer: A Gynecologic Oncology Group study, *Cancer Res.* **45**: 4447–4453.

Berek, J. S., Hacker, N. F., Lichtenstein, A., Jung, T., Spina, C., Knox, R. M., Brady, J., Greene, T., Ettinger, L. M., Lagasse, L. D., Bonnem, E. M., Spiegel, R. J., and Zighelboim, J., 1985b, Intraperitoneal recombinant α_2-interferon for "salvage" immunotherapy in persistent epithelial ovarian cancer, *Cancer Treat. Rev.* **12**:23–32.

Berek, J. S., Knapp, R. C., Hacker, N. F., Lichtenstein, A., Jung, T., Spina, C., Obrist, R., Griffiths, C. T., Berkowitz, R. S., Parker, L., Zighelboim, J., and Bast, R. C., Jr., 1985c, Intraperitoneal immunotherapy of epithelial ovarian carcinoma with *Corynebacterium parvum*, *Am. J. Obstet. Gynecol.* **152**:1003–1010.

Bogdahn, U., Fleischer, B., Hilfenhaus, J., Rothig, H. J., Krauseneck, P., Mertens, H. G., Przuntek, H., 1985, Interferon-β in patients with low-grade astrocytomas—A phase I study, *J. Neurooncol.* **3**:125–130.

Bonadonna, G., Valagussa, P., Tancini, G., Rossi, A., Brambilla, C., Zambetti, M., Bignami, P., Di Fronzo, G., and Silvestrini, R., 1986, Current status of Milan adjuvant chemotherapy trials for node-positive and node-negative breast cancer, *Natl. Cancer Inst. Monogr.* **1**:45–49.

Branca, A. A., and Baglioni, C., 1981, Evidence that types I and II interferons have different receptors, *Nature* **294**:768–770.

Brandt, S. J., Peters, W. P., Atwater, S. K., Kurtzberg, J., Borowitz, M. J., Jones, R. B., Shpall, E. J., Bast, R. C., Jr., Gilbert, C. J., and Oette, D. H., 1988, Effect of recombinant human granulocyte–macrophage colony-stimulating factor on hematopoietic reconstitution after high-dose chemotherapy and autologous bone marrow transplantation, *N. Engl. J. Med.* **318**:869–876.

Graun, D. P., Nisius, S., Hollinshead, A., and Harris, J. E., 1983, Serial immune testing in surgically resected lung cancer patients, *Cancer Immunol. Immunother.* **15**:114–120.

Brosman, S. A., 1982, Experience with bacillus Calmette–Guerin in patients with superficial bladder carcinoma, *J. Urol.* **128**:27–29.

Brown, T. D., Koeller, J., Beougher, K., Galando, J., Bonnem, E. M., Spiegel, R. J., and Von Hoff, D. D., 1987, A phase I clinical trial of recombinant DNA gamma interferon, *J. Clin. Oncol.* **5**:790–798.

Brunda, M. J., Bellatoni, D., and Sulich, V., 1987, *In vivo* anti-tumor activity of combinations of interferon alpha and interleukin-2 in a murine model. Correlation of efficacy with the induction of cytotoxic cells resembling natural killer cells, *Int. J. Cancer* **40**:365–371.

Bubenik, J., Peremann, P., Helmstain, and Moberger, G., 1970, Cellular and humoral immune responses to human urinary bladder carcinomas, *Int. J. Cancer* **5**:310–319.

Bullard, D. E., and Bigner, D. D., 1985, Applications of monoclonal antibodies in the diagnosis and treatment of primary brain tumors, *J. Neurosurg.* **63**:2–16.

Bullard, D. E., Gillespie, G. Y., Mahaley, M. S., and Bigner, D. D., 1986, Immunobiology of human gliomas, *Semin. Oncol.* **13**:94–109.

Buraggi, G. L., Callegaro, L., Turrin, A., Cascinelli, N., Attili, A., Emanuelli, H., Gasparini, M., Deleide, G., Plassio, G., and Dovis, M., 1984, Immunoscintigraphy with ^{123}I, $^{99m}Tc^{(prime)}$ and ^{111}In-labelled $F(ab^1)_2$ fragments of monoclonal antibodies to a human high molecular weight melanoma associated antigen, *J. Nucl. Med. Allied Sci.* **28**:283–295.

Buzaid, A. C., Robertone, A., Kisala, C., and Salmon, S. E., 1987, Phase II study of interferon alpha-2a, recombinant (roferon-A) in metastatic renal cell carcinoma, *J. Clin. Oncol.* **5**:1083–1089.

Bystryn, J.-C., 1985, Immunology and immunotherapy of human malignant melanoma, *Dermatol. Clin.* **3**:327–334.

Cancer Patient Survival Report Number 5, 1977, DHEW Publ. No. (NIH) 77-992, DHEW, Washington.

Carpenter, J. T., Jr., Smalley, R. V., Raney, M., Vogel, C. L., and Weiner, R. S., 1986, Ineffectiveness of levamisole in prolonging remission or survival or women treated with cyclophosphamide, doxorubicin, and 5-fluorouracil for good-risk metastatic breast carcinoma: A Southeastern Cancer Study Group trial, *Cancer Treat. Rep.* **70**:1073–1079.

Carrel, S., de Tribolet, N., and Gross, N., 1982, Expression of HLA-DR and common acute lymphoblastic leukemia antigens on glioma cells, *Eur. J. Immunol.* **12**:354–357.

Carswell, E. A., Old, L. J., Kassel, R. L., Green, S., Fiore, N., and Williamson, B., 1975, An endotoxin induced serum factor that causes necrosis of tumors, *Proc. Natl. Acad. Sci. U.S.A.* **72**:3666–3670.

Catalona, W. J., Hudson, M. A., Gillen, D. P., Andriole, G. L., and Ratliff, T. L., 1987, Risks and benefits of repeated courses of intravesical bacillus Calmette–Guerin therapy for superficial bladder cancer, *J. Urol.* **137**:220–224.

Ceriani, R. L., Peterson, J. A., and Blank, E. W., 1987, Experimental immunotherapy of breast cancer with anti-breast epithelial monoclonal antibody radioconjugates, *Proc. AACR* **28**:394.

Cheung, N.-K. V., Lazarus, H., Miraldi, F. D., Abramowsky, C. R., Kallick, S., Saarinen, U. M., Spitzer, T., Strandjord, S. E., Coccia, P. F., and Berger, N. A., 1987, Ganglioside G_{D2} specific monoclonal antibody 3F8: A phase I study in patients with neuroblastoma and malignant melanoma, *J. Clin. Oncol.* **5**:1430–1440.

Choo, Y. C., Hsu, C., Seto, W. H., Miller, D. G., Merigan, T. C., Ng, M. H., and Ma, H. K., 1985, Intravaginal application of leukocyte interferon gel in the treatment of cervical intraepithelial neolasia (CIN), *Arch. Gynecol.* **237**:51–54.

Choo, Y. C., Seto, W. H., Hsu, C., Merigan, T. C., Tan, Y. H., Ma, H. K., and Ng, M. H., 1986, Cervical intraepithelial neoplsia by perilesional injection of interferon, *Br. J. Obstet. Gynaecol.* **93**:372–379.

Clark, S. C., and Kamen, R., 1987, The human hematopoietic colony-stimulating factors, *Science* **236**:1229–1237.

Clark, W. H., Ainsworth, A. M., Bernardino, E. A., Yang, C. H., Mihm, M. C., and Reed, R. J., 1975, The developmental biology of primary human malignant melanomas, *Semin. Oncol.* **2**:83–103.

Clemens, M., 1985, Interferons and oncogenes, *Nature* **313**:531–532.

Coakham, H., 1974, Surface antigen(s) common to human astrocytoma cells, *Nature* **250**:328–330.

Coakham, H. B., and Lakshmi, M. S., 1975, Tumor-associated surface antigen(s) in human astrocytomas, *Oncology* **31**:233–243.

Coates, A., Rallings, M., Hersey, R., and Swanson, C., 1986, Phase-II study of recombinant α_2-interferon in advanced malignant melanoma, *J. Interferon Res.* **6**:1–4.

Cohen, M. H., Chretien, P. B., Ihde, D. C., Fossieck, B. E., Makuch, R., Bunn, P. A., Jr., Johnston, A. V., Shackney, S. E., Matthews, M. J., Lipson, S. D., Kenady, D. E., and Minna, J. D., 1979, Thymosin fraction V and intensive combination chemotherapy. Prolonging the survival of patients with small cell lung cancer, *J.A.M.A.* **241**:1813–1815.

Colcher, D., Esteban, J. M., Carrasquillo, J. A., Sugarbaker, P., Reynolds, J. C., Bryant, G., Larson, S. M., and Schlom, J., 1987, Quantitative analyses of selective radiolabeled monoclonal antibody localization in metastatic lesions of colorectal cancer patients, *Cancer Res.* **47**:1185–1189.

Connors, J. M., Andiman, W. A., Howarth, C. B., Liu, E., Merigan, T. C., Savage, M. E., and Jacobs, C., 1985, Treatment of nasopharyngeal carcinoma with human leukocyte interferon, *J. Clin. Oncol.* **3**:813–817.

Creagan, E. T., Ahmann, D. L., Green, S. J., Long, H. J., Rubin, J., Schutt, A. J., and Dziewanowski, Z. E., 1984a, Phase II study of recombinant leukocyte A interferon (rIFN-αA) in disseminated malignant melanoma, *Cancer* 54:2844–2849.

Creagan, E. T., Ahmann, D. L., Green, S. J., Long, H. J., Frytak, S., O'Fallon, J. R., and Itri, L. M., 1984b, Phase II study of low-dose recombinant leukocyte A interferon in disseminated malignant melanoma, *J. Clin. Oncol.* 2:1002–1005.

Creagan, E. T., Ahmann, D. L., Green, S. J., Long, H. J., Frytak, S., and Itri, L. M., 1985, Phase II study of recombinant leukocyte A interferon (IFN-rA) plus cimetidine in disseminated malignant melanoma, *J. Clin. Oncol.* 3:977–981.

Creasman, W. T., and Clarke-Pearson, D. L., 1983, Immunotherapy of ovarian cancer, *Clin. Obstet. Gynaecol.* 10:297–306.

Creasman, W. T., Gall, S. A., Blessing, J. A., Schmidt, H. J., Abu-Ghazaleh, S., Whisnant, J. K., and DiSaia, P. J., 1979, Chemoimmunotherapy in the management of primary stage III ovarian cancer: A Gynecologic Oncology Group study, *Cancer Treat. Rep.* 63:319–323.

DeKernion, J. B., Huang, M.-Y, Lindner, A., Smith, R. B., and Kaufman, J. J., 1985, The management of superficial bladder tumors and carcinoma *in situ* with intravesical bacillus Calmette–Guerin, *J. Urol.* 133:598–601.

Dellon, A. C., Potvin, C., and Chretien, P. B., 1975, Thymus-dependent lymphocyte levels in bronchogenic carcinoma; correlations with histology, clinical stage and clnical coarse after surgical treatment, *Cancer* 35:687.

Dinarello, C. A., and Mier, J. W., 1987, Lymphokines: Current concepts, *N. Engl. J. Med.* 317:940–945.

Dippold, W. G., Knuth, A., and Meyer zum Buschenfelde, K.-H., 1984, Inhibition of human melanoma cell growth *in vitro* by monoclonal anti-G_{D3}-ganglioside antibody, *Cancer Res.* 44:806–810.

DiSaia, P. J. Bundy, B. N. Curry, S. L., Schlaerth, J., and Thigpen, J. T., 1987, Phase III study on the treatment of women with cervical cancer, stage IIB, IIIB, and IVA (confined to the pelvis and/or periaortic nodes), with radiotherapy alone versus radiotherapy plus immunotherapy with intravenous *Corynebacterium parvum:* A Gynecologic Oncology Group study, *Gynecol. Oncol.* 26:386–397.

Dolei, A., Capobianchi, M. R., and Ameglio, F., 1983, Human interferon-γ enhances the expression of class I and class II major histocompatibility complex products in neoplastic cells more effectively than interferon-α and interferon-β, *Infect. Immun.* 40:172–176.

Donaldson, R. C., 1972, Methotrexate plus Bacillus Calmette–Guerin (BCG) and isoniazid in the treatment of cancer of the head and neck, *Am. J. Surg.* 124:527–534.

Douillard, J.-Y., Le Mevel, B., Curtet, C., Vignoud, J., Chatal, J. F., and Koprowski, H., 1986, Immunotherapy of gastrointestinal cancer with monoclonal antibodies, *Med. Oncol. Tumor Pharmacother.* 3:141–146.

Droller, M. J., 1987, Biologic response modifiers in genitourinary neoplasia, *Cancer* 60:635–644.

Duff, T. A., Borden, E., Bay, J., Piepmeier, J., and Sielaff, K., 1986, Phase II trial of interferon-β for treatment of recurrent glioblastoma multiforme, *J. Neurosurg.* 64:408–413.

Eggermont, A. M., Weimar, W., Marquet, R. L., Lameris, J. D., and Jeekel, J., 1985, Phase II trial of high-dose recombinant leukocyte alpha-2 interferon for metastatic colorectal cancer without previous systemic treatment, *Cancer Treat. Rep.* 69:185–187.

Eggermont, A. M., Weimar, W., and Tank, B., 1986, Clinical and immunological evaluation of 20 patients with advanced colorectal cancer treated with high dose recombinant leukocyte interferon-αA (rIFNαA), *Cancer Immunol. Imunother.* 21:81–84.

Eisenthal, A., Lafreniere, R., Lefor, A. T., and Rosenberg, S. A., 1987, Effect of anti-B16 melanoma monoclonal antibody on established murine B16 melanoma liver metastases, *Cancer Res.* 47:2771–2776.

Epenetos, A. A., Munro, A. J., Stewart, S., Rampling, R., Lambert, H. E., McKenzie, C. G.,

Soutter, P., Rahemtulla, A., Hooker, G., Sivolapenko, G. B., Snook, D., Courtenay-Luck, N., Ghokia, B., Krausz, T., Taylor-Papadimitriou, J., Durbin, H., and Bodmer, W. F., 1987, Antibody-guided irradiation of advanced ovarian cancer with intraperitoneally administered radiolabeled monoclonal antibodies, *J. Clin. Oncol.* **5**:1890–1899.

Eriksson, B., Oberg, K., Alm, G., Karlsson, A., Lundqvist, G. Magnusson, A., Wide, L., and Wilander, E., 1987, Treatment of malignant endocrine pancreatic tumors with human leukocyte interferon, *Cancer Treat. Rep.* **71**:31–37.

Erlich, P., 1906 Chemotherapy, in: *The Collection of Papers by Paul Erlich* (F. Himmelweit, ed.), Pergamon Press, London.

Eschbach, J. W., Egrie, J. C., Downing, M. R., Browne, J. K., and Adamson, J. W., 1987, Correction of the anemia of end stage renal disease with recombinant human erythropoietin, *N. Engl. J. Med.* **316**:73–78.

Estabrook, A., Yemul, S., Seldin, D., Link, M. J., and Kramer, P., 1987, Immunoimaging and biodistribution studies with ^{111}Indium labeled monoclonal antibody to breast cancer, *Proc. AACR* **28**:356(1410).

Everson, T. C., and Cole, W. H., 1966, Spontaneous regression of adenocarcinoma of the kidney (hypernephroma), in: *Spontaneous Regression of Cancer*, W. B. Saunders, Philadelphia, pp. 11–87.

Fauci, A. S., Macher, A. M., Longo, D. L., Lane, H. C., Rook, A. H., Masur, H., and Gelmann, E. P., 1984, Acquired immune deficiency syndrome: Epidemiologic, clinical, immunologic and therapeutic considerations, *Ann. Intem. Med.* **100**:92–106.

Figlin, R. A., deKernion, J. B., Maldazys, J., and Sarna, G., 1985, Treatment of renal cell carcinoma with α(human leukocyte) interferon and vinblastine in combination: A phase I–II trial, *Cancer Treat. Rep.* **69**:263–267.

Finger, H., Emmerling, P., and Bruss, E., 1970, Variable adjuvant activity of *Bordetella pertussis* with respect to the primary and secondary immunization of mice, *Infect. Immun.* **1**:251.

Fischer, S. P. Lindermuth, J., Hash, C., and Shenkin, H. A., 1985, Levamisole in the treatment of glioblastoma multiforme, *J. Surg. Oncol.* **28**:214–216.

Fischl, M., Lucas, S., Richman, S., and Koch, G., 1987, Phase II study of wellferon (WFN) and vincristine (VCR) in AIDS-related Kaposi's sarcoma (KS), *Proc. ASCO* **6**:2.

Fisher, B., Redmon, C., Fisher, E. R., and Wolmark, N., 1986, Systemic adjuvant therapy in treatment of primary operable breast cancer: National surgical adjuvant breast and bowel project experience, *Natl. Cancer Inst. Monogr.* **1**:35–43.

Fisher, R. I., Coltmlan, C. A., Doroshow, J. H., Rayner, A. A., Hawkins, M. J., Mier, J. W., Wiernik, P., McMannis, J. D., Weiss, G. R., Margolin, K. A., Gemlo, B. T., Hoth, D. F., Parkinson, D. R., and Paietta, E., 1988, Metastatic renal cancer treated with interleukin-2 and lymphokine-activated killer cells, *Ann. Intem. Med.* **108**:518–523.

Foon, K. A., Sherwin, S. A., Abrams, P. G., Stevenson, H. C., Holmes, P., Maluish, A. E., Oldham, R. K., and Herberman, R. B., 1985, A phase I trial of recombinant gamma interferon in patients with cancer, *Cancer Immunol. Immunother.* **20**:193–197.

Fossa, S. D., and de Garis, S. T., 1987, Further experience with recombinant interferon alpha-2a with vinblastine in metastatic renal cell carcinoma: A progress report, *Int. J. Cancer* (Suppl. 1): 36–40.

Fowler, J. E., Jr., 1986, Failure of immunotherapy for metastatic renal cell carcinoma, *J. Urol.* **135**: 22–25.

Frankel, A. E., Houston, L. L., and Issell, B. F., 1986, Prospects for immunotoxin therapy in cancer, *Annu. Rev. Med.* **37**:125–142.

Friedman-Kien, A. E., Laubenstein, L. J., Rubinstein, P., Buimovici-Klein, E., Marmor, M., Stahl, R., Spigland, I., Kim, K. S., and Zolla-Pazner, S., 1982, Disseminated Kaposi's sarcoma in homosexual men, *Ann. Intern. Med.* **96**:693.

Fritze, D., Massner, B., Becher, R., Kaufmann, M., Illiger, H. J., Hartlapp, J., QueiBer, W., Abel,

U., Edler, L., Mayr, A. C., Drings, P., Westerhausen, M., Jungi, W., and Senn, H. J., 1984, Combination chemotherapy (VAC/FMC) with immunostimulation in metastatic breast cancer: A randomized study comparing different times and routes of administration of *Corynebacterium parvum, Klin. Wochenschr.* **62:**162–167.

Fujimoto, S., Green, M. I., and Sehon, A. H., 1976, Regulation of the immune response to tumor antigens. I. Immunosuppressor cells in tumor bearing hosts, *J. Immunol.* **116:**791–799.

Fujisawa, T., Yamaguchi, Y., Kimura, H., Arita, M., Baba, M., and Shiba, M., 1984, Adjuvant immunotherapy of primary resected lung cancer with transfer factor, *Cancer* **54:**663–669.

Fujita, K., 1987, The role of adjunctive immunotherapy in superficial bladder cancer, *Cancer* **59:** 2027–2030.

Garfield, D. H., and Kennedy, B. J., 1972, Regression of metastatic renal cell carcinoma following nephrectomy, *Cancer* **30:**190–196.

Garnett, M. C., and Baldwin, R. W., 1986, An improved synthesis of a methotrexate–albumin–791T/36 monoclonal antibody conjugate cytotoxic to osteogenic sarcoma cell lines, *Cancer Res.* **46:**2407–2412.

Gastrointestinal Tumor Study Group, 1984, Adjuvant therapy of colon cancer: Results of a prospectively randomized trial, *N. Engl. J. Med.* **310:**737–743.

Gelmann, E. P., Preble, O. T., Steis, R., Lane, H. C., Rook, A. H., Wesley, M., Jacob, J., Fauci, A., Masur, H., and Longo, D., 1985, Human lymphoblastoid interferon treatment of Kaposi's sarcoma in the acquired immune deficiency syndrome, *Am. J. Med.* **78:**737–741.

Giacomini, P., Aguzzi, A., Pestka, S., Fisher, P. B., and Ferrone, S., 1984, Modulation by recombinant DNA leukocyte (α) and fibroblast (β) interferons of the expression and shedding of HLA- and tumor-associated antigens by human melanoma cells, *J. Immunol.* **133:**1649–1655.

Gissmann, L., Wolnik, L., Ikenberg, H., Koldovsky, U., Schnurch, H. G., and Hausen, H. Z., 1983, Human papillomavirus types 6 and 11 DNA sequences in genital and laryngeal papillomas and in some cervical cancers, *Proc. Natl. Acad. Sci. U.S.A.* **80:**560–563.

Goldberg, R. M, Ayoob, M., Silgals, R., Ahlgren, J., and Neefe, J. R., 1985, Phase II trial of lymphoblastoid interferon in metastatic malignant melanoma, *Cancer Treat. Rep.* **69:**813–816.

Goldenberg, G. J., Brandes, L. J., Lau, W. H., Miller, A. B., Wall, C., and Ho, J. H. C., 1985, Cooperative trial of immunotherapy for nasopharyngeal caricnoma with transfer factor from donors with Epstein–Barr virus antibody activity, *Cancer Treat. Rep.* **69:**761–767.

Goodman, G. E., Beaumier, P., Hellstrom, I., Fernyhough, B., and Hellstrom, K.-E., 1985, Pilot trial of murine monoclonal antibodies in patients with advanced melanoma, *J. Clin. Oncol.* **3:** 340–352.

Grimm, E. A., Mazumder, A., Zhang, H. Z., and Rosenberg, S. A., 1982, Lymphokine-activated killer cell phenomenon: Lysis of natural killer-resistant fresh solid tumor cells by interleukin 2-activated autologous human peripheral blood lymphocytes, *J. Exp. Med.* **155:**1823–1841.

Grimm, E. A., Robb, R. J., Roth, J. A., Neckers, L. M., Lachman, L. B., Wilson, D. J., and Rosenberg, S. A., 1983a, Lymphokine-activated killer cell phenomenon: III. Evidence that IL-2 is sufficient for direct activation of peripheral blood lymphocytes into lymphokine-activated killer cells, *J. Exp. Med.* **158:**1356–1361.

Grimm, E. A., Ramsey, K. M., Mazumder, A., Wilson, D. J., Djeu, J. Y., and Rosenberg, S. A., 1983b, Lymphokine-activated killer cell phenomenon: II. Precursor phenotype is serologically distinct from pheripheral T lymphocytes, memory cytotoxic thymus-derived lymphocytes, and natural killer cells, *J. Exp. Med.* **157:**884–897.

Groopman, J. E., Mitsuyasu, R. T., DeLeo, M. J., Oette, D. H., and Golde, D. W., 1987, Effect of recombinant human granulocyte–macrophage colony stimulating factor on myelopoiesis in the acquired immunodeficiency syndrome, *N. Engl. J. Med.* **317:**593–598.

Gusdon, J. P., Jr., Homesley, H. D., Muss, H. B., Heise, E. R., Herbst, G. A., Richards II, F., Spurr, C. L., Lovelace, J. V., and Di Saia, P. J., 1981, Chemotherapy of advanced ovarian epithelial carcinoma with melphalan and levamisole: A pilot study of the Gynecologic Oncology Group, *Am. J. Obstet. Gynecol.* **141:**65.

Haaff, E. O., Catalona, W. J., and Ratliff, T. L., 1986a, Detection of interleukin 2 in the urine of patients with superficial bladder tumors after treatment with intravesical BCG, *J. Urol.* **136:** 970–974.

Haaff, E. O., Dresner, S. M., Ratliff, T. L., and Catalona, W. J., 1986b, Two courses of intravesical bacillus Calmette–Guerin for transitional cell carcinoma of the bladder, *J. Urol.* **136:** 820–824.

Halpern, B. (ed.), 1975, *Corynebacterium parvum: Applications in Experimental and Clinical Oncology*, Plenum Press, New York.

Harris, D. T., 1983, Hormonal therapy and chemotherapy of renal cell carcinoma, *Semin. Oncol.* **10:** 422–430.

Hawkins, M., Horning, S., Konrad, M., Anderson, S., Sielaff, K., Rosno, S., Schiesel, J., Davis, T., DeMets, D., Merigan, T., and Borden, E., 1985, Phase I evaluation of a synthetic mutant of β-interferon, *Cancer Res.* **45:**5914–5920.

Hellstrom, I., Hellstrom, K. E., and Shepard, T. H., 1970, Cell-mediated immunity against antigens common to human colonic carcinomas and fetal gut epithelium, *Int. J. Cancer* **6:**346–351.

Hellstrom, I., Garrigues, H. J., Cabasco, L., Mosely, G. H., Brown, J. P., and Hellstrom, K. E., 1983, Studies of a high molecular weight human melanoma-associated antigen, *J. Immunol.* **130:**1467–1472.

Herberman, R. B., and Ortaldo, J. R., 1981, Natural killer cells: Their role in defenses against disease, *Science* **214:**24–30.

Herlyn, D., Lubeck, M., Sears, H., and Koprowski, H., 1985, Specific detection of anti-idiotypic immune responses in cancer patients with murine monoclonal antibody, *J. Immunol. Methods* **85:**27–38.

Herlyn, D., Sears, H., Iliopoulos, D., Lubeck, M., Douillard, J. Y., Sindelar, W., Tempero, M., Mellstedt, H., Maher, M., and Koprowski, H., 1986a, Anti-idiotypic antibodies to monoclonal antibody CO17-1A, *Hybridoma* **5:**S51–S58.

Herlyn, D., Ross, A. H., and Koprowski, H., 1986b, Anti-idiotypic antibodies bear the internal image of a human tumor antigen, *Science* **232:**100–102.

Herlyn, D., Wettendorff, M., Schmoll, E., Iliopoulos, D., Schedel, I., Dreikhausen, U., Raab, R., Ross, A. H., Jaksche, H., Scriba, M., and Koprowski, H., 1987, Anti-idiotype immunization of cancer patients: Modulation of the immune response, *Proc. Natl. Acad. Sci. U.S.A.* **84:** 8055–8059.

Herlyn, M., Stepleuski, Z., Herlyn, D., Clark, W. H., Jr., Ross, A. H., Blaszczyk, M., Pak, K. Y., and Koprowski, H., 1983, Production and characterization of monoclonal antibodies against human malignant melanoma, *Cancer Invest.* **1:**215–224.

Herlyn, M., Guerry, D., and Koproski, H., 1985, Recombinant γ-interferon induces changes in expression and shedding of antigens associated with normal human melanocytes, nevus cells, and primary and metastatic melanoma cells, *J. Immunol.* **134:**4226–4230.

Herr, H. W., Pinsky, C. M., Whitmore, W. F., Jr., Sogani, P. G., Oettgen, H. F., and Melamed, M. R., 1985, Experience with intravesical bacillus Calmette–Guerin therapy of superficial bladder tumors, *Urology* **25:**119–123.

Herr, H. W. Pinsky, C. M., Whitmore, W. F., Jr., Sogani, P. C., Oettgen, H. F., and Melamed, M. R., 1986, Long-term effect of intravesical bacillus Calmette–Guerin on flat carcinoma *in situ* of the bladder, *J. Urol.* **135:**265–267.

Hersey, P., 1985, Review of melanoma antigens recognized by monoclonal antibodies (MAbs). Their functional significance and applications in diagnosis and treatment of melanoma, *Pathology* **17:**346–354.

Hersey, P., Hasic, E., MacDonald, M., Edwards, A., Spurling, A., Coates, A.S., Milton, G. W., and McCarthy, W. H., 1985, Effects of recombinant leukocyte interferon (rIFN-αA) on tumour growth and immune responses in patients with metastatic melanoma, *Br. J. Cancer* **51:**815–826.

Hersey, P., MacDonald, M., Hall, C., Spurling, A., Edwards A., Coates, A., and McCarthy, W.,

1986, Immunological effects of recombinant interferon alpha-2a in patients with disseminted melanoma, *Cancer* **57:**1666–1674.

Hersh, E. M., Patt, Y. Z., Murphy, S. G., Dicke, K., Zander, A., Adegbite, M., and Goldman, R., 1980, Radiosensitive, thymic hormone sensitive peripheral blood suppressor cell activity in cancer patients, *Cancer Res.* **40:**3134–3140.

Herskovic, A., Bauer, M., Seydel, H. G., Yesner, R., Scotte Doggett, R. L., Pewrez, C. A., Durbin, L. M., and Zinninger, M., 1988, Post-operative thoracic irradiation with or without levamisole in non-small cell lung cancer: Results of a Radiation Therapy Oncology Group study, *Int. J. Radiat. Oncol. Biol. Phys.* **14:**37–42.

Holland, J. M., 1975, Natural history and staging of renal cell carcinoma, *Cancer J. Clin.* **25:**121–133.

Hollinshead, A. C., 1987, Antigenic epitopes of three tumor-associated antigens of well-differentiated squamous cell carcinoma of the larynx for use in monitoring patients in specific active immunochemotherapy trials, *Cancer Detect. Prevent.* **10:**153–158.

Hollinshead, A., Glew, D., Bunnag, B., Gold, P., and Herderman, R., 1970, Skin reactive soluble antigen from intestinal cancer cell membranes and relationship to carcinoembryonic antigens, *Lancet* **2:**1191–1195.

Hollinshead, A., Elias, E. G., Arlen, M., Buda, B., Mosley, M., and Scherrer, J., 1985, Specific active immunotherapy in patients with adenocarcinoma of the colon utilizing tumor-associated antigens (TAA): A phase I clinical trial, *Cancer* **56:**480–489.

Holmes, E. C., and Gail, M., 1986, Surgical adjuvant therapy for stage II and stage III adenocarcinoma and large-cell undifferentiated carcinoma, *J. Clin. Oncol.* **4:**710–715.

Holmes, E. C., Hill, L. D., Gail, M., and The Lung Cancer Study Group, 1985, A randomized comprison of the effects of adjuvant therapy on resected stages II and III non-small cell carcinoma of the lung, *Ann. Surg.* **202:**335–341.

Hong, W. K., and Bromer, R., 1983, Medical intelligence current concepts: Chemotherapy in head and neck cancer, *N. Engl. J. Med.* **308:**75–79.

Hood, A. F., Farmer, E. R., and Weiss, R. A., 1982, Kaposi's sarcoma, *Johns Hopkins Med. J.* **151:**222–230.

Hooper, J. A., McDaniel, M. C., Thurman, G. B., Cohen, G. H., Schulof, R. S., and Geldstein, A. L., 1975, Purification and properties of bovine thymosin, *Ann. N.Y. Acad. Sci.* **249:**125–144.

Hoover, H. C., Jr., Surdyke, M. G., Dangel, R. B. Peters, L. C., and Hanna, M. G., Jr., 1985, Prospectively randomized trial of adjuvant active-specific immunotherapy for human colorectal cancer, *Cancer* **55:**1236–1243.

Houghton, A.N., Mintzer, D., Cordon-Cardo, C., Welt, S., Fliegel, B., Vadhan, S., Carswell, E., Melamed, M. R., Oettgen, H. F., and Old, L. J., 1985, Mouse monoclonal IgG3 antibody detecting G_{D3} ganglioside: A phase I trial in patients with malignant melanoma, *Proc. Natl. Acad. Sci. U.S.A.* **82:**1242–1246.

Houghton, A. N., Cordon-Cardo, C., and Eisenger, M., 1986, Differentiation antigens of melanoma and melanocytes, *Int. Rev. Exp. Pathol.* **28:**217–248.

Hrushesky, W. J., and Murphy, G. P., 1977, Current status of the therapy of advanced renal carcinoma, *J. Surg. Oncol.* **9:**277–288.

Hubay, C. A., Pearson, O. H., Manni, A., Gordon, N. H., and McGuires, W. L., 1985, Adjuvant endocrine therapy, cytotoxic chemotherapy and immunotherapy in stage II breast cancer: 6-year result. III. Antiestrogens in combination with chemotherapy in early breast cancer, *J. Steroid Biochem.* **23:**1147–1150.

Humm, J. L., 1986, Dosimetric aspects of radiolabeled antibodies for tumor therapy, *J. Nucl. Med.* **27:**1490–1497.

Ikebuchi, K., Wong, G. G., Clark, S. C., Ihle, J. N., Hirai, Y., and Ogawa, M., 1987, Interleukin 6 enhancement of interleukin 3-dependent proliferation of multipotential hemopoietic progenitors, *Proc. Natl. Acad. Sci. U.S.A.* **84:**9035–9039.

Ikic, D., Maricic, Z., Oresic, V., Rode, B., Nola, P., Smidj, K., Knezevic, M., Jusic, D., and Soos, E., 1981, Application of human leukocyte interferon in patients with urinary bladder papillomatosis, breast cancer, and melanoma, *Lancet* 1:1022–1024.

Ikonopisou, R. L., 1975, The use of BCG in the combined treatment of malignant melanoma, in: *International Symposium on Immunological Reactions to Melanoma Antigens*, Vol. 56 (J. R. Kalden, ed.), Behring-werke, Hanover, pp. 206–214.

Itoh, K., Tilden, A. B., Kumagai, K., and Balch, C. M., 1985, Leu-11+ lymphocytes with natural killer (NK) activity are precursors of recombinant interleukin 2 (rIL 2)-induced activated killer (LAK) cells, *J. Immunol.* 134:802–807.

Jacobs, K., Shoemaker, C., Rudersdorf, R., Neill, S. D., Kaufman, R. J., Mufson, A., Seehra, J., Jones, S. S., Hewick, R., Fritsch, E. F., Kawakita, M., Shimizu, T., and Miyake, T., 1985, Isolation and characterization of genomic and cDNA clones of human erythropoetin, *Nature* 313:806–810.

Jacobs, S. K., Kornblith, P. L., Wilson, D. L., and Grimm, E. A., 1986a, In vitro killing of human glioblastoma by interleukin-2 activated autologous lymphocytes, *J. Neurosurg.* 64:114–117.

Jacobs, S. K., Wilson, D. J., Kornblith, P. L., and Grimm, E. A., 1986b, Interleukin-2 and autologous lymphokine-activated killer cells in the treatment of malignant glioma, *J. Neurosurg.* 64:743–749.

Jacobs, S. K., Wilson, D. J., Kornblith, P. L., and Grimm, E. A., 1986c, Interleukin-2 or autologous lymphokine-activated killer cell treatment of malignant glioma: Phase I trial, *Cancer Res.* 46:2101–2104.

Jaffers, G., Colvin, R., Cosimi, A., Giorgi, J. V., Goldstein, G., Fuller, T. C., Kurnick, J. T., Lillehei, C., and Russell, P. S., 1983, The human immune response to murine OKT3 monoclonal antibody, *Transplant Proc.* 15:646–648.

Jessup, J. M., 1987, Adjuvant active specific immunotherapy (ASIT) enhances cell mediated immunity to autologous human colorectal carcinoma, *Proc. AACR* 28:361.

Jessup, J. M., McBride, C. M., Ames, F. C., Guarda, L., Ota, D. M., Romsdahl, M. M., and Martin, R. G., 1986, Active specific immunotherapy of Dukes B₂ and C colorectal carcinoma: Comparison of two doses of the vaccine, *Cancer Immunol. Immunother.* 21:233–239.

Kaminer, B., and Murray, J. F., 1950, Sarcoma idiopathicum multiple haemorrhagicum of Kaposi with special reference to its incidence in the South African Negro, and two case reports, *South Afr. J. Clin. Sci.* 1:1–25.

Kaufmann, M., Marqverson, J., Stanley, K. E., Mouritzen, C., and Hvid-Hansen, H., 1986, Distribution of intrapleural and intravenous *Corynebacterium parvum* in humans: ⁹⁹mTc-, and ¹³¹I-labeled bacteria, *Cancer Immunol. Immunother.* 22:56–61.

Kay, R. G., Mason, B. H., Stephens, E. J. Arthur, J. F., Hitchcock, G. C., Trindall, P. L., Rodgers, R., and Mullins, P., 1983, Levamisole in primary breast cancer: A controlled study in conjunction with L-phenylalanine mustard, *Cancer* 51:1992–1997.

Kelley, D. R., Ratliff, T. L., Catalona, W. J., Shapiro, A., Lage, J. M., Bauer, W. C., Haaff, E. O., and Dresner, S. M., 1985, Intravesical bacillus Calmette–Guerin therapy for superficial bladder cancer: Effect of bacillus Calmette–Guerin viability on treatment results, *J. Urol.* 134:48–53.

Kelley, D. R., Haaff, E. O., Becich, M., Lage, J., Bauer, W. C., Dresner, S. M., Catalona, W. J., and Ratliff, T. L., 1986, Prognostic value of purified protein derivative skin test and granuloma formation in patients treated with intravesical bacillus Calmette–Guerin, *J. Urol.* 135:268–271.

Kempf, R. A., Grunberg, S. M., Daniels, J. R., Skinner, D. G., Venturi, C. L., Spiegel, R., Neri, R., Greiner, J. M., Rudnick, S., and Mitchell, M. S., 1986, Recombinant interferon α-2 (INTRON A) in a phase II study of renal cell carcinoma, *J. Biol. Resp. Mod.* 5:27–35.

Khoo, S. K., Whitaker, S. V., Jones, I. S. C., and Thomas, D. A., 1984, Levamisole as adjuvant to chemotherapy of ovarian cancer, *Cancer* 54:986–990.

Kies, M. S., Levitan, N., and Hong, W. K., 1985, Chemotherapy of head and neck cancer, *Otolaryngol. Clin. North Am.* 18:533–541.

Kirkwood, J. M., Ernstoff, M. S., Davis, C. A., Reiss, M., Ferraresi, R., and Rudnick, S. A., 1985a, Comparison of intramuscular and intravenous recombinant alpha-2 inteferon in melanoma and other cancers, *Ann. Intern. Med.* **103**:32–36.

Kirkwood, J. M., Harris, J. E., Vera, R., Sandler, S., Fischer, D. S., Khandekar, J., Ernstoff, M. S., Gordon, L., Lutes, R., Bonomi, P., Lytton, B., Cobleigh, M., and Taylor, S. J., IV, 1985b, A randomized study of low and high doses of leukocyte α-interferon in metastatic renal cell carcinoma: The American Cancer society collaborative trial, *Cancer Res.* **45**:863–871.

Kirsh, M. M., Orringer, M. B., McAuliffe, S., Schork, M. A., Katz, B., and Silva, J., Jr., 1984, Transfer factor in the treatment of carcinoma of the lung, *Ann. Thoracic Surg.* **38**:140–145.

Klefstrom, P., Holsti, P., Grohn, P., Heinonen, E., and Holsti, L., 1985, Levamisole in the treatment of stage II breast cancer: Five-year follow-up of a randomized double-blind study, *Cancer* **55**:2753–2757.

Klefstrom, P., Grohn, P., Heinonen, E., Holsti, L., and Holsti, P., 1987, Adjuvant postoperative radiotherapy, chemotherapy, and immunotherapy in stage III breast cancer. II. 5-year results and influences of levamisole, *Cancer* **60**:936–942.

Klein, E., 1967, Differential immunologic reactions in normal skin and epidermoid neoplasms, *Fed. Proc.* **26**:430.

Klein, E., 1968, Tumors of the skin. X. Immunotherapy of cutaneous and mucosal neoplasms, *N.Y. State J. Med.* **68**:900–911.

Klein, E., 1969, Hypersensitivity reactions at tumor sites, *Cancer Res.* **29**:2351–2362.

Klein, E., Holtermann, O., Milgrom, H., Case, R. W., Klein, D., Rosner, D., and Djerassi, I., 1976, Immunotherapy for accessible tumors utilizing delayed hypersensitivity reactions and separated components of the immune system, *Med. Clin. North Am.* **60**:389–418.

Kohler, G., and Milstein, C., 1975, Continuous cultures of fused cells secreting antibody of pre-defined specificity, *Nature* **256**:495–497.

Korec, S., Smith, F. P., Schein, P. S., and Phillips, T. M., 1984, Clinical experiences with extracorporeal immunoperfusion of plasma from cancer patients, *J. Biol. Resp. Mod.* **3**:330–335.

Kornblith, P. L., Walker, M. R., and Cassady, R. J., 1985, Neoplasms of the central nervous system, in: *Cancer, Principles and Practice of Oncology* (V. T. DeVita, S. Hellman, and A. Rosenberg, eds.), J. B. Lippincott, Philadelphia, pp. 1437–1510.

Krauss, S., Comas, F., Perez, C., Gordon, D., Philpott, G., Broun, G., Mill, W., Robbins, R., Smalley, R., Mendiondo, O., DeSimone, P., McLaren, J., Keller, J., Durant, J., Birch, R., and Buchanan, R., 1984, Treatment of inoperable non-small cell carcinoma of the lung with radiation therapy, with or without levamisole, *Am. J. Clin. Oncol.* **7**:405–412.

Krigel, R., Padavic, K., Comis, R., and Rudolph, A., 1987, A phase I study of recombinant interleukin-2 plus recombinant beta-interferon, *Proc. ASCO* **6**:238.

Krown, S. E., 1987, Interferon treatment of renal cell carcinoma, *Cancer* **59**:647–651.

Krown, S. E., Real, F. X., Cunningham-Rundles, S., Myskowski, P. L., Koziner, B. Fein, S., Mittelman, A., Oettgen, H. F., and Safai, B., 1983, Preliminary observations of the effect of recombinant leukocyte A interferon in homosexual men with Kaposi's sarcoma, *N. Engl. J. Med.* **308**:1071–1076.

Krown, S. E., Burk, M. W., Kirkwood, J. M., Kerr, D., Morton, D. L., and Oettgen, H. F., 1984, Human leukocyte (alpha) inteferon in metastatic malignant melanoma: The American Cancer Society phase II trial, *Cancer Treat. Rep.* **68**:723–726.

Krown, S. E., Real, F. X., Vadhan-Raj, S., Cunningham-Rundles, S., Krim, M., Wong, G., and Oettgen, H. F., 1986, Kaposi's sarcoma and the acquired immune deficiency syndrome: Treatment with recombinant interferon alpha and analysis of prognostic factors, *Cancer* **57**:1662–1665.

Krown, S. E., Mintzer, D., Cunningham-Rundles, S., Niedzwiecki, D., Krim, M., Einzig, A. I., Gabrilove, J. L., Shurgot, B., and Gessula, J., 1987, High-dose human lymphoblastoid interferon in metastatic colorectal cancer: Clinical results and modification of biological responses, *Cancer Treat. Rep.* **71**:39–45.

Lafreniere, R., and Rosenberg, S. A., 1985a, Successful immunotherapy of murine experimental hepatic metastases with lymphokine-activated killer cells and recombinant interleukin 2, *Cancer Res.* **45**:3735–3741.

Lafreniere, R., and Rosenberg, S. A., 1985b, Adoptive immunotherapy of murine hepatic metastases with lymphokine activated killer (LAK) cells and recombinant interleukin 2 (RIL 2) can mediate the regression of both immunogenic and nonimmunogenic sarcomas and an adenocarcinoma, *J. Immunol.* **135**:4273–4280.

Lamm, D. L., 1985, Bacillus Calmette–Guerin immunotherapy for bladder cancer, *J. Urol.* **134**:40–47.

Lamm, D. L., Thor, D. E. Stogdill, V. D., and Radwin, H. M., 1982, Bladder cancer immunotherapy, *J. Urol.* **128**:931–935.

Lamm, D. L., Stogdill, V. D., Stogdill, B. J., and Crispen, R. G., 1986, Complications of bacillus Calmette–Guerin immunotherapy in 1,278 patients with bladder cancer, *J. Urol.* **135**:272–274.

Larrick, J. W., and Bouria, J. M., 1986, Prospects for the therapeutic use of human monoclonal antibodies, *J. Biol. Resp. Mod.* **5**:379–393.

Larson, S. M., Brown, J. P. Wright, P. W., Carrasquillo, J. A., Hellstrom, I., and Hellstrom, K. E., 1983, Imaging of melanoma with ^{131}I labelled monoclonal antibodies, *J. Nucl. Med.* **24**:123–129.

Laurie, J., Moertel, C., Fleming, T., Wieand, H., Leigh, J., Beart, R., Cullinan, S., and Krook, J., 1987, Surgical adjuvant therapy of poor prognosis colorectal cancer with levamisole alone or combined levamisole and 5-fluorouracil (5-FU), *Proc. ASCO* **5**:81.

Lederer, E., and Chedid, L., 1982, Immunomodulation by synthetic muramyl peptides and trehalose diesters, in: *Immunologic Approaches to Cancer Therapeutics* (E. Mihich, ed.), John Wiley & Sons, New York, pp. 107–136.

Legha, S. S., Papadopoulas, N. E. J., Plager, C., Ring, S., Chawla, S. P., Evans, L. M., and Benjamin, R. S., 1987, Clinical evaluation of recombinant interferon alpha-2a (Roferon-A) in metastatic melanoma using two different schedules, *J. Clin. Oncol.* **5**:1240–1246.

Levy, R., 1987, Editorial: Will monoclonal antibodies find a place in our therapeutic armamentarium? *J. Clin. Oncol.* **5**:527–529.

Lichtenstein, A., Tuttle, R., Cantrell, J., and Zighelboim, J., 1982, Effects of different fractions of *Corynebacterium parvum* on the cytotoxic T-cell response to alloantigens in mice, *J. Natl. Cancer Inst.* **69**:495–501.

Lichtenstein, A., Berek, J., Bast, R., Spina, C., Hacker, N., Knapp, R. C., and Zighelboim, J., 1984, Activation of peritoneal lymphocyte cytotoxicity in patients with ovarian cancer by intraperitoneal treatment with *Corynebacterium parvum*, *J. Biol. Resp. Mod*, **3**:371–378.

Livingston, P. O., Albino, A. P., Chung, T. J. C., Real, F. X., Houghton, A. N., Oettgen, H. F., and Old, L. J., 1985, Serological responses of melanoma patients to vaccines prepared from VSV lysates of autologous and allogeneic cultured melanoma cells, *Cancer* **55**:713–720.

Livingston, P. O., Natoli, E. J., Calves, M. J., Stockert, E., Oettgen, H. F., and Old., L. J., 1987, Vaccines containing purified G_{M2} ganglioside elicit G_{M2} antibodies in melanoma patients, *Proc. Natl. Acad. Sci. U.S.A.* **84**:2911–2915.

Lonberg, M., Odajnyk, C., Krigel, R., Laubenstein, L., Wernz, J., Green, M., and Muggia, F., 1985, Sequential and simultaneous alpha 2 interferon (IFN) and VP-16 in epidemic Kaposi's sarcoma (EKS), *Proc. ASCO* **4**:2.

Lotze, M. T., Grimm, E. A., Mazumder, A., Strausser, J. L., and Rosenberg, S. A., 1981, Lysis of fresh and cultured autologous tumor by human lymphocytes cultured in T-cell growth factor, *Cancer Res.* **41**:4420–4425.

Lotze, M. T., Carrasquillo, J. A., Weinstein, J. N., Bryant, G. J., Perentesis, P., Reynolds, J. C., Matis, L. A., Eger, R. R., Keenan, A. M., Hellstrom, I., Hellstrom, K. E., and Larson, S. M.,

1986, Monoclonal antibody imaging of human melanoma: Radioimmunodetection by subcutaneous or systemic injection, *Ann. Surg.* **204:**223–235.

Lotzova, E., 1987, Interleukin-2-generated killer cells, their characterization and role in cancer therapy, *Cancer Bull.* **39:**30–38.

Ludwig Lung Cancer Study Group, 1985, Adverse effect of intrapleural *Corynebacterium parvum* as adjuvant therapy in resected stage I and II non-small cell carcinoma of the lung, *J. Thorac. Cardiovasc. Surg.* **89:**842–847.

Ludwig Lung Cancer Study Group, 1986, Intrapleural and intravenous *Corynebacterium parvum* in patients with resected stage I and II non-small cell carcinoma of the lung, *Cancer Immunol. Immunother.* **23:**1–4.

Lundell, G., Blomgren, H., Cedermark, B., Silfversward, C., Theve, T., and Ohman, U., 1984, High dose rDNA human alpha$_2$ interferon therapy in patients with advanced colorectal adenocarcinoma: A phase II study, *Radiother. Oncol.* **1:**325–332.

Lundquist, P.-G., Haglund, S., Carlsoo, B., Strander, H., and Lundgren, E., 1984, Interferon therapy in juvenile laryngeal papillomatosis, *Otolaryngol. Head Neck Surg.* **92:**386–391.

Magnus, K., 1977, Incidence of malignant melanoma of the skin in the five Nordic countries: Significance of solar radiation, *Int. J. Cancer* **20:**477–485.

Mahaley, M. S., Jr., Urso, M. B., Whaley, R. A., Blue, M., Williams, T. E., Guaspari, A., and Selker, R. G., 1985, Immunobiology of primary intracranial tumors. Part 10: Therapeutic efficacy of interferon in the treatment of recurrent gliomas, *J. Neurosurg.* **63:**719–725.

Mansell, P. W. A., Ichinose, H., and Reed, R. J., 1975, Macrophage mediated destruction of human malignant cells *in vivo*, *J. Natl. Cancer Inst.* **54:**571–580.

Mark, D., Brummond, R., Creasey, A., Lin, L., Khosrovi, B., Edwards, B., Groverman, D., Joseph, J., Hawkins, M., and Borden, E., 1983, A synthetic mutant of interferon beta for clinical trial, in: *Interferons, Proceedings of the International Symposium on Interferons* (T. Koshida ed.), Kyoto Prefectural University of Medicine, Kyoto, pp. 167–172.

Mark, D. F., Lu, S. D., Creasey, A. A., Yamamoto, R., and Lyn, L. S., 1984, Site specific mutagenesis of the human fibroblast interferon gene, *Proc. Natl. Acad. Sci. U.S.A.* **81:**5662–5666.

Marshall, V. F., 1952, The relation of the preoperative estimate to the pathologic demonstration of the extent of vesical neoplasms, *J. Urol.* **68:**714.

Martin, D. S., Hayworth, P., Fugmann, R. H., English, R., and McNeill, H. W., 1964, Combination therapy with cyclophosphamide and zymosan on a spontaneous mammary cancer in mice, *Cancer Res.* **24:**652–654.

Marumo, K., Murai, M., Hayakawa, M., and Tazaki, H., 1984, Human lymphoblastoid interferon therapy for advanced renal cell carcinoma, *Urology* **24:**567–571.

Mastrangelo, M. J., Baker, A. R., and Katz, H. R., 1985, Cutaneous Melanoma, in: *Cancer, Principles and Practice of Oncology* (V. T. Devita, S. Hellman, and S. H. Rosenberg, eds.), J. B. Lippincott, Philadelphia, pp. 1371–1422.

Matthay, R. A., Mahler, D. A., Beck, G. J., Loke, J., Baue, A. E., Carter, D. C., and Mitchell, M. S., 1986, Intratumoral bacillus Calmette-Guerin immunotherapy prior to surgery for carcinoma of the lung: Results of a prospective randomized trial, *Cancer Res.* **46:**5963–59–68.

Maurer, L. H., Pajak, T., Eaton, W., Comis, R., Chahinian, P., Faulkner, C., Silberfarb, P. M., Henderson, E., Rege, V. B., Balkwin, P. E., Weiss, R., Rafla, S., Prager, D., Carey, R., Perry, M., and Choi, N. C., 1985, Combined modality therapy with radiotherapy, chemotherapy, and immunotherapy in limited small-cell carcinoma of the lung: A phase III cancer and leukemia group B study, *J. Clin. Oncol.* **3:**969–976.

McLaughlin, C. A., Schwartzman, S. M., Horner, B. L., Jones, G. H., Moffatt, J. G., Nestor, J. J., Jr., and Tegg, D., 1980, Regression of tumors in guinea pigs after treatment with synthetic muramyl dipeptides and trehalose dimycolate, *Science* **208:**415–416.

McLeod, D. T., Calverley, P. M. A., Millar, J. W., and Horne, N. W., 1985, Further experience of *Corynebacterium parvum* in malignant pleural effusion, *Thorax* **40:**515–518.

McLeod, G. R. C., Thomson, D. B., and Hersey, P., 1987, Recombinant interferon alpha-2a in advanced malignant melanoma. A phase I–II study in combination with DTIC, *Int. J. Cancer (Suppl.)*1:31–35.

Medina, J. E., 1983, Commentary: The controversial role of BCG in the treatment of squamous cell carcinoma of the head and neck, *Arch. Otolaryngol.* 109:543.

Merguerian, P. A., Donahue, L., and Cockett, A. T. K., 1987, Intraluminal interleukin 2 and bacillus Calmette–Guerin for treatment of bladder cancer: A preliminary report, *J. Urol.* 137: 216–219.

Messerschmidt, G. L., Bowles, C. A., Henry, D. H., and Deisseroth, A. B., 1984, Clinical trials with *Staphylococcus aureus* and protein A in the treatment of malignant disease, *J. Biol. Resp. Mod.* 3:325–329.

Messerschmidt, G. L., Henry, D. H., Synder, J., Bertram, J., Mittelman, A., Ainsworth, S., Fiore, J., Viola, M. V., Louie, J., Ambinder, E., MacKintosh, F. R., Higby, D. J., O'Brien, P., Kiprov, D., Hamburger, M., Balint, J. P., Jr., Fisher, L. D., Perkins, W., Pinsky, C. M., and Jones, F. R., 1988, Protein A immunoadsorption in the treatment of malignant disease, *J. Clin. Oncol.* 6:203–212.

Metcalf, D., 1986, Review: The molecular biology and functions of the granulocyte–macrophage colony-stimulating factors, *Blood* 67:257–267.

Millar, J. W., Huuter, A. W., and Horne, N. W., 1980, Intrapleural immunotherapy with *Corynebacterium parvum* in recurrent malignant pleural effusions, *Thorax* 35:856–858.

Mitchell, M. S., Kempf, R. A., Harel, W., Shau, H., Boswell, W. D., Lind, S., and Bradley, E. C., 1988, Effectiveness and tolerability of low-dose cyclophosphamide and low-dose intravenous interleukin-2 disseminated melanoma, *J. Clin. Oncol.* 6:409–424.

Montie, J., Stewart, B. H., Straffon, R. A., Banowsky, L. H. W., Hewitt, C. B., and Montague, D. K., 1977, The role of adjunctive nephrectomy in patients with metastatic renal cell carcinoma, *J. Urol.* 117:272.

Morales, A., 1980, Treatment of carcinoma *in situ* of the bladder with BCG: A phase II trial, *Cancer Immunol. Immunother.* 9:69–72.

Morales, A., 1984, Long-term results and complications of intracavitary bacillus Calmette–Guerin therapy for bladder cancer, *J. Urol.* 132:457–459.

Morales, A., Eidinger, D., and Bruce, A. W., 1976, Intracavitary bacillus Calmette–Guerin in the treatment of superficial bladder tumors, *J. Urol.* 116:180–183.

Mori, K., Lamm, D. L., and Crawford, E. D., 1986, A trial of bacillus Calmette–Guerin versus adriamycin in superficial bladder cancer: A South-West Oncology Group study, *Urol. Int.* 41: 254–259.

Morton, D. L., 1971, Immunological studies with human neoplasms, *J. Reticuloendothel. Soc.* 10: 137–160.

Morton, D. L., Eilber, F. R., Malmgren, R. A., and Wood, W. C., 1970, Immunological factors which influence response to immunotherapy in malignant melanoma, *Surgery* 68:158–164.

Morton, D. L., Eiliber, F. R., Holmes, E. C., Hunt, J. S., Ketcham, A. S., Silverstein, M. J., and Sparks, F. C., 1974, BCG immunotherapy of malignant melanoma: Summary of a seven year experience, *Ann. Surg.* 180:635–643.

Mulé, J. J., Shu, S., Schwarz, S. L., and Rosenberg, S. A., 1984, Adoptive immunotherapy of established pulmonary metastases with LAK cells and recombinant interleukin-2, *Science* 225: 1487–1489.

Mulé, J. J., Shu, S., and Rosenberg, S. A., 1985, The anti-tumor efficacy of lymphokine-activated killer cells and recombinant interleukin 2 *in vivo*, *J. Immunol.* 135:646–652.

Mulé, J. J., Smith, C. A., and Rosenberg, S. A., 1987, Interleukin-4 (B-cell stimulatory factor 1) can mediate the induction of LAK activity directed against fresh tumor cells, *J. Exp. Med.* 166: 792–797.

Murray, J. L., Rosenblum, M. G., Sobol, R. E., Bartholomew, R. M., Plager, C E., Haynie, T. P., Johns, M. F., Glenn, H. J., Lamki, L., Benjamin, R. S., Papadopoulos, N., Boddie, A. W.,

Frincke, J. M., David, G. S., Carlo, D. J., and Hersh, E. M., 1985, Radioimmunoimaging in malginant melanoma with ^{111}In-labeled monoclonal antibody 96.5, *Cancer Res.* **45**:2376–2381.

Murray, J. L., Rosenblum, M. G., Lamke, L., Haynie, T. P., Glenn, H. J., Plager, C. E., Unger, M. W., Carlo, D. J., and Hersh, E. M., 1987a, Radioimmunoimaging in malignant melanoma patients with the use of indium-111-labeled antimelanoma monoclonal antibody (ZME-018) to high-molecular-weight antigen, *Natl. Cancer Inst. Monogr.* 3:3–9.

Murray, J. L., Rosenblum, M. G., Lamki, L., Glenn, H. J., Krizan, Z., Hersh, E. M., Plager, C. E., Bartholomew, R. M., Unger, M. W., Carlo, D. J., 1987b, Clinical parameters related to optimal tumor localization of indium-111-labeled mouse antimelanoma monoclonal antibody ZME-018, *J. Nucl. Med.* **28**:25–33.

Muss, H. B., Kempf, R. A., Martino, S., Rudnick, S. A., Greiner, J., Cooper, M. R., Decker, D., Grunberg, S. M., Jackson, D. V., Richars, F. II, Samal, B., Singhakowinta, A., Spurr, C. L., Stuart, J. J., White, D. R., Caponera, M., and Mitchell, M. S., 1984, A phase II study of recombinant α interferon in patients with recurrent or metastatic breast cancer, *J. Clin. Oncol.* **2**:1012–1016.

Muss, H. B., Costanzi, J. J., Leavitt, R., Williams, R. D., Kempf, R. A., Pollard, R., Ozer, H., Zekan, P. J., Grunberg, S. M., Mitchell, M. S., Caponera, M., Gavigan, N., Ernest, M. L., Venturi, C., Greiner, J., and Spiegel, R. J., 1987, Recombinant alpha interferon in renal cell carcinoma: A randomized trial of two routes of administration, *J. Clin. Oncol.* **5**:286–291.

Myers, G. H., Fehrenbaker, L. G., and Kelalis, p.p., 1968, Prognostic significance of renal vein invasion by hypernephroma, *J. Urol.* **100**:420.

Naclerio, R., 1985, Recent advances in immunology with specific reference to otolaryngology, *Otolaryngol. Clin. North Am.* **18**:821–831.

Nagai, M., and Arai, T., 1984, Clinical effect of interferon in malignant brain tumors, *Neurosurg. Rev.* **7**:55–64.

Natali, P. G., Cavaliere, R., Bigotti, A., Nicotra, M. R., Russo, C., Ng, A. K., Giacomini, P., and Ferrone, S., 1983, Antigenic heterogeneity of surgically removed primary and autologous metastatic human melanoma lesions, *J. Immunol.* **130**:1462–1466.

National Institutes of Health Consensus Development Panel on Adjuvant Chemotherapy and Endocrine Therapy for Breast Cancer, 1986, Introduction and conclusions. Adjuvant chemotherapy and endocrine therapy for breast cancer, *Natl. Cancer Inst. Monogr.* **1**:1–4.

Neidhart, J. A., 1986, Interferon therapy for the treatment of renal cancer, *Cancer* **57**:1696–1699.

Neidhart, J. A., Gagen, M. M., Young, D., Tuttle, R., Melink, T. J., Ziccarrelli, A., and Kisner, D., 1984, Interferon-α therapy of renal cancer, *Cancer Res.* 44:4140–4143.

Neifeld, J. P., Terz, J. J., Kaplan, A. M., and Lawrence, J. W., 1985, Adjuvant *Corynebacterium parvum* immunotherapy for squamous cell epitheliomas of the oral cavity, pharynx, and larynx, *J. Surg. Oncol.* **28**:137–145.

Newbill, E. T., and Johns, M. E., 1983, Immunology of head and neck cancers, *CRC Crit. Rev. Clin. Lab. Sci.* **19**:1–25.

Nicola, N. A., Metcalf, D., Matsumoto, M., and Johnson, G. R., 1983, Purification of a factor-inducing differentiation in murine myelomonocytic leukemia cells, *J. Biol. Chem.* **258**:9017–9023.

Niloff, J. M., Knapp, R. C., Jones, G., Schaetzl, E. M., Bast, R. C., Jr., 1985, Recombinant leukocyte alpha interferon in advanced ovarian carcinoma, *Cancer Treat. Rep.* **69**:895–896.

North, R. J., 1982, Cyclophosphamide-facilitated adoptive immunotherapy of an established tumor depends on elimination of tumor-induced suppressor T-cells, *J. Exp. Med.* **55**:1063–1074.

Obbens, E. A. M. T., Feun, L. G., Leavens, M. E., Savaraj, N., Stewart, D. J., and Gutterman, J. U., 1985, Phase I clinical trial of intralesional or intraventricular leukocyte interferon for intracranial malignancies, *J. Neurooncol.* **3**:61–67.

Oberg, K., Norheim, I., Lind, E., Alm, G., Lundqvist, G., Wide, L., Jonsdottir, B., Magnusson,

A., and Wilander, E., 1986, Treatment of malignant carcinoid tumors with human leukocyte interferon: Long-term results, *Cancer Treat. Rep.* **70**:1297–1304.

Odajnyk, C., and Franco, F. M., 1985, Treatment of Kaposi's sarcoma: Overview and analysis by clinical setting, *J. Clin. Oncol.* **3**:1277–1285.

Oettgen, H., Old, L., Farrow, J., Valentine, F. T., Lawrence, H. S., and Thomas, L., 1974, Effects of dialyzable transfer factor in patients with breast cancer, *Proc. Natl. Acad. Sci.* **71**:2319–2323.

Oldham, R., Weese, J. L., Herberman, R. B., Perlin, E., Mills, M. N., Heims, W., Blom, J., Green, D., Reid, J., Bellinger, S., Law, I., McCoy, J. L., Dean, J. H., Cannon, G. B., and Djeu, J., 1976, Immunologic monitoring and immunotherapy of carcinoma of the lung, *Int. J. Cancer* **18**:739.

Oldham, R. K., Foon, K. A., Morgan, A. C., Woodhouse, C. S., Schroff, R. W., Abrams, P. G., Fer, M. N., Schoenberger, C. S., Farrell, M., Kimball, E., and Sherwin, S. A., 1984, Monoclonal antibody therapy of malignant melanoma: *In vivo* localization in cutaneous metastasis after intravenous administration, *J. Clin. Oncol.* **2**:1235–1244.

Olsson, L., and Kaplan, H. S., 1980, Human-human hybridomas producing monoclonal antibodies of predefined antigenic specificity, *Proc. Natl. Acad. Sci. U.S.A.* **77**:5429–5431.

Oyama, K., Takagaki, Y., and Niki, R., 1975, Studies on the interrelation between clinical effects and immune response of a streptococcal antitumor agent OK 432, *Jpn. J. Clin. Cancer* **21**:253.

Padmanabhan, N., Balkwill, F. R., Bodmer, J. G., and Rubens, R. D., 1985, Recombinant DNA human interferon alpha 2 in advanced breast cancer: A phase 2 trial, *Br. J. Cancer* **51**:55–60.

Padmanabhan, T. K., Balaram, P., and Vasudevan, D. M., 1987, Role of levamisole immunotherapy as an adjuvant to radiotherapy in oral cancer. I. A three-year clinical follow up, *Neoplasma* **34**:627–632.

Panettiere, F. J., and Chen, T. T., 1981, Analysis of 626 patients entered on the SWOG large bowel adjuvant program, in: *Proceedings of the Third International Conference on the Adjuvant Therapy of Cancer,* (S. E. Salmon and S. E. Jones, eds.), Grune and Stratton, New York, pp. 539–546.

Papa, M. Z., Yang, J. C., Vetto, J. T., Shiloni, E., Eisenthal, A., and Rosenberg, S. A., 1988, Combined effects of chemotherapy and interleukin 2 in the therapy of mice with advanced pulmonary tumors, *Cancer Res.* **48**:122–129.

Paterson, A. H. G., Willans, D. J., Jerry, L. M., Hanson, J., and McPherson, T. A., 1984, Adjuvant BCG immunotherapy for malignant melanoma, *Can. Med. Assoc. J.* **131**:744–748.

Paul, W. E., and Ohara, J., 1987, B-cell stimulatory factor-1/interleukin 4, *Annu. Rev. Immunol.* **5**:429–459.

Paulnock, D. M., and Borden, E. C., 1985, Modulation of immune functions by interferons, in: *Immunity to Cancer,* (A. W. Reif and M. Mitchell, eds.), Academic Press, New York, pp. 545–559.

Pellegrino, M. A., Ng, A.-K., Russo, C., and Ferrone, S., 1982, Heterogenous distribution of the determinants defined by monoclonal antibodies on HLA-A and B antigens bearing molecules, *Transplantation* **34**:18–23.

Phillips, J. H., and Lanier, L. L., 1986, Dissection of the lymphokine-activated killer phenomenon: Relative contribution of peripheral blood natural killer cells and T lymphocytes to cytolysis, *J. Exp. Med.* **164**:814–825.

Pilch, Y. H., Veltman, L. L., and Kern, D. H., 1974, Immune cytolysis of human tumor cells mediated by xenogenic "immune" RNA: Implications for immunotherapy, *Surgery* **76**:23–34.

Pimm, M. V., 1987, Immunoscintigraphy: Tumor detection with radiolabeled antitumor monoclonal antibodies, in: *Immunology of Malignant Diseases* (V. S. Byers and R. W. Baldwin, eds.), MTP Press, Lancaster, pp. 21–43.

Pimm, M. V., Perkins, A. C., Armitage, N. C., and Baldwin, R. W., 1985, The characteristics of blood born radiolabels and the effect of anti-mouse IgG antibodies on localization of radiolabelled monoclonal antibody in cancer patients, *J. Nucl. Med.* **26**:1011–1023.

Pinsky, C. M., Hirshaut, Y., Wanebo, H. J., Fortner, J. G., Mike, V., Schottenfeld, D., and
    Oettgen, H. F., 1976, Randomized trial of bacillus Calmette Guerin (percutaneous administra-
    tion) as surgical adjuvant immunotherapy for patients with stage II melanoma, *Ann. N.Y. Acad.
    Sci.* **277**:187–194.
Pinsky, C. M., Camacho, F. J., Kerr, D., Geller, N. L., Klein, F. A., Herr, H. A., Whitmore, W.
    F., Jr., and Oettgen, H. F., 1985, Intravesical administration of bacillus Calmette–Guerin in
    patients with recurrent superficial carcinoma of the urinary bladder: Report of a prospective,
    randomized trial, *Cancer Treat. Rep.* **69**:47–53.
Pizza, G., Severini, G., Menniti, D., de Vinci, C., and Corrado, F., 1984, Tumour regression after
    intralesional injectin of interleukin 2 (IL-2) in bladder cancer. Preliminary report, *Int. J. Cancer*
    34:359–367.
Plowman, G. D., Brown, J. P., Enns, C. A., Schroder, J., Nikinmaa, B., Sussman, H. H.,
    Hellstrom, K. E., and Hellstrom, I., 1983, Assignment of the gene for human malanoma-
    associated antigen p97 to chromosome 3, *Nature* **303**:70–72.
Prout, G. R., 1973, The kidney and ureter, in: *Cancer Medicine* (J. F. Holland and E. Frei, eds.),
    Lea & Febiger, Philadelphia, pp. 1655–1699.
Quesada, J. R. Swanson, D. A., Trindade, A., and Gutterman, J. U., 1983, Renal cell carcinoma:
    Antitumor effects of leukocyte interferon, *Cancer Res.* **43**:940–947.
Quesada, J. R., Rios, A., Swanson, D., Trown, P., and Gutterman, J. U., 1985a, Antitumor activity
    of recombinant-derived interferon alpha in metastatic renal cell carcinoma, *J. Clin. Oncol.* **3**:
    1522–1528.
Quesada, J. R., Swanson, D. A., and Gutterman, J. U., 1985b, Phase II study of interferon alpha in
    metastatic renal-cell carcinoma: A progress report, *J. Clin. Oncol.* **3**:1086–1092.
Quesada, J. R., Kurzrock, R., Sherwin, S. A., and Gutterman, J. U., 1987, Phase II studies of
    recombinant human interferon gamma in metastatic renal cell carcinoma, *J. Biol. Resp. Mod.* **6**:
    20–27.
Rambaldi, A., Introna, M., Colotta, F., Landolfo, S., Colombo, N., Mangioni, C., and Mantovani,
    A., 1985, Intraperitoneal administration of interferon β in ovarian cancer patients, *Cancer* **56**:
    294–301.
Real, F. X., Oettgen, H. F., and Krown, S. E., 1986, Kaposi's sarcoma and the acquired immu-
    nodeficiency syndrome: Treatment with high and low doses of recombinant leukocyte A inter-
    feron, *J. Clin. Oncol.* **4**:544–551.
Reid, J. W., Cannon, G. B., Perlin, E., Blom, J., Connor, R., and Herberman, R. B., 1982,
    Immunologically defined prognostic subgroups as predictors of response to BCG immu-
    notherapy, *Recent Res. Cancer Res.* **80**:219–226.
Retsas, S., Priestman, T. J., Newton, K. A., and Westbury, G., 1983, Evaluation of human
    lymphoblastoid interferon in advanced malignant melanoma, *Cancer* **51**:273–276.
Revel, M., Kimchi, A., Shulman, L., Shuster, R., Yakobson, E., Chernajovsky, Y., Schmidt, A.,
    Shure, A., and Bendori, R., 1980, Role of interferon-induced enzymes in the antiviral and
    antimitogenic effects of interferon, *Ann. N.Y. Acad. Sci.* **350**:459–472.
Richardson, G. S., Scully, R. E., Nikrui, N., and Nelson, J. H., 1985, Common epithelial cancer of
    the ovary, *N. Engl. J. Med.* **312**:415, 474.
Richie, J., Shipley, W. U., and Yagoda, A., 1985, Cancer of the bladder, in: *Cancer, Principles and
    Practice of Oncology* (V. T. Devita, S. Hellman, and S. T. Rosenberg, eds.), J. B. Lippincott,
    Philadelphia, pp. 915–928.
Richman, S. P., Livingston, R. S., Gutterman, J. U., Suen, J. Y., and Hersh, E. M., 1976,
    Chemotherapy versus chemoimmunotherapy of head and neck cancer: Report of a randomized
    study, *Cancer Treat. Rep.* **60**:535–539.
Rinehart, J., Malspeis, L., Young, D., and Neidhart, J., 1986a, Phase I/II trial of human recombi-
    nant β-interferon serine in patients with renal cell carcinoma, *Cancer Res.* **46**:5364–5367.
Rinehart, J. J., Malspeis, L., Young, D., and Neidhart, J. A., 1986b, Phase I/II trial of human
    recombinant interferon gamma in renal cell carcinoma, *J. Biol. Resp. Mod.* **5**:300–308.

Rios, A., Mansell, P. W. A., Newell, G. R., Reuben, J. M., Hersh, E. M., and Gutterman, J. U., 1985a, Treatment of acquired immunodeficiency syndrome-related Kaposi's sarcoma with lymphoblastoid interferon, *J. Clin. Oncol.* **3**:506–512.

Rios, P., Marsell, G., and Reuben, J., 1985b, The use of lymphoblastoid interferon Hu IFNα (Ly) and vinblastine in the treatment of acquired immune deficiency syndrome (AIDS) related Kaposi's sarcoma (KS), *Proc. ASCO* **4**:6.

Robinson, E., Haim, N., Segal, R., Veseley, Z., and Mekori, T., 1985, Combined-modality treatment of inoperable lung cancer (iv immunotherapy, chemotherapy, and radiotherapy), *Cancer Treat. Rep.* **69**:251–258.

Robinson, W. A., Mughal, T. I., Thomas, M. R., Johnson, M., and Spiegel, R. J., 1986, Treatment of metastatic malignant melanoma with recombinant interferon alpha 2, *Immunobiology* **172**: 275–282.

Robustelli della Cuna, G., Pavesi, L., Knerich, R., Preti, P., and Paoletti, P., 1984, Radio-chemo-immunotherapy (CCNU plus levamisole) for treatment of metastatic brain tumors. A pilot study, *J Neuro-Oncol.* **2**:237–240.

Roitt, I. M., Thanavala, Y. M., Mule, D. K., and Huy, F. C., 1985, Anti-idiotypes as surrogate antigens: Structural considerations, *Immunol. Today* **6**:265–267.

Romics, I., Horvath, J., Feher, J., and Csontai, A., 1985, Effect of levamisole on cellular and humoral immune reactivity and on recurrences in patients with bladder papilloma, *Int. Urol. Nephrol.* **17**:323–330.

Rosenberg, S. A., 1988, Editorial: Cancer therapy with interleukin-2: Immunologic manipulations can mediate the regression of cancer in humans, *J. Clin. Oncol.* **6**:403–406.

Rosenberg, S. A., Lotze, M. T., Muul, L. M., Leitman, S., Chang, A. E., Ettinghausen, S. E., Matory, Y. L., Skibber, J. M., Shiloni, E., Vetto, J. T., Seipp, C. A., Simpson, C., and Reichert, C. M., 1985a, Observations on the systemic administration of autologous lymphokine-activated killer cells and recombinant interleukin-2 to patients with metastatic cancer, *N. Engl. J. Med.* **313**:1485–1492.

Rosenberg, S. A., Mule, J. J., Spiess, P. J., Reichert, C. M., and Schwarz, S. L., 1985b, Regression of established pulmonary metastases and subcutaneous tumor mediated by the systemic administration of high-dose recombinant IL-2, *J. Exp. Med.* **161**:1169–1188.

Rosenberg, S. A., Spiess, P., and Lafreniere, R., 1986, A new approach to the adoptive immunotherapy of cancer with tumor infiltrating lymphocytes, *Science* **233**:1318–1321.

Rosenberg, S. A., Lotze, M. T., Muul, L. M., Chang, A. E., Avis, F. P., Leitman, S., Linehan, W. M., Robertson, C. N., Lee, R. E., Rubin, J. T., Seipp, C. A., Simpson, C. G., and White, D. E., 1987, A progress report on the treatment of 157 patients with advanced cancer using lymphokine-activated killer cells and interleukin-2 or high-dose interleukin-2 alone, *N. Engl. J. Med.* **316**:889–897.

Rossi, G. A., Felletti, R., Balbi, B., Sacco, O., Cosulich, E., Risso, A., Melioli, G., and Ravazzoni, C., 1987, Symptomatic treatment of recurrent malignant pleural effusions with intrapleurally administered *Corynebacterium parvum:* Clinical response is not associated with evidence of enhancement of local cellular-mediated immunity, *Am. Rev. Respir. Dis.* **135**:885–890.

Rosso, R., Nobile, M. T., Sertoli, M. R., Giannitelli, A., Santi, P. L., Volpe, R., and Nicolo, G., 1985, Antitumoral activity of human fibroblast interferon administered intranodularly, *Oncology* **42**:86–88.

Roszkowski, K., Nozdryn-Plotnicki, B., Roszkowski, W., Ko, H. L., Jeljaszewicz, J., and Pulverer, G., 1985, Small-cell lung cancer and immunochemotherapy with *Propionibacterium granulosum* KP 45, *J. Cancer Res. Clin. Oncol.* **109**:72–77.

Roth, J. A., Grimm, E. A., Guptol, R. K., and Ames, R. S., 1982, Immunoregulatory factors derived from human tumors: Immunologic and biochemical characterization of factors that suppress lymphocyte proliferative and cytotoxic responses *in vitro*, *J. Immunol.* **128**:1955–1962.

Rowland, G. F., Axton, C. A., Baldwin, R. W., Brown, J. P., Corvalan, J. R. F., Embleton, M. J., Gore, V. A., Hellstrom, I., Hellstrom, K. E., Jacobs, E., Marsden, C. H., Pimm, M. V., Simmonds, R. G., and Smith, W., 1985, Antitumor properties of vindesine–monoclonal antibody conjugates, *Cancer Immunol. Immunother.* **19:**1–7.

Rubin, B. Y., and Gupta, S. L., 1980, Differential efficacies of human type I and type II interferons as antiviral and antiproliferative agents, *Proc. Natl. Acad. Sci. U.S.A.* **77:**5928–5932.

Sadoughi, N., Mlsna, J., Guinau, P., and Rubenstone, A., 1982, Prognostic value of cell surface antigens using immunoperoxidase methods in bladder carcinoma, *Urology* **20:**143–146.

Sahasrabudhe, D. M., deKernion, J. B., Pontes, J. E., Ryan, D. M., O'Donnell, R. W., Maarquis, D. M., Mudholkar, G. S., and McCune, C. S., 1986, Specific immunotherapy with suppressor function inhibition for metastatic renal cell carcinoma, *J. Biol. Resp. Mod.* **5:**581–594.

Sarna, G. P., and Figlin, R. A., 1985, Phase II trial of α-lymphoblastoid interferon given weekly as treatment of advanced breast cancer, *Cancer Treat. Rep.* **69:**547–549.

Sarna, G., Pertcheck, M., Figlin, R., and Ardalan, B., 1986, Phase I study of recombinant β ser 17 interferon in the treatment of cancer, *Cancer Treat. Rep.* **70:**1365–1372.

Sarna, G., Figlin, R., and de Kernion, J., 1987, Interferon in renal cell carcinoma: The UCLA experience, *Cancer* **59:**610–612.

Schantz, S. P., Skolnik, E. M., and O'Neill, J. V., 1980, Improved survival associated with postoperative wound infection in laryngeal cancer: An analysis of its therapeutic implications, *Otolaryngol. Head Neck Surg.* **88:**412–417.

Schellhammer, P. F., Ladaga, L. E., and Fillion, M. B., 1986, Bacillus Calmette–Guerin for superficial transitional cell carcinoma of the bladder, *J. Urol.* **135:**261–264.

Schiller, J. H., Storer, B., Willson, J. K. V., and Borden, E. C., 1987, Phase II trial of combined recombinant beta and gamma interferons in patients with advanced malignant melanoma, *Proc. ASCO* **6:**244.

Schreiber, M. M., Bozzo, P. D., and Moon, T. E., 1981, Malignant melanoma in Southern Arizona, *Arch. Dermatol.* **117:**6–11.

Schreml, W., Lang, M., Betzler, M., Schlag, P., Lohrmann, H. P., Heimpel, H., and Herfarth, C., 1983, Adjuvant chemo(immuno-)-therapy of primary breast cancer with adriamycin-cyclophosphamide (and levamisole)—six-year evaluation, *Eur. J. Cancer Clin. Oncol.* **19:**607–613.

Schulof, R. S., Simon, G. L., Sztein, M. B., Parenti, D. M., DiGioia, R. A., Courtless, J. W., Orenstein, J. M., Kessler, C. M., Kind, P. D., Schlesselman, S., Paxton, H. M., Robert-Guroff, M., Naylor, P. H., and Goldstein, A. L., 1986, Phase I/II trial of thymosin fraction 5 and thymosin alpha one in HTLV-III seropositive subjects, *J. Biol. Resp. Mod.* **5:**429–443.

Scorticatti, C. H., LaPena, N. C., Bellora, O. G., Mariotto, R. A., Casabe, A. R., and Comolli, R., 1982, Systemic IFN-alpha treatment of multiple papilloma grade I or II patients: Pilot study, *J. Interferon Res.* **2:**339–343.

Scott, M. T., 1974, *Corynebacterium parvum* as a therapeutic antitumor agent in mice, *J. Natl. Cancer Inst.* **53:**861–865.

Scully, C., 1983, Immunology and oral cancer, *Br. J. Oral. Surg.* **21:**136–146.

Sears, H. F., Herlyn, D., Steplewski, Z., and Koprowski, H., 1985, Phase II clinical trial of a murine monoclonal antibody cytotoxic for gastrointestinal adenocarcinoma, *Cancer Res.* **45:**5910–5913.

Sell, S. (ed.), 1980, *Cancer Markers, Diagnositic and Developmental Significance*, Humana Press, Clifton, NJ.

Sell, S., 1982, Hepatocellular carcinoma markers, in: *Human Cancer Markers* (S. Sell and B. Wahren, eds.), Humana Press, Clifton, NJ, pp. 133–164.

Sen, G. C., 1984, Biochemical pathways in interferon action, *Pharmacol. Ther.* **24:**235–257.

Sertoli, M. R., Guarneri, D., Rubagotti, A., Porcile, G., Nobile, M. T., and Rosso, R., 1987, Adjuvant immunochemotherapy in colorectal cancer Dukes C, *Oncology* **44:**78–81.

Sharpless, G. R., Davies, M. C., and Cox, H. R., 1950, Antagonistic action of certain neurotropic viruses toward a lymphoid tumor in chickens with the resulting immunity, *Proc. Soc. Exp. Biol. Med.* **73**:270–275.

Shawler, D., Bartholomew, R., Smith, L., and Dillman, R., 1985, Human immune response to multiple injections of murine monoclonal IgG, *J. Immunol.* **135**:1530–1535.

Shibata, S., Mori, K., Moriyama, T., Tanaka, K., and Moroki, J., 1987, Randomized controlled study of the effect of adjuvant immunotherapy with picibanil on 51 malignant gliomas, *Surg. Neurol.* **27**:259–263.

Shiloni, E., Eisenthal, A., Sachs, D., and Rosenberg, S. A., 1987, Antibody-dependent cellular cytotoxicity mediated by murine lymphocytes activated in recombinant interleukin 2, *J. Immunol.* **138**:1992–1998.

Shively, J. E., and Todd, C. W., 1980, Carcinoembryonic antigen A: Chemistry and biology, in: *Cancer Markers, Diagnostic and Developmental Significance* (S. Sell, ed.), Humana Press, Clifton, NJ, pp. 295–314.

Shu, S., Chou, T., and Rosenberg, S. A., 1987, Generation from tumor bearing mice of lymphocytes with *in vivo* therapeutic efficacy, *J. Immunol.* **139**:295–304.

Silgals, R. M., Ahlgren, J. D., Neefe, J. R., Rothman, J., Rudnick, S., Galicky, P., and Schein, P. S., 1984, A phase II trial of high-dose intravenous interferon alpha-2 in advanced colorectal cancer, *Cancer* **54**:2257–2261.

Silverberg, E., 1984, Cancer statistics, *Cancer J. Clin.* **34**:14.

Silverberg, E., and Lubera, J., 1986, Cancer statistics, *Cancer J. Clin.* **36**:9.

Silverberg, E., and Lubera, J., 1987, Cancer statistics, *Cancer J. Clin.* **37**:2.

Silverberg, E., and Lubera, J. A., 1988, Cancer statistics, 1988, *Cancer J. Clin.* **38**:5–22.

Sinkovics, J. G., 1986, Colorectal carcinoma, in: *Medical Oncology, an Advanced Course*, Vol. 2, Marcel Dekker, New York, pp. 981–1045.

Smith, J., Bookman, M., Carrasquillo, S., Larson, S., Reynolds, J., Dailey, V., Perentesis, P., Urba, W., McKnight, J., Clark, J., McCabe, R., Hanna, M., Haspel, M., Longo, D., and Steis, R., 1987, Evaluation of a human anti-colorectal carcinoma monoclonal antibody in patients with metastatic colorectal cancer, *Proc. ASCO* **6**:250.

Solal-Celigny, P., Simeon, J., Herrera, A., Vinci, G., Bertrand, O., Mahieu, P., Kinet, J. P., Raspaud, S., Sinegre, M., and Boivin, P., 1986, Effects of *ex-vivo* plasma adsorption over protein A sepharose in acute leukemia, *Leuk. Res.* **10**:643–649.

Soloway, M. S., and Perry, A., 1987, Bacillus Calmette–Guerin for treatment of superficial transitional cell carcinoma of the bladder in patients who have failed thiotepa and/or mitomycin C, *J. Urol.* **137**:871–873.

Spitler, L. E. Wybran, J., Fudenberg, H. H., Pirofsky, B., August, C. S., Stiehm, R., Hitzig, W. H., Gatti, R. A., 1972, Transfer factor therapy of malignant melanoma, *J. Clin. Invest.* **51**:3216–3224.

Steinitz, M., Klein, G., Koskimies, S., and Makel, O., 1977, EB virus-induced B lymphocyte cell lines producing specific antibody, *Nature* **269**:420–422.

Sterchi, J. M., Wells, H. B., Case, L. D., Spurr, C. L., White, D. R., Richards, F., Muss, H. B., Jackson, D. V., Stuart, J. J., Cooper, R., and the Piedmont Oncology Group, 1985, A randomized trial of adjuvant chemotherapy and immunotherapy in stage I and stage II cutaneous melanoma, *Cancer* **55**:707–712.

Suen, J. Y., Richman, S. P., Livingston, R. B., Hersh, E. M., Craig, R., and Tonymon, K., 1977, Results of BCG adjuvant immunotherapy in 100 patients with epidermoid carcinoma of the head and neck, *Am. J. Surg.* **134**:474–478.

Symonds, E. M., Perkins, A. C., Pimm, M. V., Baldwin, R. W., Hardy, J. G., and Williams, D. A., 1985, Clinical implications for immunoscintigraphy in patients with ovarian malignancy: A preliminary study using monoclonal antibody 791T/36, *Br. J. Obstet. Gynaecol.* **92**:270–276.

Takita, M., Hollinshead, A., Hart, J. T., Bhayana, J., Adler, R., Rao, U., Moskowitz, R., and

Ramundo, M., 1985, Adjuvant specific immunotherapy of resectable squamous cell lung carcinoma. Analysis at the eighth year, *Cancer Immunol. Immunother.* **20**:231–235.

Taylor, S. G., Sisson, G. A., Bytell, D. E., Raynor, J. W. J., 1983, A randomized trial of adjuvant BCG immunotherapy in head and neck cancer, *Arch. Otolaryngol.* **109**:544–548.

Taylor-Papadimitrous, J., 1984, Effects of interferons on cell growth and function, in: *Interferon General and Applied Aspects* (A. Billiau, ed.), Elsevier, Amsterdam, p. 139.

Terry, W. D., and Rosenberg, S. A., 1982, *Immunotherapy of Human Cancer*, Elsevier/North-Holland, New York.

Thatcher, N., Honeybourne, D., Wagstaff, J., Carroll, K. B., Barber, P. V., Morrison, J. B., and Crowther, D., 1984, Moderate to high dose cyclophosphamide and intercalated *Corynebacterium parvum* in patients with metastatic lung cancer, *Br. J. Dis. Chest* **78**:89–97.

Thatcher, N., Mene, A., Banerjee, S. S., Craig, P., Gleave, N., and Orton, C., 1986a, Randomized study of *Corynebacterium parvum* adjuvant therapy following surgery for (stage II) malignant melanoma, *Br. J. Surg.* **73**:111–115.

Thatcher, N., Wagstaff, J., Mene, A., Smith, D., Orton, C., and Craig, P., 1986b, *Corynebacterium parvum* followed by chemotherapy (actinomycin D and DTIC) compared with chemotherapy alone for metastatic malignant melanoma, *Eur. J. Cancer Clin. Oncol.* **22**:1009–1014.

Tokunaga, T., Yamamoto, S., Nakamura, R. M., and Katoaka, T., 1974, Immunotherapeutic and immunoprophylactic effects of BCG on 3-methylcholanthrene-induced autochthonous tumors in Swiss mice, *J. Natl. Cancer Inst.* **53**:459–463.

Torti, F. M., and Lum, B. L., 1984, The biology and treatment of superficial bladder cancer, *J. Clin. Oncol.* **2**:505–531.

Torti, F. M., and Lum, B. L., 1987, Superficial bladder cancer: Risk of recurrence and potential role for interferon therapy, *Cancer* **59**:613–616.

Torti, F. M, Shortliffe, L. D., Williams, R. D., Spaulding, J. T., Hannigan, J. F., Jr., Palmer, J., Meyers, F. J., Higgins, M., and Freiha, F. S., 1984, Superficial bladder cancers are responsive to alpha-2 interferon administered intravesically, *Proc. Am. Soc. Clin. Oncol.* **3**:160.

Torti, F. M., Shortliffe, L. D., Williams, R. D., Pitts, W. C., Kempson, R. L., Ross, J. C., Palmer, J., Meyers, F., Ferrari, M., Hannigan, J., Spiegel, R., McWhirter, K., and Freiha, F., 1988, Alpha-interferon in superficial bladder cancer: A Northern California Oncology Group study, *J. Clin. Oncol.* **6**:476–483.

Treurniet-Donker, A. D., Meischke-de Jongh, M. L., van Putten, W. L. J., 1987, Levamisole as adjuvant immunotherapy in breast cancer, *Cancer* **59**:1590–1593.

Trump, D. L., Elson, P. J., Borden, E. C., Harris, J. E., Tuttle, R. L., Whisnant, J. K. Oken, M. M., Carignan, J. R., Ruckdeschel, J. C., and Davis, T. E., 1987, High-dose lymphoblastoid interferon in advanced renal cell carcinoma: An Eastern Cooperative Oncology Group study, *Cancer Treat. Rep.* **71**:165–169.

Tykka, H., 1981, Active specific immunotherapy with supportive measures in the treatment of advanced palliatively nephrectomised renal adenocarcinoma. A controlled clinical study, *Scand. J. Urol. Nephrol. (Suppl.)* **63**:1.

Umeda, T., and Niijima, T., 1986, Phase II study of alpha interferon on renal cell carcinoma, *Cancer* **58**:1231–1235.

Vadhan-Raj, S., Nathan, C. F., Sherwin, S. A., Oettgen, H. F., and Krown, S. E., 1986, Phase I trial of recombinant interferon gamma by 1-hour iv infusion, *Cancer Treat. Rep.* **70**:609–614.

van der Burg, M., Edelstein, M., Gerlis, L., Liang, C.-M., Hirschi, M., and Dawson, A., 1985, Recombinant interferon-γ (immuneron): Results of a phase I trial in patients with cancer, *J. Biol. Resp. Mod.* **4**:264–272.

Veltman, L. L., Kern, D. H., and Pilch, Y. H., 1974, Immune cytolysis of human tumor cells mediated by xenogenic "immune" RNA, *Cell. Immunol.* **13**:367–377.

Vilcek, J., Kelke, H. C., Jimming, L. E., and Yip, Y. K., 1985, The structure and function of human interferon-α, in: *Mediators in Cell Growth and Differentiation* (R. J. Ford, ed.), Raven Press, New York, pp. 299–313.

Vitetta, E. S., and Uhr, J. W., 1985, Immunotoxins, *Annu. Rev. Immunol.* **3**:197–212.

Volberding, P. A., Mitsuyasu, R. T., Golando, J. P., and Spiegel, R. J., 1987, Treatment of Kaposi's sarcoma with interferon alpha-2b (Intron^{R}A), *Cancer* **59**:620–625.

Vugrin, D., Hood, L., Taylor, W., and Laszio, J., 1985, Phase II study of human lymphoblastoid interferon in patients with advanced renal carcinoma, *Cancer Treat. Rep.* **69**:817–820.

Walker, A. E., Robins, M., and Weinfeld, F. D., 1985, Epidemiology of brain tumors: The national survey of intracranial neoplasms, *Neurology* **35**:219–226.

Wallack, M. K., McNally, K. R., Leftheriotis, E., Seiger, H., Balch, C., Wanebo, H., Bartolucci, A. A., and Bash, J. A., 1986a, A Southeastern Cancer Study Group phase I/II trial with vaccinia melanoma oncolysates, *Cancer* **57**:649–655.

Wallack, M. K., McNally, K., Michaelides, M., Bash, J., Bartolucci, A., Siegler, H., Balch, C., and Wanebo, H., 1986b, A phase I/II SECSG (Southeastern Cancer Study Group) pilot study of surgical adjuvant immunotherapy with vaccinia melanoma oncolysates (VMO), *Am. Surgeon* **52**:148–151.

Weiner, R. S., Reich, S. D., Youngblood, M. W., and Witman, P. A., 1987, Phase I/II study of r-interferon-gamma and BCNU in metastatic melanoma, *Proc. AACR* **28**:377.

Weiss, D. W., 1972, Nonspecific stimulation and modulation of the immune response and of states of resistance by the MER fraction of tubercle bacilli, *Natl. Cancer. Inst. Monogr.* **35**:157–171.

Weiss, D. W., Bonhag, R. S., and Parks, J. A., 1964, Studies on the heterologous immunogenicity of a methanol-insoluble fraction of attenuated tubercle bacilli (BCG), *J. Exp. Med.* **119**:53–70.

Welander, C. E., 1987, Use of interferon in the treatment of ovarian cancer as a single agent and in combination with cytotoxic drugs, *Cancer* **59**:617–619.

Winchester, R. J., Wang, C.-Y., Gibofsky, A., Kunkel, H. G., Lloyd, K. O., and Old, L. J., 1978, Expression of Ia-like antigens on cultured human malignant melanoma cell lines, *Proc. Natl. Acad. Sci. U.S.A.* **75**:6235–6239.

Winkelhake, J. L., Stampfl, S., and Zimmerman, R. J., 1987, Synergistic effects of combination therapy with human recombinant interleukin-2 and tumor necrosis factor in murine tumor models, *Cancer Res.* **47**:3948–3953.

Woods, J. E., DeSauto, L. W., and Ritts, R. E., 1977, A controlled study of combined methotrexate, BCG, and INH therapy for squamous cell carcinoma of the head and neck, *Surg. Clin. North Am.* **57**:769–778.

Yang, Y.-C., Ciarletta, A. B., Temple, P. A., Chung, M. P., Kovacic, S., Witek-Giannotti, J. S., Leary, A. C., Kriz, R., Donahue, R. E., Wong, G. G., and Clark, S. C., 1986, Human IL-3 (multi-CSF): Identification by expression cloning of a novel hematopoietic growth factor related to murine IL-3, *Cell* **47**:3–10.

Yasumoto, K., Yaita, H., Ohta, M., Azuma, I., Nomoto, K., Inokuchi, K., and Yamamura, Y., 1985, Randomly controlled study of chemotherapy versus chemoimmunotherapy in postoperative lung cancer patients, *Cancer Res.* **45**:1413–1417.

Yasumoto, K., Miyazaki, K., Nagashima, A., Ishida, T., Kuda, T., Yano, T., Sugimachi, K., and Nomoto, K., 1987, Induction of lymphokine-activated killer cells by intrapleural instillations of recombinant interleukin-2 in patients with malignant pleurisy due to lung cancer, *Cancer Res.* **47**:2184–2187.

Zenner, H. P., Kley, W., Claros, P., Claros, A., Labas, Z., Lobe, L. P., Pavelka, R., Plath, P., Ribari, O., Niethammer, D., and Hirche, H., 1985, Recombinant interferon-alpha-2C in laryngeal papillomatosis: Preliminary results of a prospective multicentre trial, *Oncology* **42** (Suppl. 1):15–18.

Ziai, M. R., Imberti, L., Tongson, A., and Ferrone, S., 1985, Differential modulation by recombinant immune interferon of the expression and shedding of HLA antigens and melanoma associated antigens by a melanoma cell line resistant to the antiproliferative activity of immune interferon, *Cancer Res.* **45**:5877–5882.

CHAPTER 4

THE PHARMACOLOGY OF MICROBIAL MODULATION IN THE INDUCTION AND EXPRESSION OF IMMUNE REACTIVITIES

The Pharmacologically Active Effector Molecules of Immunologic Inflammation, Immunity, and Hypersensitivity

ANDOR SZENTIVANYI,
JOSEPH J. KRZANOWSKI, Jr.,
JAMES B. POLSON, and
CHRISTINE M. ABARCA

1. INTRODUCTION

Human life and development are marked by encounters with an infinite range of potentially injurious and destructive microbial agents and their products. Of the various defense systems that establish and sustain homeostasis against such agents and stimuli, this review emphasizes those that involve (1) elements that

ANDOR SZENTIVANYI and CHRISTINE M. ABARCA • Departments of Internal Medicine and Pharmacology, University of South Florida College of Medicine, Tampa, Florida 33612. JOSEPH J. KRZANOWSKI, Jr., and JAMES B. POLSON • Department of Pharmacology and Therapeutics, University of South Florida College of Medicine, Tampa, Florida 33612.

manage first encounters—the inflammatory response, and (2) elements that uti-
lize experience on reencounters—the specific immune response. These systems,
or defense functions, are anatomically, biochemically, and physiopharmacologi-
cally interrelated and interdependent. Each is in continuous interplay with elements of the internal milieu of the host as well as with elements of the host's
environment and, therefore, closely linked with neurohumoral defense
mechanisms.

Regardless of the specific microbial injury for which the inflammatory
response is set in action, the first encounter is a more or less stereotyped reaction.
Cells of predictable type are drawn into the injured area and proceed, for instance, to engulf the microbial material by phagocytosis. Vascular occlusion,
fibrin barriers, and other aspects of the inflammatory response serve to localize
infection and tissue injury and initiate repair.

The functions of the immune defense system are the properties of cells
distributed throughout the body. They include (1) free or circulating cells of the
blood, lymph, and intravascular spaces, (2) similar cells collected into units that
allow for close interaction with lymph or circulating blood—lymph nodes, spleen,
liver, and bone marrow, and (3) two major sources or control organs for the
system—the thymus gland and the hypothalamic–pituitary–adrenal complex.
Constant interchange of cells or their communicating molecules between the units
provides for rapid dissemination of information to each unit. These systems are,
therefore, dynamic, changing constantly in structure and functional capacity in
response to stimuli. Defects in genetic endowment, damage to cell lines, or factors
that alter the rate or quality of accumulation of the memory store of immunologic
experience alter the normal developmental patterns and result in clinical disorders
including immunologically based hypersensitive manifestations.

For convenience, the material currently available on the pharmacology of
microbial modulation in the induction and expression of immune reactivities is
presented in two successive parts: Part I, the present chapter, discusses the
pharmacologically active effector molecules of immunologic inflammation, immunity, and hypersensitivity, while Part II (appearing in Volume 2 of this series)
will present the pharmacological effector mechanisms involved in the microbial
modulation of the afferent and efferent limbs of the immune response.

2. THE CELLS SYNTHESIZING, STORING, SECRETING, AND/OR RELEASING THE PHARMACOLOGICALLY ACTIVE EFFECTOR MOLECULES

These cells seem to represent a continuous spectrum of related or unrelated
cell types specialized in the production and storage of various pharmacologically
active effector substances in variable proportions (i.e., of cells that might have a
common developmental origin), with differentiation being determined by the
specific requirements of the local neurohumoral regulation.

Accounting only for those mediators for which the cell type has been identified, this arbitrary spectrum of mediator-storing, -synthesizing, and -transporting cells includes lymphocytes and mononuclear cells (lymphokines, monokines, cytokines, lysosome and complement components, prostaglandins, leukotrienes, acid hydrolases, neutral proteinases, arginase, plasma proteins, nucleotide metabolites, and various neuroactive immunoregulatory peptides including ACTH, CRF-like activity, β-endorphin, TSH, SP, SOMs, etc.); neutrophil leukocytes (SRS-A, ECF-A, enzymes, PAF and other vascular permeability factors, kinin-generating substances, a complement-activating factor, histamine releasers, a neutrophil inhibitory factor, VIP, and 5-HETE); basophilic leukocytes (histamine, SRS-A, ECF-A, NCF, PAF, SP, and SOMs); murine basophilic leukocytes (histamine, serotonin, SRS-A, ECF-A, PAF, SP, and SOMs); eosinophilic leukocytes (PAF, 8,15-diHETE, and SRS-A); serosal, connective tissue, or TC mast cells (histamine, SRS-A, ECF-A, NCF, PAF, VIP, SP, SOMs); mucosal or T mast cells (histamine, SRS-A, ECF-A, NCF, PAF, VIP, SP, SOMs); "chromaffin-positive" mast cells (dopamine in ruminants; in other mammals possibly norepinephrine); the so-called P cells (histamine, serotonin); enterochromaffin cells (serotonin); chromaffin cells (catecholamines); platelets (depending on species, histamine, serotonin, catecholamines, prostaglandins, 12-HETE); neurosecretory cells (histamine, serotonin, catecholamines, acetylcholine, prostaglandins, and other eicosanoids as well as a group of neuroactive immunoregulatory peptides); the medullary thymic epithelial cells and the Hassals corpuscles (thymosins and other thymic factors); the SIF cells (dopamine); and other nerve cells (all amine mediators, prostaglandins and other eicosanoids, kinins, and other neuroactive immunoregulatory peptides) (Szentivanyi et al., 1980; Szentivanyi and Fitzpatrick, 1980; Hadden et al., 1983; Dale and Forman, 1984; Dixon and Fisher, 1983; Hadden and Szentivanyi, 1985; Gillis and Inman, 1985; Locke et al., 1985; Stites et al., 1987; Galli and Lichtenstein, 1988).

Many of these cell types possess different embryological, morphological, physiocochemical, and general biological characteristics. Nevertheless, in passing from one member of the mediator-containing cell spectrum to another, obvious transitions can be seen in all these characteristics. Furthermore, when one surveys their properties and their probable physiological function in the higher organism, certain cohesive features become apparent that set them apart from other body constituents as a distinct single class of cells that could be included in a generalized concept of neurosecretion.

3. THE PHARMACOLOGICALLY ACTIVE EFFECTOR MOLECULES OF IMMUNE, INFLAMMATORY, AND HYPERSENSITIVITY RESPONSES

Since in the design of these reviews, Section 2 serves only to introduce the remainder, we shall only discuss those agents that may have an apparent major role in the pharmacology of microbial modulation in the induction and expression of immune reactivities.

4. LYMPHOKINES, MONOKINES, AND CYTOKINES

For more than a half century, the antibody has been the focal effector molecule of immunologic thinking and investigation. Even in the era of modern immunology, the antibody molecule continued to dominate concepts that sought to explain the functioning of the immune system (Szentivanyi et al., 1987). Only in the 1970s did researchers develop an awareness and growing appreciation that lymphocytic and monocytic products other than immunoglobulins are largely responsible for a complex array of cell cooperative activities. We now know that these lymphokine and monokine activities have an essential role in the communication of immunocompetent and accessory cells and, consequently, in the regulation of the immune system (de Weck et al., 1980; Hadden and Stewart, 1981; Kahn and Hill, 1982; Hadden and Szentivanyi, 1985).

At this early point in the development of this field, it is not possible to state with any certainty the types, numbers, range, and sequence of activities in biochemical or enzymatic cascades by which this growing spectrum of effector molecules fits precisely into the multicellular network that constitutes the immune system. Therefore, the discussion that follows will have to be severely limited to a brief account of some of the best known of these effector molecules.

Furthermore, it is to be added that many of these agents, such as lymphotoxins, growth inhibitory factors, interferons, and colony-stimulating factors, are produced by a wide variety of normal, damaged, or infected cells (fibroblasts, keratinocytes, Langerhans' cells, tumor cells, etc.). In the broader sense, these substances are cytokines. They can properly be regarded as lymphokines or monokines only when produced by stimulated lymphocytes or activated macrophages; in these instances the lymphocytes and macrophages play the role of focusing and intensifying a phylogenetically ancient, traditional, nonspecific inflammatory mechanism at the site of a specific response.

This range of substances includes effector molecules that affect (1) macrophages, (2) polymorphonuclear leukocytes, (3) lymphocytes, and (4) other cell types.

4.1. Products of Activated Lymphocytes Affecting Macrophages

4.1.1. Macrophage Migration Inhibitory Factor

The first of the lymphokines to be described was the macrophage migration inhibitory factor (MIF). Human MIF has a molecular weight of 23,000 to

55,000; on electrophoresis it migrates with the albumin; it is heat stable and sensitive to chymotrypsin and neuraminidase; and its buoyant density indicates that it is a glycoprotein. Several studies demonstrate that MIF is heterogeneous, and, although there are various hypotheses, it is not yet known how MIF influences macrophage migration. Another lymphokine, originally called macrophage activation factor (MAF), is a macromolecule either very similar to or identical with MIF (Pick, 1981). Both pH3-MIF and pH5-MIF are capable of causing *in vitro* macrophage activation that is essentially identical with that produced by MAF. The changes observed include increased adherence to culture vessel, increased oxidation of glucose through the hexose monophosphate shunt together with increased levels of lactate dehydrogenase in cytoplasm, increased incorporation of glucosamine into membrane components, as well as increased ruffled membrane activity. Likewise, an enhanced bacteriostasis, phagocytosis, pinocytosis, tumoricidal, and membrane adenylate cyclase activities, and the appearance of increased numbers of cytoplasmic granules may be observable. By contrast, MAF, as does MIF, produces a decrease in electron-dense surface material and reduced levels of certain lysosomal enzymes (acid phosphatase, cathepsin-D, β-glucuronidase) (CIBA Foundation, 1985).

It is not known how the inhibition of macrophage migration is related to the late activation of these cells, especially if the two activities reside in the same lymphokine molecule. This refers to the as yet undetermined difference in time needed for the development of these two activities: inhibition of migration of macrophages may be observed within 24 hr, whereas activation of macrophages takes several days to occur. A possible explanation for this difference may lie in the observation that inhibition of macrophage migration is a reversible process, (i.e., cells initially inhibited may again migrate and actually at a higher rate than usual). In other words, the initial MIF effect on a macrophage may change its surface properties so that it becomes more sticky. Later on, as the full complement of the earlier described metabolic changes occur with the resultant macrophage activation, the overall functional capacity of the cell is enhanced (Nathan *et al.*, 1980). It may be added that the interferons (see Section 4.4.2) possess the activities of MAF and MIF, although other proteins may also have these activities. Interferon γ is more potent in its MIF activity than IFN-α or -β (Pick *et al.*, 1981; Szentivanyi and Szentivanyi, 1985).

4.1.2. Macrophage Chemotactic Factor

Antigen- or mitogen-activated lymphocytes also elaborate a chemotactic substance that selectively attracts macrophages or monocytes. This macrophage chemotactic factor (MCF), like MIF, is heterogeneous, as indicated by isoelectric focusing showing peak activities with pI of 10.1 and 5.6. Production of MCF is antigen-specific, and it is heat stable at 56°C with a molecular weight of 12,000 to 25,000 in humans. On electrophoresis, MCF migrates in the part of the gel associated with albumin, and its buoyant density is similar to that of pure protein (van Furth, 1985).

4.2. Products of Activated Lymphocytes Affecting Polymorphonuclear Leukocytes

4.2.1. Leukocyte Inhibitory Factor

Polymorphonuclear leukocytes are inhibited in their migration by a soluble material called leukocyte inhibitory factor (LIF). The LIF, which is produced by sensitized lymphocytes exposed to specific antigen or stimulation by concanavalin A, inhibits only polymorphonuclear migration but not that of macrophages (Snyderman and Goetzl, 1981). Physiocochemically, it appears to be a protease with an approximate molecular weight of 68,000, stability to heat at 56°C, a charge similar to that of albumin, and resistance to neuraminidase but not to chymotrypsin. Separately from LIF, there are chemotactic factors for neutrophils, basophils, and eosinophils produced by sensitized lymphocytes. They are similar in molecular weight, ranging from 24,000 to 55,000, and it is presently unclear whether these factors are all distinct molecular entities or the same substance with chemotactic activity for multiple cell types. Nevertheless, there is some evidence for the existence of two factors that affect the directed movement of eosinophils. One of these requires the interaction of the substance with specific antigen–antibody complexes in order to generate chemotactic activity, whereas the other is active in the absence of antigen–antibody complexes (Stites et al., 1987).

4.2.2. Histamine-Releasing Factors

Another agent that has been described specifically affects the basophil leukocytes. These factors, called histamine-releasing factors (HRFs), were originally described to be produced by sensitized human lymphocytes in response to antigen and nonspecifically by mitogens or viral agents. They have the capacity to induce histamine release from human basophils in a noncytotoxic manner, are nondialyzable, heat-stable, and have a molecular weight of 12,000 (Thueson et al., 1979; Szentivanyi et al., 1983). More recently, Lichtenstein and associates (Liu et al., 1986; Orchard et al., 1986; Schleimer et al., 1986; Warner et al., 1986) have described similar factors derived from alveolar macrophages, platelets, endothelial cells, a macrophage cell line, and in biological fluids, primarily in the course of IgE-mediated late-phase responses. The HRFs that have been described by the Lichtenstein group—but apparently not those described by other workers—activate basophils through an interaction with cell-bound IgE (Galli and Lichtenstein, 1988). Another feature of the HRFs studied by Lichtenstein and his associates is that they can initiate release only from the basophils of certain individuals, i.e., mostly of atopic asthmatic subjects of the extrinsic variety, whereas intrinsic asthmatic subjects and normal individuals are unresponsive (Fisher *et al.*, 1987). It appears from their studies that responsive individuals may have a special species of IgE molecules that can transfer sensitivity to HRF to nonresponder basophils (MacDonald *et al.*, 1987).

4.3. Products of Immunologically Activated Lymphocytes Affecting Nonsensitized Lymphocytes

Activation by specific antigen results in the release of a substance from sensitized lymphocytes that has mitogenic activity for nonsensitized lymphocytes. This factor is known by the designation of lymphocyte mitogenic factor (LMF). This material induces normal lymphocytes to undergo blast transformation and cell multiplication.

4.3.1. Lymphocyte Mitogenic Factor

Lymphocyte mitogenic factor is a nondialyzable macromolecule that is heat stable and resistant to RNase and DNase as well as to treatment with proteolytic enzymes. It has a molecular weight of approximately 20,000–30,000. When this lymphokine was first reported, it was viewed as a thymus-dependent, non-antigen-specific mediator of lymphocyte transformation, and as a probable mediator of lymphocyte cooperation in the immune response.

4.3.2. Lymphocyte-Activating Factor

A second product, "lymphocyte-activating factor" (LAF), which induced and augmented thymocyte proliferation *in vitro*, was found to be a product of macrophages. A link between these two mitogenic factors was forged when it was shown that LMP production by lymphocytes required the presence of macrophages (as does lymphocyte transformation) and that LAF production by macrophages could be stimulated by lymphokines. It appeared probable, therefore, that both macrophage-derived and lymphocyte-derived factors contributed to the activity of what had been termed LMF. When it was found that lectin-induced LMF would permit the long-term growth in culture of T cells, the active substance was termed T-cell growth factor (TCGF) and subsequently was found to allow the continuous proliferation and cloning of functional T lymphocytes able to mediate helper, cytotoxic, and suppressor activities. To direct attention to the intercellular communication role of these effector molecules, the term interleukin (IL) was coined, and LAF renamed IL-1, TCGF IL-2, and a factor promoting T-cell helper function was separately delineated as IL-3 (Dumonde and Hamblin, 1983).

4.3.3. Factors Modulating Antibody Production Released from Stimulated Lymphocytes

In this category, there are some other factors released on stimulation by specific antigen from lymphocytes that modulate antibody production. These factors have not been well characterized, and it is not known whether they are the same factor acting at a different concentrations or several distinct molecular entities. In any case, a material has been described in the mouse that triggers B cells to make IgM-class antibody to sheep red cells, and some other soluble factors have been reported that also increase IgG and IgE antibody production. In humans, an effector substance released by activated lymphocytes induces B cells to proliferate, lose their C3 receptors, and increase their protein synthesis, and it stimulates production of IgG antibody to specific antigens. Conversely, there are also factors capable of suppressing antibody production. Both the enhancing and the antibody-suppressing factors appear to be nondialyzable heat-stable macromolecules with molecular weights of 25,000 to 55,000 (Szentivanyi and Szentivanyi, 1985).

4.3.4. Transfer Factor

Sensitized lymphocytes also contain a substance that is released by either disruption of the cells or stimulation of them with a specific antigen. This material has been first described by Lawrence, and named by him transfer factor because in human beings it was possible to transfer delayed-type hypersensitivity (DTH) to previously unreactive recipients with extracts of these sensitized cells obtained from skin-test-positive donors. Transfer factor (TF) has a molecular weight of less than 4000, and although several laboratories have been successful in partially purifying the active agent, so far no one has produced a homogeneous preparation. Nevertheless, the essential functional components of the molecule appear to be a peptide, a purine base, ribose, and a phosphodiester group (Lawrence and Borkowsky, 1981; Borkowsky and Lawrence, 1981; Hitzig, 1980; Kirkpatrick and Burger, 1981).

Transfer factor can specifically transfer DTH without preparing the host to make antibody against the same antigen. The mechanism by which this is accomplished is not known, but there are two current hypotheses that may be mentioned. One suggestion is that TF enhances antigen sensitivity by potentially responsive T cells. In this view, the cytoplasmic membranes of the T cells possess receptors for antigenic determinants and for specific TFs. Activation of the cell with antigen stimulates release of the membrane-associated TF as well as other lymphokines; TF in turn interacts with membrane receptors on other cells that are potentially reactive to the antigen and renders them more responsive. This cascade effect expands the number of responding cells and thereby provides for clonal expansion, which is a requirement for transfer. A second suggested mechanism involves facilitation of antigen processing and presentation to T cells. Such an effect could occur if TF acted on macrophages or other accessory cells and facilitated cell cooperation, but it would not be antigen specific. This could explain some of the "nonspecific" effects of TF, such as amplification of DNA synthesis by antigen- and mitogen-stimulated cells *in vitro* (Kirkpatrick *et al.*, 1983; and Galbraith and Fudenberg, 1985). Although these are attractive hypotheses, the fact remains that we do not know what TF is or how it works, and immunologists have difficulties linking it with our current knowledge of immunoglobulins and T-cell receptors. The latter become critically important if TF is responsible for delayed hypersensitivity, which is a manifestation of T-cell function, and when it is taken into account that TF lacks the MHC restriction characteristic of T cells. Furthermore, it is too small to be the part of either an immunoglobulin molecule or a T cell that recognizes antigen, which raises the possibility of TF representing a third type of antigen recognition system without knowing what the structure of such a recognition system is and how its diversity is accomplished. For these reasons, at the time of this writing, the physiological significance of TF cannot be assessed (Talmage, 1986).

4.4. Effector Molecules Acting on Cell Types Other Than Lymphocytes

Additional products of activated lymphocytes include cytotoxic factors (i.e., lymphotoxins, which can kill bystander cells or tumor cells); growth inhibitory factors, which prevent the proliferation or cloning of their cells; a group of vertebrate glycoproteins with broad antiviral activity called interferons; factors capable of activating the clotting sequence; effector molecules that increase vascular permeability; colony-stimulating factors; and an agent that activates osteoclasts to solubilize bone.

4.4.1. Lymphotoxins

Thus, sensitized human lymphocytes, in response to specific antigen or mitogens, release an effector molecule or molecules that have cytotoxic effects on certain target cells. Such material or materials are generally referred to as lymphotoxin (LT). The physiochemical properties of human lymphotoxin are heterogeneous, and there are at least three distinguishable molecular species, known as α-LT, β-LT, and γ-LT. Of these, the best characterized so far is α-LT, with a molecular weight of 75,000—100,000, an isoelectric point of 6.8 to 8.0, and stability to heat at 56°C, to storage at 4°C, and to treatment with DNase, RNase, and neuraminidase. On polyacrylamide gel electrophoresis, it appears to be an $\alpha_2'\beta$-globulin. As to its mechanism of action, it is believed that the lymphocyte, having been activated by intimate contact with target cell membranes, is induced to synthesize LT, which binds to the target cell membrane, where it effects target cell lysis. Disruption or physical dislodgement of target cell membrane then promotes the lymphocyte's release from the target cell and subsequent cessation of LT secretion (Papermaster *et al.*, 1981; Pichyangkul *et al.*, 1982; Yamamoto *et al.*, 1982; Klostergard *et al.*, 1982; Dumonde and Hamblin, 1983; Stites *et al.*, 1987).

Some activities also have been described that, rather than causing lysis, inhibit the growth pattern of target cells, specifically involving inhibition of proliferation and inhibition of cloning. It is presently unclear whether the effects of lysis and the foregoing growth inhibitions reflect the activities of three separate macromolecules or of one and the same effector molecule that can exert different effects on different cells, depending on its concentration in its immediate microenvironment (Stites *et al.*, 1987).

4.4.2. The Interferons

Another category of lymphokines, the interferons, represent a group of vertebrate glycoproteins first described by Isaacs and Lindenmann as soluble factors interfering with viral multiplication. Interferons are heterogeneous in terms of both their cellular origin and mode of induction (Stewart, 1981; Merigan and Friedman, 1982). Their most recent classification, based on their antigenicities and molecular structures, defines the three antigenic types and numerous subtype interferons: (1) the antigenic type α, formerly called human leukocyte and lymphoblastoid; (2) type β, fibroblast interferon; and (3) type γ, for the type II, immune, or T-type interferons. One places the designation of the animal species from which the interferon is derived in front of the type designation, using the standard abbreviation IFN for interferon (e.g., human is HuIFN-α or HuIFN-β). Subtypings based on molecular weights are parenthetically indicated, for example, HuIFN-α(21K), and numerical subtypes refer to sequence heterogeneities such as HuIFN-α and HuIFN-β_2 (Lengyel, 1982; Faltynek and Baglioni, 1984).

All three interferon types are found in human and animal systems both *in vivo* and *in vitro*. On the basis of the sequencing of several of the interferons and their genes, α-interferons are a heterogeneous group of proteins. Similar heterogeneities are expected to be found in ongoing investigations among β- and γ-interferons. The three types of interferons are established to be distinct not only antigenically but also with respect to several other properties (e.g., molecular weights, stabilities, cross-species activities, and biological activities) (Sen, 1984).

Extensive work on α- and β-interferons as purely antiviral agents has also revealed several nonantiviral activities. Their first primary effect on interferon-pretreated cells is a better response to the inducers with production of higher levels of interferon. Many other nonantiviral properties are now known to be induced by α- and β-interferons, including inhibition of nonviral agents (bacteria, protozoans), cell multiplication inhibition, toxicity enhancement, increased or depressed cellular synthetic activities, and cell surface alterations. In addition, α- and β-interferons have become noted for their immunomodulatory actions, such as enhancement of immunocytolysis (either cell-mediated or antibody-dependent), promotion of phagocytosis, macrophage activation, inhibition of DTH and graft-versus-host reactions, and effects on humoral antibody production. Several of these associated activities have now been documented as being induced by either very highly purified or even pure interferon preparations, suggesting that interferons are pleiotypic biological response modifiers (Friedman and Vogel, 1983; Vilcek and DeMaeyer, 1984).

Essentially the same properties are possessed by γ-interferon preparations, except that this interferon type appears to have a much higher antitumor activity than the other types in general and a more potent influence on the antitumor activity of macrophages in particular. With recombinant γ-interferon, it was shown that the last-named effect of this agent involves the induction of the priming step in macrophage activation for tumor cell killing (Pace et al., 1983). With respect to its immunomodulatory activities, they include both immunosuppressive and immunoenhancing properties (National Cancer Institute, 1983; Johnson and Torres, 1983), positive regulation of class II antigen expression on macrophages (Steeg et al., 1982; Basham and Merigan, 1983), and activation of T cells for expression of interleukin 2 (IL-2) receptors (Johnson and Farrar, 1983). Interferon-γ production appears to be regulated by a dynamic interaction among various T-cell subsets involving helper cells, suppressor cells, and interferon-producing cells. The helper cell requirement for interferon-γ production is mediated by its product interleukin-2 (Torres et al., 1982), raising the question of whether other effector molecules can replace the IL-2 requirement for interferon-γ production. This issue is revisited in Section 8.7 on neuroactive immunoregulatory peptides.

4.4.3. Tissue Factor

Of the various factors capable of activating the blood-clotting sequence, the "procoagulant factor" or "tissue factor" produced by lymphocytes and monocytes is mentioned here. Mononuclear cells, stimulated by antigen or mitogen, produce a procoagulant material that, when incubated with factor-VIII-deficient plasma, is able to correct the prolonged clotting time. This substance is antigenically distinct from factor VIII and has been identified as "tissue factor." Because of the technical difficulties produced by its lability, it has not yet been well characterized, and its pathophysiological importance also has yet to be determined (Davies, 1984; Wiggins and Cochrane, 1984). Nevertheless, it is intriguing to consider its possible relation to certain manifestations characterized by both lymphocytic infiltration and pathological thrombosis, such as rejection of a transplanted kidney and the delayed hypersensitivity skin test.

4.4.4. Lymph Node Permeability Factor

A vasoactive substance that increases vascular permeability, called "lymph node permeability factor" (LNPF), could be extracted from lymph nodes of immunized animals but could also be obtained in equal amounts from nonimmune animals. The fact that it is released without an immunologic stimulus and is found in numerous nonlymphoid tissues suggests that it may not play a primary role in the delayed hypersensitivity reaction as was originally believed. It may, however, serve as one of the many secondary mediators of the inflammatory process *per se* through its release subsequent to cell or tissue injury (Morley *et al.*, 1984).

4.4.5. Colony-Stimulating Factors

Another category of effector molecules included in this section involves the "colony-stimulating factors" (CSF), which are a group of soluble effector substances that in tissue culture stimulate the differentiation of immature bone marrow precursor cells into granulocytes and macrophages (Burgess *et al.*, 1977). They were so named because they were the only macromolecular requirement, besides components in fetal calf serum, for the formation of colonies of granulocytes or macrophages or both by hemopoietic cells cultured in semisolid medium. One of these, the colony-stimulating factor for granulocytes and macrophages (GM-CSF), has been determined to derive from both IL-3 (see later) and CSF, which is selective for macrophages (Stanley and Heard, 1977). Although blood monocytes and tissue macrophages appear to be a major source of these agents, it is now established that lymphocytes may also actively produce them during immunologic reactions. Colony-stimulating factors are heat-stable glycoproteins with molecular weights in the range of 40,000–60,000 (Stanley, 1981; Ralph, 1984), and because of the discussions that follow, it may be added that CSF for monocytes (purified from a nonlymphoid line) was observed to be a potent stimulant of IL-1 production (Moore *et al.*, 1980); whether this mediator represents the same entity detected in T-cell supernatants has not yet been verified (Oppenheim *et al.*, 1986).

4.4.6. Osteoclast-Activating Factor

Osteoclast-activating factor (OAF) is an effector molecule produced by lymphocytes *in vitro* following antigenic or mitogen stimulation. It is capable of forming osteoclasts in bone and activating these cells. The OAF has a molecular weight of 13,000–25,000, is heat labile, is inactivated by proteolytic enzymes, and can be differentiated from all other established bone-resorbing substances. The nature of its role in immunobiology is unclear at the present time (Mundy, 1981).

5. THE INTERLEUKINS

Phagocytosis by macrophages has been studied since the late 1800s, but it is only since the 1970s that the importance of macrophages as secretory cells has been recognized. More than 50 secretion products of macrophages have been identified so far. Some of the secretion products of the macrophage influence the inflammatory process at its many steps. Lysosome and complement components are secreted constitutively by macrophages in all states of stimulation. Secretion of other products such as arachidonic metabolites, acid hydrolases, and neutral proteinases is triggered and regulated by engagement of specific receptors, by endocytosis, or by exposure of macrophages to membrane-active drugs, including tumor pronators, ionophores, and endotoxin. Activated lymphocytes, tissue pH, oxygen tension, and various other factors are also operative in the regulation of macrophage secretion, which in turn controls the role of macrophages in the inflammatory process (Nathan et al., 1980; van Furth, 1985; CIBA Foundation, 1985).

In this section, however, we address the macrophage not in its role as the professional phagocyte but rather in the context of the initiation of immune responses induced by mitogens or specific antigens. Such roles of the macrophage may be divided into two functional categories: (1) antigen or mitogen binding, processing, and presentation; and (2) synthesis and secretion of a class of effector molecules, the monokines, that act in conjunction with antigen or mitogen to initiate and modulate both T- and B-lymphocyte-mediated immune responses (Unanue and Rosenthal, 1980; Escobar and Friedman, 1980; Adams et al., 1981; Roubin and Benveniste, 1985; Holden and Herberman, 1985; Schultz, 1985).

5.1. Interleukin-1

As the chemical purification and characterization of the foregoing essentially lymphostimulatory factors proceeded, it became increasingly evident that many or most of the properties originally attributed to these factors by various bioassays in fact reside in the same effector molecule. Thus, a consensus was reached at the Second International Lymphokine workshop in 1979 (de Weck et al., 1980) with regard to the definition of the most extensively studied monokine, lymphocyte-activating factor (LAF). On the basis of a number of independent and collaborative studies, it was concluded that LAF is the molecular entity responsible for the biological activities associated with the terms mitogenic protein (MP), helper peaks-1 (HP-1), T-cell-replacing factor III (TRF-III), T-cell-replacing factor Mϕ (TRF$_M$), B-cell-activating factor (BAF), and B-cell differentiation factor (BDF). In order to free the terminology from the constraints associated with definitions by single bioassays, investigators accepted a revised term for LAF, interleukin-1 (IL-1) ("between leukocytes").

Macrophages stimulated with antigen, endotoxin, and other phagocytic stimulants release IL-1. This factor is active across species lines, does not support the growth of interleukin-2 (IL-2)-dependent lymphocyte lines, and is produced by monocytic rather than lymphocytic leukocytes. More recently, it has become evident that IL-1 activities can be produced by virtually every nucleated cell type (Oppenheim *et al.*, 1986, 1987). Polypeptides with molecular weights ranging from 2000 to 75,000 (17 kDa is the predominant form) have been identified to have IL-1 biological activity (Kimbal *et al.*, 1984), although it is generally accepted that the smaller-molecular-weight species are proteolytic breakdown products, and the 75-kDa species represents an aggregated form of the molecule (Dinarello *et al.*, 1984). IL-1-like activities have been reported in protein species with isoelectric points ranging from 4.0 to 8.0, with two predominant species at pI 5.0 and 7.0 (Kampschmidt, 1984; Saklatvala and Sarsfield, 1985; Simon and Willoughby, 1981; Habicht and Beck, 1985). The pI 5.0 species of IL-1 was cloned from the murine P388DI macrophage cell line by Lomedico and associates in 1984. They isolated an IL-1 complementary DNA (cDNA) clone that coded for a 270-amino acid polypeptide precursor lacking a signal peptide and with a predicted molecular weight of 31,000. Subsequently, Auron *et al.* (1984) isolated a human IL-1 cDNA clone from peripheral blood monocytes that encodes a 269-amino-acid precursor also lacking a signal peptide. The amino acid sequence of the 31-kDa precursor includes the 152 amino acids contained in the 17-kDa extracellular form of pI 7.0 IL-1 (Auron *et al.*, 1986). The 269-amino-acid recombinant human IL-1 is cleaved to produce a molecule with most of the reported biological activities of natural IL-1 (Dinarello, 1985). A second human IL-1 gene was discovered when two distinct cDNA clones encoding proteins sharing IL-1 activity from a human macrophage cDNA library were isolated (March *et al.*, 1985). These IL-1 molecules, designated IL-1α and IL-1β, show considerable homology to the murine pI 5.0 and human pI 7.0 IL-1 cDNAs, respectively. A third IL-1 subtype, derived from a B-cell line, has recently been purified to homogeneity (Bertoglio *et al.*, 1987). This molecule of 13.5 kDa displays an isoelectric point of 5, and its N-terminal amino acid sequence is different from that of either monocytic IL-1α or -β. Its serological reactivity confirms this difference, and so does Northern blot analysis using synthetic oligonucleotide as well as cDNA probes failing to reveal mRNA for IL-1α and -β in the 3B6 line. Taken together, these data indicate that IL-1γ is structurally different from Il-1α and -β. Its molecular cloning is currently in progress (Bertoglio *et al.*, 1987).

These IL-1 molecules have been demonstrated to fulfill most of the requirements for macrophages in a competent immune and inflammatory response in general (Oppenheim *et al.*, 1986). Thus, IL-1 agents stimulate T lymphocytes, fibroblasts, and synovial cells, regulate B-lymphocyte differentiation, control the growth of bone marrow cells, and effect the generation of cytotoxic T lymphocytes (Farrar *et al.*, 1982). Furthermore, they stimulate the release of acute-phase reactants by hepatocytes (Dinarello, 1984; Sarto and Mortensen, 1985), induce the release of prostaglandin and collagenase from synovial cells (Dinarello et al., 1983; Sakletvala et al., 1984; Matsushima et al., 1985), and increase the numbers of circulating neutrophils (Kampschmidt et al., 1980). There is also conclusive evidence that IL-1 is identical to "endogenous pyrogen," the elusive macrophage-derived fever-producing factor (Dinarello, 1984; Kampschmidt, 1984). Nevertheless, the IL-1 group cannot replace the functional properties of antigen processing and antigen presentation performed by macrophages. Likewise, they cannot substitute for histocompatibility antigens found on the surface of macrophages, and the aforementioned properties of IL-1 molecules may result from their ability to initiate the release of a lymphokine, termed interleukin II (IL-2) (previously known as T-cell growth factor) from helper T lymphocytes.

5.2. Interleukin-2

During the years since its discovery (Morgan et al., 1976), the perception of IL-2 (formerly called T-cell growth factor) as an in vitro novelty has given way to an appreciation of its crucial role both in the immune response and in the etiology and potential therapy of a number of diseases. In addition to playing a pivotal role in the culturing and cloning of T cells (Gillis and Smith, 1977; Schreier et al., 1980), IL-2 potentiates the release of a number of other important lymphokines, including γ-interferon (Farrar et al., 1981; Kasahara et al., 1983), B-cell growth factor (Howard et al., 1983), and B-cell differentiation factor (Inaba et al., 1983). Moreover, IL-2 or defects in its production or function have been implicated in such pathological states as congenital and acquired immunodeficiency (Palladino et al., 1984; Flomenberg et al., 1983; Harel-Bellan et al., 1983), autoimmunity (Linker-Israeli et al., 1983), and cancer (Rey et al., 1983).

Efforts to purify IL-2 were handicapped for years both by the minute quantities secreted by stimulated normal peripheral blood cells and by the tendency of this hydrophobic protein to adsorb to various surfaces as its purity approached homogeneity. Two developments made it possible to overcome these difficulties: (1) the discovery by Gillis and Watson (1980) that a human T-leukemia cell line, named Jurkat, was capable of releasing 100 times more IL-2 after stimulation than normal lymphocytes, making the preparation of milligram quantities of the substance feasible (Robb et al., 1983); and (2) the cloning of a cDNA corresponding to IL-2 mRNA by Taniguchi et al. (1983) using stimulated Jurkat cells and by Devos et al. (1983) employing stimulated human splenocytes. Together with protein sequence information obtained from purified IL-2, the cDNA data provided the primary amino acid sequence of the entire molecule.

Consequently, the molecular properties of IL-2 can be summarized as follows. Human, primate, and murine IL-2 have been purified to homogeneity. Human IL-2 is a 133-amino-acid single protein with a molecular weight of

15,000 that is variably glycosylated. The pressure of significant amounts of carbohydrates results in higher molecular weights and lower-pI forms of IL-2. Since recombinant IL-2, which lacks carbohydrate groups, is as active as "natural" IL-2, carbohydrates are unnecessary for IL-2 activity, at least *in vitro* (Greene and Robb, 1985; Paetkau *et al.*, 1985; Oppenheim *et al.*, 1987). Mapping of genomic DNA from various human sources and other species indicates that there is only a single gene for IL-2 (Maeda *et al.*, 1983; Seigal *et al.*, 1984). Its genomic structure has the coding region present in three exons. Chromosome mapping using hybrids between a mouse and the human line showed that the IL-2 gene is on the long arm of chromosome 4 at q 26–28 (Sykora *et al.*, 1984). Physical studies of recombinant IL-2 (Liang *et al.*, 1985) show that the secondary structure of the protein is predominantly α-helix; it has a sedimentation velocity of 1.865 and a pI of 7.7. A comparison of human recombinant IL-2 from *E. coli* and highly purified human IL-2 from the Jurkat cell line (Doyle *et al.*, 1985) shows the two proteins to be identical except at cysteine 125, which is replaced by a serine residue in the recombinant form. Both species have a specific activity of 2–4×10^6 U/mg as measured by their ability to induce DNA synthesis in the murine cell line HT2 (Fletcher and Goldstein, 1987). There is little or no homology between the sequence of IL-2 and that of other sequenced growth factors (Oppenheim *et al.*, 1987).

5.2.1. Effector Molecules with IL-2-like Activity

Among these, there are two factors with IL-2-like activity that are structurally and functionally distinct from IL-2 and need to be mentioned here. These two factors, designated leukemic T-cell growth factors I and II (L-TCGF I and II) and produced by a human T-cell lymphoma line, will, like IL-2, support the growth of activated but not resting T-lymphocytes (Gootenberg *et al.*, 1982; Gootenberg, 1984; Gootenberg and Wallace, 1987). The L-TCGF I has a molecular weight of 45,000 and a pI of 5.5, is resistant to temperatures of 56°C, and is unaffected by a variety of proteolytic enzymes that inactivate IL-2. The L-TCGF II, with a molecular weight of 27,000 and a pI of 4.5, exhibits marked stability at temperatures up to 80°C and is resistant to degradation by trypsin. Human IL-2 subjected to similar studies yields an estimated molecular weight of 24,000 and a pI of 6.5 to 8.0 and is inactivated by incubation at 56°C and by exposure to chymotrypsin, trypsin, pronase II, and staphylococcal V8 protease. Unlike IL-2, L-TCGF I and II do not support the proliferation of cloned mouse CTLL cells and provide a growth advantage to Leu 3+ ("helper") human lymphocytes. Anti-IL-2 monoclonal antibodies do not cross react with either L-TCGF. These factors may therefore represent a new family of interleukins distinct from IL-2 whose actions are not mediated through the IL-2 cell-surface receptors (Gootenberg and Wallace, 1987).

5.2.2. IL-1 and IL-2 Immunoregulatory Interactions

Both IL-1 and IL-2 exhibit a number of common biological properties, including the enhancement of thymocyte mitogenic response to phytohemagglutinin and concanavalin A as well as the stimulation of antigen-dependent, cell-mediated, and humoral immune responses. The functional relationship between IL-1 and IL-2 in the context of macrophage and T-cell interactions in the expression and regulation of immunity may be stated as follows. Activation of helper and delayed-hypersensitivity (DH)-reactive T cells by antigen requires two signals, each of which is mediated by the macrophage. The first signal requires the presentation of antigen in a manner suitable for recognition by T cells. The second signal is associated with the synthesis of IL-1 by macrophage and is necessary for full T-cell activation to proceed. The precise events involved in the ability of macrophages to present antigen to T cells are not completely understood. Nevertheless, activation of helper and DH-reactive T cells requires that they recognize antigen in conjunction with self-Ia determinants. Therefore, display of Ia determinants by macrophages constitutes a minimal requirement for their antigen-presenting capabilities (Oppenheim *et al.*, 1986, 1987).

The second signal required for activation of helper and DH-reactive T cells involves the synthesis of IL-1 by the macrophage. IL-1 exerts its effect by stimulating the production of IL-2 by T cells, and it is IL-2 that then acts in concert with the first signal mediated by antigen plus Ia to allow full T-cell activation to proceed. It is unclear whether the T cells that are sensitive to the action of IL-2 actually synthesize IL-2. To date, only malignant T-cell lines have been shown to be capable of both synthesizing and responding to IL-2. In any case, the sequence in which the two signals act on reactive T cells to induce their activation appears to be as follows. First, T cells interact with antigen presented in conjunction with Ia, resulting in an increase in the expression of receptors for IL-2. Second, synthesis of IL-1 by macrophages induces synthesis of IL-2 by T cells, and it is the action of IL-2 that then allows full T-cell activation to proceed. An obvious missing link in these interactions is represented by the signal that induced IL-1 production by macrophages. It is possible that no signal is required and that synthesis of sufficient amounts of IL-1 is a constitutive function of macrophages and other accessory cells (see Oppenheim *et al.*, 1987).

Conditioned media from activated T cells contain a factor that induces 20α-hydroxysteroid dehydrogenase (20αSDH) activity in cultures of *nu/nu* splenic lymphocytes. The enzyme is uniquely allied with the T-cell lineage, and in mice it is associated predominantly with Thy-1-positive functional T cells. It appears, therefore, that the factor in conditioned media causes a precursor cell from *nu/nu* lymphocytes to differentiate, becoming Thy 1^+, hydrocortisone resistant, and 20αSDH-positive. On the basis of this assay as a measure of early T-cell differentiation (Ihle *et al.*, 1981) as well as the T-cell origin of the factor and some biochemical characteristics (Ihle *et al.*, 1982a,b,c; 1983), the factor was named interleukin-III (IL-3). In a recent comprehensive review of the biochemical and biological properties of IL-3, it appears that this lymphokine is a 28,000-dalton protein that mediates the differentiation of a lineage of cells that includes prothymocytes and mastlike cells (Ihle, 1985).

5.3. The Interleukin-3 Family

In the context of IL-3 and its biological activities, it is necessary to mention at least three other factors: the P-cell-stimulating factor (PSF), the histamine-producing cell-stimulating factor (HCSF), and the mast cell growth factor (MCGF). These are clearly members of a closely related family of effector molecules.

5.3.1. The P Cells

The so-called P cells were first observed in the course of attempts to grow suppressor T cells from a subpopulation of spleen cells using cultures supplemented with medium conditioned by Con-A-stimulated spleen cells (Schrader *et al.*, 1980; Schrader and Nossal, 1980; Schrader, 1981). After several weeks, the cultures were dominated by a homogeneous population of cells that appeared to share many morphological and cytochemical properties with mast cells. Present on the cell surface were Fc receptors for IgE, IgG, IgG2a, IgG2b, and the cells contained histamine, serotonin, acid phosphatase, and chloroacetate esterase. Although many of these features are shared with mast cells, until there was definitive evidence that they were related to mast cells, these investigators elected to use an operational title "persisting" cell (P cell) based on the characteristic pattern of persistent *in vitro* growth. Furthermore, since the growth of P cells was absolutely dependent on a specific factor produced by Con-A-stimulated spleen cells, this substance was named P-cell-stimulating factor (PSF). This requirement of P cells for PSF could not be replaced by the addition of either of two distinct T-cell-derived factors, IL-2 or T-cell GM-CSF. Nor could PSF be replaced by other polypeptides such as macrophage-CSF (CSF-1), mouse lung-derived GM-CSF, epidermal growth factor, nerve growth factor, or fibroblast growth factor (Schrader *et al.*, 1985).

5.3.2. The Histamine-Producing Cell-Stimulating Factor

The histamine-producing cell-stimulating factor (HCSF) has been first described as a factor, produced during secondary mixed-lymphocyte culture, able to induce an increase in histamine synthesis by hematopoietic cells (Dy *et al.*, 1981). In a subsequent study, this group has shown that another factor, differing from IL-3, semipurified from P388D1 cell-line-conditioned medium (P388D1 CM), also induces an increase in histamine synthesis by hematopoietic cells, and the term HCSF has been assigned specifically to this factor (Dy *et al.*, 1986). Most recently, evidence was obtained that this HCSF is identical to GM-CSF. This has been demonstrated by (1) the similarity of the physicochemical characteristics of HCSF from P388D1 CM and those of GM-CSF already described in the literature (heat stability, molecular weight, isoelectric point, and behavior following reverse phase HPLC); (2) the coelution of a CSF activity with HCSF all through various biochemical purification procedures (gel filtration, ion exchange chromatography, chromatofocusing, and RP-HPLC); (3) the HCSF activity of a commercial GM-CSF semipurified from mitogen-induced supernatants of the murine T-lymphoma LBRM-33-5 A4 (preparation devoid of IL-3, IL-2, and IL-1 activities); and (4) the inhibition of HCSF-induced histamine synthesis by an anti-GM-CSF antiserum. Furthermore, Northern analyses of poly-A$^+$ RNA from P388D1 cells (HCSF-producing cells), from WEHI-3 cells (IL-3-producing cells), from P815 cells (HCSF- or IL-3-nonproducing cells), and from lung after endotoxin injection (GM-CSF-producing cells) were conducted with GM-CSF cDNA and IL-3 cDNA probes. The findings obtained in these studies have collectively demonstrated that (1) the P388D1 cell line can spontaneously produce GM-CSF and (2) HCSA is a property of two distinct hematopoietic growth factors: IL-3 and GM-CSF (Dy *et al.*, 1987).

In a complementary series of experiments, Pluznik and associates (1987) have examined the regulatory aspects of murine T-lymphocyte production of GM-CSF, IL-2, and IL-3. Their experimental design was guided by the following considerations: GM-CSF, IL-2, and IL-3 are produced by mitogen- or antigen-stimulated T lymphocytes, raising the possibility that the coordinated expression of these lymphokines is based on common regulatory mechanisms of synthesis. Since, furthermore, cyclosporin A (CsA) inhibits the production of IL-2 and IL-3, possibly at the transcriptional level, whereas its effects on the production of GM-CSF have not been defined, these workers have chosen CsA together with other approaches to differentiate between the regulatory mechanisms involved in the production of these three effector molecules. Thus, murine spleen cells were stimulated with Con A in the presence or absence of CsA, and the supernatants were assayed on lymphokine-dependent cell lines: IL-2 on the CTLL line, IL-3 on the DA-1 line, and GM-CSF and/or IL-3 on the PT-18 line. In accord with the foregoing, IL-2 and IL-3 activities could not be detected in the supernatants of cultures treated with CsA. In order to rule out derivation of GM-CSF from another cell type in the spleen cell cultures, the studies were repeated with a homogeneous T-cell population using the EL-4 thymoma cell line stimulated with mitogen in the presence of CsA, resulting in the same findings as before. To confirm that the activity resistant to CsA was GM-CSF, supernatants from the IL-4 preparations were fractionated by chromatography, showing two peaks of activity corresponding to IL-3 and GM-CSF in the absence of CsA, whereas only a single peak identified as GM-CSF was detectable in the presence of CsA. Monospecific antibodies against recombinant GM-CSF neutralized the biological activity retained after CsA exposure. Northern analysis of poly-A$^+$ RNA from EL-4 cells with IL-2 and GM-CSF cDNA probes showed that CsA inhibited the expression of the IL-2 gene, but GM-CSF mRNA was detectable even in the presence of CsA. This pattern of findings indicates that CsA selectively blocks IL-2 and IL-3 but not GM-CSF gene expression, suggesting that differential control mechanisms exist for the production of these substances.

5.3.3. Mast Cell Growth Factor

Mast cell growth factor (MCGF) derived from mitogen-stimulated splenic leukocyte-conditioned medium is a glycoprotein with low affinity for DEAE-cellulose. Macrophages are unnecessary for its production, and, provided a T-cell mitogen is used, T cells alone are adequate for MCGF production. This effector molecule activates mast cells (immature and committed precursors), has a molecular weight in the range of 28,000–35,000, is heterogeneous with respect to pI on isoelectric focusing, is sensitive to trypsin and neuraminidase–sialic acid-containing glycoprotein, and is relatively resistant to heat (boiling temperature, 5 min). It induces differentiation of mast cell precursors into immature granulated mastoblast (Yung and Moore, 1985). Although molecular purity of MCGF preparations is as yet unattainable, available data provide evidence that MCGF is distinct from granulocyte and macrophage CSFs. For possible relationship between cultured MCGF-dependent mast cells and the so-called "mucosal" mast cells (see Guy-Grand et al., 1978; Ginsburg et al., 1981, 1982; Haig et al., 1982; Befus et al., 1982; Razin et al., 1982; Galli et al., 1982.)

5.4. Interleukin-4

The proliferation and differentiation of B cells is mediated in part by effector molecules produced by antigen- or mitogen-activated T-cells (Kehrl et al., 1984; Kishimoto et al., 1984; Vitetta et al., 1984; Howard et al., 1984). In the mouse system, at least two distinct B-cell growth factors (BCGFs), B-cell stimulatory factor 1 (BSF-1, previously called BCGF1) and BCGFII (now called interleukin-V and discussed below), have been described (Howard et al., 1984; Swain et al., 1983). Although BSF-1 was originally reported as a glycoprotein required for proliferation of anti-IgM-activated B cells (Howard et al., 1982), recent studies established that multiple biological activities are associated with this lymphokine. Several groups of investigators have recently described the isolation of cDNA clones encoding a polypeptide that has BSF-1 activity from a cDNA library made with mRNA from mitogen-activated mouse helper T-cell clones (Lee et al., 1986; Noma et al., 1986; Yokota et al., 1986, 1987). This cDNA clone encodes a polypeptide with three activities of BSF-1, including (1) costimulation of anti-IgM-activated B cells, (2) induction of Ia antigen on resting B cells (Roehm et al., 1984), and (3) enhancement of IgE (Coffman and Carty, 1986) as well as IgG1 production (Vitetta et al., 1985). This agent also possesses T-cell growth factor (TCGF) and mast-cell growth factor (MCGF) activities distinct from IL-2 and IL-3 (Lee et al., 1986). On the basis of these multiple biological activities, it was proposed that this lymphokine be called interleukin 4 (IL-4) rather than BSF-1 (Lee et al., 1986; Noma et al., 1986; Yokota et al., 1987; Takebe et al., 1987).

Most recent investigations have clarified additional features of the pleiotropic effects of IL-4 on B lymphocytes using recombinant human IL-4 (Banchereau et al., 1987). The latter is a short-term BCGF that synergizes with the cellular products BCGF for the long-term proliferation of preactivated B cells, but it does not induce the proliferation of resting B lymphocytes. Interleukin IV specifically induces the expression of low-affinity receptor for IgE ($FcER_L$) on 40–70% of tonsil B cells. This induction of $FcER_L$ is enhanced by the polyclonal B-cell activators (SAC, anti-IgM, TPA) but is inhibited by γ-interferon. The amount of IL-4 necessary to induce the $FcER_L$ on B cells is 10- to 50-fold lower than the amount necessary to induce the proliferation of the same cells. Interleukin IV is also able to induce $FcER_L$ expression on six of eight Burkitt lymphoma cell lines as well as of the class II HLA antigens on resting B lymphocytes. Furthermore, it induces the expression of class II MHC antigens on an EBV-transformed B-cell line but not expression of class II MHC antigens, which was established from a bare-lymphocyte-syndrome patient (Banchereau et al., 1987).

New information is also available on the capacity of IL-4 to induce proliferation of different T-cell subsets and on its role in the response of T helper (T_H) cells to antigen (Fernandez-Botran et al., 1987). Purified IL-4 induces proliferation in the IL-2-dependent T-cell line HT-2 and in three other T_H-cell lines but not in alloreactive or cytotoxic T-cell lines. The IL-4-induced proliferation of T cells can be completely inhibited by monoclonal anti-IL-4 antibodies but not by anti-IL-2 receptor antibodies, which block IL-2-mediated T-cell proliferation, suggesting that the proliferation induced by IL-4 is not mediated by IL-2 or its receptor. Antigenic stimulation of a keyhole-limpet hemocyanin-specific T_H cell line or two clones in the context of B lymphocytes or adherent cells resulted in secretion of IL-4 but not IL-2. Induction of IL-4 secretion was antigen specific and major histocompatibility complex restricted. Antigenic stimulation resulted also in increased responsiveness of the T_H cells to exogenously added or endogenously produced IL-4 (Fernandez-Botran et al., 1987). Moreover, the antigen-induced proliferation of the T_H cells could be blocked by an anti-IL-4 antibody but not by an anti-IL-2 receptor antibody, suggesting that IL-4 mediates the proliferation of some T_H cells by an antigen-induced autocrine mechanism.

This combination of data indicates that during T–B interactions involving some soluble protein antigens, IL-4 and not IL-2 is the critical lymphokine for activating resting B cells and inducing proliferation of the T_H cells (Fernandez-Botran et al., 1987). Compared to the effect of IL-2, however, the effect of IL-4 is relatively short lasting, since T cells stop to proliferate after approximately 7 days after stimulation but could be maintained in culture for prolonged periods (ca. 3 weeks) without significant cell death, indicating that under these conditions IL-4 acts as a maintenance factor (Spits et al., 1987). Also, the proliferation induced by IL-4 is considerably weaker than that by IL-2, but in contrast to IL-2, which selects for T8$^+$ T cells, the T4 : T8 ratios remain 2 : 1 in the presence of IL-4. Another feature of the interaction between these interleukins is that IL-4 acts in synergy with IL-2, particularly at suboptimal IL-2 concentrations; IL-4 also induces proliferation of T3$^-$ NK clones, but it does not induce the generation of LAK cells and does not synergize with IL-2 in the generation of these cells (Spits et al., 1987). In all these activities, at least over the range of concentrations tested, IL-4 appears to be species specific, whereas IL-2 is not (Mosmann et al., 1987).

The precise role of IL-4, or indeed if it has any role in the regulation of macrophage effector function, is not known. However, in addition to the identification of macrophage receptors for IL-4, recent reports document that IL-4 exerts a broad range of regulatory effects on the macrophage, which includes induction of macrophage-mediated tumor cytotoxicity, Ia antigen expression, and increased Fc-dependent binding of IgG immune complexes to bone-marrow-derived macrophages (Meltzer et al., 1987). By all these criteria, IL-4 qualifies to be one of the established "macrophage-activating factors" (interferons, colony-stimulating factors, bacterial cell-wall components, etc.).

5.5. Interleukin-5

The study of interleukin-V (IL-5) began with the description of a T-cell-derived, antigen-nonspecific B-cell differentiation factor originally called T-cell-replacing factor (TRF, also TRF-1, and B151-K12 TRF; Takatsu et al., 1980a,b). In subsequent experiments, both B-cell differentiation and proliferation factors were demonstrated in various T-cell supernatants, leading to the characterization of a B-cell proliferation factor, BCGF-II, displaying proliferation-inducing properties on activated B cells (dextran sulfate-treated cells or BCL tumor cells; Swain et al., 1981, 1983; Swain and Dutton 1982). In contrast to the previously discussed BCGF-I (later renamed BSF, or IL-4), BCGF-II was shown not to enhance anti-µ antibody activation of B cells, whereas BCGF-I was ineffective on dextran sulfate-treated B cells. Finally, TRF and BCGF-II were found to be identical in their proliferative and differentiative activities (Harada et al., 1985; Swain, 1985) and distinct from all other lymphokines (Swain and Dutton, 1982; Swain, 1985; O'Garra, 1986). At this point, the literature began to refer to TRF/BCGF-II as IL-5 (Harriman and Strober, 1987).

By conventional biochemistry as well as gene-cloning techniques, the structure of IL-5 has been determined (Harada *et al.*, 1985; Swain, 1985; Takatsu *et al.*, 1985; Kinashi *et al.*, 1986; Azuma *et al.*, 1986). The primary molecule consists of a single-chain 112 or 113-amino-acid polypeptide (mol.wt. 12,300) that is heavily glycosylated. It usually occurs as a 45- to 6-kDa oligomer with evidence, however, that it is also active as a much lower-weight monomer (Harada *et al.*, 1985).

Current studies on the various aspects of IL-5 activity are mainly targeted to clarify the following points: (1) whether its proliferative and differentiative effects are the result of a single activity or the two effects are partially or entirely separable; (2) the issue of the IgA isotype specificity of IL-5 activity and the molecular events associated with IgA-specific B-cell switching; (3) the relationship between IL-5 activities and those of other lymphokines; (4) identification of the subpopulation of helper T (T_H) cells that is most involved in the secretion of IL-5 and consequently in the regulation of IgA B cells; and (5) whether IL-5 is capable of acting on cells other than B cells.

We do not have conclusive evidence on the identity or separateness of the proliferative versus differentiative effects of IL-5. On the other hand, considerable experimental material is available on the IgA isotype specificity of IL-5 action. Thus, recent experiments have shown that IL-5 acts on endotoxin-stimulated B cells to induce a significant increase in IgA secretion without a concurrent increase in the synthesis of any of the IgG subclasses or IgM (Coffman *et al.*, 1987; Bond *et al.*, 1987). Likewise, in the mucosa (Peyer patches), IgM B cells undergo a series of differentiative steps leading to an isotype switch to IgA B cells brought about by the so-called switch T cells as well as T cells that mediate postswitch IgA B-cell expansion (Kawanishi *et al.*, 1983a,b; Murray *et al.*, 1987). Although the molecular events associated with IgA-specific B-cell switching are incompletely understood, recent studies of switching in certain B-cell lines such as the 1.29 or 70Z/3 B-cell lymphoma lines suggest that the initial step in the molecular sequence involves an opening up (activation) of a particular Ig switch region followed by a step characterized by gene rearrangement and deletion (Stavnezer-Nordgren and Sirlin, 1986; Harriman and Strober, 1987). It appears, furthermore, that IL-5 may act either quite early on the B cell during isotype differentiation (Snapper and Paul, 1987) or on postswitch IgA B cells by promoting proliferation of these cells (BCGF-II activity) or by causing their terminal differentiation into IgA-producing plasma cells (TRF activity; Harriman and Strober, 1987).

Moreover, important functional interrelationships are shown by earlier (Swain, 1985) as well as current (Coffman *et al.*, 1987; Bond *et al.*, 1987; Murray and Kagnoff, 1987) studies between IL-5 and other lymphokines, including IL-5's capacity to induce the development of IL-2 receptors on B cells (Loughnan *et al.*, 1987). In all these studies, the effects of IL-5 are most manifest when other lymphokines are also present and acting in concert. The activity of IL-5 is not limited to B cells. It also acts on eosinophil precursors to produce eosinophil colony formation (Sanderson et al., 1986) and is capable of inducing cytotoxic T lymphocytes (Takatsu et al., 1987).

With respect to the cellular source of IL-5, recent observations (Mosmann and Coffman, 1987) indicate the existence of two classes of helper T (T_H) cells that secrete different groups of effector molecules. Thus, the T_{H1} cell secretes IL-2 and interferon-γ, whereas the T_{H2} cell secretes IL-4, IL-5, and granulocyte–macrophage colony-stimulating factor. In light of the preceding discussion, it is likely that the T_{H2} cell will prove to be the most involved in the regulation of IgA B cells (Harriman and Strober, 1987).

5.6. Interleukin-6

This substance, formerly referred to as $IFN\beta_2$ or BSF-2 (see above), is a glycoprotein of 184 amino acids that was originally identified in human fibroblasts induced by poly(I)–poly(C) to produce IFN-β (Weissenbach et al., 1980). Subsequently, a number of other factors identified on the basis of biological activities were found to be the same substance (Sehgal et al., 1987). These agents include the 25-kDa protein (Content et al., 1982; Haegeman et al., 1986; Poupart et al., 1987) BSF-2 (Hirano et al., 1987), the "hybridoma/plasmacytoma" growth factor (HPGF; Van Damme et al., 1987), and a hepatocyte-stimulating factor (Gauldie et al., 1987; Nijsten et al., 1987). There is evidence that IFN-β_2/BSF-2/IL6 can be produced by a variety of cell types either constitutively or on stimulation (Tosato et al., 1988). Interleukin 6 appears to have a number of biological functions including antiviral activity (May et al., 1986), inhibition of human fibroblast growth (Kohase et al., 1986), induction of growth of myeloma cells and certain mouse–rat hybridomas (Van Damme et al., 1987), induction of acute-phase proteins as a hepatocyte-stimulating factor (Gauldie et al., 1987; Nijsten et al., 1987), activation of hematopoietic stem cells as multi-CSF (Kishimoto et al., 1988), induction of cytotoxic T cells as killer helper factors (Herrmann et al., 1988), NCF-like activity on PC12 cells (Kishimoto et al., 1988), and induction of B-cell differentiation for the terminal maturation of activated B cells into antibody production cells (Hirano et al., 1987). High- and low-affinity receptors are demonstrable on a wide variety of cells such as EBV-transformed B-cell lines, hepatoma cells, myeloma cells, and a macrophage cell line. Of the normal lymphocytes, resting T cells and activated B cells express IL-6 receptors (Kishimoto et al., 1988).

Proliferation of Epstein–Barr virus (EBV)-immortalized human B cells is dependent on the presence of growth factors that are produced either by the same EBV-infected B cells (autocrine factors) or by activated monocytes (paracrine factors). One such monocyte-derived growth factor has been identified as IL-6. In examining the spectrum of B-cell growth factor activities of IL-6, it has been shown that IL-6 functions not as an autocrine but as a paracrine growth factor for human B cells activated by EBV (Tosato et al., 1988b). There are, furthermore, either qualitative or quantitative differences in IL-6 requirements in antigen-driven responses of primary versus secondary B lymphocytes (Cancro *et al.*, 1988).

6. THE AMINE MEDIATORS

In this group, we find the physiologically and pharmacologically familiar, chemically defined, small molecular amine mediators such as histamine, serotonin, and acetylcholine.* In addition to these three *bona fide* amine mediators of antigen–antibody responses, i.e., histamine, serotonin, and acetylcholine, the catecholamines (epinephrine, norepinephrine, and dopamine) are also considered in the discussion that follows. Several reasons justify their inclusion. (1) They are prominent members of this group of pharmacologically active substances, a review of which would be incomplete without them. (2) Since they are the principal natural antagonists of the other three amines as well as many, if not most, of the other effector substances, their interplay is likely to be operative in determining the ultimate nature of reactivity of the target cells to these mediators. (3) An understanding of this interplay can be most meaningfully approached through an analysis of the manifold interrelationships between catecholamines and their amine adversaries. (4) Each of the three amine mediators and most of the other effector molecules releases or is capable of releasing the catecholamines, and potentially, therefore, they are among the participants in the induction and expression of the immune reactivity in question. (5) Although in this capacity, they usually do not have any untoward effect, under certain conditions, their entry into the reaction may be harmful, and thus they may sometimes be regarded on their own right as fully accredited mediators of a pathological immune reaction (i.e., in various infectious and respiratory and cutaneous disorders of atopic allergy).

Each of these mediators possesses different physicochemical and biological properties. Nevertheless, when one surveys their characteristics and their probable physiological function in a higher animal organism, certain cohesive features become apparent that set them apart from other body constituents as a distinct, single class of natural substances. These cohesive features include similarities in chemical structure, metabolic derivation and degradation, cellular storage and release, and the basic identity of their principal target cells as well as some degree of overlapping specificities in their membrane receptor sites.

6.1. Histamine (β-Imidazolylethylamine)

Basophils, mast cell subsets, the so-called P cells, platelets (depending on species), and certain neurosecretory and nerve cells contain histamine that is formed from L-histidine by decarboxylation, and it may reside in and be released

*It is convenient to refer to acetylcholine herein as an amine.

by secretory granules, or it may be generated in other subcellular compartments in its activated storage cells. The biological effects of histamine include the production of leaking venules attributed to partial disconnection of endothelial cells, increase in airway resistance with a concomitant reduction in compliance (contraction of bronchial smooth muscle, activation of irritant receptors, bronchial edema), the so-called "triple response" in skin, activation of certain sensory neurons (itch and pain), cardiac stimulation, and alterations in some cell functions, including motility. These pathobiological effects as well as others are carried out via H_1 and H_2 receptors as defined by their respective inhibition by distinct groups of antihistamines (Rocha e Silva, 1978; Uvnas and Tasaka, 1982; Ganellin and Parsons, 1982).

Histamine *in vitro* expresses several important activities that have yet to be fully evaluated *in vivo* (Schwartz, 1987). Down-regulation of T-lymphocyte-mediated cytotoxicity and release of lymphokines, proliferation of lymphocytes, and secretion of granule mediators by neutrophils, basophils, and mast cells along with augmentation of T-lymphocyte suppressor activity occur with activation of H_2 receptors (Melmon *et al.*, 1981; Plaut and Lichtenstein, 1982; Marquart, 1983; Rocklin and Beer, 1983; Schwartz and Austen, 1984; Beer and Rocklin, 1984). Migration of eosinophils and neutrophils is enhanced by H_1-receptor together with H_2-receptor activation (Anwar and Kay, 1978). The expression of C3b receptors on eosinophils (not on monocytes and neutrophils) is increased, as is the complement-dependent killing of schistosomula by eosinophils *in vitro* (Anwar *et al.*, 1980).

6.2. Serotonin (5-Hydroxytryptamine)

Before the identification of 5-hydroxytryptamine (5-HT), it was known that when blood is allowed to clot, a vasoconstrictor substance is released; this substance was called "serotonin" (Page, 1968). Independent studies established the existence of a smooth muscle stimulant in intestinal mucosa, which was called enteramine (Erspamer, 1966). Subsequent synthesis of 5-hydroxytryptamine permitted the identification of serotonin and enteramine as the same decarboxylated metabolite of the amino L-tryptophan (Lewis, 1958).

In humans, more than 90% of the serotonin in the body is stored in secretory granules of enterochromaffin cells in the gastrointestinal tract. In the blood, serotonin is found in rodent mast cells (but not in humans) and in platelets. The latter lack the enzymes required for 5-HT synthesis but are able to concentrate the amine by means of an active carrier mechanism (Ciba Foundation, 1975; deGaetano and Garattini, 1978). Serotonin is present in a variety of sites in the brain contained in tryptaminergic (serotoninergic) neurons that synthesize, store, and release serotonin as a neurotransmitter (Garattini and Valzelli, 1965; Kandel and Schwartz, 1985; Shepherd, 1983; Snyder, 1984). Serotoninergic neurons are also found in the enteric nervous system of the gastrointestinal tract and around blood vessels. In this connection, it is noted that the function of 5-HT in the enterochromaffin cells is still unclear. These cells show a basal release of 5-HT that is augmented by mechanical stimulation, hypertonicity, acidity, by norepinephrine and vagal influences, apparently mediated by adrenergic fibers (De-Clerck and Vanhoutte, 1982).

Two subsets of serotonin receptors have been identified and designated 5-HT$_1$ and 5-HT$_2$. Most peripheral serotonin receptors (in platelets and smooth muscle) appear to be of the 5-HT$_2$ variety (Brukhalter and Frick, 1987). Both 5-HT$_1$ and 5-HT$_2$ types have been identified in the brain (Peroutka and Snyder, 1983). Serotonin produces both arterial as well as venous vasoconstriction except in skeletal muscle and heart, where vessels are dilated. The venoconstriction, with a resulting increased capillary filling, appears responsible for the flush that is observed following serotonin exposure (Vanhoutte, 1985). Serotonin also contracts nonvascular smooth muscle. In the gastrointestinal tract, it contracts gastrointestinal smooth muscle, increasing tone and facilitating peristalsis, and in the airways it has a small direct stimulant effect on bronchiolar smooth muscle in normal humans (Cohen et al., 1985), which is considerably enhanced in asthmatics (Szentivanyi and Fishel, 1966; Szentivanyi and Fitzpatrick, 1980). Likewise, in patients with carcinoid tumor, episodes of asthmatic bronchiolar obstruction occur in response to elevated levels of the amine (Essman, 1978). Like histamine, serotonin is a potent stimulant of pain and itch sensory nerves together with chemosensitive nerve endings in the coronary vascular bed, and it causes aggregation of blood platelets by activating surface 5-HT$_2$ receptors. This response is not accompanied by release of serotonin stored in the platelets (Burkhalter and Frick, 1987).

6.3. Acetylcholine

Acetylcholine (ACh) is synthesized by combination of choline and acetyl-coenzyme A (acetyl-CoA) catalyzed by the enzyme choline-O-acetyltransferase (ChAc). The ChAc transfers the acetyl radical from active acetate (acetyl-CoA) to choline (Tucek, 1982). This process takes place in the axoplasm and most actively in the region of the nerve terminal. The ChAc is at its highest concentration in the terminal, and it accumulates above and disappears below ligature sites on neurons. These findings are consistent with the formation of the enzyme in the perykaryon and its axoplasmic transport to the terminals (Kandel and Schwartz, 1985). This does not, however, imply the predominant or exclusive occurrence of ACh in neural structures or that its presence in these areas represents a universal characteristic of nerve cells.

For instance, ACh is present in high concentrations in the nettle sting, aneural placenta of humans and primates, ciliated tissues of the sea mussel *Mytilus edulis,* and certain other animal tissues where it is assumed to be of nonnervous origin, such as in the spleen of oxen and horses, intestinal wall, auricular tissue, and tracheal mucous membrane (Szentivanyi et al., 1988). Although as its natural distribution implies, ACh may have other as yet unknown functions, its function as a neurotransmitter is the one that can be most certainly identified and still compels the greatest interest. That it is a neurotransmitter released by certain groups of neurons, which by this release are defined as cholinergic neurons, is now generally accepted, and although other ideas about the function of ACh in the nervous system continue to be moot, no critical evidence has emerged that requires the original concept of chemical transmission to be modified. Instead, it receives increasingly more support as time passes, and the separate events of transmission, both presynaptic and postsynaptic, are analyzed in more detail (Stjarne et al., 1981).

6.4. Catecholamines

The term catecholamine refers generically to all compounds containing a catechol nucleus (benzene with two adjacent hydroxy groups, i.e., dihydroxybenzene, also known as catechol) and an amine group (Fig. 17-4 in Szentivanyi et al., 1988). However, use of this term is usually reserved for dihydroxyphenylethylamine (dopamine) and its metabolic products norepinephrine and epinephrine. Of these compounds, norepinephrine has been established as the neurotransmitter of most sympathetic postganglionic neurons and probably of certain tracts in the central nervous system. Dopamine is emerging as an important transmitter in the extrapyramidal and possibly mesolimbic systems, and epinephrine is the acknowledged major hormone of the adrenal medulla (Kohsaka et al., 1982).

With the exception of the adrenal medullae, in all peripheral tissues the predominant catecholamine is norepinephrine. Its concentration in a given tissue reflects the density of adrenergic innervation and thus varies considerably. Most of the norepinephrine in peripheral tissues is localized in adrenergic nerve terminals, but small amounts are also found along the entire length of such neurons and in their perikarya in the sympathetic ganglia. In the adrenal medullae, norepinephrine and epinephrine are stored in separate cells. There are considerable species differences in medullary distribution of the two cell types and consequently in the relative proportions of the two amines. Of the total catecholamine contents of human medullary tissues, norepinephrine accounts for about 20% and epinephrine for almost 80%, with dopamine being present only in trace amounts (Izumi et al., 1982). With respect to the last-named catecholamine, the same statement could apply to most tissues, since dopa and dopamine exist only as transient intermediates in catecholamine synthesis. However, in peripheral tissues of some ruminant animals, dopamine has been demonstrated to account for as much as 80% of the total catecholamine content. This dopamine is stored not in adrenergic neurons but in a specialized type of mast cell, which is chromaffin-positive and occurs in abundance in dopamine-rich tissues (Falck et *al.*, 1959; Szentivanyi and Fishel, 1966; Coupland, 1972; Szentivanyi and Fitzpatrick, 1980; Kohsaka *et al.*, 1982). In the rat, dopamine has also shown to be present in duodenal mucosa and gastric secretion (Szabo *et al.*, 1982).

The central nervous system (CNS) of mammals contains significant amounts of both norepinephrine and dopamine, distributed in well-defined and distinct regional patterns. The two amines are stored in different neurons, and a distinct class of adrenergic neurons in which dopamine is the transmitter rather than norepinephrine exists in certain regions of the central nervous system. Highest levels of norepinephrine are found in the hypothalamus and other areas of central sympathetic representation, whereas dopamine is concentrated in the neostriatum, nucleus accumbens, and tuberculum olfactorium (Szentivanyi and Fishel, 1966; Kandell and Schwartz, 1985; Szentivanyi *et al.*, 1988). Dopamine is also present in the superior cervical ganglion, which has at least three distinct populations of neurons: cholinergic, noradrenergic, and small intensely fluorescent (SIF) cells. The SIF cells are small interneurons that contain dopamine (Eranko *et al.*, 1980). Release of the amine from these interneurons is responsible for hyperpolarization of the ganglion (Neff *et al.*, 1983).

7. THE LIPID-DERIVED MEDIATORS

These highly potent effector molecules have a critically important role in the pharmacology of immunologic (allergic) as well as nonimmunologic inflammatory reactions and produce many of the long-recognized hallmarks of the clinical inflammatory response. Any time a cell membrane is perturbed, its environment is enriched selectively by the various products of the oxidative metabolism of arachidonic acid. The program for selection largely resides in the enzymatic capabilities of the particular cell membrane (Austen, 1983). In addition to the prostaglandins, more recent investigations have revealed the existence of other pharmacologically active lipids and peptidolipids biosynthesized from the same precursors as the prostaglandins through interrelated enzymatic pathways. These other lipids include the thromboxanes, hydroperoxyeicosatetraenoic acids (HPETEs), hydroxyeicosatetraenoic acids (HETEs), the lipoxins, the leukotrienes, and platelet-activating factor (PAF). The remarkable expansion in the number of these interrelated substances has led to the introduction of the all-inclusive term "eicosanoids," since they all derive from the same eicosaenoic (*eicosa*, 20-carbon; enoic, containing double bonds) acid precursors.

Eicosanoids are the cyclooxygenase- and lipoxygenase-oxygenated products of arachidonic acids. Arachidonic acid is released from the 2 position of specific glycerophospholipids (that constitute part of the lipid bilayer of the cell membrane) by phospholipase A_2 and/or phospholipase C in conjunction with diacylglycerol lipase after appropriate cell activation by immunologic (i.e., immune complexes, complement fragments, and IgE-mediated) and nonimmunologic (i.e., hypoxia and trauma) stimuli (Samuelsson, 1983). Depending on the nature of the stimulus and the type of cell that is activated, the free, un-esterified arachidonic acid is converted to effector molecules of either the cyclooxygenase or lipoxygenase pathway.

The first enzyme, cyclooxygenase, converts arachidonic acid to unstable endoperoxide intermediates (PGG$_2$ and PGH$_2$). These can then be further metab-olized through enzymatic activity to either the prostaglandins (PGD$_2$ through PGF$_{2\alpha}$ and PGI$_2$, also called prostacyclin) or to the thromboxanes. The E pros-taglandins can be further metabolized to the B prostaglandins *in vivo* or to the A or B prostaglandins *in vitro*. The second enzyme, lipoxygenase, converts arachi-donic acid to a series of HPETEs, which are then further metabolized to either a series of corresponding HETEs or to the leukotrienes (Goldyne, 1987).

7.1. The Prostaglandins

In the 1930s, three laboratories independently described a uterine smooth-muscle-contracting activity deriving from semen. Von Euler named this sub-stance prostaglandin because of its assumed origin from the prostate gland. In the 1960s Bergstrom and associates showed that prostaglandin activity derived from several related agents and named the first two prostaglandins E and F (PGE and PGF) because of their respective solvent partitioning into ether and phosphate buffer (*fosfat* in Swedish).

"Prostanoic acid" is the name given to the molecular skeleton common to all prostaglandins, which consists of a cyclopentane ring with two aliphatic side chains. Today, nine prostaglandin groups are recognized that, with the exception of the initially discovered E and F groups, are arbitrarily assigned the letter designations A through I. All prostaglandins have a Δ^{13} double bond, but they differ from each other by the substitutions on the carbon-9 and carbon-11 posi-tions of the pentane ring and, in the case of PGG, on carbon 15. The substitutions on the pentane ring are responsible for the qualitative activities of the different groups, whereas the Δ^{13} bonding and carbon-15 hydroxyl group are required for full activity. Each prostaglandin group except PGI can be classified in one of three series, designated by a subscript 1, 2, or 3 following the group designation. This subscript indicates the total number of double bonds in the two side chains of the prostaglandin molecule and reflects the fact that prostaglandins can be synthesized from three different eicosaenoic acids (Goldyne, 1987).

All mammalian cell types studied so far (with the exception of the erythro-cyte) have microsomal enzymes for the synthesis of prostaglandins. The latter are not preformed but newly generated mediators that are synthesized *de novo* and released whenever cells are damaged. They can be detected in increased concentrations in inflammatory exudates and contribute importantly to the ex-pression of the signs and symptoms of inflammation (Larsen and Henson, 1983). Although prostaglandins do not have direct effects on the vascular permeability (leakage) of the postcapillary and collecting venules, both PGE$_2$ and PGI$_2$ enhance edema formation and leukocyte infiltration by promoting blood flow in the inflamed area. Interestingly, however, PGEs inhibit (1) secretion of mast cell mediators in anaphylaxis, (2) participation of lymphocytes in delayed hypersensitivity reactions, and (3) release of hydrolases and lysosomal enzymes from human neutrophils as well as from mouse peritoneal macrophages (Moncada et al., 1985).

Several of the earlier mentioned pharmacological mediators of the allergic response release prostaglandins from areas where manifestations of immediate hypersensitivity occur. For instance, histamine is released from lung mast cells after antigen challenge of passively sensitized lung fragments in vitro; the released histamine, by an H_1-receptor-mediated effect, stimulates the production of PGF_2 (Platshon and Kaliner, 1978). In this effect, however, some other mediators have also been implicated, one of which is the so-called "prostaglandin-generating factor of anaphylaxis" (PGF-A). This mediator is not preformed in lung tissue but is newly generated after lung anaphylaxis. Since it is a peptide, it is mentioned further in the discussion of peptide mediators below (Section 8.2).

Prostaglandins are also associated with two other hallmarks of inflammation, the development of pain and fever. With respect to the first characteristic, prostaglandins have the ability to sensitize pain receptors to mechanical and chemical stimulation. This has been confirmed by electrophysiological measurement of sensory nerve discharge in the presence of prostaglandins. The prostaglandin-induced hyperalgesia results from a lowering of the threshold of the polymodal nociceptors of C fibers (Flower et al., 1985). In this context, fever assumes major importance as one of the sequelae of tissue damage and inflammation in general and of infection in particular. Although a multitude of microorganisms can cause fever, the one that is best investigated is caused by bacterial endotoxins. In this capacity endotoxins act by stimulating the synthesis and release of the so-called "endogeneous pyrogen" (EP) from neutrophils, macrophages, and other cells. As stated earlier, there is conclusive evidence that EP is identical with IL-1 (Dinarello, 1984; Kampschmidt, 1984), and in the current view EP is believed to pass from the circulation into the central nervous system, where it acts on discrete sites, especially the preoptic hypothalamic area (Bernheim et al., 1979; Dinarello and Wolff, 1982). The evidence that the resultant elevation of body temperature is mediated by the release of prostaglandins includes the following: (1) prostaglandins, especially PGE_2, produce fever when infused into the cerebral ventricles or injected into the hypothalamus; (2) fever is a frequent side effect of prostaglandins when used as abortifacients; (3) prostaglandinlike substances have been demonstrated in cerebrospinal fluid when EP is injected intravenously; and (4) EP but not prostaglandin-induced fever is reduced by aspirinlike drugs (Milton, 1982).

Prostaglandins exhibit immunoregulatory activity. Prostaglandin$_1$ has a suppressive effect on B-lymphocyte function including the humoral antibody response, and PGEs inhibit both production and release of lymphokines by sensitized T lymphocytes. The T ("killer") lymphocyte, active in killing malignant cells, in inhibited by PGEs in its ability to reject allogeneic thymus cells *in vitro*, and exogenously administered prostaglandins have been reported to prolong skin allograft survival. In view of the pivotal role of macrophages in the initiation and subsequent regulation of both cell-mediated and humoral immunity, it is to be noted that several studies demonstrate that PGE_2 is involved in the autoregulation of macrophage function. Prostaglandins do not appear to initiate but rather modulate responses in macrophages induced by some other stimulus. Moreover, this prostaglandin-mediated modulation is variable, depending on the stage of differentiation of the macrophage and its state of functional activation (Schultz, 1985).

Because of the nature of the microbial modulation of the immunopharmacology of human asthma, it is important to review briefly the major prostaglandins formed by stimulated human lung tissues from the endoperoxide precursors. These are PGI_2, PGD_2, PGE_2, and $PGF_{2\alpha}$. A PGI_2 synthase located in the plasma and nuclear membranes converts PGH_2 to PGI_2. In addition to its earlier mentioned vasodilatory activity, PGI_2 inhibits intrapulmonary platelet aggregation and is a bronchodilator. A PGH–PGE isomerase converts PGH_2 to another prostaglandin with bronchodilator activity, PGE_2. The latter relaxes both pulmonary smooth muscle and vascular beds (Henderson, 1987). On the other hand, the major bronchoconstrictor prostaglandins are PGD_2 and $PGF_{2\alpha}$. Prostaglandin$_2$ formed by the action of a PGH–PGD isomerase enzyme is the predominant arachidonate product released by human lung mast cells after either immunologic or nonimmunologic (calcium ionophore A23187) stimulation (Peters *et al.*, 1984). A reductase catalyzes the formation of a $PGF_{2\alpha}$ from PGH_2. Although it is a substrate for PGDH, $PGF_{2\alpha}$ is less completely metabolized than PGH_2 after passage through the lung. The bronchoconstrictor activities of PGD_2, $PGF_{2\alpha}$, and histamine after bronchial inhalation have been compared in patients with asthma. Prostaglandin$_2$ was 3.5 times more potent than $PGF_{2\alpha}$ and 30 times more potent than histamine as a bronchoconstrictor. When PGD_2 and $PGF_{2\alpha}$ were inhaled by normal individuals, only PGD_2 was found to constrict airways as determined by a fall in specific airway conductance (Hardy *et al.*, 1984). It is to be added that human lung parenchyma and airway tissues present different profiles of released prostaglandins as a consequence of IgE-mediated stimulation. Pulmonary parenchyma releases the following prostaglandins *in vitro*: $PGD_2 \simeq PGI_2 \gg PGF_{2\alpha} > PGE$. After comparable stimulation, airway tissue generates a qualitatively different profile of agents: $PGI_2 > PGE \simeq PGF_{2\alpha} > PGD_2$. The total amount of prostaglandins generated by immunologically stimulated airway tissue is also much less than that released by the parenchyma (Schulman *et al.*, 1982).

7.2. The Thromboxanes

In 1975, Hamberg *et al.* described substances released by aggregating platelets (thrombocytes) that derived from the same precursors as the prostaglandins but differed in that they contained an oxane ring; thus, the name thromboxane was coined. The structure common to all thromboxanes is the presence of the oxane ring with the same two aliphatic side chains common to prostaglandins. Two thromboxane groups are recognized, designated TXA and TXB. Thromboxane A is a highly unstable oxane : oxetane substance with an aqueous half-life of 45 sec. Thromboxane is the stable spontaneous hydration derivative of TXA. Thromboxanes can also exist in any one of three series designated by a subscript 1, 2, or 3, depending, as with the prostaglandins, on the fatty acid precursor (Goldyne, 1987).

There are two important areas of thromboxane activity that need to be mentioned in this section. One involves platelet, and the other smooth muscle function. It is established that stimulation of platelets to aggregate leads to activation of membrane phospholipases with the resultant release of arachidonic acid and its transformation into prostaglandin endoperoxides and TXA_2. The latter serves as a signal that induces platelet aggregation and the platelet-release reaction. Although this is not the only mechanism in the physiopathology of platelet aggregation, the significance of the thromboxane pathway is reflected by the fact that aspirin inhibits the second phase of platelet aggregation (Jobim, 1978; see also Fishel et al., 1973; Klein et al., 1974). Since PGI_2 generated in the vessel wall appears to be an antagonist to the thromboxane effect, it is postulated that PGI_2 and TXA_2 represent functionally opposing components in regulating platelet–vessel wall interaction and the formation of hemostatic plugs and intraarterial thrombi (Moncada and Vane, 1979; Whittle and Moncada, 1983).

With respect to smooth muscle function, TXA_2 contracts all vascular smooth muscle strips tested so far, and it is a powerful vasoconstrictor both in the whole animal as well as in isolated vascular beds (Dusting et al., 1979; Whittle et al., 1981). Thromboxane$_2$ is inactive when effects on the cardiovascular system are tested (Moncada et al., 1985). Thromboxane$_2$, however, is one of the most potent of the eicosanoids as a bronchoconstrictor. It can be released from human lung following immunologic stimulation and may also participate with other eicosanoids in the physiology and physiopathology of respiratory smooth muscle reactivity (Goldyne, 1987).

7.3. The HPETEs and HETEs

At the same time when Hamberg et al. (1975) described the thromboxanes, they also identified another series of products synthesized from the prostaglandin precursor arachidonic acid. These substances lacked a cyclic structure and contained a hydroperoxy or hydroxyl substitution on the eicosatetraenoic (arachidonic) acid backbone and were accordingly labeled hydroperoxyeicosatetraenoic acids (HPETEs) and hydroxyeicosatetraenoic acids (HETEs).

The HPETEs derive from a different enzymatic pathway (lipoxygenase) than the prostaglandins and thromboxanes and are not cyclic compounds. Their structure consists of the parent fatty acid with a hydroperoxy substituent. The position of this group is designated by a numerical prefix indicating the carbon position of the substitution (e.g., 12-HPETE). The HPETEs are relatively unstable and are reduced enzymatically or nonenzymatically to the corresponding HETEs (e.g., 12-HPETE → 12-HETE).

In terms of smooth muscle pharmacology, HPETEs and HETEs do not appear to significantly affect vascular smooth muscle tone, but 5-HETE does produce slow contractions of isolated human bronchial smooth muscle with a potency comparable to that of histamine. If given at subthreshold doses, 5-HETE potentiates histamine-induced contractions; 15-HETE is somewhat less potent than either 5-HETE or histamine, and 12-HETE is inactive (Goldyne, 1987).

These lipoxygenase metabolites are important participants in the inflammatory process. The 5-, 12-, or 15-HETE, when applied to human skin, produces local erythema and some extravasation of plasma proteins. 12-HETE was the first lipoxygenase product reported to have chemotactic activity for human PMN (Turner et al., 1975). The other mono-HETEs and, more significantly, the HPETEs are also potent chemotactic agents for rabbit and human PMN (Goetzl and Sun, 1979). 5-HPETE and 5-HETE may be required for the release of histamine and other substances from mast cells, reflecting another feature of their involvement in inflammatory mechanisms (Moncada et al., 1985).

The HPETEs and HETEs also contribute to the regulation of lymphocyte function. Thus, in 1980 it was reported for the first time that a 15-lipoxygenase metabolite of arachidonic acid, tentatively identified as 15-HPETE, inhibited the proliferative response of mouse splenocytes to several mitogens (Goodman and Weigle, 1980). Subsequently, 15-HETE was reported to inhibit mitogen-induced [^{3}H]thymidine incorporation into mouse splenocytes (Bailey et al., 1982), and in vivo administration of 15-HETE was also shown to reduce the proliferative response of murine splenocytes to PHA, Con A, or allogeneic cells (Aldigier et al., 1984). The expression of lymphocytic surface markers is also affected by these substances, with possible phenotypic correlation with functional effects. For example, 15-HPETE inhibits rosette formation with sheep erythrocytes (Gualde et al., 1982), decreases the density of Fc receptors on human T cells and monocytes (Goodwin et al., 1984), and enhances the expression of the Lyt-2$^+$ antigen on mouse splenocytes after a 48-hr culture (Aldigier et al., 1984).

These effector molecules also influence natural killer or natural cytotoxic cell activity against certain tumors or virus-infected target cells. The generation of murine T_c cells is inhibited by the in vivo administration of 15-HETE (Aldigier et al., 1984), and 14,15-diHETE reduces natural killer function but does not affect antibody-dependent cell-mediated cytotoxicity or T_c-cell responses (Ramstedt et al., 1984). Finally, complex interactions have been demonstrated to occur between the products of various lipoxygenases. Thus, 12-HPETE from platelets enhances the activity of 5-lipoxygenase of human leukocytes, whereas 12-HETE is inactive in this capacity (Maclouf et al., 1982). In contrast, 15-

HPETE and its more stable product 15-HETE are inhibitors of 5- and 12-lipoxygenases (Vanderhoek et al., 1980).

7.4. The Lipoxins

Recent research has uncovered yet another group of structurally unique metabolites of arachidonic acid generated by human leukocytes from 15-HPETE. Structurally they are trihydroxytetraenes and have been given the name lipoxins. So far two members of the group have been described: 5,6,15-triHETE or lipoxin A, and 5,14,15-triHETE or lipoxin B. Their discovery suggests interactions between the 5- and 15-lipoxygenase pathways in human leukocytes (Serhan et al., 1984a,b). At the time of this writing there is not enough information available about their endogenous synthesis, function, and physiopathological significance, but there is evidence that lipoxin A enhances NK-cell function (Rola-Pleszczynski, 1985a).

7.5. The Leukotrienes

In 1978, Parker demonstrated that the smooth-muscle-contracting principle called "slow-reacting substance of anaphylaxis" (SRS-A) was a derivative of the prostaglandin precursor arachidonic acid. Subsequently, Borgeat et al. isolated arachidonic acid derivatives from rabbit leukocytes that contained a conjugated triene bonding—hence the name leukotrienes. The work that followed showed that SRS-A was in fact a mixture of three of these leukotrienes.

Five groups of leukotrienes have currently been identified, designated LTA through LTE. As is the case with prostaglandins, there are three series of leukotrienes; they are designated by a subscript 3, 4, or 5 since, unlike the other eicosanoids, all the double bonds in the parent trienoic, tetraenoic, and pentaenoic acids are retained (Borgeat et al., 1985; Rouzer and Samuelsson, 1985). These agents represent a group of pharmacologically active effector molecules that are readily synthesized by leukocytes and by several other cell types following immune or nonimmune stimulation. In addition to their initially described myotropic activities, they strongly affect several leukocyte functions and play a significant role in immunoregulation during inflammatory processes in general (Sirois, 1985; Rola-Pleszczynski, 1985).

The pivotal intermediate in the formation of leukotrienes (LTs) is 5-hydroperoxy-6,8,11,14-eicosatetraenoic acid, which results from the oxygenation of arachidonic acid at the C-5 position. This reaction is catalyzed by 5-lipoxygenase, the only enzyme in the cyclooxygenase and lipoxygenase pathways of arachidonic acid metabolism whose activity is stimulated by calcium; 5-hydroperoxy-6,8,11,14-eicosatetraenoic acid is either reduced to form 5-hydroxy-6,8,11,14-eicosatetraenoic acid or converted to an unstable epoxide derivative, 5-(S),6-(S)-oxido-7,9-*trans*-11,14-*cis*-eicosatetraenoic acid (LTA$_4$) (Radmark *et al.*, 1984). The enzymatic addition of water to LTA_4 by a cytosolic hydrolase forms the biologically potent dihydroxy acid, LTB_4 (Henderson, 1987).

A second group of leukotrienes that constitute the SRS-A is the sulfidopeptide leukotrienes (LTC_4, LTD_4, and LTE_4). The parent compound of this group is LTC_4 [5-(*S*)-hydroxy-6-(*R*)-S-glutathionyl-7,9-*trans*-11,14-*cis*-eicosatetraenoic acid], which is formed by the addition of glutathione to the epoxide ring of LTA_4. Once secreted, LTC_4 can be metabolized sequentially to the two other major slow-reacting substances by extracellular enzymes, LTD_4 by removal of glutamine and LTE_4 by removal of glycine.

Several cell types are known to contain lipoxygenases and to produce leukotrienes. They include polymorphonuclear leukocytes (Henderson and Klebanoff, 1983; Rola-Pleszczynski, 1985), monocytes and macrophages (Fels *et al.*, 1982; Hsueh and Sun, 1982; Goldyne *et al.*, 1984; Williams *et al.*, 1984; Rouzer *et al.*, 1982), normal and leukemic basophils (MacGlashan *et al.*, 1986; Jakschik and Lee, 1980), various mast cell subsets (Razin *et al.*, 1982; Katz *et al.*, 1985; Peters *et al.*, 1984), which produce mainly 5-lipoxygenase and 15-lipoxygenase metabolites, and eosinophils, which produce mainly 15-lipoxygenase metabolites (Turk *et al.*, 1982; Weller *et al.*, 1983; Jorg *et al.*, 1982; Henderson *et al.*, 1984; Shaw *et al.*, 1985; Henderson, 1985). These and possibly other cell types may be responsible for leukotriene formation in the lung (Stimler *et al.*, 1982), the spleen (Malik and Wang, 1981), the kidney (Van Praag and Farber, 1981), the synovium (Klickstein *et al.*, 1980), or the epidermis (Brain *et al.*, 1982).

With respect to the pharmacology of the leukotrienes, it was their myotropic activities that first attracted major interest because of the historical background of SRS-A. Briefly stated, Feldberg and Kellaway (1938) introduced the descriptive term "SRS" for material obtained from lung during perfusion with cobra venom. The occurrence of a slow-reacting substance following challenge of a sensitized tissue with the appropriate antigen was first reported in 1940 by Kellaway and Trethewie. When the perfusate obtained during anaphylactic shock from a sensitized guinea pig lung was assayed on the guinea pig ileum, these workers recognized that the contraction differed from that of histamine in that the gut was slower to relax; they ascribed this modification of the characteristic histamine effect to the presence of SRS. This problem was reexamined by Brocklehurst (1953, 1960) when potent and specific antihistamines had been developed. It then became possible to abolish the response to histamine, allowing the contraction caused by SRS to be obtained separately, since the more specific antihistamines do not depress such contraction even at a concentration of 10^{-6} M. Since, furthermore, this at that time unidentified agent produced by the anaphylactic reaction in guinea pig lung had a different pattern of pharmacological activity from that of any known substance, it was named "SRS-A," "slow-reacting substance of anaphylaxis," to avoid confusion with other substances in the SRS group (Brocklehurst, 1955). When finally the long-elusive structure of

SRS-A was found to be a mixture of LTC_4, LTD_4, and LTE_4, the possible role of these agents in the pathogenesis of human asthma became a major natural target of inquiry.

Although some conflicting data do exist (Griffin et al., 1983), there is consensus in the literature that the sulfidopeptide leukotrienes are potent constrictors of human bronchi and pulmonary vascular smooth muscle, increase vascular permeability, and stimulate airway mucus secretion (Dahlen et al., 1980; Samuelsson, 1983; Farrukh et al., 1985). In general, LTC_4 and LTD_4 are more active pharmacologically than LTE_4. The first two sulfidopeptides are about 1000 times more active than histamine in contracting bronchial smooth muscle in vitro (Hanna et al., 1981), and there is evidence that patients with asthma are hyperresponsive to the sulfidopeptide leukotrienes (Smith et al., 1985; Adelroth et al., 1986). It is to be noted, however, that asthmatics who appeared to be most reactive to acetylcholine were the least responsive to bronchial inhalation of LTC_4 and LTD_4. These observations suggest that leukotrienes may have unique bronchoconstrictor activities, since other bronchospastic agents, such as histamine and $PGF_{2\alpha}$, have the same relative potency in comparison to methacholine in either normal or asthmatic patients (Adelroth et al., 1986).

In view of the excessive mucus production in the airways, a major component in the pathology of bronchial obstruction in asthma, it is important that lung fluid obtained from human pulmonary tissue after in vitro anaphylaxis shows the release of mucus glycoproteins. In fact, the most potent mucus secretagogues are the sulfidopeptide leukotrienes in the anaphylactic lung, with a rank order of $LTD_4 \geq LTC_4$ (picomolar) > mono-5-hydroxy-6,8,11,14-eicosatetraenoic acid (nanomolar) > $PGF_{2\alpha} = PGD_2 = PGI_2 = PGE_1 = PGA_2$ (micromolar) > histamine (H_2 receptor mediated; micromolar) (Shelhamer et al., 1982). Other possible effector molecules may also be involved in the release of airway mucus glycoproteins. Thus, human peripheral blood monocytes (Marom et al., 1985) and alveolar macrophages (Marom et al., 1984a) have been shown to secrete a mucus secretagogue through complement or Fc receptor-mediated activation. The macrophage-derived mucus secretagogues are newly generated acidic molecules of approximately 2000 mol. wt. and are either similar or identical substances, but they are unlikely to be derived from arachidonic acid (Marom et al., 1984, 1985). Finally, in patients with allergic disorders, tear fluid from the eye, when exposed to the appropriate allergen, shows increased levels of the sulfidopeptide leukotrienes (Ford-Hutchinson, 1984). Also, allergen challenge of lung tissue from asthmatics elicits the release of these agents in good correlation with bronchial obstruction, underlining again the great potential importance of these substances in human asthma (Dahlen et al., 1983).

Another prominent member of the leukotriene family is LTB_4. It is the primary eicosanoid formed by human neutrophils, monocytes, and alveolar macrophages, and it is also produced by passively sensitized pulmonary parenchyma and airway tissue after incubation with the corresponding allergen (Salari et al.,

1985). Airway epithelial tissue generates LTB_4 after stimulation with either the calcium ionophore A23187 (Holtzman et al., 1983) or PGF-A (Marom et al., 1984b). Leukotriene B_4 plays a critical role in the pharmacology of both immunologic and nonimmunologic inflammation as well as in that of lymphocyte function.

Thus, LTB_4 is a highly potent chemotactic and chemokinetic agent for neutrophils, eosinophils, and monocytes, and it is the predominant neutrophil chemoattractant produced by resident alveolar macrophages on activation by either soluble or phagocytic stimuli (Martin et al., 1985). In these capacities LTB_4 is about 100 times more potent than any of the HETEs or HPETE, and these activities of LTB_4 are stereospecific for the cis-trans-trans triene structure (Rola-Pleszczynski, 1985a). Leukotriene B_4 is also more active than 5-, 12-, or 15-HETE in inducing extravasation of plasma proteins, an effect that can be significantly potentiated by coadministration of PGE_1, PGE_2, PGD_2, or bradykinin. Other inflammatory activities of LTB_4 include induction of leukocyte aggregation (Ford-Hutchinson et al., 1980), accumulation (Higgs et al., 1981; Lewis et al., 1981; Soter et al., 1983; Smith et al., 1980), increased leukocyte adherence to vascular endothelial cells (Bray et al., 1981; Dahlen et al., 1981; Gimbrone et al., 1984), and increase in the secretion of lysosomal enzymes (Hafstrome et al., 1981; Showell et al., 1982).

Leukotrienes, primarily LTB_4, play a significant role in the regulation of the immune response through numerous and varied effects on several cell types. Proliferation of the T4+ (helper/inducer) subset of human T cells is inhibited by LTB_4, whereas proliferation of the T8+ (suppressor/cytotoxic) subset is enhanced (Payan et al., 1984; Gualde et al., 1985). Although suppressor cell activity resides in the T8+ subset of T cells, it is inducible from both T4+ and T8+ subsets (Atluru and Goodwin, 1984; Rola-Pleszczynski, 1985b). However, T4+ lymphocytes are inducible to become suppressors only when monocytes are present in the responder population, in contrast to T8+ cells, which do not require the presence of monocytes to become active suppressor cells (Rola-Pleszczynski, 1985b). Furthermore, LTB_4 also induces the appearance of T8+ cells in a T8-depleted lymphocyte population (Atluru and Goodwin, 1984; Rola-Pleszczynski, 1985b). Leukotriene B_4 also regulates monocyte function by stimulating them to produce prostaglandins and IL-1 (Dinarello et al., 1984; Rola-Pleszczynski et al., 1986).

With respect to other cell functions, the implication of lipoxygenase products in cytotoxic processes is indicated by the following observations: (1) natural killer (NK) or natural cytotoxic (NC) activity is markedly enhanced by LTB_4 and to a lesser extent by LTA_4 (Rola-Pleszczynski et al., 1983, 1984), including increased binding of effector molecules to target cells as well as the rate of target cell killing (Gagnon et al., 1984); (2) LTB_4 augments neutrophil- and eosinophil-mediated, complement-dependent killing of schistosomula (Moqbel et al., 1983); (3) selective depletion of T8+ cells before stimulation with poly I:C and

LTB_4 results in enhanced, and depletion of $T4^+$ cells in suppressed, γ-interferon production by LTB_4 (Rola-Pleszczynski, 1985a); and (4) LTB_4, LTC_4, and LTD_4 are capable of replacing T_H cells or IL-2 in inducing the production of γ-interferon (Johnson and Torres, 1984).

In closing this section, it should be added that *in vitro* immunoglobulin production by murine splenocytes is inhibited when these cells are cultured in the presence of LTD_4 and LTE_4 (Bailey et al., 1982; Webb et al., 1982), whereas in humans the same effect can only be produced with LTB_4 (Atluru and Goodwin, 1984).

7.6. Platelet-Activating Factor

The last lipid-derived mediator included in this section is platelet-activating factor (PAF), which represents a new class of pharmacologically potent lipids that are active in the subnanomolar range with important implications in the inflammatory response in general and immunologic inflammation in particular.

The historical background of its discovery could be briefly stated as follows. Barbaro and Zvaifler (1966) described a leukocyte-dependent histamine-releasing mechanism that was followed up by the proposal of Henson (1971) suggesting that there was an interaction between leukocytes and platelets whereby a soluble "fluid-phase mediator" was released from leukocytes of immunologically hypersensitive rabbits. This hypothetical mediator was then believed to activate platelets, resulting in the release of amine mediators. Subsequently, two groups of investigators, Siraganian and Osler (1971) and Benveniste et al. (1972), independently reported a confirmation of that earlier observation. The latter group also coined the term platelet-activating factor, demonstrated its release from IgE-sensitized rabbit basophils, and began studies targeted to the chemical identification of the substance. Finally, two separate groups, Benveniste and associates in Paris (1979) and Demopoulos et al. (1979) in San Antonio, reported its chemical structure as being a 1-O-alkyl-2-acetyl-*sn*-glyceryl-3-phosphorylcholine, or more briefly an alkylacetylglycerophosphocholine (AGEPC). An entirely different but parallel line of research culminated in the simultaneous description and semisynthesis of an identical molecule, which had an antihypertensive effect. This observation followed studies of antihypertensive molecules from the renal medulla, which led to evidence that the biological activity resided in a polar lipid (Blank et al., 1979). It is now well established that the hypotensive agent and the platelet-activating factor are the same compound (Hanahan, 1986).

The continuing uncertainty of the final spectrum of biological activities of PAF, together with questions of its physiological role, have led to the concurrent use of different names for the material: antihypertensive polar renomedullary lipid (APRL); acetyl-glyceryl-ether-phosphorylcholine (AGEPC); PAF-acether; alkylacetyl-GPC. Since a unifying term is not yet available, for the purpose of this discussion, the original PAF will be employed, but with emphasis that the activity of the molecule is not confined to the platelet.

The cellular sources of PAF include monocytes, alveolar macrophages, mast cells, basophils, eosinophils, neutrophils, platelets, and endothelial cells (Roubin and Benveniste, 1985; Henson, 1985; Hanahan, 1986). This list is probably not complete, and investigators in the field believe that given the appropriate stimulus, PAF may be generated from a broad variety of cells as yet undetermined. Considering, however, only the foregoing list of cells, it is noted that PAF is not found preformed in these cells but is extractable from stimulated cells before release to the outside can be detected. Although there are some unresolved issues surrounding the mechanisms involved in the cellular generation of PAF (Hanahan, 1986), the current view is that the PAF precursor in cells is composed of lyso-PC and long-chain fatty acids, including arachidonic acid. Cell stimulation leads to the sequential influx of calcium intracellularly, phospholipase A_2 activation, and liberation of the long-chain fatty acids and arachidonic acid from the PAF precursor. The resulting lyso-PC is acetylated in the presence of calcium to form PAF. This last step in the biosynthesis of PAF is catalyzed by an acetyltransferase and occurs within an intracellular membrane, possibly the endoplasmic reticulum (Ribbes et al., 1985). An acetylhydrolase inactivates PAF to form 1-alkyl-2-lyso-GPC. In platelets and other cells, the inactive lyso-PAF compound in reacylated primarily with arachidonic acid, indicating the close relationship between PAF and arachidonic acid metabolism (Malone et al., 1985).

Platelet-activating factor is an intriguing substance in several ways: (1) it is the first established pharmacologically active phosphoglyceride; (2) it has an O-alkyl ether residue at the sn-1 position and a short-chain acyl moiety, i.e., acetyl, at the sn-2 position; and (3) at the sn-3 position, the polar head group in all naturally formed PAFs is that of an O-phosphocholine group (Hanahan, 1986). With the structure known and semisynthetic material available, studies on the structure–function relationship of PAF have been actively pursued. So far these studies indicate that three portions of the PAF molecule are critical for its pharmacological activities: the acetyl group in the 2 position, the ether-linked alkyl chain in the 1 position, and the polar head group of the phosphorylcholine (Hanahan, 1986). Knowledge of the structure and of structure–activity relationships and availability of the synthetic preparation have paved the way for a new and extensive surge of investigations into the biology and physiopharmacology of this effector molecule. Nevertheless, its short biological half-life (Farr et al., 1980) and the concurrent release of other mediators in both physiological and pathological conditions (Snyder, 1985) have continued to impede the definition of the role and significance of PAF in these situations, reflecting a critical need for the availability of highly specific PAF antagonists.

With respect to the development of PAF antagonists on platelet responses, studies on isolated platelets have revealed that a chemically diverse group of agents show properties consistent with competitive PAF receptor antagonism on this test system. Among these, CV3988 (a structural analogue of PAF), RD48740 (pyrrolothiazole agent), $L652_1731$ (a trimethoxyphenyltetrahydrofuran), BN52021 (ginkgolide B), and WEB2086 (a thienotriazolodiazepine) were tested. Dose ratios were calculated, and Schild plots generated and analyzed with computer programs. The pA_2s obtained were 7.74, 7.29, 6.04, 5.55, and 5.08 for WEB2086, BN52021, $L652_1731$, CV3988, and RP48740, respectively. Schild slot slopes were not significantly different from unity (Levy and Ezzet, 1987). In a separate series of experiments, the potency and selectivity of these same substances where evaluated *ex vivo* by impedance aggregometry on human whole blood, showing that the rank order of potencies is similar for whole blood and for isolated platelets (Chan and Levy, 1987). Another group of compounds that are established α-adrenergic antagonists, such as phenoxybenzamine and phentolamine, were also found to inhibit the PAF-induced platelet and neutrophil aggregation and degranulation, whereas yohimbine and prazosin showed little or no activity (Chesney *et al.*, 1985). With respect to WEB2086, recent studies reported (Kornecki *et al.*, 1984) that two psychotropic triazolobenzodiazepine drugs, alprazolam and triazolam, inhibited PAF-induced shape, aggregation, and secretion patterns in human platelets. The most challenging facet of this study is that PAF may play a role in neuronal functions, and this may explain the mechanism by which these psychotropic drugs act on cells. For a more comprehensive discussion of PAF antagonists, the reader is referred to the articles by Hanahan (1986) and Saunders and Handley (1987).

The currently available PAF antagonists may be considered as only first-generation agents, since the most potent antagonist is still less than 1/100 as potent as PAF is as an agonist, and the wide diversity of physiological and pathological conditions may require antagonists with selective attributes such as delivery route or biological half-life. The same applies to the lack of highly potent inhibitors of PAF synthesis. Furthermore, the currently available receptor antagonists or synthesis inhibitors possess multiple sites of action along the arachidonate cascade or pathways of phospholipid metabolism. They also have various pharmacological actions unrelated to the arachidonate cascade. Until more potent and selective receptor antagonists and synthesis inhibitors are developed, the interpretation of results obtained by less selective compounds may be misleading. Despite these handicaps, even the current state of development of receptor antagonists together with the knowledge of chemical structure as well as structure–activity relationships resulted in significant progress in our understanding of the pharmacology of this agent.

Summarily stated, the pharmacological activities of PAF include activation of platelets, neutrophils, and eosinophils to degranulate, aggregate, and/or generate oxygen radicals, chemotaxis of eosinophils, increased postcapillary venular permeability, a wheal and flare response after intradermal injection in human subjects, and contraction of bronchial and intestinal smooth muscle (Schwartz,

1987). Many of these activities occur by binding of PAF to stereospecific cell membrane receptors (Valone, 1984). Although this introduction adequately sums up the essentials of PAF pharmacology, it is necessary to discuss further these and some other features of PAF activities.

Across species lines, the most prominent pharmacological effect of PAF is increased vascular permeability (Wedmore and Williams, 1981; Humphrey et al., 1984; Handley et al., 1984), which occurs at postcapillary venules (Bjork and Smedegard, 1983; Humphrey et al., 1984). At low doses, the effect of PAF is direct and does not require leukocyte (Bjork and Smedegard, 1983; Pirotzky et al., 1984) or platelet (Pirotzky et al.,1984) involvement. The concentration of PAF required to produce extravasation is severalfold less than that needed for the same effect by leukotrienes or histamine (Hwang et al., 1985; Handley et al., 1986).

Activation of platelets (Valone et al., 1982; Hwang et al., 1983), eosino-phils (Numao and Makino, 1986), and neutrophils (Hwang et al.,1983; Valone and Goetzl, 1983) occurs by specific, saturable binding of PAF to cell-surface membrane receptors. Platelet sensitivity to PAF varies greatly among species and also appears related to the capacity of this agent to induce bronchoconstriction (Vargaftig et al., 1980). With respect to the latter effect, pulmonary tissue does exhibit a direct contractile response to exposure to PAF (Hwang et al., 1983; Stimler et al., 1981; Stimler and O'Flaherty, 1983; Touvay et al., 1987). The PAF binds specifically to the smooth muscle membrane (Hwang et al., 1983), and blockade of PAF-induced intracellular calcium mobilization in smooth mus-cle cells by a PAF receptor antagonist has been reported (Doyle et al., 1986). This contractile effect on bronchial smooth muscle may be more apparent when PAF is administered by aerosol inhalation (Patterson and Harris, 1983) than after intravenous infusion (Saunders et al., 1985). Indeed, after aerosol administra-tion, nonspecific bronchial reactivity, as measured by methacholine aerosol chal-lenge, appears to be enhanced for as long as 2 weeks after a single PAF inhala-tion (Saunders and Handley, 1987).

Although PAF does possess a direct contractile effect on airway smooth muscle, the presence of polymorphonuclear neutrophil leukocytes and eosino-phils in the lung (Lellouch-Tubiana, 1985; McManus et al., 1985) after PAF infusion suggests that all these cells contribute to the overall pulmonary response induced by PAF. In addition to bronchoconstriction, the pulmonary response to PAF also includes increased pulmonary artery pressure, pulmonary vascular resistance, and pulmonary edema formation (Lichey et al., 1984; Camussi et al., 1983); PAF mediates these effects both by direct action on airway tissue and secondarily by stimulating the release of prostaglandins, leukotrienes, and com-plement fragments. Thus, PAF perfusion of isolated lungs releases LTC_4 and LTD_4, and, conversely, these 5-lipoxygenase products increase the production of both PAF and thromboxane A_2 (Voelkel et al., 1982; Engineer et al., 1978; Parker, 1987). Similarly, in neutrophils stimulated with A-23187, the production of PAF is greatly augmented by 5-HETE, 5-HPETE, and LTB_4 (Billah et al., 1985), and in endothelial cells LTC_4 and LTD_4 generally stimulate arachidonic and metabolism as well as increase PAF, possibly through augmenting phospholipase A_2 activation (McIntyre, 1986). The 5-lipoxygenase products also stimulate PAF production in macrophages (Saito et al., 1985). Potentiation of PAF formation as well as its activities by these lipoxygenase products could be expected to markedly enhance local tissue responses. It may be added that PAF also stimulates the release of arachidonic acid and LTB_4 from neutrophils (Lin et al., 1982; Chilton et al., 1982), which could serve as an additional means for amplifying reactions of immunologic inflammation.

As stated earlier, PAF is a major effector molecule of IgE-mediated anaphylaxis in rabbits. Intravenous challenge with the homologous antigen of specifically sensitized rabbits produces a significant depression of circulating levels of basophils, neutrophils, and platelets within 1 min of antigen administration, and within the same time the presence of PAF can be demonstrated in plasma (Pinckard et al., 1979; Stimler et al., 1981). Intravenous infusion of nanomolar concentrations of PAF in rabbits and baboons reproduces the entire clinical syndrome of anaphylactic shock (McManus et al., 1980), including the manifestation of renal failure during systemic anaphylaxis and serum sickness. The role of PAF in renal failure is further supported by observations that PAF can induce a loss of glomerular anionic charges (Camussi et al., 1984) and fibrogen accumulation in the perfused kidney (Pirotzky et al., 1985) and is released from sensitized animals to participate in hyperacute renal allograft rejection (Ito et al., 1984).

Immunoglobulin E is not the only immunoglobulin that mediates reactivities that are accompanied by endogenous PAF production leading to lethal systemic anaphylaxis: IgG can also mediate the same manifestations, but IgG-mediated models of PAF release are not as severe as the IgE or endotoxin models in terms of resulting pathology. The IgG responses can be induced with soluble aggregates of IgG (Inarrea et al., 1983; Sanchez-Crespo et al., 1985) and by passive sensitization to nonspecific (Touvay et al., 1985; Page et al., 1984) or pulmonary specific (Camussi et al., 1983) antigens.

The clinically dramatic development of IgE-mediated, usually lethal anaphylactic shock raises the issue of PAF's significance in the pathophysiology of various shock states. Emergence of this issue is based on the demonstration that administration of PAF to several species (guinea pig, rat, rabbit, dog, pig) produced severe hypotension, shock, and death (Feuerstein et al., 1982, 1985; Bessin et al., 1983; Goldstein et al., 1987). Indeed, PAF is the single most potent agent to cause shock when administered systemically (Feuerstein and Hallenbeck, 1987). One of the critically important features of these shock states is the severe hypotension induced by PAF, an activity that is similar to the vascular permeability-increasing effect of PAF in that it occurs in all species tested (Saunders et al., 1985; McManus et al., 1981; Tanaka et al., 1983) and is a non-platelet-mediated occurrence (Sanchez-Crespo et al., 1981). It is to be noted, however, that in the pharmacology of PAF, permeability increase and hypotension are independent events, since hypotension occurs at lower doses and is immediate and reversible (Handley et al., 1986), whereas the extravasation response requires 4–10 min to peak and several hours to reverse (Handley and Saunders, 1986; Handley et al., 1986; McManus et al., 1981). The vascular endothelium has been suggested to be required for the hypotensive activity of PAF in the rat (Cervoni et al., 1983; Kasuva et al., 1984) but not in the rabbit (Lefer and Lefer, 1986). Some recent studies suggest that the hypotensive effect may be the result of arteriolar dilation, especially in the splanchnic vascular bed (Struyker-Boudier et al., 1985). Investigations of the nature of the hypotensive action have ruled out renin inhibition, CNS influences, and α-adrenergic antagonism as possible mechanisms (Kamitani et al., 1984).

In addition to the permeability and vasodilatory actions, the other effects that may be contributory to the development of the various shock states are as follows. Pulmonary circulation is affected by the earlier mentioned increase in pulmonary vascular resistance (PVR; Voelkel et al., 1982; Goldstein et al., 1987) and bronchoconstriction, both of which contribute to hypoxemia and the increase in PVR to right heart failure. The heart is also affected by reduction in cardiac input from coronary constriction, reduction in myocardial contractility, and cardiac preload (Feuerstein and Hallenbeck, 1987). All these actions ultimately result in a very significant contraction of blood and plasma volume. In fact, no other vasoactive lipid is known to date that can produce the degree and breadth of sustained derangements in organ blood flow that is caused by PAF.

Before leaving this section on lipid-derived mediators, we need to refer briefly to a group of phospholipase A_2 inhibitory proteins, collectively called lipocortin. By blocking phospholipase A_2, lipocortin both inhibits the release of arachidonic acid, which is, as mentioned earlier, the precursor for prostaglandins and leukotrienes, and prevents the formation of the lysophospholipid precursor of PAF. Lipocortinlike proteins have been isolated from various cell types including monocytes, neutrophils, and renal medullary cell preparations. The predominant active form is a protein with an apparent relative molecular mass (M_r) of 40,000 (40K). Using amino acid sequence information obtained from purified rat lipocortin, Wallner et al. (1986) have now cloned human lipocortin complementing DNA and expressed the gene in E. coli. Based on these findings, it appears that lipocortin may play a critical role in the regulation of the release and generation of highly potent lipid-derived mediators of immunologic inflammation. In accord with this, corticosteroids at least in part are now thought to exert their antiinflammatory activity through their induction of lipocortin (Parente and Flower, 1985).

8. THE PEPTIDE MEDIATORS

8.1. Thymic Peptides

Primarily as a result of the pioneering contributions of Robert A. Good and many of his associates in the 1960s and 1970s, it became recognized that the thymus participates in the normal maturation of many different functional sub-classes of T lymphocytes (e.g., helper, suppressor, and cytotoxic effector cells). The thymus exerts its influence by the release of various effector molecules both within its own microenvironment and at distant target tissue sites (e.g., peripheral lymphoid tissues) via these molecules secreted into the blood. In this sense, the thymic-derived effector molecules behave like hormones, and the thymus itself as an endocrine organ. Several chemically defined thymic peptides produced by the thymic epithelium now fulfill this definition. They have been isolated from thymic extracts, characterized, eventually sequenced, and synthesized. The four thymic peptides best characterized so far are thymosin α_1, thymopoietin, THF, and thymulin.

8.1.1. The Thymosins

A standardized procedure for the isolation of thymosin fraction V was reported by Hooper *et al.* in 1975, and this fraction was found to consist of a heterogeneous mixture of more than 25 heat-stable small polypeptides with molecular weight ranging from 1000 to 12,000. On isoelectric focusing gel, fraction V is separated into many peptides components. Of these, thymosin α_1 was the first to be isolated and sequenced. It consists of 28 amino acid residues and has a molecular weight of 3108 (Goldstein *et al.*, 1983). Thymosin α_1 increases mitogenic responses of murine lymphocytes, stimulates antibody production, enhances production of the macrophage migration inhibitory factor, and augments the number of Thy 1^+ Lyt $1,2,3^+$ cells (Ahmed *et al.*, 1979; Goldstein *et al.*, 1983). It also increases the expression of terminal deoxynucleotidyltransferase (Tdt), which catalyzes the formation of DNA sequences without template involvement. The Tdt is the earliest marker of lymphocyte differentiation, and it is present in mice and humans within bone marrow lymphoid precursors as well as in the majority of cortical thymocytes but not in medullary lymphocytes (Bollum, 1979; Hu *et al.*, 1981).

The second thymosin peptide to be sequenced (Low and Goldstein, 1979), and synthesized (Wang *et al.*, 1982) is thymosin β_4. In addition to stimulating the expression of Tdt in T cells (Hu *et al.*, 1981) and having MIF-like activity (Thurman *et al.*, 1981), thymosin β_4 is a potent inducer of luteinizing hormone-releasing factor (LRF) and luteinizing hormone (LH) (see below; Rebar *et al.*, 1981; Hall *et al.*, 1985). Thymosin β_4 was also shown to be produced by monocytes (Xu *et al.*, 1982) and, therefore, cannot be regarded as thymus-specific. Two additional β_4-like molecules, termed β_8 and β_9, have been sequenced (Hannapel *et al.*, 1982). There is a significant amino acid sequence homology among thymosins β_4, β_8, and β_9 (Goldstein *et al.*, 1983).

A 74-amino-acid polypeptide has been isolated from thymosin fraction 5 by Low and co-workers (Low and Goldstein, 1979; Low *et al.*, 1979) and named thymosin β_1. The yield of β_1 from fraction 5 ranges from 1.5% to 6.2% and represents the major single component of thymosin fraction 5 (Low *et al.*, 1979).

Thymosin β_1 turned out to be chemically identical with a polypeptide that had been isolated by Goldstein et al. (1975) from a variety of animal and plant sources, including calf thymus, with lymphocyte-differentiating properties, which they termed "ubiquitin" (UB) (Schlesinger et al., 1975, 1978).

Of thymosins α_2 through β_8, we do not have detailed biological or chemical information available for further characterization here. Nevertheless, there is now a substantial body of evidence that the so far partially purified thymosin fraction 5 is active in all three major compartments of the lymphoid system (bone marrow, thymus, and peripheral lymphoid tissue) in influencing the maturation and differentiation of helper T cells (Ahmed et al., 1979; Frasca et al., 1982) and suppressor T cells (Asherson et al., 1976; Ahmed et al., 1979). Furthermore, several of the thymosins appear to have selective sites of action. Thus, α_1 induces helper T cells (Ahmed et al., 1979; Frasca et al., 1982) and phenotypic T-cell markers (Twomey and Kouttab, 1982), whereas thymosin α_7 may be an inducer of suppressor T cells (Ahmed et al., 1979). Thymosins β_3 and β_4 appear to act at an earlier stage in T-cell differentiation, particularly at low doses (Pazmino et al., 1978).

In the human thymus, there appears to be a rather segregated localization of the thymosin producing cells. This has been shown with antibodies developed against α_1, β_4, and α_7 for the purpose of identifying the thymic cells that are producing these peptides. Thymosin α_1 is found in the rim of subcapsular cortical epithelial cells and in the medullary epithelial cells; β_4 is found in cells in the subcapsular rim; and α_7 is found primarily in epithelial cells surrounding Hassall's corpuscles and in a few isolated cells in the medullary epithelium (Goldstein et al., 1983). It may be added that Haynes et al. (1983) have found that the cells that are making α_1, β_4, and α_7 are also the cells that react with monoclonal antibodies directed against neuroendocrine-secreting cells. Complementary to these observations is the mounting evidence of recent years that certain thymosin peptides are neuroactive immunoregulatory substances that modulate the hypothalamic–pituitary–adrenal and gonadal axes and represent a component of the immune–neuroendocrine circuitry subserving immune homeostasis.

In one of the approaches used to explore such a relationship, it was shown that thymosin fraction 5 (TF5) causes increased serum corticosterone levels in rodents in vivo (McGillis et al., 1985). In a related study, ACTH, β-endorphin, cortisol, LH, FSH, prolactin, growth hormone, and thyroid-stimulating hormone levels were determined in prepubertal female macaque monkeys following the administration of TF5, thymosin α_1 (Tα_1), or thymosin β_4 (Tβ_4). The last two thymosins did not have any effect on any of the hormones, whereas TF5 caused an elevation in plasma ACTH, β-endorphin, and cortisol, an effect that was dose and time dependent (Healy et al., 1983). Conversely, following thymectomy circulating levels of the same hormones were found to be reduced.

In an attempt to identify the possible sites of action where the thymosin effects may be exerted, it was shown in cultured adrenal fasciculata cells treated with either TF5, α_1, β_4, or α_7 that the plasma corticosterone increases does not result from direct stimulation of the adrenal glands (Vahouny et al., 1983), suggesting that the site of thymosin action might be at the pituitary level. Experiments designed to answer this question utilized pituitary tissue superfused with TF5 or thymosin α_1 (McGillis et al., 1985) or cultured monolayers of pituitary cells (McGillis et al., 1987). In the latter system, TF5 was shown to be capable of directly stimulating ACTH release, but the superfusion model was ineffective. On the other hand, in the superfusion approach TF5 and $T\beta_4$ were each found to stimulate LH release in both males and females. This effect was dose dependent and occurred only when the pituitary was superfused in sequence with the medial basal hypothalamus. Simultaneous measurements of LH-releasing hormone indicated that secretion of this substance was also stimulated. These findings are interpreted to mean that thymosins may act at the CNS level in modulating the reproductive axis (Rebar et al., 1981). In a further exploration of the interrelationships between thymosins and the CNS, both hormonal changes following intracerebral injection of thymosins as well as the localization of thymosin peptides in subcortical nuclei were studied (Hall et al., 1985a). Administration of $T\alpha_1$ resulted in a significant increase of corticosterone but not serum LH levels, whereas $T\beta_4$ increased LH but not corticosterone levels, indicating that the thymosins may exert differential effects on neuroendocrine circuits. From use of the radioimmunoassay for CNS localization of thymosins, it appears that $T\alpha_1$ is present in highest concentrations in the arcuate nucleus and in the median eminence, whereas $T\beta_4$ does not seem to show selective localization in the brain (Hannappel et al., 1981; Palaszynski et al., 1983). Since thymosin stimulation of lymphocytes is known to produce several pharmacologically active effector molecules including some neuroactive immunoregulatory peptides, it has been suggested that they might also stimulate directly other lymphocytic production of ACTH and β-endorphin, but no conclusive evidence exists at present for such an activity (Hall et al., 1985; Deschaux and Rouabhia, 1987; Geenen et al., 1987; Spangelo et al., 1987).

The full significance of these findings with respect to immune–neuroendocrine circuits (Szentivanyi et al., 1952–1960; Filipp and Szentivanyi, 1985; Szentivanyi, 1987; Goetzl, 1985, 1987; Goetzl et al., 1985; Besedovsky et al., 1985; Felten et al., 1985; Roszman et al., 1985; Johnson and Torres, 1985; Smith et al., 1982, 1985; Payan and Goetzl, 1985; O'Dorisio et al., 1985; O'Dorisio, 1987; Hall et al., 1985; Blalock et al., 1985; Shavit et al., 1985, 1986; Golub, 1986; Spector, 1986) is discussed in the section on neuroactive immunoregulatory peptides below (Section 8.7).

8.1.2. The Thymopoietins

The recognition of thymopoietin (initially named thymin) resulted from experimental studies related to the human disease myasthenia gravis. This disease is characterized by a deficit in neuromuscular transmission and thymic malfunction. On the basis of a biological assay measuring impairment of neuromuscular transmission, researchers first isolated thymopoietin by following its capacity to induce blockage, as is seen in patients with myasthenia gravis (Goldstein and Lau, 1980). Subsequently, two factors were identified on the basis of their ability to induce the differentiation of bone marrow cells into mature T cells *in vitro,* and the peptides have been designated thymopoietin I and thymopoietin II. Since they are immunologically cross-reactive and have indistinguishable biological activities, they appear to be closely related polypeptides, which is also reflected by the fact that thymopoietins I and II differ by only two amino acid residues (Schlesinger *et al.,* 1975). Thus, the two thymopoietins probably represent isohormonal variation. Thymopoietin II has a molecular weight of 5562, and the synthesis of its entire chain of 49 amino acids has been accomplished (Laroche and Bach, 1985). A tridecapeptide corresponding to thymopoietin residues 29–41 has been synthesized and demonstrated to have biological activity similar to that of the native molecule (Schlesinger *et al.,* 1975). Within this sequence, a pentapeptide called thymopoietin 32–36 (TP-5) was shown to be the smallest active synthetic fragment. The amino acid sequences of thymopoietin I and II have recently been revised, and a thymopoietin III peptide has also been isolated from spleen (Audhya *et al.,* 1981). The three peptides have largely identical sequences except for the amino acid residues at positions 1, 2, 34, and 43 (Incefy, 1983). Some of the most important biological properties of the thymopoietins include (1) induction of differentiation of prothymocytes to thymocytes, as detected by cell surface markers and functional characteristics (i.e., responsiveness to T cell mitogens), (2) enhancement of lymphoid cell transcription and translation of DNA, (3) inhibition of early-stage and induction of late-stage of B-cell differentiation, and (4) induction of complement receptors on human granulocytes (Stutman, 1983; Incefy, 1983).

8.1.3. Thymic Humoral Factor

Thymic humoral factor (THF) was discovered through the demonstration that thymic tissue in Millipore® chambers implanted into neonatally thymectomized mice led to the restoration of specific immunologic competence in these animals (Kook and Trainin, 1974). The THF consists of 30 amino acid residues, its purification to homogeneity has been achieved, and, based on leucine as unity, the minimal molecular weight is 3220 (Trainin *et al.,* 1980). This effector molecule has been reported to have many effects and to lead to differentiation of young thymus-derived T cells, promoting them to maturation and acquisition of full immunocompetence. Thus, THF could increase the responses of splenocytes and thymocytes from intact mice as well as thymectomized animals in the mixed lymphocyte reaction (MLR). It can also strongly enhance the responses to phytohemagglutinin (PHA) and concanavalin A (con A) of human lymphocytes from peripheral blood (PBL) or umbilical cord blood (Trainin *et al.,* 1980; Incefy, 1983).

8.1.4. Thymulin

In the course of studies assessing the immunologic status and the relative likelihood of kidney rejection in patients with renal transplants, another thymic-hormone-like activity has been detected in the serum of these patients. Initially, the active agent has been isolated directly from serum; hence, its first name, *"facteur thymique serique"* (Bach and Dardenne, 1973). It is only recently, when its production by thymic epithelial cells was directly demonstrated by immunofluorescence (Savino *et al.*, 1982) and after the presence of zinc in the molecule was revealed (Dardenne *et al.*, 1982), that it was given the name of thymulin. The agent has a molecular weight of 847 and has been characterized as a nonapeptide with the following amino acid composition: Glu-Ala-Lys-Ser-Glu-Gly-Gly-Ser-Asn. Synthesis of the molecule has been achieved, and the synthetic and natural substances show comparable biological activities. Some of the more significant of the latter include (1) restoration of responsiveness of adult thymectomized animals to mitogens and of their capacity to generate cytotoxic lymphoid cells to restrain the growth of virus-induced sarcoma, (2) inhibition of antibody production to thymic-independent antigen and of the development of contact sensitivity, (3) delay of allogeneic skin graft rejection through the generation of suppressor T cells and prevention of appearance of autoimmune hemolytic anemia and Sjogren syndrome in animal models, and (4) transformation of cortisone-sensitive into cortisone-resistant thymocytes (Laroche and Bach, 1985).

Although thymic epithelial cells and the foregoing thymic effector molecules probably represent the major regulatory signals of intrathymic differentiation, other agents secreted by the thymic epithelium as well as other thymic cell types may play roles in T-cell processing, at least as amplifying mechanisms. For instance, by using a system for long-term culture of human thymic epithelial cells (TE cells), it was recently found that human TE cells produce an IL-1-like molecule that augments the proliferation of C3H/HeJ mouse thymocytes to mitogen. This TE IL-1 is a substance of 18,000–20,000 relative molecular mass and in gel electrophoresis migrates at 15,000–17,000 M_r. With electrofocusing, charge heterogeneity is demonstrable with two major isoelectric points of 5.7–5.8 and 6.9–7.0. Polyclonal antibody to human monocyte IL-1 markedly inhibits the TE IL-1 activity, and rabbit anti-IL-1 antibody reacts with TE cells in human thymic cortex and medulla. Thus, TE cells are capable of providing an intrathymic source of IL-1 that affects thymocyte proliferation (Singer *et al.*, 1985, 1986; Denning *et al.*, 1986; Le *et al.*, 1987).

There is, however, a recently described subpopulation of phagocytic cells of the thymic reticulum that can be isolated from *in vitro* secondary cultures serving as another thymic source of IL-1 (Papiernik and Nabarra, 1981; Papiernik *et al.*, 1983). These cells, which represent a macrophage phenotype (Thy 1$^-$, Ig$^-$, Ia$^+$, Fc$^+$, phagocytosis), exert both positive and negative controls on T-cell proliferation by secreting, respectively, IL-1 and prostaglandins (Papiernik and Homo-Delarche, 1983). Furthermore, several lines of argument favor the notion that mature thymic medullary lymphocytes also play a role in the maturation of T-cell precursors: (1) they appear early in ontogeny; (2) their majority resides permanently in the thymus; and (3) they are essentially Lyt 1$^+$ associated with a helper function and are expected to produce IL-2 in response to IL-1 release or autologous stimulation. On the other hand, since IL-2 is produced only by T cells that themselves had to differentiate from precursor stem cells (with thymic epithelial contact and under the influence of thymic effector molecules), IL-2 may not be a requisite stimulus in the intrathymic circuit of T-cell maturation (Laroche and Bach, 1985).

In closing this section, it should be added that many other less well-defined thymic effector molecules have been described. At the time of this writing, their chemical and biological characterization has not progressed to the point that they could be included here.

8.2. Prostaglandin-Generating Factor of Anaphylaxis

As stated earlier various pharmacologically active effector molecules promote the anaphylactic release of prostaglandins from lung or other tissues. One such agent is the so-called "prostaglandin-generating factor of anaphylaxis" (PGF-A) (Steel and Kaliner, 1981; Steel et al., 1982). This substance is not preformed and intracellularly stored but is newly synthesized in the course of the anaphylactic response. PGF-A is an oligopeptide composed of 13 amino acids with a molecular weight of 1450. It stimulates the production of $PGF_{2\alpha}$, PGE_2, and TXB_2 by human lung fragments. So far the pulmonary arteries have been identified as the source of release of TXB_2, and the pulmonary veins, parenchyma, and airway tissues as the source of $PGF_{2\alpha}$ release (1984). The relative significance or contribution of PGF-A to anaphylaxis cannot be assessed as yet.

8.3. Eosinophil Chemotactic Factor of Anaphylaxis

One of the clinical hallmarks of manifestations of anaphylactic allergy is the accumulation of eosinophils in the local area of antigen–antibody reactions or in the body fluids. Originally, these examples of eosinophilia were accounted for by the associated phenomenon of histamine release (Szentivanyi and Fishel, 1966) as well as the subsequent recognition of β-adrenergic functional deficits existing in these conditions (Szentivanyi, 1968; Szentivanyi and Fitzpatrick, 1980; Szentivanyi and Szentivanyi, 1985). Although both histamine and a genetically determined or acquired β-adrenergic impairment (Szentivanyi et al., 1986) may, and in fact do, produce eosinophil accumulation, there are also one or several chemotactic factors distinct from histamine and unrelated to β-adrenergically induced mechanisms. This has been chemically identified and designated "eosinophil chemotactic factor of anaphylaxis" (ECF-A; Goetzl and Austen, 1975), with a molecular weight of about 400. In lung, about 50% of ECF-A activity is contained in two tetrapeptides: Val-Gly-Ser-Glu and Ala-Gly-Ser-Glu. The ECF-A in human lung mast cells is preformed, but not that in basophils, where it is newly generated after cell stimulation (Czarnetzki *et al.*, 1976).

Other eosinophil chemotactic factors of low molecular weight have been described but not as yet completely structurally characterized. Cells other than basophils and mast cells can synthesize and/or release ECF-A. These include neutrophils and eosinophils, which respond to various stimuli, and importantly for this discussion to phagocytic stimuli, with the synthesis of an ECF physicochemically similar to ECF-A, and neutrophils also release a material that inactivates ECF (Plaut and Lichtenstein, 1983). Some of these are selective for eosinophils, and, in addition to chemotaxis, they stimulate the hexose-monophosphate shunt, release granular enzymes, and induce rapid increases in C3b receptors (Anwar and Kay, 1978).

Elevated blood levels of ECF-A have been shown in human anaphylaxis and experimental cold urticaria (Soter *et al.*, 1976). Although allergic eosinophil accumulations are thought to be caused by histamine, defective β-adrenergic mechanisms, and several ECF-like molecules, other agents such as C5a and lymphocyte products may also have eosinophil-directed chemotactic activity (Plaut and Lichtenstein, 1983).

8.4. Complement-Derived "Anaphylatoxins" C3a, C4a, and C5a

The complement system consists of a series of serum glycoproteins that possess many effector functions. Two distinct routes exist for complement activation: the classical and the alternative pathways. Both pathways result in sequential activation of the complement components. For several reactions in these pathways, the product of one step is the enzyme that catalyzes the next step. Consequently, the amount of activated complement components can be significantly amplified in each succeeding step. The intermediate products of the complement pathways possess several types of biological activity, including chemotaxis of cells, activation of cells for mediator release, and smooth muscle contraction. Activation of the entire complement sequence results in cell lysis. The steps in the activation of the complement systems initiated by immune reactions are called the classical pathway of complement activation. This may be contrasted with the alternative pathway, which involves nonimmune activation of the complement and serum properdin systems. For a more detailed account of the various aspects of the complement system in health and disease, the reader is referred to Szentivanyi and Szentivanyi (1985). This section is limited to the discussion of the complement-derived anaphylatoxins C3a, C4a, and C5a.

The low-molecular-weight fragments of C3, C4, and C5, that is, C3a, C4a, and C5a, respectively, are known as "anaphylatoxins." Originally, the term "anaphylatoxin" was coined by C. Richet early this century to explain the onset of anaphylaxis as the result of a "poison" generated by the union of antigen with antibodies. This assumption has proved to be no more tenable than the later interpretation of the clinical syndrome of anaphylactic shock, primarily by E. Friedberger but also by J. Bordet, that the "poison" that elicits the shock is set free from the precipitate (in the course of the antigen–antibody interaction) by the influence of the complement, or the hypothesis by V. Vaughan that it is derived from protein by proteolytic processes in the course of parenteral digestion (Szentivanyi and Fishel, 1966).

As histamine gradually came to occupy center stage in the interpretation of the clinical syndrome of anaphylaxis, and as the complement system came to be recognized as an important requirement for precipitating the development of shock, attention was directed increasingly to the role of complement with special regard to its relationship to histamine release (Szentivanyi and Fitzpatrick, 1980). These studies ultimately led to the clarification of the elusive nature of anaphylatoxins and identified them as three complement fragments, C3a, C4a, and C5a.

C3a, C4a, and C5a have molecular weights of 9038, 8740, and 11,200, respectively. They are basic peptides formed by limited proteolysis of C3, C4, and C5 as a consequence of activation of either the classic or alternative complement pathways (Hugli, 1975; Fernandez and Hugli, 1978). Analyses of their primary structures indicate that they are genetically related. C3a and C4a both are 77-amino-acid peptides with C-terminal arginines, whereas C5a is a 74-amino-acid peptide with a C-terminal arginine and an oligosaccharide side chain (Plaut and Lichtenstein, 1983). They share a number of the same pharmacological activities such as inducing noncytotoxic histamine release from mast cells and basophils, lysosomal enzyme release from granulocytes, smooth muscle contraction, and increased capillary vascular permeability (Hugli, 1975; Fernandez and Hugli, 1978; Stimler et al., 1980; Hellewell and Williams, 1986). The anaphylatoxins derived from later complement components are more potent than those derived from early components (i.e., C5a, C3a). Also, C3a and C4a appear to act on the same cell surface receptors, whereas C5a uses a separate receptor (Plaut and Lichtenstein, 1983). The carboxy-terminal arginine of the anaphylatoxins is required for pharmacological activity.

In harmony with its distinct cell membrane receptors, one of the pharmacological effects of C5a that is not shared by the other anaphylatoxins is its chemotactic capacity for inflammatory cells. This effector molecule is chemotactic for neutrophils, eosinophils, monocytes, and basophils and acts synergistically with a lymphocyte-derived chemotactic factor for basophils (Boetcher and Leonard, 1973; Lett-Brown et al., 1976). Other chemotactic factors can also activate the cells that they are attracting. For instance, C5a activates basophils for mediator release and neutrophils for lysosomal enzyme release. C5a also has other properties including granulocyte aggregation and activation of intracellular processes in certain cells leading to effects such as release of oxygen metabolites, SRS-A, or histamine (Cooper, 1987).

Many of the C3a and C4a effects seem to be mediated by histamine released by their interaction with mast cells and basophils. These effects are abrogated by antihistamines and by the action of an anaphylatoxin inactivator or carboxypeptidase N, a serum enzyme that removes the C-terminal arginine residue from these peptides. C5a retains slightly more than 10% of its chemotactic activity after cleavage to [des-Arg]C5a by carboxypeptidase N. However, its abilities to increase vascular permeability and to induce smooth muscle contractions are reduced by 1000-fold and 10,000-fold, respectively (Bokisch and Muller-Eberhard, 1970). C5a is also irreversibly inactivated in human sera by an α-globulin termed chemotactic factor inactivator activity (Berenberg and Ward, 1973).

The anaphylatoxins and other complement-derived molecules may also promote immunologic inflammation by their effects on eicosanoid formation and mucus secretion. Thus, C3a induces the release of TXB_2 from macrophages (Hartung et al., 1983) and mucus glycoproteins from cultured human airway tissue (Marom et al., 1985), whereas C5a stimulates the production of both LTB_4 from exogenous arachidonic acid by neutrophils (Clancy et al., 1983) and LTD_4 by lung tissue (Stimler et al., 1982). The arachidonate metabolism in phagocytes is also affected by complement-derived molecules other than C3a and C5a. Thus, the terminal complement complex, C5b–9, stimulates the release of arachidonic acid, 6-keto-$PGF_{1\alpha}$, PGE_2, and LTC_4 from macrophages (Imagawa et al., 1983, 1986).

Another consequence of the activation of the complement system is the generation of a vasoactive substance called C-kinin, possibly a product of C2, which increases vascular permeability and contracts smooth muscle. This molecule is believed to be formed by cleavage, by serum plasmin, of either C2a or C2b (Muller-Eberhard, 1978), and it does not appear to function through release of histamine. It is thought to be involved in the clinical symptomatology of hereditary angioedema. Functional C1 inactivator is genetically lacking in this disease characterized by uncontrolled activation of the complement system. This kinin leads us to the issue of the role of plasma kinins in immunologic inflammation and hypersensitivity.

8.5. The Kinins

Kinins are a group of potent vasoactive peptides that are formed enzymatically by the action of enzymes known as kallikreins or kininogenases on protein substrates called kininogens. Their discovery can be traced back to an old observation at the turn of the century that urine, injected intravenously, lowers blood pressure (Bouchard, 1900). This finding has been rediscovered and gained new significance in the course of research on the relationship between myocardial work load and kidney function by E. K. Frey (1926). Frey with his associates Kraut and Werle characterized this hypotensive substance and showed its presence in plasma, saliva, and a variety of tissues. The pancreas was found to be an important source of this agent, and therefore the name "kallikrein" was coined after the ancient Greek name of the pancreas, "*kallikreas.*" By 1937, Werle and associates determined that kallikrein is an enzyme that is responsible for splitting off the *de facto* hypotensive agent from an inactive precursor in the plasma. Subsequently, Werle and Berek (1948) named the active substance "kallidin" and found it to be a polypeptide cleaved from a plasma globulin that they termed "kallidinogen."

In an entirely separate line of investigation in Brazil, Rocha e Silva and associates (1949) demonstrated that the venoms of certain snakes (i.e., *Bothrops jararaca*) as well as trypsin acting on plasma globulin produce a hypotensive polypeptide that also causes a slowly developing contraction of the gut. Because of the latter activity, they named the substance "bradykinin" after the Greek words "*bradys,*" meaning "slow," and "*kinein,*" meaning "to move." Chemical characterization of bradykinin was accomplished by Elliot (1960); it was found to be a nonapeptide and was synthesized by Boissonnas *et al.* (1960a,b,c, 1963). This nonapeptide was then shown to be a constituent of kallidin. The two pharmacologically active effector molecules are two of a large number of polypeptides with similarities in chemical structure and pharmacological properties. For the whole group, the generic term "kinins" has been adopted, and kallidin and bradykinin are referred to as plasma kinins (Bertaccini, 1976; Erdos, 1979; Schachter and Barton, 1979; Fritz *et al.*, 1983; Douglas, 1985). Included in this group is the cleavage product of basophil kallikrein of anaphylaxis (BK-A) that is probably one or more of these kinins, or it could be a new kinin that is immunochemically similar to bradykinin.

Thus, kinins are small polypeptide molecules that have many pharmacological properties including those of contracting or relaxing smooth muscle, increasing vascular permeability, and producing pain. In general, there are three major groups: the bradykinins, the leukokinins, and the nonmammalian kinins. This discussion concentrates on bradykinins and only briefly mentions the latter two types of kinins at the end of this section.

As stated earlier, two separate lines of investigation (in Germany and Brazil) have ultimately led to the identification of plasma kinins, a circumstance that resulted in a confusing terminology. At present, the term kallidin (which formerly referred to both the nonapeptide and decapeptide) is now limited to the decapeptide, and the term bradykinin applies to the nonapeptide. Bradykinin is a nine-amino-acid peptide (Arg-Pro-Pro-Gly-Phe-Ser-Pro-Phe-Arg), kallidin has an additional lysine residue in the N-terminal position (lysyl-bradykinin; Lys-bradykinin; Lys-Arg-Pro-Pro-Gly-Phe-Ser-Pro-Phe-Arg), and methionyllysyl-bradykinin an additional methionyl residue (Met-Lys-Arg-Pro-Pro-Gly-Ser-Pro-Phe-Arg). Bradykinin is released by plasma kallikrein, lysylbradykinin by glandular kallikrein, and methionyllysylbradykinin by pepsin and pepsinlike enzymes. All three are present in plasma and urine, but bradykinin is predominant in plasma, whereas lysylbradykinin (kallidin) is the major urinary kinin (Reid, 1987).

The kinins are rather evanescent molecules (half-life of about 15 sec in the plasma) that are catabolized by nonspecific exo- or endopeptidases, referred to as kininases. Two plasma kininases are well characterized. The principal catabolizing enzyme in the lung and other vascular beds is a dipeptidyl carboxypeptidase known in the context of this section as kininase II and in another as angiotensin-converting enzyme. This zinc-containing metalloenzyme, with an approximate molecular weight of 150,000, cleaves the C-terminal two amino acids (Phe-Arg) from bradykinins, thereby inactivating them. The active enzyme is present in the plasma and on the luminal surface of vascular endothelial cells throughout the body. Approximately half of the identifiable kininase II in the mammalian body is in the pulmonary tissues, which makes it likely that the lung is the principal site of kinin catabolism. This is in agreement with findings that in a single passage through the pulmonary vascular bed about 80% to 90% of the kinins may be destroyed, and as many as five peptide bonds may be cleaved (Ryan, 1982). Kininase II is also active in the conversion of angiotensin I to angiotensin II by cleaving the C-terminal two amino acids from angiotensin I. Furthermore, since the affinity of kinins for kininase II is approximately 100 times that of angiotensin I (K_m 10^{-7} versus 10^{-5}), one might consider the possibility bradykinin to be capable of influencing vascular tone indirectly by successfully competing with angiotensin I for the kininase II enzyme.

A slower-acting enzyme, called kininase I (carboxypeptidase-N), is an arginine carboxypeptidase that also participates in the catabolism of plasma kinins. This enzyme, apparently synthesized in the liver, removes the C-terminal arginine. Like kininase II, it is also a metalloprotease and is inhibited by edetate and o-phenanthroline (Reid, 1987). Although kininase I usually also abolishes kininlike activity, the des-Arg kinins that are so produced may remain active in some damaged tissues in which the physicochemical characteristics of the receptors are altered (Marceau et al., 1983). In addition to plasma kinins, this metalloenzyme with a molecular weight of 300,000 and a plasma concentration of 30–40 μg/ml is also capable of cleaving C-terminal basic amino acids from other pharmacologically active peptides including fibrinopeptides, C3a, C4a, and C5a. As stated earlier, it is probably the major inactivator of the complement-derived anaphylatoxins in plasma but inactivates kinins less rapidly. Other cellular peptidases may also destroy the plasma kinins, but their possible importance is unclear.

The plasma kinins possess a broad spectrum of potent pharmacological activities on autonomic effector cells, and they also stimulate the proliferation of a wide variety of other cells in vivo and in vitro, including thymocytes (Wiggins and Cochrane, 1984). In all these respects, bradykinin and kallidin behave very similarly. They appear to have these direct effects, but they also act indirectly through arachidonic acid metabolites, histamine, serotonin, vasopressin, and catcholamines. For instance, the interaction of kinins with cell surface receptors activates acylhydrolases (i.e., phospholipase A_2), which liberate arachidonic acid from phospholipids. Kinins also act further along the arachidonic acid pathway, since they selectively increase production of PGE_2 and PGI_2 (vasodilator) in arteries and $PGF_{2\alpha}$ (vasoconstrictor) in veins. This difference is believed to result from activation of PGE 9-ketoreductase by kinins in veins. Whatever the responsible molecular mechanisms may be, however, the plasma kinins are the most potent currently known vasodilator substances in the mammalian organism. Indeed, on a molar basis, kinins are about ten times more potent than histamine in causing vasodilation (Regoli and Barabe, 1980; Szentivanyi and Fitzpatrick, 1980), and they are among the pharmacologically active effector molecules that induce endothelium-dependent vasodilation (Fritz et al., 1983).

With respect to their vasodilatory effects, it is a fair assumption that intravascular kinins must reach the vascular smooth muscle cells directly to effect vasodilation. However, no evidence is available for this, and because of the earlier described high concentration of kininase II in the plasma as well as on the luminal surface of vascular endothelial cells, the latter would be expected to form a relatively impermeable layer for the penetration of kinins. On the other hand, there are close contacts between endothelial cells and the underlying smooth muscle cells, making it conceivable that kinins could cause smooth muscle contraction or relaxation via intercellular signals such as the prostaglandins mentioned before. Prostaglandins as well as other messenger molecules could then affect cyclic-nucleotide-dependent protein kinases, which regulate the actin–myosin–ATP interaction under the influence of calmodulin (Kakiuchi et al., 1982).

Plasma kinins also produce a significant increase in vascular permeability. This effect is very similar to that of histamine and serotonin, since it is exerted at the level of postcapillary venules as determined by tracer studies and electron microscopy (Ganellin and Parsons, 1982). Increased permeability is the result of endothelial cell contraction and widening of intercellular junctions and may be prevented by β-adrenergic agonists (Szentivanyi et al., 1985). It is an energy-requiring process and appears to be mediated by prostaglandins. The combination of arteriolar dilation, venous contraction, and increased permeability of postcapillary venules results in an increased pressure and flow in the capillary bed, i.e., an increased hydrostatic pressure gradient. As a result of these changes, water and solutes pass from the blood to the extracellular fluid, lymph flow increases, and edema develops. In addition to vascular smooth muscle it is the tracheobronchial smooth muscle that is most relevant to this discussion. Tracheobronchial constriction is prominent in the guinea pig, but both dilatation and constriction may be observed in other species. In man, airway obstruction manifested in respiratory distress is demonstrable in asthmatics, especially when the kinins are inhaled. Furthermore, asthmatics show an exquisite hypersensitivity to kinins in the same quantitative and qualitative pattern as they do to other pharmacologically active effector molecules (Szentivanyi, 1968; Szentivanyi et al., 1985).

When the abovementioned kinin-produced edema is coupled with stimulation of sensory nerve endings, a typical "wheal and flare" response to intra-dermal injections in man ensues, which is the cutaneous hallmark of the inter-mediate type of hypersensitivities (Szentivanyi and Szentivanyi, 1985). Stimulation of sensory nerve endings is connected with the pain-producing ca-pacity of kinins. They are powerful algesic agents that can produce intense pain. Sensory nerve endings, however, are not the only neurons that can be activated by kinins. In relatively high concentrations, kinins are able to stimulate ganglion cells and elicit catecholamine release from adrenal medulla through depolariza-tion of chromaffin cells. Injection of bradykinin into cerebral ventricles also causes a broad spectrum of behavioral, autonomic, and EEG effects.

Kinin formation can be brought about through at least three distinct path-ways: (1) Hageman factor activation, (2) the process of phagocytosis of immune complexes by polymorphonuclear cells, and (3) the release of an acid protease resembling cathepsin D by normal white cells or neoplastic cells. Although it is the first two mechanisms that represent immediate interest for the purposes of this review, the third mechanism is quite intriguing and may turn out also to be significant at some point for our understanding of immunologic phenomena.

The first of these occurs following cell or tissue injury in which the blood-clotting pathway is triggered. A key event is the formation of active Hageman factor. Several high-molecular-weight Hageman factor pathway-associated pro-teolytic enzymes are found preformed in some human tissues such as lung and in cells such as basophils and mast cells; that the latter is a cellular source has been confirmed by using highly purified (99%) human lung mast cells. There are at least three enzymatic activities associated with Hageman factor pathways in antigen-challenged lung: kinin-generating activity (i.e., kallikreinlike), pre-kallikrein activating, and Hageman factor cleaving (and activating). These en-zymes were originally identified as arginine esterases, including a kallikreinlike activity, that after antigen-IgE interaction are released in a dose-dependent man-ner from basophils and mast cells. This original kinin-generating activity associ-ated with basophils has been named BK-A or basophil kallikrein of anaphylaxis (Plaut and Lichtenstein, 1983).

A second pathway of kinin generation occurs during the process of phago-cytosis of immune complexes by polymorphonuclear leukocytes (PMN). During phagocytosis of immune complexes by PMN, a neutral protease that is capable of cleaving kininlike peptides was first described in lysosomal lysates (Movat et al., 1973). The enzyme was subsequently isolated and purified (Movat et al., 1976). This enzyme appeared to be identical to elastase, with which it cochromato-graphed, but subsequent data with specific elastase inhibitors indicated that the kinin-forming enzyme is distinct from elastase and is not kallikrein either (Wasi et al., 1978). In any case, what can be stated is that during phagocytosis of immune complexes a methionyl-lysyl-bradykinin-generating enzyme is released into the surrounding medium. The significance of these findings lies in the fact that (1) although immune complexes per se are harmless, their deposition in tissues is associated with complement fixation and generation of complement fragments that can induce vascular injury and are chemotactic to PMN leukocytes; and (2) a considerable body of evidence has accumulated over the past two decades that implicates the PMN leukocyte as the effector of the tissue and vascular injury associated with the deposition of immune complexes (Ranadive and Movat, 1979; Espinoza and Osterland, 1983).

Immune complex deposition occurs in the wall and lumen of venules in the local Arthus reaction, in small arteries, glomeruli, joints, and pulmonary vessels in acute and chronic serum sickness or immune complex disease (Fox and Lockey, 1983), in pulmonary vessels in systemic aggregate anaphylaxis, and in the connective tissue in local aggregate anaphylaxis (Movat, 1979). There is some similarity between the pathological changes in experimental serum sickness and those in certain human diseases, and there is growing evidence that implicates immune complexes in the pathogenesis of a number of human diseases, such as systemic lupus erythematosus (Dixon, 1983; Kunkel, 1983), poststreptococcal glomerulonephritis (Nissenson, 1979; Wilson and Dixon, 1983; Villareal et al., 1983), rheumatoid arthritis (Karsh, 1983; Krane, 1981), and Churg–Strauss syndrome (Lanham et al., 1984).

A third pathway for kinin generation is activated when white cells or neoplastic cells release a cellular acid proteinase that by all available information is the lysosomal enzyme cathepsin D. This proteinase catalyzes the formation of high-molecular-weight kinins that have been originally referred to as "PMN-kinin" and later termed "leukokinins" (Greenbaum, 1976). They are 21- to 25-amino-acid hypotensive polypeptides that contract or relax preparations of smooth muscle in vitro and cause increased vascular permeability. The leukokinins are formed from the substrate "leukokininogen" (41,000 molecular weight), which is found in ascites fluid but not in normal plasma or other normal body fluids, although it can be generated in normal plasma by heating to 57°C for 30 min (Wiggins and Cochrane, 1984) or by cell and tissue injury.

The notion that leukokinin is a pharmacologically significant effector molecule is inferred by studies on ascitic fluid in tumor-bearing mice in which administration of pepstatin inhibited ascites accumulation. Pepstatin is a polypeptide that inhibits cathepsin-D-like proteases (Umezawa, 1972). It does not inhibit the generation of bradykinin by kallikrein but is highly potent in inhibiting in vitro leukokinin formation (10^{-6} M). When mice were injected with 10^6 mastocytoma or L-1210 cells and 3 days later with pepsatin, it was unequivocally demonstrated that this agent markedly reduced the ascites accumulation in the animals (Greenbaum, 1976).

Kinins that resemble bradykinin and other mammalian kinins are found in the venom sacs of wasps, hornets, and yellow jackets. In addition, comparative studies have led to the discovery of many pharmacologically active peptides in diverse lower vertebrates and invertebrates. Among these, amphibian skin is extremely rich in apparently active bradykinins, and it has been shown that nonmammalian kinins have partial sequence homology with bradykinin (Fritz *et al.*, 1983). Also, several of the peptides have a close structural resemblance to substance P and are grouped with it as tachykinins (Erspamer, 1981).

8.6. The Tachykinin Peptides: Substance P

There are five peptides currently classified as members of the tachykinin family: substance P, kassinin, substance K, eledoisin, and neuromedin K. They exhibit significant structural homologies, but despite the structural similarities, it is only substance P that has been extensively investigated and is most relevant to the discussion below.

In 1931, von Euler and Gaddum discovered a pharmacologically active substance in extracts of brain and intestine, which they later named substance P because it was present in the dried acetone powder of the extract. Substance P (SP) is an undecapeptide with the following structure: Arg-Pro-Lys-Pro-Gln-Gln-Phe-Phe-Gly-Leu-Met. It is present in neurons projecting into the substantia gelatinosa of the spinal cord from the dorsal root ganglia and has been proposed as the transmitter for primary afferent sensory fibers. This proposal is unlikely, however, in view of its long duration of action. Alternatively, because of the presence of Glu in dorsal root ganglion cells, it is possible that SP serves as a cotransmitter with Glu for some sensory fibers, providing a complementary factor that is prolonging and intensifying the transmission into the cord (Palkovits, 1984). Brain regions other than the spinal cord that are rich in SP include the substantia nigra, caudate–putamen, amygdala, hypothalamus, and cerebral cortex. Of these, the substantia nigra appears to be a structure that is rich in both SP and its stereospecific receptors (Jessel and Womack, 1985). The full functional significance of this, however, remains to be determined.

For the purposes of this review, the role of SP may be conveniently discussed in two related major areas of immune reactivities: (1) immunologic inflammatory manifestations (i.e., immediate hypersensitivities) primarily with respect to SP's relationship to antidromic vasodilation and axon reflex mechanisms as well as its effect on inflammatory cells, and (2) immunoregulation through its lymphocytic modulatory function.

As far as immunologic inflammation is concerned, SP and some other neuropeptides released from sensory nerve endings have direct effects on the functions of smooth muscles, blood vessels, leukocytes, and secretory gland cells of epithelial surfaces and have indirect effects through the actions of pharmacologically active effector molecules released from mast cells by the peptide. The application of substituent peptides of SP and antagonists of secondarily released mediators has permitted the definition of two determinants in SP. The carboxy-terminal sections account for the direct actions, and the amino-terminal tetrapeptide for the stimulation of mast cells, which consequently releases mediators of the indirect effects of SP (Mazurek *et al.*, 1981; Erspamer, 1981;

Pernow, 1983; Payan et al., 1987). The diverse cutaneous, pulmonary, and other in vivo reactions evoked by SP and some other neuropeptides released from sensory nerve endings resemble qualitatively and temporally the cutaneous and pulmonary immediate hypersensitivity responses elicited by administration of the homologous antigen to previously sensitized allergic individuals (Goetzl et al., 1985). Thus, vascular or aerosol administration of SP at picomolar (pM) concentrations to humans induces directly profound flushing, diaphoresis, rhinorrhea (increased secretion of nasal epithelial cells), hypotension, and various bronchial reactions from coughing to bronchospasm (Lundberg and Saria, 1982; Pernow, 1983). In human skin, amounts of SP as small as 10 pmole per intradermal site can rapidly produce a typical flare and wheal reaction indicating that the potency of SP to trigger such a reactivity is about 100–400 times greater than that of histamine (Hagermark et al., 1978; Foreman and Jordan, 1983; Bernstein and Hamill, 1981). Nevertheless, the dependence of both early cutaneous vasodilation and in vitro release of histamine from mast cells on the amino-terminal substituent tetrapeptide of SP suggests that histamine release is responsible for some or for much of the indirect flare response to SP. Conversely, the later wheal is attributable largely to a direct increase in capillary–venular permeability by the carboxy-terminal octapeptide substituent of SP and only minimally to the effect of mast cell derived histamine (Foreman and Jordan, 1983).

The ability of SP to degranulate mast cells in vivo led to an inquiry into the cellular requirements and other features of the process. Thus, at micromolar (μM) concentrations SP evokes substantial release of histamine by rat serosal or connective tissue-type mast cells through a noncytotoxic mechanism. Unlike histamine release by other basic peptides, the activity of SP exhibits cell specificity and includes enhanced generation of unstored mediators, such as the leukotrienes (LT-S). Mouse mast cells obtained from bone marrow precursors exposed to interleukin-3 (IL-3), which serve as a model for mucosal-type mast cells, are activated to release histamine, LTC_4 and LTB_4, by 1/1000–1/100 the concentration of SP required to release histamine from connective tissue-type mast cells (Goetzl et al., 1986). On the other hand, basophils fail to release histamine in vitro by SP even at concentrations as high as 10^{-5} M (Goetzl and Payan, 1984), and mast cell releases by SP may be distinguished from those related to IgE because of the lack of requirement for extracellular calcium and of any effect of prior desensitization that prevents activation by IgE-mediated mechanisms (Payan et al., 1987).

With respect to the relationship of SP to antidromic vasodilation and axon reflex mechanisms, we need to return to the characteristic cutaneous expression of immediate hypersensitivities, the flare and wheal response. This manifestation was originally described and termed by Sir Thomas Lewis (1927) the "triple response." As defined by Lewis, the triple response is a triad of reactions. In the first reaction, the red point produced in the site of injection of histamine by pricking the skin with a fine needle represents the immediate effect on the vessels of the skin directly attained by the drug or by the traumatic stimulus (i.e., immunologic release of histamine). Second, the flare, or erythema, that develops 30–45 sec after the initial cell injury is produced by the reflex dilation of the small cutaneous vessel in a large area around the point of attack; it is abolished by anesthetizing the skin with cocaine or degeneration of sensory fibers such as occurs in leprosy, for instance. The flare is caused by an axon reflex due to the histamine stimulation of afferent sensory nerve endings with the resultant impulses that travel through other branches of the same axon producing an antidromic vasodilatory response. Third, a wheal or edema develops as a consequence of the increased permeability of the vessels of the microcirculation, especially the postcapillary vessels. The increased permeability itself is directly due to the separation of the endothelial cells, permitting the transduction of fluid and molecules as well as small proteins in the perivascular tissue. Through recent and extensive analysis of the triple response, it has now been determined that SP is specifically associated with pain sensory fibers that are actively involved in antidromic vasodilation and axon reflex mechanisms. Indeed, SP is released by peripheral endings of sensory neurons through antidromic stimulation, and close-arterial administration of SP causes vasodilation and plasma extravasation, mimicking the effects of antidromic stimulation. When SP is depleted by capsaicin from these chemosensitive primary afferents, both antidromic vasodilation and plasma extravasation are blocked. The same can be accomplished by specific SP receptor antagonists (Pernow, 1985).

Another regulatory influence of SP on inflammatory responses in general, and on immunologic inflammation in particular, is reflected by its activities on inflammatory cells. Thus, SP stimulates human monocyte chemotaxis *in vitro*, an effect that is blocked by D-amino acid analogues of SP but that is inhibited by fMLP antagonists (Ruff *et al.*, 1985). Not only mononuclear leukocyte chemotaxis, but also the generation of thromboxane A_2, $O_2^- \cdot$ and H_2O_2 by activated macrophages has been shown to be produced by this neuropeptide (Hartung and Toyka, 1983). Other macrophage reactivities triggered by SP include down-regulation of membrane-associated 5'-nucleotidase and stimulation of synthesis and release of lysosomal enzymes and metabolites of arachidonic acid, such as LTC_4, prostaglandin D_2, and thromboxane B_2 (Payan *et al.*, 1987).

The capacity of SP to precipitate chemotactic responses of PMN leukocytes is attributed to binding to fMLP receptors. While the required dose of SP to elicit this effect may be unphysiological, other PMN leukocyte responses have been demonstrated to be producible by nanomolar concentrations of SP. These include induction of lysosomal enzyme release (Marasco *et al.*, 1981), and phagocytosis of yeast cells (Bar-Shavit *et al.*, 1980), effects connected with distinct molecular domains of the SP molecule, i.e., the chemotactic activity residing in the carboxy terminal substituent peptide, whereas the phagocytosis activity residing in the N-terminal tetrapeptide (Bar-Shavit *et al.*, 1980). The latter is also important for the stability of the native undecapeptide by retarding the enzymatic degradation of SP (Blumberg and Teichberg, 1979). Another leukocyte that participates in immunologic inflammation is the eosinophil. In recent experiments, it has been shown that *in vitro* SP significantly increased FcIgG and FcIgE receptor expression on the surface of human eosinophils together with antibody-dependent cytotoxicity against nucleated target cells (DeSimone et al., 1987). In these studies, enhancement of optimal receptor expression was achieved with a 60-min incubation period, suggesting that this effect is not based on the production of new receptors, but on either the unmasking or an increased activity of existing Fc receptors on the surface of circulating blood eosinophils.

A part of the inflammatory response is tissue repair. Substance P participates in the repair process by the enhancement of the proliferation of fibroblasts, smooth muscle, and endothelial cells (Nilsson et al., 1985; Payan, 1985). The proliferative effect of SP on smooth muscle cells is diminished by preincubation with its specific antagonists or the concurrent stimulation with platelet-derived growth factor reflecting important interactions between sensory neuropeptides and polypeptide growth factors. A possible chemical basis for such interaction may be explained by the recent demonstration of homologies between the amino acid sequences of polypeptide growth factors for fibroblasts, which show potent mitogenic and angiogenic activities, and those of neuropeptides of the tachykinin family, such as SP (Gimenez-Gallego et al., 1985).

The second major immunoregulatory role of SP is reflected by its effects on lymphocyte function and the attendant issue of antibody production. Proliferation of both human (Payan et al., 1983) and murine (Stanisz et al., 1986) T lymphocytes is significantly increased by nanomolar concentrations of SP; in human T lymphocytes, SP and SP (4–11) generate increases at up to 60–70% as measured by [^{3}H]leucine uptake *in vitro* (Payan et al., 1983). Similar effects of SP were observed in murine lymphocytes from spleen, mesenteric lymph nodes, and Peyer's patches. Biochemical analysis of these effects shows that SP enhances the incorporation of ^{32}P into membrane phospholipids through the activation of the phosphatidylinositol pathway and the increase of cytosolic Ca^{2+} (Payan et al., 1987). In accord with these findings are the observations showing that SP enhances *in vitro* immunoglobulin synthesis by spleen lymphocytes. The effect was found to be isotype specific, and greatest on IgA synthesis, slightly less on IgM with an unaltered IgG response (Stanisz et al., 1987).

8.7. Other Neuroactive Immunoregulatory Peptides

8.7.1. Neurotensin

Neurotensin (NT) is not a member of the tachykinin family of peptides. Nevertheless, this agent is frequently associated with the tachykinin family because of the historical relationship, in that Carraway and Leeman (1975) isolated and sequenced this peptide immediately after their success with SP.

NT is a tridecapeptide, first isolated from the CNS, but subsequently found to be present in the gastrointestinal tract and in the circulation (Nemeroff and Prange, 1982). It has the following structure: Glu-Leu-Tyr-Glu-Asn-Lys-Pro-Arg-Arg-Pro-Tyr-Ile-Leu. Largest amounts in this peptide are to be found in the anterior and basal hypothalamus, in the nucleus accumbens and septum, and in the spinal cord and brainstem within small interneurons of the substantia gelatinosa and motor trigeminal nucleus. Neurotensin colocalizes to, and may be the cotransmitter of, some dopamine and some adrenergic neurons (Cooper et al., 1986).

In the peripheral circulation, NT produces hypotension, vasodilatation, increased vascular permeability, hyperglycemia, inhibition of gastric secretion and motility. In these manifestations, the blood pressure receptors, and the hyperglycemia receptors appear to read the Arg-Arg dipeptide near the middle of neurotensin. Administered into the cerebrospinal fluid, it produces hypothermia and analgesia, whereas in case of intracisternal administration, it accentuates barbiturate sleeping time and stimulates the release of growth hormone and prolactin. Structure activity studies indicate that the 5–6-amino acid residues at the carboxy terminal of the molecule are required for biologic activity (Reid, 1987).

So far, we have more information on the role of NT in the induction and expression of inflammatory reactions rather than in immunoregulation per se. Thus, cutaneous flushing in humans may be elicited by intracutaneous neuroten-sin and it is attributable principally to the mediators released from degranulating mast cells and other inflammatory cells (Foreman et al., 1982; Casale et al., 1984; Goetzl et al., 1985). Any inflammatory stimulus to the skin may result in the discharge of SP from bipolar sensory neurons. Because of its ability to stimulate phagocytosis by neutrophils and also to enhance lymphocyte proliferation, SP may, induce an inflammatory response. NT released in the same manner would induce vasodilation to permit influx of inflammatory cells. In addition to mast cell degranulation with release of histamine, NT also stimulates neutrophil chemotaxis and phagocytosis (Goldman et al., 1983; Sagi-Eisenberg et al., 1983). Thus, NT and SP, acting in concert, may initiate the inflammatory response. Somatostatin may be envisioned to act centrally in blocking SP· or NT release from primary sensory neurons.

8.7.2. Somatostatin (Somatotropin Release-Inhibiting Factor)

Vale, Brazeu, Guillemin, and their associates (1975) in studying the potency of their hypothalamic extracts for releasing growth hormone from long-term cultured anterior pituitary cells found a substance that inhibited even basal growth-hormone release in minute amounts that they named somatostatin (SOM).

Although SOM immunoreactive cells and fibers are also present in dorsal root ganglia, in the autonomic plexi of the intestine, in the amygdala and neo-cortex, SOM is largely concentrated in the mediobasal hypothalamus (Johansson *et al.*, 1984; Morrison *et al.*, 1983; Cooper *et al.*, 1986). Outside the nervous system, SOM is found in the gastrointestinal tract and the pancreatic islets, localized in the latter to the delta cells. In the islets, SOM can suppress the release of both glucagon and insulin. The mechanism of this suppression is not known but may be similar to the effect of SOM on growth hormone release from the pituitary, an action that is also accompanied by suppression of TSH release (Reichlin, 1983).

Somatostatin is a tetradecapeptide with an amino acid sequence of Ala-Gly-Cys-Lys-Asn-Phe-Phe-Trp-Lys-Thr-Phe-Thr-Ser-Cys and with a disulfide bridge between Cys^3 and Cys^{14}. A 28-amino acid peptide called prosomotostatin, isolated from the hypothalamus and intestine, is believed to be the precursor of somatostatin and is much more potent in many of the established pharmacologic activities of SOM. Peptides have been synthesized that partially separate the various properties of SOM. A 7-amino heptanoic acid derivative containing only four of the 14 amino acids of SOM has been found to block the effect of SOM (Klonoff and Karam, 1987).

Somatostatin modulates several immune functions acting at different levels of the organization of the immune response. Among these is the capacity of SOM to modify lymphocyte growth and function. Inhibition of the spontaneous proliferation of lymphocytes *in vitro* by low concentrations of SOM seems to be connected with the more general antiproliferative action of SOM. This is indicated by SOM-induced abolition of the mitogenic effects of TRH on the anterior pituitary (Pawlikowski *et al.*, 1978), and of the epidermal growth factor (EGF) on HeLa and gerbil fibroma cells (Mascardo and Sherline, 1982). More recently, it was found that SOM induced dephosphorylation of a membrane protein whose phosphorylation is promoted by EGF (Hierowski *et al.*, 1985). Also, the antiproliferative activity of SOM is responsible, at least in part, for the antitumor effect of SOM analogues (Schally *et al.*, 1984).

The immunomodulatory role of SOM also involves a counterregulatory interplay with SP in many of the immunologic parameters studied (Stanisz *et al.*, 1987). Lymphocyte proliferation is enhanced by SP but inhibited by SOM. These results are similar to those obtained from studies using human PBL (Payan *et al.*, 1983, 1984a; Pawlikowski *et al.*, 1985) and lymphoblastoid cell lines (Payan *et al.*, 1984b,c). The effects of SP and SOM on immunoglobulin also reveal antagonistic features such as the enhancement of IgA and IgM synthesis of SP and inhibition of the same by SOM (Stanisz *et al.*, 1987). An interesting exception to this so far is that both SP as well as SOM stimulate histamine release, at least from rat peritoneal mast cells (Piotrowski and Foreman, 1985).

Another aspect of lymphocyte function of immunologic interest with respect to SOM involves the formation of a lymphokine—leukocyte migration inhibiting factor (MIF). As described earlier in this chapter, in the presence of specific antigens, sensitized lymphocytes are known to produce among other lymphokines, a factor inhibiting the migration of leukocytes. This can also be induced with nonspecific mitogens like phytohemagglutinin (PHA) or concanavalin A (Con A). Recently reported information shows that SOM and SOM analogs enhance the migration inhibition of human leukocytes induced by myocardial antigen or PHA (Pawlikowski *et al.*, 1987). Furthermore, there is evidence that SOM reduces the release of colony-stimulating activity (CSA) from PHA-activated mouse spleen lymphocytes (Hinterberger *et al.*, 1978).

8.7.3. Vasoactive Intestinal Peptide

Originally isolated from porcine intestine and named for its ability to alter enteric blood flow, vasoactive intestinal peptide (VIP) is a 29 amino acid peptide, related structurally to glucagon, secretin, and another peptide of gastric origin that inhibits gastric muscular contraction (GIP). Its structure is as follows: His-Ser-Asp-Ala-Val-Phe-Thr-Asp-Asn-Tyr-Thr-Arg-Leu-Arg-Lys-Gln-Met-Ala-Val-Lys-Lys-Tyr-Leu-Asn-Ser-Ile-Leu-Asn-NH_2.

Vasoactive intestinal peptide is prominently present in many regions of the autonomic and central nervous systems, but it appears most abundant in the CNS and in presynaptic vesicles of neurons that innervate the intestines. Immunohistochemical studies have established that VIP is also localized in secretory granules of nerve terminals in pancreatic, uterine, cardiac, and salivary gland tissues (Said, 1982). In the parasympathetic nerves of the last-named tissue, VIP coexist with acetylcholine and is released with ACh apparently as part of an integrated command to activate secretion and to increase blood flow through the gland (Lundberg *et al.*, 1982). In the CNS, VIP-containing neurons are among the most numerous of the chemically defined cells of the neocortex (Morrison *et al.*, 1984).

This peptide is also present in the circulation; it produces marked vasodilation in most vascular beds. The vasodilatory action of VIP is not a mediated, but a direct, action on the VIP receptors on vascular smooth muscle cells. In addition, VIP relaxes tracheobronchial and gastrointestinal smooth muscle together with a broad spectrum of other effects, including stimulation of growth hormone, prolactin, somatostatin, and renin release (Tapia-Arancibia and Reichlin, 1985; Reid, 1987).

Indications of the nature of the participation of VIP in immunoregulation are suggested by the demonstration of VIP-mediated inhibition of mitogen stimulation (Ottaway and Greenberg, 1984). Proliferation of T-lymphocytes in response to Con A or PHA is inhibited by VIP, whereas proliferation of lymphocytes from mesenteric and subcutaneous lymph nodes, or spleen is unaffected by VIP when induced by LPS. These findings are in accord with earlier observations that T lymphocytes, but not B cells, possess high-affinity receptors for VIP (Ottaway *et al.*, 1983). Another possible feature of the role of VIP in the organization of the immune response is its modulation of lymphocyte migration. Studies on the effect of VIP on the passage of cells out of popliteal lymph nodes indicate that

VIP inhibits egress of small lymphocytes suggesting that peptidergic neurons in the intestine may regulate migration of small lymphocytes in Peyer's patches or in intestinal lamina propria (Moore, 1984). The role of cyclic nucleotides (O'Dorisio et al., 1985) in these VIP-induced lymphocytes reactivities will be discussed in Part II of this review, to appear in Volume 2 of the *Immunopharmacology Reviews* series.

8.7.4. The Endogenous Opioid Peptides

During the mid-1970s, the first collective term used for this group of substances was "endorphin." In that phase of development, "endorphin" simply referred to any "endogenous substance" that exhibits the pharmacological properties of morphine. In the subsequent years, in a massive effort, research has succeeded in greatly clarifying the molecular and genomic relationships between the three major groups of the opioid peptide family: the pro-opiomelanocortin (POMC)-derived peptides, the pro-enkephalin-derived peptides, and the pro-dynorphin-derived peptides. In an incredible explosion of work on these substances as well as the rapidly developing inherent inconsistencies in the terminology have persuaded the leading investigators in the field to give to the entire family of these agents a more general name, such as "endogenous opioid peptides," which is the adopted term of this review.

In discussing this growing family of immunopharmacologically pertinent peptides, an appropriate point of departure would seem to be a brief statement of our current understanding of the chemical and cellular relationships among the opioid peptides. Thus, the pro-opiomelanocortin (POMC) peptides are expressed independently in the anterior pituitary, intermediate lobe of the pituitary, and one main group of neurons in the arcuate nucleus area of the hypothalamus. The major opioid agonist produced from POMC is the 31-amino acid C-terminal fragment, β-endorphin, the most potent of the natural opioids. The neurons containing β-endorphin represent long neuronal projection systems that fall within the general endocrine-oriented systems of the medial hypothalamus, diencephalon, and pons (Swanson and Sawchenko, 1983). With respect to the second group, the enkephalin pentapeptides, Met^5-enkephalin and Leu^5-enkephalin, are expressed in entirely separate neuronal systems from the POMC neurons and are more pervasively distributed throughout the central and peripheral nervous systems including the adrenal medulla and enteric nervous system. The third group, the pro-dynorphin peptides, consist of C-terminally extended forms of Leu^5-enkephalin arising from a different gene (Civelli et al., 1985) and from a different mRNA that encodes for production of four major peptides termed Dynorphin A, Dynorphin B, and two neoendorphins, α and β. On mapping, they were found to represent a third separated series of generally distributed central and peripheral neurons (Paklovits, 1984). The pro-enkephalin and pro-dynorphin-derived peptides are found in neurons with nodes to short projections and show important neuroanatomical interrelationships (Cooper et al., 1986).

Although the physiological significance of all these peptides remains open to more comprehensive analysis, it appears that among the proposed physiological properties that may be regulated by one or another of the endogenous opioid peptides are blood pressure, temperature, feeding, sexual activity, pain perception and memory, and the functions of the immune cells.

The problem of the interrelationships between immune cells and endogenous opioid peptides as well as other neuroactive immunoregulatory molecules is a rather complex one, since immune and inflammatory cells serve both as a peripheral source and as the targets of these agents. The discovery of the capacity of immune cells to produce these substances can be traced back to the finding that virus infection of human peripheral blood cells was observed to elicit the coordinate expression of α-interferon (IFN-α), corticotropin (ACTH), and endorphins (Blalock and Smith, 1980; Smith and Blalock, 1981). Other IFN-α inducers, such as tumor cells (Smith and Blalock, 1981) and bacterial lipopolysaccharide (LPS), have also been shown to cause the production of these peptides by both human leukocytes and mouse spleen cells. Subsequently, a subpopulation of the latter (probably macrophages) was shown to constitutively produce adrenocorticotrophic hormone (ACTH), β-endorphin, and their POMC precursor (Lolait et al., 1984). The leukocyte-derived ACTH and endorphins are identical to their pituitary counterparts in terms of bioactivity, antigenicity, molecular weight, and retention time on reverse-phase HPLC (Blalock et al., 1985). In fact, it has now been demonstrated at the level of both the polypeptide (Lolait et al., 1984; Blalock and Smith, 1985), and mRNA (Westly et al., 1986; Lolait et al., 1986), that leukocytes synthesize POMC-related polypeptides such as ACTH and endorphin. Production of these substances by the immune system is not limited to POMC-related peptides but includes thyrotropin (TSH) (Smith et al., 1983), vasoactive intestinal peptide (VIP) (Giachetti et al., 1978; O'Dorisio et al., 1980; Lygren et al., 1984) somatostatin (SOM) (Lygren et al., 1984), and prolactin (Hiestand et al., 1986; Montgomery et al., 1987; Russell et al., 1987). Furthermore, depending on the stimulus, human leukocytes and mouse spleen cells may have the potential to produce chorionic gonadotropin (CG), growth hormone (GH), follicle-stimulating hormone (FSH), and lutenizing hormone (LH) (Blalock et al., 1985).

Besides producing endogenous opioid peptides, lymphocyte functions are modulated by the same peptides. Thus, β-endorphin enhances the proliferative response of lymphocytes to T-cell mitogens (Gilman et al., 1982), cytolytic activity, and γ-interferon production by human NK cells (Mathews et al., 1983; Mandler et al., 1986) and stimulates chemotaxis of human peripheral blood mononuclear cells (Van Epps and Saland, 1984). The studies of Gilman et al. (1982) are supported by the work of Plotnikoff and Miller (1983), indicating that β-endorphin 1–31 enhances human T-cell proliferation. In contrast to these data, McCain et al. (1982) found that this peptide decreases the proliferation of human peripheral blood T cells. In an attempt to interpret these contradictory findings, two more recent studies need to be mentioned here. One is the study by Claas et *al.* (1986) showing that γ-endorphin (i.e., β-endorphin 1–17) can bind preferentially to certain HLA class I antigens (HLA-A10,11, HLA-B13,15,22, and HLA-C6), which could reflect a mechanism by which MHC antigens interfere in the interactions between ligand and cell membrane receptors. This finding suggests the possibility that not only genetic factors, but also factors regulating receptor expression for β-endorphin, are involved in the ultimate outcome of the response. The second study, by Heijnen *et al.* (1987), shows that β-endorphin 10–16 mirrors the activity of β-endorphin 1–31. Both the enhancing as well as the inhibitory action of β-endorphin 1–31 are affected by the lymphocyte recognition of the amino acid site 10–16. When the N-terminal amino acid tyrosine is removed (β-endorphin 2–31) the response pattern to β-endorphin is seen again indicating that the opioid-binding site on the lymphocyte is not decisive for the magnitude of the response. It appears possible that the final outcome of the response may be determined by a combined action of multiple binding sites on the membrane of the lymphocytes (Heijnen *et al.*, 1987).

Of the enkephalins, met-enkephalin was shown to be recognized by T lymphocytes through opiate receptors. This recognition appears to activate a series of intracellular molecular events, resulting probably in the induction of various surface receptors linked to lymphocyte activation (the active sheep T RBC receptors, the OKT 10 receptor, and the IL-2 receptor). Met-enkephalin will also induce the production of IL-2, which in turn may recruit and activate a number of other T-cell subsets (OKT 3, OKT 4). Met-enkephalin also enhances NK activity, both directly and indirectly (Wybran *et al.*, 1987), and the T-cell rosettes from lymphoma patients (Miller *et al.*, 1983) and from normal volunteers (Miller *et al.*, 1984). However, similar to endorphins, enkephalins appear both to suppress and to potentiate a number of parameters of immune responsiveness, depending on the concentration of immunologic reactants and other experimental conditions used. This applies to *in vivo* and *in vitro* modulation of both humoral and cell-mediated immune reactivities (Jakovic and Maric, 1987; Maric and Jakovic, 1987) as well as to the interactions of enkephalins with granulocytes (Fischer and Falke, 1987; Foris *et al.*, 1987) and the macrophage (Peck, 1987).

8.7.5. Vasopressin and Oxytocin

Vasopressin and oxytocin are produced in the perikarya of the magnocellular neurons of the supraoptic and paraventricular nuclei of the hypothalamus. These peptides are synthesized as high-molecular-weight precursors, which are then cleared during axonal transport into the nonapeptides, vasopressin and oxytocin, and their associated "carrier" proteins, neurophysins. They are released into the blood stream from the axons of these neurons in the neurohypophysis. These magnocellular neurons of the supraoptic and paraventricular nuclei have also been shown to give off axon collaterals that project within the nuclei, between the nuclei, and to the median eminence. It may be added that some parvocellular neurons in these hypothalamic nuclei also contain oxytocin or vasopressin. Their circuits project either to the median eminence where vasopressin appears to act as a co-releasing hormone of ACTH or to other more distant sites in the brain (Swanson and Sawchenko, 1983; Doris, 1984).

These two highly similar molecules are nonapeptides with internal 1,6-disulfide bridges and with the following amino acid sequences:

Vasopressin: Cys-Tyr-Phe-Gln-Asn-Cys-Pro-Arg-Gly
Oxytocin: Cys-Tyr-Ile-Gln-Asn-Gys-Pro-Leu-Gly

In addition to their long-established roles in mammalian physiology, i.e., homeostasis of water metabolism for vasopressin, and induction of uterine contractions and milk ejection for oxytocin, more recently two other major functions came to be recognized. Of these, one involves the behavioral action of vasopressin, and the other the immunoregulatory properties of both peptides. The behavioral actions of vasopressin as they were originally described in rats consist of delaying the extinction of learned aversive or appetitive tasks. Humans given vasopressin analogues also show enhanced performance of attention-related memory tasks (de Wied, 1983; Gash and Thomas, 1983). Osmotic stress mimicks these effects of vasopressin on learned behavior (Koob *et al.*, 1985). The mechanisms accounting for these effects are unclear.

The recognition of the potential importance of the two peptides in immunoregulation may be traced back to two independent findings: (1) the capacity of vasopressin and oxytocin to replace interleukin 2 (IL-2) in the T-helper cell requirement for IFN-γ production, and (2) the synthesis of vasopressin and oxytocin by human thymic epithelium.

γ-Interferon production is regulated by interactions between various T-cell subsets involving helper cells, suppressor cells, and IFN-γ-producing cells. Until now, it was viewed as conclusively established that the helper cell requirement for IFN-γ production is mediated solely by its product IL-2. Recently, however, it was found that vasopressin and oxytocin as well as structurally related peptides at extremely low concentrations are capable of replacing the IL-2 requirement for T-cell mitogen induction of IFN-γ in mouse spleen cell cultures (Johnson and Torres, 1985). While both peptides are efficient in providing the accessory signal for IFN-γ production, or in fact completely replace it, vasopressin is about 10 times more effective than oxytocin on a molar basis. Vasotocin, which is the nonmammalian vertebrate counterpart of vasopressin and oxytocin shows a similar potency to oxytocin in the capacity of the helper signal. This may be related to the fact that both oxytocin and vasotocin have isoleucine at structural position three. On the other hand, another related peptide, pressionic acid, which comprises the six N-terminal amino acids of vasopressin, is as effective as vasopressin in replacing the IL-2 helper signal for IFN-γ production. This suggests that the N-terminal end of vasopressin is the binding site for the membrane receptor on the lymphocyte. Furthermore, from studies with a competitive antagonist of the vasopressor (and not antidiuretic) activity of vasopressin, it is apparent that this antagonist blocks the vasopressin helper signal for IFN-γ production, while having no effect on IL-2 help (Johnson and Torres, 1985). This indicates that the vasopressin helper signal operates through binding to a "vasopressor"-type receptor of vasopressin on lymphocytes. In view of current knowledge about vasopressin receptors, it would seem that this lymphocytic vasopressin receptor may be similar to the so-called V_1-receptors that mediate vasopressin responses on arteriolar walls and not the V_2-receptors that mediate vasopressin responses on renal tubules (Cooper et al., 1986). So far no other immune function has been identified in which vasopressin or oxytocin or both, can replace IL-2 requirements (Johnson and Torres, 1985; Geenen et al., 1987).

Another indication of the potential importance of vasopressin and oxytocin in immunoregulation is connected with the demonstration of these peptides in the thymus. Their presence in the thymus was first reported by Gennen et al. (1986), who found the thymic contents of oxytocin and neurophysin to be far greater than those expected from their known circulating levels and the molar ratio of thymic oxytocin to neurophysin was compatible with that found in the hypothalamus. The coexistence of almost equimolar amounts of neurophysin appeared to reflect an intrathymic synthesis of oxytocin by cleavage from a common precursor, as demonstrated in the hypothalamus (Land et al., 1983) and in the bovine corpus luteum (Ivell and Richter, 1984). Indeed, subsequent studies have detected mRNA for oxytocin and vasopressin in high quantities, indicating that their genes are actively expressed in the young human thymus and that the presence of oxytocin and vasopressin in this tissue must be attributed to local synthesis. Calculation of relative amounts shows that human thymus can produce levels of oxytocin and vasopressin mRNA comparable to those in the adult male hypothalamus.

Although thymic vasopressin and oxytocin may participate in the usual physiological functions established for these peptides, it is entirely possible, in fact likely, that they may also have intrathymic paracrine actions on thymocytes. Thus, they possess IL-2-like activities that could be of importance in view of the observation that IL-2 receptor expression is a differentiation marker on intrathymic stem cells (Ceredig et al., 1985; Raulet et al., 1985). Furthermore, vasopressin stimulates DNA synthesis in bone marrow cells and oxytocin enhances glucose oxidation in thymocytes (Goren et al., 1984). These peptides, therefore, may have some co-mitogenic, inductive, or repressive actions during lymphocyte differentiation (Geenan et al., 1987).

Another possible physiological role for thymic vasopressin and oxytocin could be some regulatory influence on lymphocytic hormone production. For instance, Smith et al. (1986) showed that vasopressin enhances the number of lymphocytes containing immunoreactive ACTH in the presence of corticotropin-releasing factor (CRF). The significance of this finding lies in the fact that CRF is co-expressed within distinct subsets of oxytocin, vasopressin, and neurotensin immunoreactive neurons in the hypothalamus (Sawchenko *et al.*, 1984), and vasopressin and oxytocin modulate the action of CRF on ACTH secretion in the pituitary (Antoni *et al.*, 1984). Thus, the regulatory mechanisms of ACTH secretion in the anterior pituitary are similar to the same at the lymphocyte level. Furthermore, from what we know today about the neuroanatomy of the thymus and other lymphoid tissues with respect to their innervation by cholinergic, adrenergic, and VIP-immunoreactive fibers (Bulloch, 1985; Felten *et al.*, 1985), it appears that thymic cells would translate a neural input to neuropeptide secretion. These neuropeptides could then modulate lymphocyte production of both lymphokines (i.e., IFN-γ) and hormones (i.e., ACTH and β-endorphin).

9. OTHER MEDIATORS

We conclude this review by listing some other mediators that are under active investigation. Among those mediators we have selected for listing, bodies of research are consolidating and the immunopharmacological implications seem strong. This list includes, but is not limited to, the new interleukins-7 and -8, various leukocytes and mast cell products, angiotensins, prolactin, calcitonin gene-related peptides, CRF, T-cell derived, macrophage/monocyte-derived, B-cell derived, and other suppressor factors detectable in the circulation of patients with infection, malignant disease, and following inflammation. We shall structure a discussion of these agents in the framework of microbial modulation of immune reactivities in Part II of this review, appearing in Volume 2 of the *Immunopharmacology Reviews* series, that will also include a reexamination of the ACTH–corticosteroid system as it relates to immunopharmacology.

10. THE RELATIVE SIGNIFICANCE OF THE PHARMACOLOGICALLY ACTIVE EFFECTOR MOLECULES IN THE INDUCTION AND EXPRESSION OF IMMUNE REACTIVITIES

There is much disagreement regarding the relative importance of many of the known pharmacologically active effector molecules in immune reactivities. Opinions differ even further on the question of what other, potentially important, active substances are involved in a given manifestation or in an immunoregulatory role. It would seem that no two normal or abnormal situations would be indeed strictly comparable and, in the final analysis, the relative significance of a given effector molecule will depend on a multitude of various determinants. Schematically, the following circumstances or factors would seem to determine the relative significance of any one of the currently known pharmacologically active effector molecules and, thus, the nature of the ultimate response at any one time:

1. The species
2. The physicochemical and biological character as well as the quantities of immunological reactants participating in the immune response and/or the immunoregulatory event
3. The tissue site of the immunological event
4. Susceptibility of the mediator or their precursor-storing cells to the activating stimulus
5. Types and relative amounts of active mediators present in the local area of the immunological event
6. The occurrence in a pre-existing store, or the presence of precursors or substrates which can give rise to the active principles
7. Availability of appropriate enzymes or other biochemical mechanisms required for such activation
8. Relative efficiency of the primarily released mediator to mobilize another active agent
9. Factors, such as diffusibility, rate of inactivation of the pharmacologically active effector molecules and the proximity of the target cells to the site of release or activation
10. The types of target cells within the sphere of influence of the released or activated mediator
11. The functional state of these target cells and that of their mediator-specific receptors
12. The capacity of the primarily released mediator to up-regulate, down-regulate, or otherwise influence the target cells to the action of the secondarily mobilized or otherwise activated agent
13. Persistence of the manifestation (the number of active agents entering into the reaction is increasing with time, and the relative significance of any of these is varying with the biochemical stage that the process has reached)
14. If there is a selectively altered reactivity to any of these pharmacologically active effector molecules, the types of target cells to which this altered reactivity is localized

With these qualifications in mind, Part II of this review that will appear in Volume 2 of the *Immunopharmacology Reviews* series shall discuss the biochemical mechanisms that are involved in the normal cellular actions of these pharamcologically active effector molecules and how these activities are modulated by microbial cells or their products thereof.

REFERENCES

Adams, D. O., Edelson, P. J., and Koren, H. S., 1981, *Methods for Studying Mononuclear Phagocytes*, Academic, New York.

Adelroth, E., Morris, M. M., Hargreave, F. E., and O'Byrne, P. M., 1986, Airway responsiveness to leukotrienes C_4 and D_4 and to methacholine in patients with asthma and normal controls, *N. Engl. J. Med.* **315**:480.

Ahlquist, R. P., 1948, A study of the adrenotropic receptor, *Am. J. Physiol.* **153**:586.

Ahmed, A., Wong, D. M., Thurman, G. B., Low, T. L., Goldstein, A. L., Sharkis, S. J., and Goldschneider, I., 1979, T-lymphocyte maturation: cell surface markers and immune function induced by T lymphocyte cell-free products and thymosin polypeptide, *Ann. N.Y. Acad. Sci.* **332**:81.

Aiuti, F., and Businco, L., 1983, Effects of thymic hormones on immunodeficiency, *Clin. Immunol. Allergy* **3**:187.

Akahoshi, T., Oppenheim, J. J., and Matsushima, T., 1987, Induction of high affinity functional receptors for interleukin 1 by glucocorticoid hormones on human peripheral blood lymphocytes, *Lymphokine Res.* **6**:1240 (abst.)

Aldigier, J. C., Gualde, N., Mexmain, S., Chable-Rabinovitch, H., Ratinand, M. H., and Rigaud, M., 1984, Immunosuppression induced in vivo by 15-hydroxyeicosatetraenoic acid (15-HETE), *Prostaglandins Leukotrienes Med.* **13**:99.

Alter, S. C., Margolius, H. S., and Schwartz, L. B., 1986, The effect of tryptase from human mast cells on human urinary prekallikrein, *Fed. Proc.* **45**:626.

Antoni, F. A., Holmes, M. C., and Jones, M. T., 1984, Oxytocin as well as vasopressin potentiate ovine CRF in vitro, *Peptides* **4**:411.

Anwar, A. R. E., and Kay, A. B., 1978, Enhancement of human eosinophil complement receptors by pharmacologic mediators, *J. Immunol.* **121**:1245.

Anwar, A. R. E., McKean, J. R., Smithers, S. R., and Kay, A. B., 1980, Human eosinophil and neutrophil-mediated killing of schistosomula of *Schistosoma mansoni* in vitro. I. Enhancement of C'-dependent damage by mast cell-derived mediators and formyl methionyl peptides, *J. Immunol.* **124**:1122.

Appleman, M. M., Allan, E. J., Ariano, M. A., Ong, K. K., Tusang, C. A., Weber, H. W., and Whitson, R. H., 1984, Insulin control of cyclic AMP phosphodiesterase, in: *Advances in Cyclic Nucleotide and Protein Phosphorylation Research* (S. J. Strada and W. J. Thompson, eds.), Vol. 16, pp. 149–158, Raven, New York.

Apte, R. N., Durum, S. K., and Oppenheim, J. J., 1987, Beta-endorphin enhances IL-1 production in bone marrow macrophages, *Lymphokine Res.* **6**:1125 (abst.).

Asano, T., Brandt, D. R., Pedersen, S. E., and Ross, E. M., 1985, Beta-adrenergic receptors and regulatory GTP-binding proteins: Reconstitution of coupling in phospholipid vesicles, in: *Advances in Cyclic Nucleotide and Protein Phosphorylation Research* (D. M. F. Cooper and K. B. Seamon, eds.), Vol. 19, pp. 47–56, Raven, New York.

Asherson, C. L., Zembala, M., Mayhew, B., and Goldstein, A. L., 1976, Adult thymectomy prevention of appearance of suppressor T cells which depress contact sensitivity to picryl chloride and reversal of adult thymectomy effect by thymus extract, *Eur. J. Immunol.* **6**:699.

Askenase, P. W., and Van Loveren, H., 1983, Delayed-type hypersensitivity: Activation of mast cells by antigen-specific T-cell factors initiates the cascade of cellular interactions, *Immunol. Today* **4**:259.

Atluru, D., and Goodwin, J. S., 1984, Control of polyclonal immunoglobulin production from human lymphocytes by leukotrienes—Leukotriene B4 induces an OKT8[+], radiosensitive suppressor cell from resting human OKT8[−] T cells, *J. Clin. Invest.* **74**:1444.

Audhya, T. K., Schlesinger, D. H., and Goldstein, G., 1981, Complete amino acid sequences of bovine thymopoietin I, II and III: Closely homologous polypeptides, *Biochemistry* **20**:6195.

Auron, P. E., Webb, A. C., Rosenwasser, L. J., Mucci, S. F., Rich, A., Wolff, S. M., and Dinarello, C. A., 1984, Nucleotide sequence of human monocyte interleukin 1 precursor cDNA, *Proc. Natl. Acad. Sci. U.S.A.* **81**:7907.

Auron, P. E., Rosenwasser, L. J., Matsushima, K., Copeland, T., Dinarello, C. A., Oppenheim, J. J., and Webb, A. C., 1985, Human and murine interleukin-1 possess sequence and structural similarities, *J. Mol. Cell. Immunol.* **2**(3):169.

Austen, K. F., 1983, Tissue mast cells in immediate hypersensitivity, in: *The Biology of Immunologic Disease* (F. J. Dixon and D. W. Fisher, eds.), pp. 223–233, Sinauer, Sunderland, Massachusetts.

Azuma, C., Tanabe, T., Konishi, M., Kinashi, T., Noma, T., Matsuda, F., Yaoita, Y., Takatsu, K., Hammarstrom, L., Smith, C. I. E., Severinson, E., and Honjo, T., 1986, Cloning of cDNA for human T-cell replacing factor (interleukin-5) and comparison with the murine homologue, *Nucleic Acids Res.* **14**:9149.

Babior, B. M., 1984, The respiratory burst of phagocytes, *J. Clin. Invest.* **73**:599.

Bach, J.-F. (ed.), 1983, Thymic hormones, *Clin. Immunol. Allergy* **3**:1.

Bach, J.-F., 1983, Conclusions: The plurality of thymic hormones, *Clin. Immunol. Allergy* **3**:196.

Bach, J.-F., 1983, Thymulin (FTS-Zn), *Clin. Immunol. Allergy* **3**:133.

Bach, J.-F., and Dardenne, M., 1973, Studies on thymus products. 2. Demonstration and characterization of a circulating thymic hormone, *Immunology* **25**:353.

Bailey, J. M., Bryant, R. W., Low, C. E., Pupilla, M. B., and Vanderhoek, J. W., 1982, Regulation of lymphocyte T mitogenesis by the leukocyte product 15-hydroxyeicosatetraenoic acid (15-HETE), *Cell. Immunol.* **67**:112.

Banchereau, J., DeFrance, T., Rousset, F., Aubry, J. P., Vanbervliet, T., Bonnefoy, J. Y., Arai, N., Takebe, Y., Yokota, T., Lee, F., Arai, K., and DeVries, J. E., 1987, The pleiotropic effectors of recombinant human IL-4 on B lymphocytes, *Lymphokine Rs.* **6**:1816.

Bandouvakis, J., Cartier, A., Roberts, R., Ryan, J. G., and Hargreave, F. E., 1981, The effect of ipratropium and fenoterol on methacholine- and histamine-induced bronchoconstriction, *Br. J. Dis. Chest* **75**:295.

Barbaro, J. F., and Zvaifler, N. J., 1966, Antigen-induced histamine release from platelets of rabbits producing homologous PCA antibody, *Proc. Soc. Exp. Biol. Med.* **122**:1245.

Barnes, P. J., 1987, Neuropeptides in the lung: Localization, function, and pathophysiologic implications, *J. Allergy Clin. Immunol.* **79**:285.

Barrett, K. E., and Metcalfe, D. O., 1984, Mast cell heterogeneity: Evidence and implications, *J. Clin. Immunol.* **4**:253.

Bar-Shavit, Z., Goldman, R., Stabinsky, Y., Gottlieb, P., Fridkin, M., Teichberg, V. I., and Blumberg, S., 1980, Enhancement of phagocytosis—A newly found activity of substance P residing in its N-terminal tetrapeptide sequence, *Biochem. Biophys. Res. Commun.* **94**:1445.

Barton, B. E., and Wheeler, L. A., 1987, Inhibition of arachidonic acid metabolism does not inhibit proliferation due to IL-3 in DA-1 cells, *Lymphokine Res.* **6**:1308 (abst.).

Basham, T. Y., and Merigan, T. C., 1983, Recombinant interferon-gamma increases HLA-DR synthesis and expression, *J. Immunol.* **130**:1492.

Basten, A., and Beeson, P. B., 1970, Mechanism of eosinophilia. II. Role of the lymphocyte, *J. Exp. Med.* **131**:1288.

Beasley, C. R. W., Featherstone, R. L., Church, M. K., and Holgate, S. T., 1986, 11-Epiprostaglandin F2alpha is a potent contractile agonist of human airways, *J. Allergy Clin. Immunol.* **77**:155.

Becker, S. K., 1987, Inhibition of LAK cell differentiation by prostaglandin E, *Lymphokine Res.* **6**:1709 (abst.).

Beckner, S. K., and Farrar, W. L., 1987, Biochemical mechanisms of LAK cell differentiation, *Lymphokine Res.* **6**:1503.

Beer, D. J., and Rocklin, R. E., 1984, Histamine-induced suppressor-cell activity, *J. Allergy Clin. Immunol.* **73**:439.

Beer, D. J., Osband, M. E., McCaffrey, R. P., et al., 1982, Abnormal histamine induced suppressor cell function in atopic individuals, *N. Eng. J. Med.* **306:**454.

Befus, A. D., Johnston, N., and Bienenstock, J., 1979, *Nippostrongylus brasiliensis:* Mast cells and histamine levels in tissues of infected and normal rats, *Exp. Parasitol.* **48:**1.

Befus, A. D., Pearce, F. L., Gouldie, J., Horsewood, P., and Bienenstock, J., 1982, Mucosal mast cells. I. Isolation and functional characteristics of rat intestinal mast cells, *J. Immunol.* **128:** 2475.

Befus, A. D., Bienenstock, J., and Denburg, J. A., 1986, *Mast Cell Differentiation and Heterogeneity,* Raven, New York.

Befus, A. D., Dyck, N., Goodacre, R., and Bienenstock, J., 1987, Mast cells from the human intestinal lamina propria, *J. Immunol.* **138:**2604.

Bennett, V., O'Keefe, E., and Cuatrecasas, P., 1975, Mechanism of action of cholera toxin and the mobile receptor theory of hormone receptor–adenylate cyclase interactions, *Proc. Natl. Acad. Sci. U.S.A.* **72:**33.

Benveniste, J., Henson, P. M., and Cochrane, C. G., 1972, Leukocyte-dependent histamine release from rabbit platelets: The role of IgE, basophils and a platelet-activating factor, *J. Exp. Med.* **136:**1356.

Benveniste, J., Tence, M., Varenne, P., Bidault J., Boullet, C., and Polonsky, J., 1979, Semisynthèse et structure proposée du facteur activant les plaquettes (PAF): PAF-acether, un alkylether analogue de la lysophosphatidylcholine, *C.R. Acad. Sci. Ser. D* **289:**1037.

Berenberg, J. L., and Ward, P. A., 1973, The chemotactic factor inactivator in normal human serum, *J. Clin. Invest.* **52:**1200.

Bernheim, H. A., Block, L. H., and Atkins, E., 1979, Fever: Pathogenesis, pathophysiology, and purpose, *Ann. Intern. Med.* **91:**261.

Bernheim, H. A., Jensen, M. C., and Dinarello, C. A., 1987, Role of phosphoinositides in the interleukin-1 induction of prostaglandins from human neuroblastoma cells, *Lymphokine Res.* **6:** 1235.

Bernstein, J. E., and Hamill, J. R., 1981, Substance P, *J. Invest. Der.* **77**(2):250.

Bertaccini, G., 1976, Active polypeptides of nonmammalian origin, *Pharmacol. Rev.* **28**(2): 127.

Bertoglio, J., Wakasugi, H., Rimsky, L., Wollman, E., Fradelizi, D., and Tursz, T., 1987, B cell line interleukin 1: Further assessment of the uniqueness of IL-1 gamma and of its biological activities, *Lymphokine Res.* **6:**1122.

Besedovsky, H. O., Del Rey, A. E., and Sorkin, E., 1985, Immune–neuroendocrine interactions, *J. Immunol.* **135:**750s.

Bessin, P., Bonnet, J., Apffel, D., Soulard, C., Desgroux, L., Pelos, I., and Benveniste, J., 1983, Acute circulating collapse caused by platelet activating factor (PAF acether) in dogs, *Eur. J. Pharmacol.* **86:**403.

Betz, S. H., and Henson, P. M., 1980, Production and release of platelet-activating factor (PAF): Dissociation from degranulation and superoxide production in the human neutrophil, *J. Immunol.* **125:**2756.

Billah, M. M., Bryant, R. W., and Siegel, M. I., 1985, Lipoxygenase products or arachidonic acid modulate biosynthesis of platelet-activating factor (1-*O*-alkyl-2-acetyl-*sn*-glycero-3-phosphocholine) by human neutrophils via phospholipase A2, *J. Biol. Chem.* **260:**6899.

Bjork, J., and Smedegard, G., 1983, Acute microvascular effects of PAF-acether, as studied by intravital microscopy, *Eur. J. Pharmacol.* **96:**87.

Blalock, J. E., and Smith, E. M., 1980, Human leukocyte interferon: Structural and biological relatedness to adrenocorticotropic hormone and endorphins, *Proc. Natl. Acad. Sci. U.S.A.* **77:** 5972.

Blalock, J. E., and Smith, E. M., 1982, Human lymphocyte production of neuroendocrine hormone-related substances, in: *Human Lymphokines—The Biological Immune Response Modifiers,* pp. 323–330, (A. Khan and N. Hill, Academic, New York.

Blalock, J. E., and Smith, E. M., 1985, A complete regulatory loop between the immune and neuroendocrine systems, *Fed. Proc.* **44**:108.

Blalock, J. E., Harbour-McMenamin, D., and Smith, E. M., 1985, Peptide hormones shared by the neuroendocrine and immunologic sytems, *J. Immunol.* **135**:858s.

Blank, M. L., Snyder, F., Byers, L. W., Brooks, B., and Muirhead, E. E., 1979, Antihypertensive activity of an alkyl ether analog of phospholidylcholine, *Biochem. Biophys. Res. Commun.* **90**:1194.

Bloom, F. E., 1985, Neuropeptides and other mediators in the central nervous system, *J. Immunol.* **135**:743s.

Blumberg, S., and Teichberg, V. I., 1979, Biological activity and enzymic degradation of substance P analogs—implications for studies of the substance P receptor, *Biochem. Biophys. Res. Commun.* **90**:347.

Bockman, D. E., and Kirby, M. L., 1985, Neural crest interactions in the development of the immune system, *J. Immunol.* **135**:766s.

Boetcher, D. A., and Leonard, E. J., 1973, Basophil chemotaxis—Augmentation by a factor from stimulated lymphocyte cultures, *Immunol. Commun.* **2**:421.

Boissonnas, R. A., Guttmann, S., and Jaquenoud, P.-A., 1960a, Synthèse de la L-arginyl-L-prolyl-L -prolyl-glycyl-L-phenylalanyl-L-seryl-L-phenyl-alanyl-L-arginine. Distinction entre cet octapeptide et la bradykinine, *Helv. Chim. Acta* **43**:1481.

Boissonnas, R. A., Guttmann, S., and Jaquenoud, P.-A., 1960b, Synthèse de la L-arginyl-L-prolyl-L -prolyl-glycyl-L-phenylalanyl-L-seryl-prolyl-L-phenylalanyl-L-arginine, un nonapeptide présentant les proprietes de la bradykinine, *Helv. Chim. Acta* **43**:1349.

Boissonnas, R. A., Guttmann, S., Jaquenoud, P.-A., Konzett, H., and Sturmer, E., 1960c, Synthesis and biological activity of peptides related to bradykinin, *Experientia* **16**:326.

Boissonnas, R. A., Guttmann, S., Jaquenoud, P.-A., Pless, J., and Sandrin, E., 1963, The synthesis of bradykinin and of related peptides, *Ann. N.Y. Acad. Sci.* **104**:5.

Bokisch, V. A., and Muller-Eberhard, H. J., 1970, Anaphylatoxin inactivator of human plasma: Its isolation and characterization as a carboxypeptidase, *J. Clin. Invest.* **49**:2427.

Bollum, F. J., 1979, Terminal deoxynucleotidyl transferase as a hematopoietic cell marker, *Blood* **54**:1203.

Bond, M. W., Shrader, B., Mosmann, T. R., and Coffman, R. L., 1987, A mouse T cell product that preferentially enhances IgA production. II. Physiochemical characterization, *J. Immunol.* **139**:3691.

Borgeat, P., Nadeau, M., Salari, H., Poubelle, P., and Delaclos, B. F., 1985, Leukotrienes: Biosynthesis, metabolism, and analysis, *Adv. Lipid Res.* **21**:47.

Borish, L. C., and Rocklin, R. E., 1987, Effects of leukocyte inhibitory factor (LIF) on neutrophil (PMN) phagocytosis and bactericidal activity, *Lymphokine Res.* **6**:1450 (abst.).

Borkowsky, W., and Lawrence, H. S., 1981, Deletion of antigen-specific activity from leukocyte dialysates containing transfer factor by antigen-coated polystyrene, *J. Immunol.* **126**:486.

Bourne, H. R., Lichtenstein, L. M., Melmon, K. L., Henney, C. S., Weinstein, V., and Shearer, J., 1974, Modulation of inflammation and immunity by cyclic AMP, *Science* **184**:19.

Brain, S. D., Camp, R. D. R., Dowd, P. M., Black, A. K., Woollard, P. M., Mallet, A. I., and Greaves, M. W., 1982, Psoriasis and leukotriene B4, *Lancet* **2**:762.

Braude, S., Coe, C., Royston, D., and Barnes, P. J., 1984, Histamine increases lung permeability by an H-2 receptor mechanism, *Lancet* **2**:372.

Bradley, B., Collins, K., McDonald, B., Alexander, S., Auron, E., Webb, A. C., and Rosenwasser, L. J., 1987, Pharmacologic modulation and molecular characterization of endothelial cell production of interleukin-1, *Lymphokine Res.* **6**:1137 (abst.).

Bray, M. A., Ford-Hutchinson, A. W., and Smith, M. J. H., 1981, Leukotriene B4 an inflammatory mediator in vivo, *Prostaglandins* **22**:213.

Brocklehurst, W. E., 1953, Occurrence of an unidentified substance during anaphylactic shock in calf lung, *J. Physiol. (Lond.)* **120**:16.

Brocklehurst, W. E., 1955, Response of the calf ileum to SRS-A from lung of man and of calf, *J. Physiol. (Lond.)* **128**:1.

Brocklehurst, W. E., 1960, Release of histamine and formation of a slow-reacting substance (SRS-A) during anaphylactic shock, *J. Physiol. (Lond.)* **151**:416.

Broder, S., Uchiyama, T. T., Muul, L., Goldman, C., Sharrow, S., Poplack, D., and Waldman, T., 1981, Activation of leukemic presuppressor cells to become suppressor effector cells, *N. Engl. J. Med.* **304**:1382.

Broderick, G., Osinski, J., Lenhardt, R., and Rajfer, S., 1987, Effects of guanine nucleotides on beta-adrenergic agonist binding in human myocardium, *Fed. Proc.* **46**:1309.

Brooks, C. G., and Henney, C. S., 1985, Interleukin-2 and the regulation of natural killer activity in cultured cell populations, *Contemp. Top. Mol. Immunol.* **10**:63.

Bulloch, K., 1985 Neuroanatomy of lymphoid tissue: A review, in: *Neural Modulation of Immunity* (R. Guillemin, M. Cohn, and T. Melnechuk, eds.), pp. 111–141, Raven, New York.

Burgess, A. W., Camarakis, J., and Metcalf, D., 1977, Purification and properties of colony stimulating factor from mouse lung-conditioned medium, *J. Biol. Chem.* **252**:1998.

Burkhalter, A., and Frick, O., 1987, Histamine, serotonin, and the ergot alkaloids, in: *Basic and Clinical Pharmacology*, 3rd ed. (B. G. Katzung, ed.), pp. 183–200, Appleton & Lange, E. Norwalk, Connecticut.

Burt, D. S., and Stanworth, D. R., 1983, The effect of ribose and purine modified adenosine analogues on the secretion of histamine from rat mast cells induced by ionophore A23187, *Biochem. Pharmacol.* **32**:2729.

Busse, W. W., and Lee, T. P., 1976, Decreased adrenergic responses in lymphocytes and granulocytes in atopic eczema, *J. Allergy Clin. Immunol.* **58**:586.

Busse, W. W., Cooper, W., Warshaver, D. M., Dick, E. C., Wallow, I. H. L., and Albrecht, R., 1979, Impairment of isoproterenol, H_2 histamine, and prostaglandin E_1 response of human granulocytes after incubation in vitro with live influenza vaccines, *Am. Rev. Respir. Dis.* **119**:561.

Butler, J. M., Chan, S. C., Stevens, S. R., and Hanifin, J. M., 1983, Increased leukocyte histamine release with elevated cyclic AMP-phosphodiesterase activity in atopic dermatitis, *J. Allergy Clin. Immunol.* **71**:490.

Campbell, P. A., Schuffler, C., and Rodriguez, C. E., 1976, Listeria cell wall fraction: A B cell adjuvant, *J. Immunol.* **116**:590.

Camussi, G., Aglietta, M., Malavasi, F., Tetta, C., Piacibelo, W., Sanavio, F., and Bussolino, F., 1983a, The release of platelet activating factor from human endothelial cells in culture, *J. Immunol.* **131**:2397.

Camussi, G., Paulowski, I., Bussolino, F., Caldwell, P. R. B., Brentjens, J., and Andres, G., 1983b, Release of platelet-activating factor in rabbits with antibody-mediated injury of the lung: The role of leukocytes and of pulmonary injury, *J. Immunol.* **131**:1802.

Camussi, G., Tetta, C., Coda, R., Segoloni, G. P., and Vercellone, A., 1984, Platelet-activating factor-induced loss of glomerular anionic charges, *Kidney Int.* **25**:73.

Cancro, M. P., Hilbert, D. M., Nordan, R., and Rudikoff, S., 1988, Differential IL-6 requirements in antigen-driven responses of primary versus secondary B-lymphocytes, *FASEB J.* **2**:A899 (abst. 3509).

Cannon, J. G., Tatro, J. B., Reichlin, S., and Dinarello, C. A., 1987, Inhibition of interleukin-1-mediated lymphocyte activation by alpha-melanocyte stimulating hormone involves a novel melanotropin receptor, *Lymphokine Res.* **6**:1104 (abst.)

Carraway, R., and Leeman, S. E., 1975, The amino acid sequence of a hypothalamic peptide, neurotensin, *J. Biol. Chem.* **250**:1907.

Casale, J. B., Bowman, S., and Kaliner, M., 1984, Induction of human cutaneous mast cell degranulation by opiates and endogenous opioid peptides: Evidence for opiate and non-opiate receptor participation, *J. Allergy Clin. Immunol.* **73**:775.

Ceredig, R., Lowenthal, J. W., Nabholz, M., and MacDonald, H. R., 1985, Expression of interleukin-2 receptor as a differentiation marker on intrathymic stem cells, *Nature (Lond.)* **314:** 98.

Cervoni, P., Herzlinger, H. E., Lai, F. M., and Tanikella, T. K., 1983, Aortic vascular and atrial responses to (1)-1-*O*-octadecyl-2-acetyl-glyceryl-3-phosphorylcholine, *Br. J. Pharmacol.* **79:** 667.

Chan, W., and Levy, J. V., 1987, Comparative potency of platelet activating factor (PAF) receptor antagonists on platelet aggregation response in human whole blood, *The Pharmacologist* **29:** 219.

Cheever, M. A., and Greenberg, P. D., 1985, In vivo administration of interleukin-2, *Contemp. Top. Mol. Immunol.* **10:**263.

Chen, M., Pasanen, V., Hammerling, N., Hammerling, G., and Hoffmann, M. K., 1979, Tumor necrosis serum induces a serologically distinct population of NK cells, *J. Exp. Med.* **150:**426.

Chernov-Rogan, T., Leed, J., Payan, D. G., and Goetzl, E. J., 1985, Endogeneous somatostatin-like peptides of rat basophilic leukemia cells, *Clin. Res.* **33:**515A.

Chesney, C. M., Pifer, D. D., and Huch, K. M., 1985, Desensitization of human platelets by platelet activating factor, *Biochem. Biophys. Res. Commun.* **127:**24.

Chilton, F. H., O'Flaherty, J. T., Walsh, C. E., Thomas, M. J., Wykle, R. L., DeChatelet, L. R., and Waite, B. M., 1982, Platelet-activating factor. Stimulation of the lipoxygenase pathway in polymorphonuclear leukocytes by 1-*O*-alkyl-2-*O*-acetyl-*sn*-glycero-3-phosphocholine, *J. Biol. Chem.* **257:**5402.

Chu, A. C., Patterson, J. A., Goldstein, G., Berger, C. L., Takezaki, S., and Edelson, R. L., 1983, Thymopoietin-like substance in human skin, *J. Invest. Dermatol.* **81:**194.

CIBA Foundation, 1975, *Symposium No. 35, Biochemistry and Pharmacology of Platelets*, Elsevier, Amsterdam.

CIBA Foundation, 1985, *Symposium No. 118, Biochemistry of Macrophages*, Pitman, New York.

Civelli, O., Douglass, J., Goldstein, A., and Herbert, E., 1985, Sequence and expression of the rat prodynorphin gene, *Proc. Natl. Acad. Sci. U.S.A.* **82:**4291.

Claas, F. H. J., Van Ree, J. M., Verhoeven, W. M. A., Van Den Poel, J. J., Verduyn, W., De Wied, D., and Van Rood, J. J., 1986, The interaction between gamma-type endorphins and HLA class I antigens, *Human Immunol.* **15:**347.

Clancy, R. M., Dahinden, C. A., and Hugli, T. E., 1983, Arachidonate metabolism by human polymorphonuclear leukocytes stimulated by *N*-formyl-met-leu-phe or complement C5a is independent of phospholipase activation, *Proc. Natl. Acad. Sci. U.S.A.* **80:**7200.

Clark-Lewis, I., Schrader, J. W., Ziltener, H., Lopez, A., Vadas, M., Hood, L., and Kent, S. B. H., 1987, Structure–function studies of lymphokines by total chemical synthesis, *Lymphokine Res.* **6:**1318 (abst.).

Coffman, R. L., and Carty, J., 1986, A T-cell activity that enhances polyclonal IgE production and its inhibition of interferon gamma, *J. Immunol.* **136:**949.

Coffman, R. L., Shrader, B., Carty, J., Mosmann, T. R., and Bond, M. W., 1987, A mouse T cell product that preferentially enhances IgA production. I. Biologic characterization, *J. Immunol.* **139:**3685.

Cohen, J. J., 1987, Immunity and behavior, *J. Allergy Clin. Immunol.* **79:**2.

Cohen, M. L., Schenck, K. W., Colbert, W., and Wittenauer, L., 1985, Role of 5-HT$_2$ receptors in serotonin-induced contractions of nonvascular smooth muscle, *J. Pharamcol. Exp. Ther.* **232:** 770.

Cohen, S., Berrih, S., Dardenne, M., and Bach, J.-F., 1983, Regulation in vitro de la secretion de thymuline par les cellules epitheliales thymiques humaines, *C.R. Acad. Sci.* **297:**63.

Content, J., Dewit, L., Pierard, D., Derynck, R., DeClercq, E., and Fiers, W., 1982, Secretory proteins induced in human fibroblasts under conditions used for the production of interferon beta, *Proc. Natl. Acad. Sci. U.S.A.* **79:**2768.

Cooper, J. R., Bloom, R. E., and Roth, R. H. (eds.), 1986, *The Biochemical Basis of Neuropharmacology*, 5th ed., Oxford University Press, Oxford.

Cooper, N. R., 1987, The complement system, in: *Basic and Clinical Immunology* (D. P. Stites, J. D. Stobo, and J. V. Wells, eds.), Vol. 6, pp. 114–127, Appleton and Lange, E. Norwalk, Connecticut.

Coupland, R. E., 1972, The chromaffin system, in: *Handbook of Experimental Pharmacology* (H. Blascko and E. Muscholl, eds.), Vol. 33, pp. 16–45, Springer-Verlag, Berlin.

Craig, S. S., DeBlois, G., and Schwartz, L. B., 1986, Mast cells in human keloid, small intestine and lung by an immunoperoxidase technique using a murine monoclonal antibody against tryptase, *Am. J. Pathol.* **124:**4270.

Creticos, P. S., Peters, S. P., Adkinson, N. F., Naclario, R. M., Hayes, E. C., Norman, P. S., and Lichtenstein, L. M., 1984, Peptide leukotriene release after antigen challenge in patients sensitive to ragweed, *N. Engl. J. Med.* **310:**1626.

Czarnetzki, B. M., Konig, W., and Lichtenstein, L., 1976, Antigen-induced eosinophil chemotactic factor release by human leukocytes, *Inflammation* 1:201.

Dahlen, S.-E., Hedqvist, P., Hammarstrom, S., and Samuelsson, B., 1980, Leukotrienes are potent constrictors of human bronchi, *Nature (Lond.)* **288:**484.

Dahlen, S.-E., Bjork, J., Hedqvist, P., Afors, K.-E., Hammarstrom, S., Lindgren, J.-A., and Samuelsson, B., 1981, Leukotrienes promote plasma leakage and leukocyte adhesion in postcapillary venules: In vivo effects with relevance to the acute inflammatory response, *Proc. Natl. Acad. Sci. U.S.A.* **78:**3887.

Dahlen, S.-E., Hansson, G., Hedqvist, P., Bjork, T., Granstrom, E., and Dahlen, B., 1983, Allergen challenge of lung tissue from asthmatics elicits bronchial contraction that correlates with the release of leukotrienes C_4, D_4, and E_4, *Proc. Natl. Acad. Sci. U.S.A.* **80:**1712.

Dale, M. M., and Foreman, J. C. (eds.), 1984, *Textbook of Immunopharmacology*, Blackwell Scientific Publications, Oxford.

Dardenne, M., 1983, Evaluation of thymic hormone serum levels in health and disease, *Clin. Immunol. Allergy* **3:**157.

Dardenne, M., Pleau, J. M., and Bach, J.-F., 1980, Evidence of the presence in normal serum of a carrier of the serum thymic factors, *Eur. J. Immunol.* **10:**83.

Dardenne, M., Pleau, J. M., Nabarra, B., LeFrancier, P., Derrien, M., Choay, J., and Bach, J.-F., 1982, Contribution of zinc and other metals to the biological activity of the serum thymic factors, *Proc. Natl. Acad. Sci. U.S.A.* **79:**5370.

Davies, P., 1984, The mononuclear phagocyte, in: *Textbook of Immunopharmacology* (M. M. Dale and J. C. Foreman, eds.), pp. 79–92, Blackwell Scientific Publications, Oxford.

DeClerck, F. F., and Vanhoutte, M. (eds.), 1982, *5-Hydroxytryptamine in Peripheral Reactions*, Raven, New York.

deGaetano, G., and Garattini, S. (eds.), 1978, *Platelets: A Multidisciplinary Approach*, Raven, New York.

Demopoulos, C. A., Pinckard, R. N., and Hanahan, D. J., 1979, Platelet-activating factor: evidence for 1-O-alkyl-2-acetyl-sn-glyceryl-3-phosphorylcholine as the active component (a new class of lipid chemical mediators), *J. Biol. Chem.* **254:**9355.

Denning, S. T., Tuck, D. T., Singer, K. H., and Haynes, B. F., 1986, Human thymic epithelial cells function as accessory cells for autologous mature thymocyte activation, *Clin. Res.* **34:**669A.

Deschaux, P. and Rouabhia, M., 1987, The thymus. Key organ between endocrinologic and immunologic systems, in: *Neuroimmune Interactions* (B. D. Jankovic, B. M. Markovic, and N. H. Spector, eds.), *Ann. N.Y. Acad. Sci.* **496:**49.

De Simone, C., Ferrari, M., Ferrarelli, G., Rumi, C., Pugnaloni, L., and Sorice, F., 1987, The effects of substance P on human eosinophil receptors and functions, in: *Neuroimmune Interactions* (B. D. Jankovic, B. M. Markovic, and N. H. Spector, eds.), *Annals N.Y. Acad. Sci.* **496:** 226.

Devos, R., Plaetinck, G., Cheroutre, H., Simons, G., DeGrave, W., Tavernier, J., Remaut, E., and Fiers, W., 1983, Molecular cloning of human interleukin 2 carrier DNA and its expression in *Escherichia coli, Nucl. Acid. Rev.* **11:**4307.

de Weck, A., Kristensen, F., and Landy, M. (eds.), 1980, *Biochemical Characterization of Lymphokines. Proceedings of the Second International Lymphokine Workshop*, Academic, New York.

de Wied, D., 1983, The importance of vasopressin memory, *Trends Neurosci.* **7**:62.

Diel, F., Bethge, N., and Opree, W., 1983, Histamine secretion in leukocyte incubates of patients with allergic hypersensitivity induced by somatostatin-14 and somatostatin-28, *Agents Actions* **13**:216.

DiMicco, J. A., and Aprison, M. H., 1986, Distribution and function of amino acid neurotransmitters: Roles in central modulation of the autonomic, neuroendocrine and immune systems, in: *Neuroregulation of Autonomic, Endocrine and Immune Systems* (R. C. A. Frederickson, H. C. Hendrie, J. N. Hingtgen, and M. H. Aprison, eds.), Kluwer Academic, Hingham, MA, pp. 29–60.

Dinarello, C. A., 1984, Interleukin-1, *Rev. Infect. Dis.* **6**:51.

Dinarello, C. A., 1985, New perspectives in the study of human interleukin-1: Contribution from molecular biology, *J. Leukocyte Biol.* **36**:696.

Dinarello, C. A., and Wolff, S. M., 1982, Molecular basis of fever in humans, *Am. J. Med.* **72**:799.

Dinarello, C. A., Marnoy, S. O., and Rosenwasser, L. J., 1983, Role of arachidonate metabolism in the immunoregulatory function of human leukocytic pyrogen lymphocyte-activating factor interleukin 1, *J. Immunol.* **130**:890.

Dinarello, C. A., Clowes, G. H. A., Jr., Gordon, A. H., Saravis, C. A., and Wolff, S. M., 1984, Cleavage of human interleukin 1—Isolation of a peptide fragment from plasma of febrile humans and activated monocytes, *J. Immunol.* **133**:1332.

Dinarello, C. A., Bishai, I., Rosenwasser, L. J., and Coceani, F., 1984, The influence of lipoxygenase inhibitors on the in vitro production of human leukocytic pyrogen and lymphocyte activating factor (IL-1), *Int. J. Immunopharmacol.* **6**:43.

Dinarello, C. A., Cannon, J. G., Oroncle, S. F., Lisi, P., Warner, S. J. C., and Libby, P. L., 1987a, Recombinant human interleukin-1-alpha (rIL-1A) induces IL-1-beta, *Lymphokine Res.* **6**:1202 (abst.).

Dinarello, C. A., Maxwell, R., Saijo, T., Ikejima, T., and Mier, J. W., 1987b, Mechanisms of interleukin 1 production and activity: Role of the 5-lipoxygenase pathway, *Lymphokine Res.* **6**:1138 (abst.).

Dixon, F. J., 1983, Murine SLE models and autoimmune disease, in: *The Biology of Immunologic Disease* (F. J. Dixon and D. W. Fisher, eds.), pp. 235–245, Sinauer, Sunderland, Massachusetts.

Dixon, F. J., and Fisher, D. W. (eds.), 1983, *The Biology of Immunologic Diseases*, Sinauer, Sunderland, Massachusetts.

Doebber, T. W., Wu, M. S., Robbins, J. C., Choy, B. M., Chang, M. N., and Shen, T., 1985, Platelet activating factor (PAF) involvement in endotoxin induced hypotension in rats: Studies with PAF-receptor antagonist kadsurenone, *Biochem. Biophys. Res. Commun.* **127**:799.

Doris, P. A., 1984, Vasopressin and central integrative processes, *Neuroendocrinology* **38**:75.

Douglas, W. W., 1985, Polypeptides—Angiotensin, plasma kinins and others, in: *The Pharmacological Basis of Therapeutics*, (A. G. Gilman, L. S. Goodman, T. W. Rall, and F. Murad, eds.), pp. 639–659, Macmillan, New York.

Doyle, M. V., Lee, M. T., and Fong, S., 1985, Comparison of the biological activities of human recombinant interleukin 2125 and native interleukin 2, *J. Biol. Response Mod.* **4**:96.

Doyle, V. M., Creba, J. A., and Ruegg, U. T., 1986, Platelet-activating factor mobilizes intracellular calcium in vascular smooth muscle cells, *FEBS Lett.* **197**:13.

Dumonde, D. C., and Hamblin, A., 1983, Lymphokines, in: *Immunology in Medicine* (E. J. Holborow and W. G. Reeves, eds.), pp. 121–150, Grune & Stratton, Orlando, Florida.

Durum, S. K., Schmidt, J. A., and Oppenheim, J. J., 1985, Interleukin-1: An immunological perspective, *Annu. Rev. Immunol.* **3**:263.

Dusting, G. J., Moncada, S., and Vane, J. R., 1979, Prostaglandins, their intermediates, and precursors, their cardiovascular actions, and regulatory roles in normal and abnormal circulatory systems, *Prog. Cardiovascular Dis.* **21**:405.

Dy, M., Lebel, B., Kamoun, P., and Hamburger, J., 1981, Histamine production during the anti-allograft responses: Demonstration of a new lymphokine enhancing histamine synthesis, *J. Exp. Med.* **153**:293.

Dy, M., Lebel, B., and Schneider, E., 1986, Histamine-producing cell stimulating factor (HCSF) and interleukin 3 (IL-3): Evidence for two distinct molecular entities, *J. Immunol.* **136**:208.

Dy, M., Schneider, E., Auffray, C., and Gastinel, L. N., 1987, Interleukin 3 (IL-3) and granulocyte macrophage colony-stimulating factor (GM-CSF) both express histamine-producing cell-stimulating activity (HCSA), *Lymphokine Res.* **6**:1325 (abst.).

Eliakim, R., Gilead, L., Ligumsky, M., Okon, E., Rachmilewitz, D., and Razin, E., 1986, Histamine and chondroitin sulfate E proteoglycan released by cultured human colonic mucosa: Indication for possible presence of E mast cells, *Proc. Natl. Acad. Sci. U.S.A.* **83**:461.

Elliott, D. F., 1960, Discussion, in: *Polypeptides Which Affect Smooth Muscles and Blood Vessels* (M. Schachter, ed.), pp. 266–271, Pergamon, New York.

Elsas, P., Lee, T., David, J. R., Austen, K. F., Lewis, R. A., and Dessein, A. J., 1987, Monokine(s) enhance Ca^{++} ionophore stimulated arachidonic acid metabolism in human eosinophils, *Lymphokine Res.* **6**:1453 (abst.).

Engineer, D. M., Morris, H. R., Piper, P. J., and Sirois, P., 1978, The release of prostaglandins and thromboxanes from guinea pig lung by slow reacting substance of anaphylaxis and its inhibition, *Br. J. Pharmacol.* **64**:211.

Eranko, O., Sonila, S., and Paiverinta, M., 1980, *Histochemistry and Cell Biology of Autonomic Neurons, SIF Cells and Paraneurons*, Academic, New York.

Erdos, E. (ed.), 1979, *Bradykin, Kallidin, and Kallikrein, Handbook of Experimental Pharmacology*, Vol. XXV, Springer-Verlag, Berlin.

Erspamer, V., 1966, *5-Hydroxytryptamine and Related Indolealkylamines, Handbook of Experimental Pharmacology*, Vol. XIX, Springer-Verlag, Berlin.

Erspamer, V., 1981, The tachykinin peptide family, *Trends Neurosci.* **4**:267.

Escobar, M. R., and Friedman, H., 1980, *Macrophages and Lymphocytes*, Parts A and B, Plenum, New York.

Espinoza, L. R., and Osterland, C. K. (eds.), 1983, *Circulating Immune Complexes. Their Clinical Significance*, Futura, Mt. Kisco, New York.

Essman, W. B., 1978, *Serotonin in Health and Disease*, Vols. 1–4, Spectrum, Jamaica, NY.

Etienne, A., Hecquet, F., Soulard, C., Spinnewy, B., Clostre, F., and Broquet, P., 1985, In vivo inhibition of plasma protein leakage and *Salmonella enteritidis*-induced mortality in the rat by specific PAF acether antagonist BN 52021, *Agents Actions* **17**:368.

Falck, B., Hillard, N. A., and Torp, A., 1959, Some observations on the histology and histochemistry of chromaffin cells probably storing dopamine, *J. Histochem. Cytochem.* **7**:323.

Faltynek, C. R., and Baglioni, C., 1984, Interferon is a polypeptide hormone, *Microbiol. Sci.* **1**(4):81.

Farr, R. S., Cox, C. P., Wardlow, M., and Jorgensen, R., 1980, Preliminary studies of an acid-labile factor (ALF) in human sera that inactivates platelet-activating factor (PAF), *Clin. Immunol. Immunopathol.* **15**:318.

Farrar, W. L., Johnson, H. M., and Farrar, J. J., 1981, Regulation of the production of immune interferon and cytotoxic lymphocytes by interleukin 2, *J. Immunol.* **126**:1120.

Farrar, J. J., Benjamin, W. R., Hilfiker, M. L., Howard, M., Farrar, W. L., and Fuller-Farrar, A., 1982, The biochemistry, biology, and role of interleukin 2 in the induction of cytotoxic T-cell and antibody forming B-cell responses, *Immunol. Rev.* **63**:129.

Farrar, W. L., Kilian, P., Hill, J. M., Ruff, M. R., and Pert, C. B., 1987, Visualization of cytokine and virus receptors common to the immune and central nervous system, *Lymphokine Res.* **6**(1): 29.

Farrukh, I. S., Spannhake, E. M., Scinto, A. M., Michael, J. R., and Gurtner, G. H., 1985,

Mechanisms by which LTD₄ increases fluid infiltration, vascular and airway pressure in the isolated perfused rabbit lung, *Am. Rev. Respir. Dis.* **131**:A423.

Feldberg, W., and Kellaway, C. H., 1938, The liberation of histamine by staphylococcal toxin and mercuric chloride, *Aust. J. Exp. Biol. Med. Sci.* **16**:249.

Feldberg, W., and Keogh, E. V., 1937, Liberation of histamine from the perfused lung by staphylococcal toxin, *J. Physiol.* (Lond.) **90**:280.

Fels, A.O.S., Pawlowski, N. A., Cramer, E. B., King, T.K.C., Cohn, Z. A., and Scott, W. A., 1982, Human alveolar macrophages produce leukotriene B4, *Proc. Natl. Acad. Sci. U.S.A.* **79**:7866.

Felten, D. L., Felten, S. Y., Carlson, S. L., Olschowka, J. A., and Livnat, S., 1985, Noradrenergic and peptidergic innervation of lymphoid tissue, *J. Immunol.* **135**: 755s.

Fernandez, H. N., and Hugli, T. E., 1978, Primary structural characterization of the polypeptide portion of human C5a anaphylatoxin: Polypeptide sequence of determination and assessment of the oligosaccharide attachment site in C5a, *J. Biol. Chem.* **253**:6955.

Fernandez-Botran, R., Sanders, V. M., Oliver, K., Chen, Y.-W., Krammer, P. H., Uhr, J. W., and Vitetta, E. S., 1987, The role of interleukin 4 in the response of helper T cells to antigen, *Lymphokine Res.* **6**:1625(abst.)

Feuerstein, G., and Hallenbeck, J. M., 1987, Prostaglandins, leukotrienes and platelet-activating factor in shock, *Annu. Rev. Pharmacol. Toxicol.* **27**:301.

Feuerstein, G., Zukowska-Groject, A., Krausz, M. M., Blank, M. L., Snyder, F., and Kopin, I. J., 1982, Cardiovascular and sympathetic effects of 1-*O*-hexadecyl-2-acetyl-*sn*-glycero-3-phosphorylcholine in conscious SHR and WKY rats, *Clin. Exp. Hypertension* **A4**:1335.

Feuerstein, G., Lux, W. E., Jr., Erza, D., Hayes, E. C., Snyder, F., and Faden, I., 1985, Thyrotropin releasing hormone blocks the hypotensive effect of platelet activating factor in unanesthetized guinea pig, *J. Cardiovasc. Pharmacol.* **7**:335.

Filipp, G., and Szentivanyi, A., 1956, Experimentelle data zur regulativen rolle des neuroendokriniums in experimenteller anaphylaxie. I. Relazioni e communicazioni, Rome Il Pansiero Scientifico 237.

Filipp, G., and Szentivanyi, A., 1957, Die wirkung von hypothalamuslasionen auf den anaphylaktischen schock des meerschweinchens, *Allergie Asthmaforsch.* **1**:23.

Filipp, G., and Szentivanyi, A., 1985, Anaphylaxis and the nervous system. Part III, in: *Foundations of Psychoneuroimmunology* S. Locke, R. Ader, H. O. Besedovsky, N. R. Hall, G. Solomon, and T. Strom, eds., pp. 1–12, Aldine, Hawthorne, New York.

Filipp, G., Szentivanyi, A., and Mess, B., 1952, Anaphylaxis and nervous system, *Acta Med. Hung.* **2**:163.

Fischer, E. G., and Falke, N. E., 1987, Interaction of met-enkephalin with human granulocytes, in: *Neuroimmune Interactions* (B. D. Jankovic, B. M. Markovic, and N. H. Spector, eds.), *Ann. N.Y. Acad. Sci.* **496**:146.

Fishel, C. W., Szentivanyi, A., and Talmage, D. W., 1964, Adrenergic factors in *Bordetella pertussis*-induced histamine and serotonin hypersensitivity of mice, in: *Bacterial Endotoxins*, (M. Landy and W. Braun, eds.), pp. 414–481, Rutgers University Press, New Brunswick, New Jersey.

Fishel, C. W., Szentivanyi, A., and Klein, T., 1973, Effect of epinephrine on plasma cyclic adenosine monophosphate levels of *B. pertussis*-vaccinated and of adrenergically blocked mice, *Fed. Proc.* **32**:1009.

Fisher, R. H., Kagey-Sobotka, A., Proud, D., Orchard, M. A., Lichtenstein, L. M., 1987, Platelet–basophil interactions: Clinical correlates, *J. Allergy Clin. Immunol.* **79**:196.

Fletcher, M., and Goldstein, A. L., 1987, Recent advances in the understanding of the biochemistry and clinical pharmacology of interleukin-2, *Lymphokine Res.* **6**:45.

Flomenberg, N., Welte, L., Mertelsmann, R., Kernan, N., Ciobanu, N., Venuta, S., Feldman, S., Kruger, G., Kirkpatrick, D., DuPont, B., and O'Reilly, R., 1983, Immunological effects of interleukin 2 in primary immunodeficiency diseases, *J. Immunol.* **130**:2644.

Flower, R. J., Moncada, S., and Vane, J. R., 1985, Analgesic-antipyretics and anti-inflammatory agents; drugs employed in the treatment of gout, in: *The Pharmacological Basis of Therapeutics*, 7th ed. (A. G. Gilman, L. S. Goodman, T. W. Rall, and F. Murad, eds.), pp. 674–715, Macmillan, New York.

Ford-Hutchinson, A. W., 1984, Leukotriene involvement in pathologic processes, *J. Allergy Clin. Immunol.* **74**(suppl.):437.

Ford-Hutchinson, A. W., Bray, M. A., Doig, M. V., Shipley, M. E., and Smith, A., 1980, Leukotriene B: A potent chemokinetic and aggregating substance released from polymorphonuclear leukocytes, *Nature (Lond.)* **286**:264.

Foreman, J. C., and Jordan, C. C., 1983, Histamine release and vascular changes induced by neuropeptides, *Agents Actions* **13**:105.

Foreman, J. C., Jordan, C. C., and Piotrowski, W., 1982, Interaction of neurotensin with the substance P receptor mediating histamine release from rat mast cells and the flare in human skin, *Br. J. Pharmacol.* **77**:531.

Foris, G., Medgyesi, G. A., Nagy, J. T., and Varga, Z., 1987, Concentration-dependent effect of met-enkephalin on human polymorphonuclear leukocytes, in: *Neuroimmune Interactions* (B. D. Jankovic, B. M. Markovic, and N. H. Spector, eds.), *Ann. N.Y. Acad. Sci.* **496**:56.

Fornet, B., Filipp, G., Vegh, L., and Szentivanyi, A., 1954, Beeinflussung der experimentellen anaphylaxie durch zisternal verabreichten farbstoff, *Acta Med. Hung.* **4**:115.

Fox, R. W., and Lockey, R. F., 1983, Immediate hypersensitivity and immune complex disease, in: *Circulating Immune Complexes. Their Clinical Significance* (L. R. Espinoza and C. K. Osterland, eds.), pp. 295–319, Futura, Mt. Kisco, New York.

Frasca, D., Garavini, M., and Doria, G., 1982, Recovery of T-cell functions in aged mice injected with synthetic thymosin alpha₁, *Cell. Immunol.* **72**:384.

Frederickson, R. C. A., Hendrie, H. C., Hingtgen, J. N., and Aprison, M. H., eds., 1986, *Neuroregulation of Autonomic, Endocrine, and Immune Systems*, Martinus Nijhoff, Boston.

Frei, K., Bodmer, S., Siepl, C., and Fontant, A., 1987, Astrocyte-derived interleukin 3 as growth factor for microglial cells and peritoneal macrophages, *Lymphokine Res.* **6**:1310 (abst.).

Frey, E. K., 1926, Zusammenhange zwischen Herzarbeit und Nierentatigkeit, *Langenbecks Arch. Klin. Chir.* **142**:663.

Friedman, R. M., and Vogel, S. N., 1983, Interferons with special emphasis on the immune system, *Adv. Immunol.* **34**:97.

Fritz, H., Back, N., Dietze, G., and Haberland, G. L. (eds.), 1983, Kinins. III, *Adv. Exp. Med. Biol.* **156A**:1, **156B**:706.

Fuller, R. W., 1986, Brain monoaminergic neurons: Distribution and function in relation to regulation of autonomic, neuroendocrine and immune systems, in: *Neuroregulation of Autonomic, Endocrine and Immune Systems* (R. C. A. Frederickson, H. C. Hendrie, J. N. Hingtgen and M. H. Aprison, eds.), pp. 9–28, Kluwer Academic, Hingham, MA.

Gagnon, L., Sirois, P., and Rola-Pleszczynski, M., 1984, Leukotriene B4 augments natural cytotoxicity by increasing effector to target binding and by inducing the production of a cytotoxic lymphokine, *Fed. Proc.* **43**:1989.

Galbraith, G. M. P., and Fudenberg, H. H., 1985, Transfer factor, in: *Dermatologic Immunology and Allergy* (J. Stone, ed.), pp. 889–898, C. V. Mosby, St. Louis.

Galli, S. J., and Lichtenstein, L. M., 1988, Biology of mast cells and basophils, in: *Allergy—Principles and Practice*, 3rd ed. (E. Middleton, C. E. Reed, and E. F. Ellis, eds.), pp. 106–134, C. V. Mosby, St. Louis.

Galli, S. J., Dvorak, A. M., Marcum, J. A., Ishizaka, T., Nabel, G., Dersimonian, H., Pyne, K., Goldin, J. M., Rosenberg, R. D., and Cantor, H., 1982, Mast cell clones—A model for the analysis of cellular maturation, *J. Cell Biol.* **95**:435.

Ganellin, C. R., and Parsons, M. E. (eds.), 1982, *Pharmacology of Histamine Receptors*, Wright-PSG, Bristol.

Garattini, S., and Valzelli, L., 1965, *Serotonin*, Elsevier, Amsterdam.

Garland, J. M., 1987, Specific protein phosphorylation stimulated by different growth factors in different IL-3 dependent cell lines and its relationship to protein kinases, *Lymphokine Res.* **6:** 1319.

Gash, D. M., and Thomas, F. J., 1983, What is the importance of vasopressin in memory processes, *Trends Neurosci.* **6:**197.

Gauldie, J., Sauder, D. N., McAdam, K. P., and Dinerello, C. A., 1987, Purified interleukin 1 from human monocytes stimulates acute-phase protein synthesis by rodent hepatocytes in vitro, *Immunology* **60:**203.

Genan, V., Legros, J.-J., Franchimont, P., Baudrihaye, M., Defresne, M. P., and Boniver, J., 1986, The neuroendocrine thymus: Coexistence of oxytocin and neurophysin in the human thymus, *Science* **232:**508.

Geenan, V., Legros, J.-J., and Franchimont, P., 1987, The thymus as a neuroendocrine organ. Syntheses of vasopressin and oxytocin in human thymic epithelium, in: *Neuroimmune Interactions* (B. D. Jankovic, B. M. Markovic, and N. H. Spector, eds.), *Ann. N.Y. Acad. Sci.* **496:**56.

Gery, I., and Lepezuniga, J. L., 1984, Interleukin-1: Uniqueness of its production and spectrum of activities, in: *Lymphokines,* Academic, Orlando, Florida.

Giachetti, A., Goth, A., and Said, S. I., 1978, Vasoactive intestinal polypeptide (VIP) in rabbit platelets and rat mast cells, *Fed. Proc.* **37:**657.

Gillis, S., Baker, P. E., Ruscetti, F. W., and Smith, K. A., 1978, Long-term culture of human antigen specific cytotoxic T cell lines, *J. Exp. Med.* **148:**1093.

Gillis, S. J., and Inman, F. P. (eds.), 1985, *Contemporary Topics in Molecular Immunology. The Interleukins,* Plenum, New York.

Gillis, S., and Smith, K. A., 1977, Long-term culture of tumor-specific cytotoxic T-cells, *Nature (Lond.)* **268:**154.

Gillis, S., and Watson, J., 1980, Biochemical and biological characterization of lymphocyte regulatory molecules. 5. Identification of an interleukin 2-producing human leukemia T-cell line, *J. Exp. Med.* **152:**1709.

Gilman, S. C., Schwartz, J. M., Milner, R. J., Bloom, F. E., and Feldman, J. R., 1982, Beta-endorphin enhances lymphocyte proliferative responses, *Proc. Natl. Acad. Sci. U.S.A.* **79:** 4226.

Gilman, S. C., Berner, P. R., and Chang, J., 1987, Phospholipase A_2 activation: A mechanism for the proinflammatory actions of interleukin 1, *Lymphokine Res.* **6:**1220 (abst.)

Gimbrone, M. A., Jr., Brock, A. F., and Schafer, A. I., 1984, Leukotriene B_4 stimulates polymorphonuclear leukocyte adhesion to cultured vascular endothelial cells, *J. Clin. Invest.* **74:** 1552.

Gimenez-Gallego, G., Rodkey, J., Bennett, C., Rios-Candelone, M., DiSalvo, J., and Thomas, K., 1985, Brain-derived acidic fibroblast growth factor—complete amino acid sequence and homologies, *Science* **230:**1385.

Ginsburg, H., Olson, E. C., Huff, T. F., Okudaira, H., and Ishizaka, T., 1981, Enhancement of mast-cell differentiation in vitro by T-cell factors, *Int. Arch. Allergy Appl. Immunol.* **66:**447.

Ginsburg, H., Ben-Shahan, D., and Ben-David, E., 1982, Mast cell growth on fibroblast monolayers—two cell entities, *Immunology* **45:**371.

Giulian, D., Young, D. G., and Woodward, J., 1987, Interleukin 1 and brain development, *Lymphokine Res.* **6:**1206 (abst.).

Goetzl, E. J., 1985, Forward, *J. Immunol.* **135**(2):is.

Goetzl, E. J., 1987, Leukocyte receptors for lipid and peptide mediators, *Fed. Proc.* **46:**190.

Goetzl, E. J., and Austen, K. F., 1975, Purification and synthesis of eosinophilotactic tetrapeptides of human lung tissue: Identification as eosinophilotactic factor of anaphylaxis (ECF-A), *Proc. Natl. Acad. Sci. U.S.A.* **72:**4123.

Goetzl, E. J., and Payan, D. G., 1984, Inhibition of somastatin, *J. Immunol.* **133:**3255.

Goetzl, E. J., and Sun, F. F., 1979, Generation of unique mono-hydroxyeicosatetraenoic acids from arachidonic acid by human neutrophils, *J. Exp. Med.* **150:**406.

Goetzl, E. J., Chernov, T., Renold, F., and Payan, D. G., 1985, Neuropeptide regulation of the expression of immediate hypersensitivity, *J. Immunol.* **135:**802s.

Goetzl, E. J., Chernov-Rogan, T., Furuichi, K., Goetzl, L. M., Ule, J. Y., and Renold, F., 1986, in: *Mast Cell Differentiation and Heterogeneity* (J. Bienenstock, A. D. Befus, and J. A. Denberg, eds.), p. 223, Raven, New York.

Goldman, D. W., Gifford, L. A., Marotti, T., Koo, C. H., and Goetzl, E. J., 1987, Molecular and cellular properties of human polymorphonuclear leukocyte receptors for leukotriene B_4, *Fed. Proc.* **46:**200.

Goldman, R., Bar-Shavit, Z., and Romeo, D., 1983, Neurotensin modulates human neutrophil locomotion and phagocytic capability, *FEBS Lett.* **159:**63.

Goldstein, A. L., Low, T. L. K., Zatz, M. M., Hall, N. R., and Naylor, P. H., 1983, Thymosins, *Clin. Immunol. Allergy* **3:**119.

Goldstein, G., and Lau, C., 1980, Thymopoietin and immunoregulation, in: *Polypeptide Hormones* (F. Beers and E. G. Bassett, eds.), pp. 459–466, Raven, New York.

Goldstein, G., Scheid, M., Hammerling, U., Boyse, E. A., Schlesinger, D. H., and Niall, H. D., 1975, Isolation of a polypeptide that has lymphocyte-differentiating properties and is probably represented universally in living cells, *Proc. Natl. Acad. Sci. U.S.A.* **72:**11.

Goldstein, R. E., Laurindo, F. R. M., Erza, D., and Feuerstein, G., 1987, Mechanism of circulating collapse induced by PAF-acether, in: *Lipid Mediators in Immunology of Burn and Sepsis* (M. Braquet, ed.), pp. 211–221, Plenum, New York.

Goldyne, M. E., 1987, Prostaglandins and other eicosanoids, in: *Basic and Clinical Pharmacology*, 3rd ed., (B. G. Katzung, ed.), Appleton & Lange, E. Norwalk, Connecticut.

Goldyne, M. E., Burrish, G. F., Poubelle, P., and Borgeat, P., 1984, Arachidonic acid metabolism among human mononuclear leukocytes: Lipoxygenase-related pathways, *J. Biol. Chem.* **259:** 8815.

Golub, E. S., 1986, An overview of the immune response or an immunologist's view of the nervous system control of the immune system, in: *Neuroregulation of Autonomic, Endocrine, and Immune Systems* (R. C. A. Frederickson, H. C. Hendrie, J. N. Hingtgen, and M. H. Aprison, eds.), pp. 323–341, Martinus Nijhoff, Boston.

Good, R. A., 1983, The thymus and its hormones, *Clin. Immunol. Allergy* **3:**3.

Goodman, M. G., and Weigle, W. O., 1980, Modulation of lymphocytes activation. 1. Inhibition of an oxidation product of arachidonic acid, *J. Immunol.* **125:**593.

Goodwin, J. S., Gualde, N., Aldigier, J., Rigaud, M., and Vanderhoek, J. Y., 1984, Modulation of FC-gamma receptors on T-cells and monocytes by 15 hydroperoxyeicosatetraenoic acid, *Prostaglandins Leukotrienes Med.* **13:**109.

Gootenberg, J. E., 1984, Biochemical variants of human T-cell growth factor produced by malignant cell lines, *Lymphokine Res.* **3:**33.

Gootenberg, J. E., and Wallace, B. D., 1987, Factors with IL-2-like activity which are structurally and functionally distinct from IL-2, *Lymphokine Res.* **6:**1620 (abst.).

Gootenberg, J. E., Ruscetti, F. W., and Gallo, R. C. 1982, A biochemical variant of human T-cell growth factor produced by a cutaneous T-cell lymphoma cell line, *J. Immunol.* **129:**1499.

Goren, H., Okabe, T., Lederis, K., and Hollenberg, R. D., 1984, Oxytocin stimulates glucose oxidation in rat thymocytes, *Proc. West. Pharmacol. Soc.* **27:**461.

Grabstein, K., Reed, S., Shanebeck, K., and Morrissey, P., 1987, Induction of macrophage microbicidal activity by granulocyte–macrophage colony stimulating factor (GM-CSF), *Lymphokine Res.* **6:**1707 (abst.).

Greaves, M. F., Owen, J. J. T., and Raff, M. C., 1974, *T and B Lymphocytes: Origins, Properties, and Roles in Immune Responses*, Elsevier, New York.

Greenbaum, L. M., 1976, Kinins and immunity, in: *Immunopharmacology* (M. E. Rosenthale and H. C. Mansmann, eds.), pp. 73–77, Spectrum, New York.

Greene, W. C., and Robb, R. J., 1985, Receptors for T cell growth factor: Structure, function, and expression on normal and neoplastic cells, *Contemp. Top. Mol. Immunol.* **10:**1.

Griffin, M., Weiss, J. W., Leitch, A. G., McFadden, E. R., Jr., Corey, E. J., Austen, K. F., and Drazen, J. M., 1983, Effects of leukotriene D on the airways in asthma, *N. Engl. J. Med.* **308**: 346.

Gualde, N., Rabinovitch, H., Fredon, M., and Rigaud, M., 1982a, Effects of 15-hydroperoxy-eicosatetraenoic acid on human lymphocyte sheep erythrocyte rosette formation and response to Concanavalin A associated with HLA system, *Eur. J. Immunol.* **12**:773.

Gualde, N., Rigaud, M., and Bach, J.-F., 1982b, Stimulation of prostaglandin synthesis by the serum factor (FTS), *Cell. Immunol.* **70**:362.

Gualde, N., Atluru, D., and Goodwin, J. S., 1985, Effect of lipoxygenase metabolites of arachidonic-acid on proliferation of human T cell subsets, *J. Immunol.* **134**:1125.

Guy-Grand, D., Griscelli, C., and Vassalli, P., 1978, Mouse gut T-lymphocyte: Novel type of T-cell—nature, origin, and traffic in mice in normal and graft versus host conditions, *J. Exp. Med.* **148**:1661.

Habicht, G. S., and Beck, G., 1985, Inflammation and interleukin-1, *J. Leukocyte Biol.* **36**:709.

Hadden, J. W., and Stewart, W. E., 1981, *The Lymphokines: Biochemistry and Biological Activity*, Humana Press, Clifton, New Jersey.

Hadden, J. W., and Szentivanyi, A. (eds.), 1985, *The Pharmacology of the Reticuloendothelial System*, Plenum, New York.

Hadden, J. W., Chedid, L., Dukor, P., Spreafico, F., and Willoughby, D. (eds.), 1983, *Advances in Immunopharmacology*, Vol. 2, Pergamon, Oxford.

Haegeman, G., Content, J., Volckaert, G., Derynck, R., Tavernier, J., and Fiers, W., 1986, Structural analysis of the sequence coding for an inducible 26-kDa protein in human fibroblasts, *Eur. J. Biochem.* **159**:625.

Hafstrom, I., Palmblad, J., Malmsten, C. L., Radmark, O., and Samuelsson, B., 1981, Leukotriene B4—a stereospecific stimulator for release of lysosomal enzymes from neutrophils, *FEBS Lett.* **130**:146.

Hagermark, O., Hokfelt, T., and Pernow, B., 1978, Flare and itch induced by substance P in human skin, *J. Invest. Dermatol.* **71**:233.

Haig, D. M., McKee, T. A., Jarrett, E. E. R., Woodbury, R., and Miller, H. R. P., 1982, Generation of mucosal mast cells is stimulated in vitro by factors derived from T cells of helminth-infected rats, *Nature (Lond.)* **300**:188.

Hall, N. R., McGillis, J. P., Spangelo, B. L., and Goldstein, A. L., 1985a, Evidence that thymosins and other biologic response modifiers can function as neuroactive immunotransmitters, *J. Immunol.* **135**:806s.

Hall, N. R., McGillis, J. P., Spangelo, B. L., and Goldstein, A. L., 1985b, Thymosin peptides: Modulation of host defense by neuroendocrine circuits, in: *Contributions of Modern Biology to Medicine* (G. Bertazzoni, F. J. Bollum, and M. Ghione, eds.), Serono Symposia, Vol. 17, pp. 57–69, Raven, New York.

Hamberg, M., Svensson, J., and Samuelsson, B., 1975, Thromboxane: A new group of biologically active compounds derived from prostaglandin endoperoxides, *Proc. Natl. Acad. Sci. U.S.A.* **72**: 2994.

Hanahan, D. J., 1986, Platelet-activating factor: A biologically active phosphoglyceride, *Annu. Rev. Biochem.* **55**:483.

Handley, D. A., and Saunders, R. N., 1986, Platelet activating factor and inflammation in atherosclerosis: Targets for drug development, *Drug Dev. Res.* **7**:361.

Handley, D. A., Arbeeny, C. M., Lee, M. L., Van Valen, R. G., Saunders, R. N., 1984, Effect of platelet-activating factor on endothelial permeability to plasma macromolecules, *Immunopharmacology* **8**:137.

Handley, D. A., Farley, C., Deacon, R. W., and Saunders, R. N., 1986a, Evidence for distinct systemic extravasation effects of platelet activating factor, leukotrienes B_4, D_4, D_4 and histamine in the guinea pig, *Prostaglandins Leukotrienes Med.* **21**:269.

Handley, D. A., Van Valen, R. G., Melden, M. K., Flury, S., Lee, M. L., and Saunders, R. N., 1986b, Inhibition and reversal of endotoxin-, aggregated IgG- and PAF-induced hypotension in the rat by SRI 63-072, a PAF receptor antagonist, *Immunopharmacology* **12**:11.

Hanna, C. J., Bach, M. K., Pare, P. D., and Schellenberg, R. R., 1981, Slow-reacting substances (leukotrienes) contract human airway and pulmonary vascular smooth muscle in vitro, *Nature (Lond.)* **290**:343.

Hannappel, E., Xu, C.-J., Morgan, J., Hempstead, J., and Horecker, B. L., 1981, Thymosin beta 4: A ubiquitous peptide in rat and mouse tissues, *Proc. Natl. Acad. Sci. U.S.A.* **79**:2172.

Hannappel, E., Davoust, S., and Horecker, B. L., 1982, Thymosin beta-8 and thymosin beta-9— two new peptides isolated from calf thymus homologous to thymosin beta-4, *Proc. Natl. Acad. Sci. U.S.A.* **79**:1708.

Harada, N., Kikuchi, Y., Tominaga, A., Takaki, S., and Takatsu, K., 1985, BCGFII activity on activated B cells of a purified murine T cell-replacing factor (TRF) from a T cell hybridoma (B151K12), *J. Immunol.* **134**:3944.

Hardy, C. C., Robinson, C., Tattersfield, A. E., Holgate, S. T., 1984, The bronchoconstrictor effect of inhaled prostaglandin D_2 in normal and asthmatic men, *N. Engl. J. Med.* **311**:209.

Harel-Bellan, A., Joskowicz, M., Fradelizi, D., and Eisen, H., 1983, Modification of T-cell proliferation and interleukin 2 production in mice infected with *Trypanosoma cruzi*, *Proc. Natl. Acad. Sci. U.S.A.* **80**:3466.

Harriman, G. R., and Strober, W., 1987, Interleukin 5, a mucosal lymphokine, *J. Immunol.* **139**:3553.

Hartung, H. P., and Toyka, K. V., 1983, Activation of macrophages by substance P. Induction of oxidative burst and thromboxane release, *Eur. J. Pharmacol.* **89**:301.

Hartung, H. P., Suermann, D. B., and Hadding, U., 1983, Induction of thromboxane release from macrophages by anaphylatoxic peptide C3a of complement and synthetic hexapeptide C3a 72–77, *J. Immunol.* **130**:1345.

Haynes, B. F., Scearce, R. M., and Hensley, L. L., 1983, Production of monoclonal antibodies that selectively define neuroendocrine, nonneuroendocrine and Hassall body components of human thymic epithelium, *Clin. Res.* **31**(2):A346.

Healy, D. L., Hodgen, G. D., Schultz, H. M., Chrousos, G. P., Loriaux, D. L., Hall, N. R., and Goldstein, A. L., 1983, The thymus–adrenal connection: Thymosin has corticotropin-releasing activity in primates, *Science* **222**:1353.

Heijnen, C. J., Croiset, G., Zijlstra, J., and Ballieux, R. E., 1987, Modulation of lymphocyte function by endorphins, in: *Neuroimmune Interactions* (B. D. Jankovic, B. M. Markovic, and N. H. Spector, eds.), *Ann. N.Y. Acad. Sci.* **496**:161.

Hellewell, P. G., and Williams, T. J., 1986, A specific antagonist of platelet-activating factor suppresses oedema formation in an Arthus reaction but not oedema induced by leukocyte chemoattractants in rabbit skin, *J. Immunol.* **137**:302.

Henderson, W. R., 1985, Formation and oxidative degradation of leukotrienes by eosinophils and neutrophils, in: *Drugs Affecting Leukotrienes and Other Eicosanoid Pathways*, (B. Samuelsson, F. Berti, G. C. Folco, and G. P. Velo, eds.), pp. 339–350, Plenum, New York.

Henderson, W. R., 1987, Lipid-derived and other chemical mediators of inflammation in the lung, *J. Allergy Clin. Immunol.* **79**:543.

Henderson, W. R., and Kaliner, M., 1978, Immunologic and nonimmunological generation of superoxide from mast cells and basophils, *J. Clin. Invest.* **61**:187.

Henderson, W. R., and Kaliner, M., 1979, Mast cell granule peroxidase: Location, secretion, and SRS-A inactivation, *J. Immunol.* **122**:1322.

Henderson, W. R., and Klebanoff, S. J., 1983, Leukotriene production and inactivation by normal, chronic granulomatous disease and myeloperoxidase-deficient neutrophils, *J. Biol. Chem.* **258**:13522.

Henderson, W. R., Harley, J. B., and Fauci, A. S., 1984, Arachidonic acid metabolism in normal and hypereosinophilic syndrome eosinophils: Generation of leukotrienes B_4, C_4, D_4, and 15-lipoxygenase products, *Immunology* **51**:679.

Henderson, W. R., Chi, E. Y., Jong, E. C., and Klebanoff, S. J., 1986, Mast cell-mediated toxicity to schistosomula of *Schistosoma mansoni:* Potentiation by exogeneous peroxidase, *J. Immunol.* **137**:2695.

Henney, C. S., and Gillis, S., 1984, Cell mediated cytotoxicity, in: *Fundamental Immunology* (W. Paul, ed.), Raven, New York.

Henson, P. M., 1970, Release of vasoactive amines from rabbit platelets induced by sensitized mononuclear leukocytes and antigen, *J. Exp. Med.* **131**:287.

Henson, P. M., 1971, The immunologic release of constituents from neutrophil leukocytes. I. The role of antibody and complement on nonphagocytosable surfaces or phagocytosable particle, *J. Immunol.* **107**:1525.

Henson, P. M., 1985, Platelet-activating factor, in: *Textbook of Pharmacology* (M. M. Dale and J. C. Foreman, eds.), pp. 187–195, Blackwell Scientific Publications, Oxford.

Herberman, R. B., 1981, Significance of natural killer (NK) cells in cancer research, *Hum. Lymphocyte Diff.* **1**:63.

Hermann, S., Takai, Y., Clark, S., Wong, G., Stringfellow, M., and Burakoff, S., 1988, IL-6 (BSF-2) is a cytotoxic differentiation factor, *FASEB J.* **2**:A877 (abst. 3379).

Hierowski, M. T., Liebow, C., DuSapin, K., and Schally, A. V., 1985, Stimulation by somatostatin of dephosphorylation of membrane proteins in pancreatic cancer MIA PACA-2 cell line, *FEBS Lett.* **179**:252.

Hiestand, P. C., Mekler, P., Nordmann, R., Grieder, A., and Perminongkok, C., 1986, Prolactin as a modulator of lymphocyte responsiveness provides a possible mechanism of action for cyclosporin, *Proc. Natl. Acad. Sci. U.S.A.* **83**:2599.

Higgs, G. A., Salmon, J. A., and Spayne, J. A., 1981, The inflammatory effects of hydroperoxy and hydroxy acid products of arachidonate lipoxygenase in rabbit skin, *Br. J. Pharmacol.* **74**:429.

Hinterberger, W., Cerny, C., Kinast, H., Pointner, H., and Tragl, K. H., 1978, Somatostatin reduces the release of colony-stimulating activity (CSA) from PHA-activated mouse spleen lymphocytes, *Experientia* **34**:860.

Hirano, T., Taga, T., Yasukawa, K., Nakajima, K., Nakano, N., Takatsuki, F., Shimizu, M., Murashima, A., Tsunasawki, S., and Sakiyama, F., 1987, Human B-cell differentiation factor defined by an antipeptide antibody and its possible role in autoantibody production, *Proc. Natl. Acad. Sci. U.S.A.* **84**:228.

Hirokawa, K., McClure, J., and Goldstein, A. L., 1982, Age-related changes in localization of thymosin in the human thymus, *Thymus* **4**:19.

Hitzig, W. H., 1980, Transfer factor: Characterization and clinical application—a critical review, in: *The Immune System: Functions and Therapy of Dysfunction Proceedings of the Symposia,* Vol. 27, pp. 227–240, Academic, Orlando, Florida.

Hojima, Y., Cochrane, C. G., Wiggins, R. C., Austen, K. F., and Stevens, R. L., 1984, In vitro activation of the contact (Hageman Factor) system of plasma by heparin and chondroitin sulfate E, *Blood* **63**:1453.

Hokfelt, T., Melander, T., Staines, W., Wiesenfeld-Hallin, S., Hulting, A.-L., Werner, S., Eneroth, P., Lindgren, J.-A., Samuelsson, B., Patrono, C., Kokaeus, A., Fahrenkrug, J., Joseph, S. A., and Fischer, J. A., 1986, Neuropeptides and their possible role as auxiliary messengers, in: *Neuroregulation of Autonomic, Endocrine and Immune Systems* (R. C. A. Frederickson, H. C. Hendrie, J. N. Hingtgen and M. H. Aprison, eds.), pp. 61–87, Kluwer Academic, Hingham, MA.

Holden, H. T., and Herberman, R. B., 1985, Modulation of immunity by macrophages, *Pharmacol. Ther.* Suppl. No. 15.

Holgate, S. T., Burns, G. B., Robinson, C., and Church, M. K., 1984, Anaphylactic- and calcium-dependent generation of prostaglandin D_2 (PGD_2) thromboxane B_2, and other cyclooxygenase products of arachidonic acid by dispersed human lung cells and relationship to histamine, *J. Immunol.* **133**:2138.

Holtzman, M. J., Aizawa, H., Nadel, J. A., and Goetzl, E. J., 1983, Selective generation of leukotriene B$_4$ by tracheal epithelial cells from dogs, *Biochem. Biophys. Res. Commun.* **114**:1071.

Hooper, J. A., McDaniel, M., Thurman, G. B., Cohen, G. H., Schulof, R. S., and Goldstein, A. L., 1975, Purification and properties of bovine thymoxin, *Ann. N.Y. Acad. Sci.* **249**:125.

Howard, M., 1985, Soluble factor induction of B-cell growth, *Contemp. Top. Mol. Immunol.* **10**:181.

Howard, M., Farrar, J., Hilfiker, M., Johnson, B., Takatsu, K., Hamaoka, K., and Paul, W. E., 1982, Identification of a T-cell-derived B-cell growth factor distinct from interleukin-2, *J. Exp. Med.* **155**:914.

Howard, M., Matis, L., Malek, T. R., Shevach, E., Kell, W., Cohen, D., Nakanishi, K., and Paul, W. E., 1983, Interleukin 2 induces antigen-reactive T-cell lines to secrete BCGF-1, *J. Exp. Med.* **158**:2024.

Howard, M., Nakanishi, K., and Paul, W. E., 1984, B-cell growth and differentiation factors, *Immunol. Rev.* **78**:185.

Hsueh, W., and Sun, F. F., 1982, Leukotriene B4 biosynthesis by alveolar macrophages, *Biochem. Biophys. Res. Commun.* **106**:1085.

Hu, S. K., Low, T. L. K., and Goldstein, A. L., 1981, Modulation of terminal deoxynucleotidyl transferase activity by thymosin, *Mol. Cell. Biochem.* **41**:49.

Hugli, T. E., 1975, Human anaphylatoxin (C3a) from the third component of complement. Primary structure, *J. Biol. Chem.* **250**:8293.

Humphrey, D. M., McManus, L. M., Hanahan, D. J., and Pinckard, R. N., 1984, Morphological basis of increased vascular permeability induced by acetyl glyceryl ether phosphorylcholine, *Lab. Invest.* **50**:16.

Hwang, S. B., Lee, C.-S. C., Cheah, M. J., and Shen, T. Y., 1983, Specific receptor sites for 1-*O*-alkyl-2-*O*-acetyl-*sn*-glycero-3-phosphocholine (platelet activating factor) on rabbit platelet and guinea pig smooth muscle membranes, *Biochemistry* **22**:4756.

Hwang, S. B., Li, C.-H., Lam, M. H., and Shen, T. Y., 1985, Characterization of cutaneous vascular permeability induced by platelet-activating factor in guinea pigs and rats and its inhibition by a platelet-activating factor receptor antagonist, *Lab. Invest.* **52**:617.

Ihle, J., 1985, Biochemical and biological properties of interleukin-3: A lymphokine mediating the differentiation of a lineage of cells that includes prothymocites and mast-like cells, *Contemp. Top. Mol. Immunol.* **10**:93.

Ihle, J. N., Pepersack, L., and Rebar, L., 1981, Regulation of T-cell differentiation—In vitro induction of 20-alpha-hydroxysteroid dehydrogenase in splenic lymphocytes from athymic mice by a unique lymphokine, *J. Immunol.* **126**:2184.

Ihle, J. N., Lee, J. C., and Hapel, A. J., 1982a, Interleukin 3: Biochemical and biological properties and possible role in the regulation of immune responses, in: *Lymphokines* (S. B. Mizel, ed.), Vol. 6, Academic, Orlando, Florida.

Ihle, J. N., Keller, J., Henderson, L., Klein, F., and Palaszynski, E. W., 1982b, Procedures for the purification of interleukin 3 to homogeneity, *J. Immunol.* **129**:2431.

Ihle, J. N., Rebar, L., Keller, J., Lee, J. C., and Hapel, A., 1982c, Interleukin 3—Possible roles in the regulation of lymphocyte differentiation and growth, *Immunol. Rev.* **63**:5.

Imagawa, D. K., Osifehin, N. E., Paznekas, W. A., Shin, M. L., and Mayer, M. M., 1983, Consequences of cell membrane attack by complement: Release of arachidonate and formation of inflammatory derivatives, *Proc. Natl. Acad. Sci. U.S.A.* **80**:6647.

Imagawa, D. K., Osifehin, N. E., Ramm, L. E., Koga, P. G., Hammer, C. H., Shin, H. S., and Mayer, M. M., 1986, Release of arachidonic acid and formation of oxygenated derivatives after complement attack on macrophages: Role of channel formation, *J. Immunol.* **136**:4637.

Inaba, K., Granelli Piperno, A., and Steinman, R. M., 1983, Dendritic cells induce lymphocytes to release B-cell stimulating factors by an IL-2 dependent mechanism, *J. Exp. Med.* **158**:2040.

Inarrea, P., Alonso, F., and Sanchez-Crespo, M., 1983, Platelet-activating factor: An effector substance of the vasopermeability changes induced by the infusion of immuno aggregates in the mouse, *Immunopharmacology* 6:7.

Inarrea, P., Gomez-Cambronero, J., Pascual, J., del Carmen-Ponte, M., Hernando, L., and Sanchez-Crespo, M., 1985, Synthesis of PAF acether and blood volume changes in gram negative sepsis, *Immunopharmacology* 9:45.

Incefy, G. S., 1983, Effect of thymic hormones on human lymphocytes, *Clin. Immunol. Allergy* 3: 95.

Irani, A. A., Craig, S. S., DeBlois, G., Hutchinson, L., Sismanis, A., Schechter, N. M., 1986, Distribution of mast cell subsets in human tissues, *Clin. Res.* 34:277A.

Irani, A. A., Schechter, N. M., Craig, S., DeBlois, G., and Schwartz, L. B., 1986, Two human mast cell subsets with different neutral protease compositions, *Proc. Natl. Acad. Sci. U.S.A.* 83:4464.

Irani, A. A., Schechter, N. M., and Schwartz, L. B., 1987, Deficiency of the tryptase-positive, chymase-negative mast cell type in gastrointestinal mucosa of patients with defective T lymphocyte function, *J. Immunol.* 138:4381.

Ito, S., Camussi, G., Tetta, C., Milgrom, F., and Andres, G., 1984, Hyperacute renal allograft rejection in the rabbit, *Lab. Invest.* 51:148.

Ivell, R., and Richter, D., 1984, The gene for the hypothalamic peptide hormone oxytocin is highly expressin in the bovine corpus luteum, *EMBO J.* 3:2351.

Izumi, F., Oka, M., and Kumakura, K., 1982, Synthesis, storage, and secretion of adrenal catecholamines, in: *Adv. Biosci.* 36.

Jakschik, B. A., and Lee, L. H., 1980, Enzymatic assembly of slow reacting substance, *Nature (Lond.)* 287:51.

Jambon, B., Montagne, P., Bene, M. C., Brayer, M. P., Faure, G., and Duheille, J., 1981, Immunohistologic localization of "factueur thymique serique" (FTS) in human thymic epithelium, *J. Immunol.* 127:2055.

Janeway, C., Jr., Bottomly, K., Horowitz, J., Kaye, J., Jones, B., and Tite, J., 1985, Modes of cell : cell communication in the immune system, *J. Immunol.* 135:739s.

Jankovic, B. D., and Maric D., 1987, Enkephalins and immunity, in: *Neuroimmune Interactions* (B. D. Jakovic, B. M. Markovic, and N. H. Spector, eds.), *Ann. N.Y. Acad. Sci.* 496:115.

Jessel, T. M., 1985, Cellular interactions at the central and peripheral terminals of primary sensory neurons, *J. Immunol.* 135:746s.

Jessel, T. M., and Womack, M. D., 1985, Substance P and the novel mammalian tachykinins: A diversity of receptors and cellular actions, *Trends Neurosci.* 8:43.

Jobim, F., 1978, Acetylsalicylic acid, hemostasis and human thromboembolism, *Semin. Thromb. Hemost.* 4:199.

Jobling, S. A., Auron, P. E., Webb, A. C., McDonald, B., Rosenwasser, L. J., and Gehrke, L., 1987, Biological activity of human prointerleukin 1 beta and subpeptides defined by enhanced in vitro translation of SP6 transcripts, *Lymphokine Res.* 6:1105 (abst.).

Johansson, O., Hokfelt, T., and Elde, R. P., 1984, Immunohistochemical distribution of somatostatin-like immunoreactivity in the central nervous system of the adult rat, *Neuroscience* 13:265.

Johnson, H. M., and Farrar, W. L., 1983, The role of a gamma interferon-like lymphokine in the activation of T cells for expression of interleukin 2 receptors, *Cell. Immunol.* 75:154.

Johnson, H. M., and Torres, B. A., 1983, Recombinant mouse gamma interferon regulation of antibody production, *Infect. Immun.* 41:546.

Johnson, H. M., and Torres, B. A., 1984, Leukotrienes—positive signals for regulation of gamma interferon production, *J. Immunol.* 132:413.

Johnson, H. M., and Torres, B. A., 1985, Regulation of lymphokine production by arginine vasopressin and oxytocin: Modulation of lymphocyte function by neurohypophyseal hormones, *J. Immunol.* 135:773s.

Jorg, A., Henderson, W. R., Murphy, R. C., and Klebanoff, S. J., 1982, Leukotriene generation by eosinophils, *J. Exp. Med.* **155**:390.

Jurado, A., Severson, E., and Heusser, C., 1987, TCGH-like activity of interleukin-4 on CTC/L is inhibited by anti-IL-2 and IL-2 receptor antibodies, *Lymphokine Res.* **6**:1822 (abst.).

Kadish, A. S., Doyle, A. T., Steinhauser, E. H., and Ghossein, N. A., 1981, Natural cytotoxicity and interferon production in human cancer: Deficient natural killer activity and normal interferon production in patients with advanced disease, *J. Immunol.* **127**:1817.

Khan, A., and Hill, N. O. (eds.), 1982, *Human Lymphokines*, Academic, Orlando, Florida.

Kaliner, M., Orange, R. P., and Austen, K. F., 1972, Immunological release of histamine and slow reacting substance of anaphylaxis from human lung. IV. Enhancement of cholinergic and alpha adrenergic stimulation, *J. Exp. Med.* **136**:556.

Kalland, T., 1987, Regulation of natural killer cell precursors by interleukin 3, *Lymphokine Res.* **6**: 1701.

Kamitani, T., Katamoto, M., Tatsumi, M., Katsuta, K., Ono, T., Kikuchi, H., and Kumada, S., 1984, Mechanism(s) of the hypotensive effect of synthetic 1-*O*-octadecyl-2-*O*-acetyl-glycero-3-phosphorylcholine, *Eur. J. Pharmacol.* **93**:357.

Kampschmidt, R. F., 1984, The numerous postulated biological manifestations of interleukin-1, *J. Leukocyte Biol.* **36**:341.

Kampschmidt, R. F., Pulliam, L. A., and Upchurch, H. F., 1980, The activity of partially purified leukocytic endogenous mediators in endotoxin-resistant C3H/H3J mice, *J. Lab. Clin. Med.* **95**: 616.

Kandel, E. R., and Schwartz, J. H., 1985, *Principles of Neural Science*, 2nd ed. Elsevier, New York.

Karsh, J., 1983, The role of immune complexes in the pathogenesis of rheumatoid arthritis and the genesis of its complications, in: *Circulating Immune Complexes. Their Clinical Sigificance*, (L. R. Espinoza, and C. K. Osterland, eds.), pp. 87–104, Futura, Mt. Kisco, New York.

Kasahara, T., Hooks, J. J., Dougherty, S. F., and Oppenheim, J. J., 1983, Interleukin 2 mediated immune interferon (IFN gamma) production by human T-cells and T-cell subsets, *J. Immunol.* **130**:1784.

Kastin, A. J., Galina, Z. H., Horvath, A., and Olson, R. D., 1987, Some principles in the peptide field, *J. Allergy Clin. Immunol.* **79**:6.

Kasuya, Y., Masuda, Y., and Shigenobu, K., 1984, Possible role of endothelium in the vasodilator response of rat thoracic aorta to platelet-activating factor (PAF), *J. Pharmacol. Dyn.* **7**:138.

Kato, K., Ikeyama, S., Takaoki, M., Shino, A., Takeuchi, M., and Kakinuma, A., 1981, Epithelial cell components immunoreact with antiserum thymic factor antibodies: Possible association with intermediate sized filaments, *Cell* **24**:885.

Kakiuchi, J. S., Yasuda, J. S., Yamazaki, R., Teshima, Y., Kanda, K., Kakiuchi, R., and Sobue, K., 1982, Quantitative determinations of calmodulin in the supernatant and particulate fractions of mammalian tissues, *J. Biochem.* **92**:1041.

Katz, H. R., Stevens, R. L., and Austen, K. F., 1985, Heterogeneity of mammalian mast cells differentiated in vivo and in vitro, *J. Allergy Clin. Immunol.* **76**:250.

Kawanishi, H., Saltzman, L., and Strober, W., 1983a, Mechanisms regulating IgA class-specific immunoglobulin production in murine gut-associated lymphoid tissues. I. T cells derived from Peyer's patches that switch sIgM B cells to sIgA B cells in vitro, *J. Exp. Med.* **157**:437.

Kawanishi, H., Saltzman, L., and Strober, W., 1983b, Mechanisms regulating IgA class-specific immunoglobulin production in murine gut-associated lymphoid tissues. II. Terminal differentiation of post-switch sIgA-bearing Peyer's patch B cells, *J. Exp. Med.* **158**:649.

Kehrl, J. H., Muraguchi, A., Butler, J. L., Calkoff, R. J. M., and Fauci, A. S., 1984, Human B cell activation, proliferation, and differentiation, *Immunol. Rev.* **78**:75.

Kellaway, C. V. H., and Trethewie, E. R., 1940, Liberation of a slow reacting smooth muscle stimulating substance in anaphylaxis, *Q. J. Exp. Physiol.* **30**:121.

Kendall, M. D., 1983, The cells of thymus, in: *The Thymus Gland* (M. D. Kendall, ed.), pp. 63–84, Academic, Orlando, Florida.

Kimball, E. S., Pickeral, S. F., Oppenheim, J. J., and Rossio, J. L., 1984, Interleukin 1 activity in normal human urine, *J. Immunol.* **133:**256.

Kinashi, T., Harada, N., Severinson, E., Tanabe, T., Sideras, P., Konishi, M., Azuma, C., Tominaga, A., Bergstedt-Lindqvist, S., Takahashi, M., Matsuda, F., Yaoita, Y., Takatsu, K., and Honjo, T., 1986, Cloning of complementary DNA encoding T-cell replacing factor and identity with B-cell growth factor II, *Nature (Lond.)* **324:**70.

Kirkpatrick, C. H., and Burger, D. R., 1981, Transfer factor. Progress toward isolation and chemical characterization, in: *The Lymphokines. Biochemistry and Biological Activity* (J. W. Hadden and W. E. Stewart II, eds.), pp. 261–274, Humana Press, Clifton, New Jersey.

Kirkpatrick, C. H., Lawrence, H. S., and Burger, D. R. (eds.), 1983, *Fourth International Transfer Factor Workshop*, Academic, Orlando, Florida.

Kishimoto, T., Yoshizaki, K., Kimoto, M., Okada, M., Kuritani, T., Kikutani, H., Shimizu, K., Nakagawa, T., Nakagawa, N., Miki, Y., Kishi, H., Fukanaga, K., Yoshikubo, T., and Taga, T., 1984, B-cell growth and differentiation factors and mechanism of B-cell activation, *Immunol. Rev.* **78:**97.

Klebanoff, S. J., Jong, E. C., and Henderson, W. R., 1980, The eosinophil peroxidase: Purification and biological propertiess, in: *The Eosinophil in Health and Disease* (A. F. F. Mahmoud and K. F. Austen, eds.), pp. 99–106, Grune & Stratton, Orlando, Florida.

Klein, T., Szentivanyi, A., and Fishel, C. W., 1974, Effects of serotonin on platelets of normal and *B. pertussis*-injected mice, *Proc. Soc. Exp. Biol. Med.* **147:**681.

Klickstein, L. B., Shapleigh, C., and Goetzl, E. J., 1980, Lipoxygenation of arachidonic acid as a source of polymorphonuclear leukocyte chemotactic factors in synovial fluid and tissue in rheumatoid arthritis and spondyloarthritis, *J. Clin. Invest.* **66:**1166.

Klonoff, D. C., and Karam, J. H., 1987, Hypothalamic and pituitary hormones. in: *Basic and Clinical Pharmacology* (B. G. Katzung, ed.), pp. 423–435, Appleton & Lange, E. Norwalk, Connecticut.

Klostergaard, J., Orr, S. L., and Granger, G. A., 1982, Purification of the alpha-heavy class of human lymphotoxin to electrophoretic homogeneity, in: *Human Lymphokines* (A. Kahn and N. O. Hill, eds.), pp. 199–208, Academic, Orlando, Florida.

Kluger, M. J., Oppenheim, J. J., and Powanda, M. C. (eds.), 1985, *The Physiologic, Metabolic, and Immunologic Actions of Interleukin-1*, Vol. 2, Alan R. Liss, New York.

Kohase, M., Henriksen-DeStefano, D., May, L. T., Vilcek, J., and Sehgal, B. P., 1986, Induction of beta$_2$-interferon by tumor necrosis factor: A homeostatic mechanism in the control of cell proliferation, *Cell* **45:**659.

Kohsaka, M., Shohmori, T., Tsukada, Y., and Woodruff, G. N., 1982, *Advances in Dopamine Research, Advances in the Biosciences*, Vol. 37, Pergamon, New York.

Koob, G. F., Dantzer, R., Rodriguez, F., Bloom, F. E., and LeMoal, M., 1985, Osmotic stress mimics the effects of vasopressin on learned behavior, *Nature (Lond.)* **315:**750.

Kook, A. I., and Trainin, N., 1974, Hormone-like activity of a thymus humoral factor on the induction of immune competence in lymphoid cells, *J. Exp. Med.* **139:**193.

Kornecki, E., Ehrlich, Y., H., and Lenox, R. H., 1984, Platelet-activating factor induced aggregation of human platelets specifically inhibited by triazolobenzodiazepines, *Science* **226:**1454.

Krane, S. M., 1981, Aspects of cell biology of the rheumatoid synovial lesion, *Ann. Rheum. Dis.* **40:**433.

Kunkel, H. G., 1983, The immunopathology of SLE, in: *The Biology of Immunologic Disease* (F. J. Dixon and D. W. Fisher, eds.), pp. 247–256, Sinauer, Sunderland, Massachusetts.

Kupfermann, I., 1981a, Hypothalamus and limbic system. I. Peptidergic neurons, homeostasis, and emotional behavior, in: *Principles of Neural Science* (E. R. Kandel and J. H. Schwartz, eds.), pp. 443–449, Elsevier/North-Holland, New York.

Kupfermann, I., 1981b, Hypothalamus and limbic system. II. Motivation, in: *Principles of Neural*

Science (E. R. Kandel and J. H. Schwartz, eds.), pp. 450–460, Elsevier/North-Holland, New York.

Lagunoff, D., and Rickard, A., 1983, Evidence for control of mast cell granule protease in situ by low pH, *Exp. Cell Res.* **144**:353.

Land, H., Grez, S., Ruppert, S., Schmale, H., Rehbein, H., Richter, D., and Schutz, G., 1983, Deduced amino acid sequence from the bovine oxytocin–neurophysin I precursor cDNA, *Nature (Lond.)* **302**:342.

Lanham, J. G., Elkon, K. B., Pusey, C. D., and Hughes, G. R., 1984, Systemic vasculitis with asthma and eosinophilia—a clinical approach to the Churg–Strauss syndrome, *Medicine (Baltimore)* **63**(2):65.

Laroche, L., and Bach, J.-F., 1985, Thymus and regulatory factors, in: *Dermatologic Immunology and Allergy* (J. Stone, ed.), pp. 15–25, C. V. Mosby, St. Louis.

Larsen, G. L., and Henson, P. M., 1983, Mediators of inflammation, *Annu. Rev. Immunol.* **1**:335.

Lawrence, H. S., and Borkowsky, W., 1981, Tranfer factor: Recent developments in the pursuit of an idea, *Cell. Immunol.* **62**:301.

Le, P. T., Tuck, D. T., Dinarello, C. A., Haynes, B. F., and Singer, K. H., 1987, Human thymic epithelial cells produce interleukin 1, *J. Immunol.* **138**:2520.

Lee, C. W., Lewis, R. A., Tauber, A. I., Methrotra, M., Corey, E. J., and Austen, K. F., 1983, The myeloperoxidase-dependent metabolism of leukotrienes C4, D4, and E4, to 6-trans-leukotriene B4 diastereoisomers and the subclass specific S-diastereoisomeric sulfoxides, *J. Biol. Chem.* **258**:15004.

Lee, F., Yokota, T., Otsuka, T., Meyerson, P., Villaret, D., Coffman, R., Mosmann, T., Rennick, D., Roehn, N., Smith, C., Zlotnik, A., and Arai, K.-I., 1986, Isolation and characterization of a mouse interleukin cDNA clone that expresses B-cell stimulatory factor 1 activities and T-cell and mast-cell stimulating activities, *Proc. Natl. Acad. Sci. U.S.A.* **83**:2061.

Lee, T. C., Lenihan, D. J., Malone, B., Roddy, L. L., and Wasserman, S. I., 1984, Increased biosynthesis of platelet-activating factor in activated human eosinophils, *J. Biol. Chem.* **259**:5526.

Lefer, D. J., and Lefer, A. M., 1986, Failure of endothelium to mediate potential vasoactive action of platelet activating factor (PAF), *Int. Res. Commun. Syst. Med. Sci.* **14**:356.

Lellouch-Tubiana, A., Lefort, J., Pirotzky, E., Vargiftig, B. B., and Pfister, A., 1985, Ultrastructural evidence for extravascular platelet recruitment in the lung upon intravenous injection of platelet-activating factor (PAF-acether) to guinea pigs, *Br. J. Exp. Pathol.* **66**:345.

Lengyel, P., 1982, Biochemistry of interferons and with actions, *Annu. Rev. Biochem.* **51**:251.

Lett-Brown, M. A., Boetcher, D. A., and Leonard, E. J., 1976, Chemotactic response to normal human basophils to C5a and to lymphocyte derived chemotactic factor, *J. Immunol.* **117**:246.

Levy, B., 1966, The adrenergic blocking activity of *N*-terbutylmethoxamine (butoxamine), *J. Pharmacol. Exp. Ther.* **151**:413.

Levy, J. V., and Ezzet, K., 1987, Schild plot analysis of six putative antagonists of platelet activating factor (PAF) on human platelets, *Pharmacologist* **29**:219.

Lewis, G. P., (ed.), 1955, *5-Hydroxytryptamine*, Pergamon, New York.

Lewis, R. A., and Austen, K. F., 1984, The biologically active leukotrienes, biosynthesis, metabolism, receptors, functions and pharmacology, *J. Clin. Invest.* **73**:889.

Lewis, R. A., Drazen, J. M., Austen, K. F., Toda, M., Brion, F., Marfat, A., and Corey, E. J., 1981, Contractile activities of structural analogs of leukotriene C and leukotriene D—Role of the polar substituents, *Proc. Natl. Acad. Sci. U.S.A.* **78**:4579.

Lewis, R. A., Soter, N. A., Diamond, P. T., Austen, K. F., Oates, J. A., Roberts, L. J., 1982, Prostaglandin D_2 generation after activation of rat and human mast cells with anti-IgE, *J. Immunol.* **129**:1627.

Lewis, T., 1927, *The Blood Vessels of the Human Skin and Their Response*, Shaw, London.

Liang, S. M., Allet, B., Rose, K., Hirschi, M., Liang, C. M., and Thatcher, D. R., 1985, Characterization of human interleukin 1 derived from *Escherichia coli*, *Biochem. J.* **229**:429.

Lichey, J., Friedrich, T., Franke, J., Nigam, S., Priesnitz, M., and Oeff, K., 1984, Pressure effects and uptake of platelet-activating factor in isolated rat lung, *J. Appl. Physiol.* **57**:1039.

Lin, A. H., Morton, D. R., and Gorman, R. R., 1982, Acetyl glyceryl ether phosphorylcholine stimulates leukotriene B_4 synthesis in human polymorphonuclear leukocytes, *J. Clin. Invest.* **70**:1058.

Lindstron, J., 1985, Techniques for studying the biochemistry and cell biology of receptors, in: *Neurotransmitter Receptor Binding*, 2nd ed., (H. I. Yamamura, S. J. Enna, and M. J. Kuhar, eds.), pp. 91–111, Raven, New York.

Linker-Israeli, M., Bakker, A. C., Kitridou, R. C., Gendler, S., Gillis, S., and Horwitz, D. A., 1983, Defective production of interleukin 1 and interleukin 2 in patients with systemic lupus erythromatosus (SLE), *J. Immunol.* **130**:2651.

Lipsky, P. E., 1985, Role of interleukin-1 in human B-cell activation, *Contemp. Top. Mol. Immunol.* **10**:195.

Liu, M. C., Proud, D., Lichtenstein, L. M., MacGlashan, D. W., Schleimer, R. P., Adkinson, N. F., Kagey-Sobotka, A., Schulman, E. S., and Plaut, M., 1986, Human lung macrophage-derived histamine releasing activity is due to an IgE-binding factor(s), *J. Immunol.* **136**:2588.

Locke, S., Ader, R., Besedovsky, H., Hall, N., Solomon, G., and Strom, T. (eds.), 1985, *Foundations of Psychoneuroimmunology*, Aldine, New York.

Lolait, S. J., Lim, A. T. W., Toh, B. H., and Funder, J. W., 1984, Immunoreactive beta-endorphin in a subpopulation of mouse spleen macrophages, *J. Clin. Invest.* **73**:277.

Lolait, S. J., Clements, J. A., Markwick, A. J., Cheng, C., McNally, M., Smith, A. I., and Funder, J. W., 1986, Proopiomelanocortin messenger ribonucleic acid and posttranslational processing of endorphin in spleen macrophages, *J. Clin. Invest.* **77**:1776.

Lomedico, P. T., Gubler, U., Hellmann, C. P., Dukovich, M., Giri, J. G., Pan, Y., Collier, K., Semionow, R., Chua, A. O., and Mizel, S. B., 1984, Cloning and expression of murine interleukin 1 cDNA in *Escherichia coli, Nature (Lond.)* **312**:458.

Loughnan, M. S., Takatsu, K., Harada, N., and Nossal, G. J. V., 1987, T-cell-replacing factor (interleukin 5) induces expression of interleukin 2 receptors on murine splenic B cells, *Proc. Natl. Acad. Sci. U.S.A.* **84**:5399.

Low, T. L. K., and Goldstein, A. L., 1979, The chemistry and biology of thymosin. II. Amino acid sequence analysis of thymosin alpha$_1$ and polypeptide beta$_1$, *J. Biol. Chem.* **254**:987.

Low, T. L. K., and Goldstein, A. L., 1982, The chemistry and biology of thymosin. III. Chemical characterization of thymosin beta-4, *J. Biol. Chem.* **257**:1000.

Low, T. L. K., Thurman, C. B., McAdoo, M., McClure, J., Rossio, J. L., Naylor, P. H., and Goldstein, A. L., 1979, The chemistry and biology of thymosin. I. Isolation, characterization and biological activities of thymosin alpha$_1$ and polypeptide beta$_1$ from calf thymus, *J. Biol. Chem.* **254**:981.

Lundberg, J. M., and Saria, A., 1982, Bronchial smooth muscle contraction induced by stimulation of capsaicin-sensitive vagal sensory neurons, *Acta Physiol. Scand.* **116**:473.

Lundberg, J. M., Hedlund, B., and Bartfai, T., 1982, Vasoactive intestinal polypeptide enhances muscarinic ligand binding in cat submandibular gland, *Nature (Lond.)* **295**:147.

Lundberg, J. M., Saria, A., Brodin, E., Rosell, S., and Folkara, K., 1983, A substance P antagonist inhibits vagally induced inflammation and bronchial smooth muscle contraction in the guinea pig, *Proc. Natl. Acad. Sci. U.S.A.* **80**:1120.

Lygren, I., Revhaug, A., Burhol, P. G., Giercksky, K. E., and Jenssen, T. G., 1984, Vasoactive intestinal peptide and somatostatin in leukocytes, *Scand. J. Clin. Lab. Invest.* **44**:347.

MacDonald, S. M., Lichtenstein, L. M., Proud, D., Plaut, M., Naclerio, R. M., MacGlashan, D. W., and Kagey-Sobotka, A., 1987, Studies of IgE-dependent histamine releasing factors: heterogeneity of IgE, *J. Immunol.* **139**:506.

MacGlashan, D. W., Jr., Peters, S. P., Warner, J., and Lichtenstein, L. M., 1986, Characteristics of human basophil sulfidopeptide leukotriene release: Releasability defined as the ability of basophils to respond to dimeric cross-links, *J. Immunol.* **136**:2231.

Mackaness, G. B., and Blanden, R. V., 1967, Cellular immunity, *Prog. Allergy* **11**:89.

Maclouf, J., Fruteau-de-Laclos, B., and Borgeat, P., 1982, Stimulation of leukotriene biosynthesis in human blood leukocytes by platelet-derived 12-hydroperoxyeicosatetraenoic acid, *Proc. Natl. Acad. Sci. U.S.A.* **79**:6042.

MacSween, J. M., 1987, Histamine as a mediator of MIF and migration stimulation factor (MStF) responses, *Lymphokine Res.* **6**:1441 (abst.).

Maeda, S., Nishino, N., Obaru, K., Mita, S., Nomiyama, H., Shimada, K., Fujimoto, K., Teranishi, T., Hirano, T., and Onoue, K., 1983, Cloning of interleukin 2 messenger RNAs from human tonsils, *Biochem. Biophys. Res. Commun.* **115**:1040.

Maier, M., Spragg, J., and Schwartz, L. B., 1983, Inactivation of human high molecular weight kininogen by human mast cell tryptase, *J. Immunol.* **130**:2352.

Malik, K. U., and Wong, P. Y., 1981, Leukotriene C4—The major lipoxygenase metabolite of arachidonic acid in dog spleen, *Biochem. Biophys. Res. Comun.* **103**:511.

Malone, B., Lee, T.-C., and Synder, F., 1985, Inactivation of platelet-activating factor by rabbit platelets: Lyso-platelet-activating factor as a key intermediate with phosphatidylcholine as the source of arachidonic acid in its conversion to a tetraenoic acylated product, *J. Biol. Chem.* **260**:1531.

Mandler, R. N., Biddison, W. E., Mandler, R., and Serrate, S. A., 1986, Beta-endorphin augments the cytolytic activity and interferon production of natural killer cells, *J. Immunol.* **136**:934.

Mannel, D., Falk, W., and Northoff, H., 1987, Thermoregulatory activity of tumor necrosis factor independent of macrophage IL-1 production, *Lymphokine Res.* **6**:1424.

Marasco, W. A., Showell, H. J., and Becker, E. L., 1981, Substance P binds to the formylpeptide chemotaxis receptor on the rabbit neutrophil, *Biochem. Biophys. Res. Commun.* **99**:1065.

Marceau, F., Lussier, A., Regoli, D., and Giroud, J. P., 1983, Pharmacology of kinins—their relevance to tissue injury and inflammation, *Gen. Pharmacol.* **14**:209.

March, C., Mosley, B., Larsen, A., Cerretti, D. P., Braedt, G., Price, V., Gillis, S., Henney, C. S., Kronheim, S. R., and Grabstein, K., 1985, Cloning, sequence and expression of two distinct human interleukin 1 complementary DNAs, *Nature (Lond.)* **315**:641.

Maric, D., and Janokovic, B. D., 1987, Enkephalins and immunity. II. In vivo modulation of cell-mediated immunity. in: *Neuroimmune Interactions* (B. D. Jankovic, B. M. Markovic, and N. H. Spector, eds.), *Ann. N.Y. Acad. Sci.* **496**:126.

Marom, Z., Shelhamer, J. H., and Kaliner, M., 1984a, Human pulmonary macrophage-derived mucus secretagogue, *J. Exp. Med.* **159**:844.

Marom, Z., Shelhamer, J. H., Steel, L., Goetzl, E. J., and Kaliner, M. A., 1984b, Prostaglandin-generating fctor of anaphylaxis induces mucous glycoprotein release and formation of lipoxygenase products of arachidonate from human airways, *Prostaglandins* **28**:79.

Marom, Z., Shelhamer, J. H., Berger, M., Frank, M., and Kaliner, M., 1985a, Anaphylatoxin C3a enhances mucuous glycoprotein release from human airways in vitro, *J. Exp. Med.* **161**:657.

Marom, Z., Shelhamer, J. H., and Kaliner, M., 1985b, Human monocyte-derived mucus secretagogue, *J. Clin. Invest.* **75**:191.

Marone, G., Sobotka, A. K., and Lichtenstein, L. M., 1979, Effects of arachidonic acid and its metabolites on antigen-induced histamine release from human basophils in vitro, *J. Immunol.* **123**:1669.

Marquardt, D. L., 1983, *Clin. Rev. Allergy* **1**:343.

Marquardt, D. L., Gruber, H. E., and Wasserman, S. I., 1984, Adenosine release from stimulated mast cells, *Proc. Natl. Acad. Sci. U.S.A.* **81**:6192.

Martin, T. R., Altman, L. C., Albert, R. K., and Henderson, W. R., 1984, Leukotriene B4 production by the human alveolar macrophage: A potential mechanism for amplifying inflammation in the lung, *Am. Rev. Respir. Dis.* **129**:106.

Martin, T. R., Merritt, T. L., Raughi, G., and Henderson, W. R., 1985, Leukotriene B4 is the predominant neutrophil chemotoxin produced by the human alveolar macrophage, *Am. Rev. Respir. Dis.* **131**:A37.

Mascardo, R. N., and Sherline, P., 1982, Somatostatin inhibits rapid centrosomal separation and cell proliferation induced by epidermal growth factor, *Endocrinology* **111**:1394.

Mathews, P. M., Froelich, C. J., Sibbitt, W. L., and Bankhurst, A. D., 1983, Enhancement of natural cytotoxicity by beta-endorphin, *J. Immunol.* **130**:1658.

Matsushima, K., Apella, E., and Oppenheim, J. J., 1987, Phosphorylation of the intracellular precursor of human interleukin 1, *Lymphokine Res.* **6**:1127 (abst.).

Matsushima, K., Bano, M., Kidwell, W. R., and Oppenheim, J. J., 1985, Interleukin 1 increases collagen type IV production by murine mammary epithelial cells, *J. Immunol.* **134**:904.

May, L. T., Helfgott, D. C., and Sehgal, P. B., 1986, Anti-beta interferon antibodies inhibit the increased expression of HLA-B7 mRNA in tumor necrosis factor-treated human fibroblasts: Structural studies of the beta$_2$ interferon involved, *Proc. Natl. Acad. Sci. U.S.A.* **83**:8957.

Mazurek, N., Pecht, I., Teichburg, V. I., and Blumberg, S., 1981, The role of the N-terminal tetrapeptide in the histamine releasing action of substance P, *Neuropharmacology* **20**:1025.

McCain, H. W., Lamster, I. B., Bozzone, J. M., and Grbic, J. T., 1982, Beta-endorphin modulates human immune activity via non-opiate receptor mechanisms, *Life Sci.* **31**:1619.

McGillis, J. P., Hall, N. R., Vahouny, G. V., and Goldstein, A. L., 1985, Thymosin fraction 5 causes increased serum corticosterone in rodents in vivo, *J. Immunol.* **134**:3952.

McGillis, J. P., Organist, M. L., and Payan, D. G., 1987, Substance P and immunoregulation, *Fed. Proc.* **46**:196.

McIntyre, T. M., Zimmerman, G. A., and Prescott, S. M., 1986, Leukotrienes C$_4$ and D$_4$ stimulate human endothelial cells to synthesize platelet-activating factor and bind neutrophils, *Proc. Natl. Acad. Sci. U.S.A.* **83**:2204.

McManus, L. M., and Pinckard, R. N., 1985, Kinetics of acetyl glyceryl ether phosphorylcholine (AGEPC)-induced acute lung alterations in the rabbit, *Am. J. Pathol.* **121**:55.

McManus, L. M., Hanahan, D. M., Demopoulos, C. A., and Pinckard, R. N., 1980, Pathobiology of the intravenous infusion of acetyl glyceryl ether phosphorylcholine (AGEPC), a synthetic platelet-activating factor (PAF), in the rabbit, *J. Immunol.* **124**:2929.

McManus, L. M., Pinckard, R. N., Fitzpatrick, F. A., O'Rourke, R. A., Crawford, M. H., and Hanahan, D. J., 1981, Acetyl glyceryl ether phosphorylcholine (AGEPC): intravascular alterations following intravenous infusion in the baboon, *Lab. Invest.* **45**:303.

Meier, H. L., Kaplan, A. P., Lichtenstein, L. M., Revak, S., Cochrane, C. G., and Newball, H. H., 1983, Anaphylactic release of a prekallikrein activator from human lung in vitro, *J. Clin. Invest.* **72**:574.

Meier, H. L., Heck, L. W., Schulman, E. S., and MacGlashan, D. W., 1985, Purified human mast cells and basophils release human elastase and cathepsin G by an IgE-mediated mechanism, *Int. Arch. Allergy Appl. Immunol.* **77**:179.

Melder, R. J., and Ho, M., 1982, Modulation of natural killer cell activity in mice after interferon induction: Depression of activity and depression of in vitro enhancement by interferon, *Infect. Immun.* **36**:990.

Melmon, K. L., Rocklin, R. E., and Rosenkranz, R. P., 1981, Autacoids as modulators of the inflammatory and immune response, *Am. J. Med.* **71**:100.

Meltzer, M. S., Crawford, R. M., Finbloom, D. S., Ohara, J., and Paul, W. E., 1987, BSF-1: A macrophage activation factor, *Lymphokine Res.* **6**:1719 (abst.).

Mencia-Huerta, J. M., Roubin, R., Morgat, J., and Benveniste, J., 1982, Biosynthesis of platelet-activating factor (PAF-acether). III. Formation of PAF-acether from synthetic substrates by stimulated murine macrophages, *J. Immunol.* **129**:804.

Mencia-Huerta, J. M., Razin, E., Ringel, E. W., Corey, E. J., Hoover, D., Austen, K. F., and Lewis, R. A., 1983, Immunologic and ionophore-induced generation of leukotriene B$_4$ from mouse bone marrow-derived mast cells, *J. Immunol.* **120**:1885.

Merigan, T. C., and Friedman, R. M. (eds.), 1982, *Interferons. UCLA Symposia on Molecular and Cellular Biology*, Vol. 25, Academic, Orlando, Florida.

Metcalfe, D. D., Bland, C. E., and Wasserman, S. I., 1984, Biochemical and functional characterization of proteoglycans isolated from basophils of patients with chronic myelogenous leukemia, *J. Immunol.* **132:**1943.

Mier, J. W., Dinarello, C. A., Atkins, M. B., and Perlmutter, D. H., 1987, Induction of hepatic acute phase protein synthesis by products of interleukin-2-stimulated human mononuclear cells, *Lymphokine Res.* **6:**1128 (abst.).

Miles, K., Chelmicka-Schorr, E., Atweh, S., Otten, G., and Arnason, B. G. W., 1985, Sympathetic ablation alters lymphocyte membrane properties, *J. Immunol.* **135**(suppl.):797s.

Miller, G. C., Murgo, A. J., and Plotnikoff, N. P., 1983, Enkephalin-enhancement of active T cell rosettes from lymphoma patients, *Clin. Imunol. Immunopathol.* **26:**446.

Miller, G. C., Murgo, A. J., and Plotnikoff, N. P., 1984, Enkephalins: Enhancement of active T cell rosetts from normal volunteers, *Clin. Immunol. Immunopathol.* **31:**132.

Milton, A. S., 1982, Prostaglandins in fever and the mode of action of antipyretic drugs, in: *Pyretics and Antipyretics, Handbook of Experimental Pharmacology*, Vol. 60, (A. S. Milton, ed.), pp. 257–303, Springer-Verlag, Berlin.

Moncada, S., and Vane, J. R., 1979, Pharmacology and endogenous roles of prostaglandin endoperoxides, thromboxane A_2, and prostacyclin, *Pharmacol. Rev.* **30:**293.

Moncada, S., Flower, R. J., and Vane, J. R., 1985, Prostaglandins, prostacyclin, thromboxane A_2, and leukotrienes, in: *The Pharmacological Basis of Therapeutics*, 7th ed. (A. G. Gilman, L. S. Goodman, T. W. Rall, and F. Murad, eds.), pp. 660–674, Macmillan, New York.

Monier, J. C., Dardenne, M., Pleau, J. M., Schmitt, D., DesChaux, P., Bach, J.-F., 1980, Characterization of the facteur thymique serique (FTS) in the thymus. I. Fixation of anti-FTS antibodies on thymic reticuloepithelial cells, *Clin. Exp. Immunol.* **42:**470.

Montgomery, D. W., Zukoski, C. F., Shah, G. N., Buckley, A. R., Pacholczyk, T., and Russell, D. H., 1987, Concanavalin A-stimulated murine splenocytes produce a factor with prolactin-like bioactivity and immunoreactivity, *Biochem. Biophys. Res. Commun.* **145:**692.

Moore, R. N., Oppenheim, J. J., Farrar, J. J., Carter, C. S., Waheed, A., and Shadduck, R. K., 1980, Production of lymphocyte activating factor (IL-1) by macrophages activated with colony-stimulating factors, *J. Immunol.* **125:**1302.

Moore, T. C., 1984, Modification of lymphocyte traffic by vasoactive neurotransmitter substances, *Immunology* **52:**511.

Moqbel, R., Sass-Kuhn, S. P., Goetzl, E. J., and Kay, A. B., 1983, Enhancement of neutrophil- and eosinophil-mediated complement-dependent killing of schistosomula of *Schistosoma mansoni* in vitro by leukotriene B4, *Clin. Exp. Immunol.* **52:**519.

Morgan, D. A., Ruscetti, F. W., and Gallo, R., 1976, Selective in vitro growth of T lymphocytes from normal human bone marrows, *Science* **193:**1007.

Morice, A., Univin, R., and Sever, P. S., 1983, Vasoactive intestinal peptide causes bronchodilatation and protects against histamine-induced bronchoconstriction in asthmatic subjects, *Lancet* **2:**1225.

Morley, J., Hanson, J. M., and Rumjanek, V. M., 1984, Lymphokines, in: *Textbook of Immunopharmacology* (M. M. Dale and J. C. Foreman, eds.), pp. 170–186, Blackwell Scientific Publications, Oxford.

Morrison, J. H., Benoit, R., Magistretti, P. M., and Bloom, F. E., 1983, Immunohistochemical distribution of pro-somatostatin related peptides in cerebral cortex, *Brain Res.* **262:**344.

Morrison, J. H., Magistretti, P. J., Benoit, R., and Bloom, F. E., 1984, The distribution and morphological characteristics of the intracortical VIP-positive cell: An immunohistochemical analysis, *Brain Res.* **292:**269.

Mosmann, T. R., and Coffman, R. L., 1987, Two types of mouse helper T-cell clone. Implications for immune regulation, *Immunol. Today* **8:**223.

Mosmann, T. R., Yokota, T., Kastelein, R., Zurawski, S. M., Arai, N., and Takebe, Y., 1987, Species-specificity of T-cell stimulating activities of IL-2 and BSF-1 (IL-4): Comparison of normal and recombinant mouse and human IL-2 and BSF-1 (IL-4), *J. Immunol.* **138:**1813.

Movat, H., 1979, The acute inflammatory reaction, in: *Inflammation, Immunity and Hypersensitivity* (H. Z. Movat, ed.), pp. 1–161, Harper & Row, Hagerstown, Maryland.

Movat, H. Z., Habal, F. M., and Macmorine, D. R. L., 1976, The cleavage of a methionyl lysylbradykinin-like peptide from kininogen by a protease of human neutrophil leukocyte lysosomes, in: *Kinins, Pharmacodynamics and Biological Role* (F. Sicuteri, N. Back, and G. L. Haberland, eds.), Plenum, New York.

Movat, H., Steinberg, S., Habal, F., and Ranadive, N., 1973, Demonstration of a kinin-generating enzyme in the lysosomes of human polymorphonuclear leukocytes, *Lab. Invest.* **29:**669.

Muller-Eberhard, H. J., 1978, Complement: Molecular mechanisms, regulation and biologic function, in: *Molecular Basis of Biological Degradative Processes: Proceedings of the Dedication Symposium of the University of Connecticut,* (R. Berlin, H. Herrmann, I. H. Lepow, and I. M. Tanzerr, eds.), pp. 65–114, Academic, New York.

Mundy, G. R., 1981, Control of osteoclast function by lymphokines in health and disease, *Lymphokines* **4:**395.

Munoz, J. J., 1963, Symposium on relationship of structure of microorganisms to their immunological properties. I. Immunological and other biological activities of *Bordetella pertussis* antigens, *Bacteriol. Rev.* **27:**325.

Murray, P. D., and Kagnoff, M. F., 1987, Regulation of the anti-alpha (1,3) dextran response: two populations of dextran-reactive B cells that differ in their T cell requirements for induction to antibody synthesis, *J. IMmunol.* **138:**2439.

Murray, P. D., McKenzie, D. T., Swain, S. L., and Kagnoff, M. F., 1987, Interleukin 5 and interleukin 4 produced by Peyer's patch T cells selectively enhanced immunoglobulin A expression, *J. Immunol.* **139:**2669.

Nathan, C. F., Murray, H. W., and Cohn, Z. A., 1980, The macrophage as an effector cell, *N. Engl. J. Med.* **303:**622.

National Cancer Institute, 1983, *Monograph 63: Biological Response Modifiers,* U.S. Department of Health and Human Services, National Institutes of Health, National Cancer Institute, Bethesda, Maryland.

Neff, N. H., Karoum, F., and Hadjiconstantinov, M., 1983, Dopamine-containing small intensely fluorescent cells and sympathetic ganglion function, *Fed. Proc.* **42:**3009.

Nemeroff, C. B., and Prange, A. J. (eds.), 1982, Neurotensin: A brain and Gastrointestinal Peptide, *Ann. N.Y. Acad. Sci.* **400.**

Nijsten, M. W. N., DeGrout, E. R., Tenduis, H. J., Klasen, H. J., Hack, C. E., and Aarden, L. A., 1987, Serum levels of interleukin 6 and acute phase responses, *Lancet* **2:**921.

Nilsson, J., von Euler, A. M., and Dalsgaard, C.-J., 1985, Stimulation of connective tissue cell growth by substance P and substance K, *Nature (Lond.)* **315:**61.

Nissenson, A. R., Baraff, L. J., Fine, R. N., and Knutson, D W., 1979, Post-streptcoccol acute glomeruloenphritis—fact and controversy, *Ann. Intern. Med.* **91:**76.

Noma, Y., Sideras, P., Naito, T., Bergstedt-Lindquist, S., Azuma, C., Severinson, E, Tanabe, T., Kinashi, T., Matsuda, F., Yaoita, Y., and Honjo, T, 1986, Cloning of cDNA encoding the murine IgGl induction factor by a novel strategy using SP6 promoter, *Nature (Lond.)* **319:**640.

Numao, T., and Makino, S., 1986, Specific binding of AGEPC by human eosinophils, presented at the *Symposium on Platelet Activating Factor, Pulmonary Hyperreactivity and Asthma, L'Esterel, Quebec, 1986.*

O'Dorisio, M. S., 1987, Biochemical characteristics of receptors for vasoactive intestinal polypeptide in nervous, endocrine, and immune systems, *Fed. Proc.* **45:**192.

O'Dorisio, M. S., O'Dorisio, T. M., Cataland, S., and Blacerzak, S. P., 1980, Vasoactive intestinal peptide as a biochemical marker for polymorphonuclear leukocytes, *J. Lab. Clin. Med.* **96:**666.

O'Dorisio, M. S., Wood, C. L., and O'Dorisio, T. M., 1985, Vasoactive intestinal peptide and neuropeptide modulation of the immune response, *J. Immunol.* **135**(suppl.):792.

O'Flaherty, J. T., and Wykle, R. L., 1983, Biology and biochemistry of platelet-activating factor, *Clin. Rev. Allergy* **1:**535.

O'Garra, A., Warren, D. J., Holman, M., Popham, A. M., Sanderson, C. J., and Klaus, G. G. B., 1986, Interleukin 4 (B-cell growth factor II/eosinophil differentiative factor) is a mitogen and differentiation factor for preactivated murine B lymphocytes, *Proc. Natl. Acad. Sci. U.S.A.* **83:** 5228.

Oppenheim, J. J., 1985, Antigen non-specific lymphokines: An overview, *Methods Immunol.* **116** (part H):357.

Oppenheim, J. J., and Cohen, S., 1983, *Interleukins, Lymphokines and Cytokines,* Academic, Orlando, Florida.

Oppenheim, J. J., 1984, The role of cytokines in promoting accessory cell functions, *Prog. Immunol.* **5:**285.

Oppenheim, J. J., Kovacs, E. J., Matsushima, K., and Durum, S. K., 1986, There is more than one interleukin 1, *Immunol. Today* **7**(2):45.

Oppenheim, J. J., Ruscetti, F. W., and Faltynek, C. R., 1987, Interleukins and interferons, in: *Basic and Clinical Immunology* (D. P. Stites, J. D. Stobo, and J. V. Wells, eds.), Vol. 6, pp. 82–95, Appleton & Lange, E. Norwalk, Connecticut.

Orchard, M. A., Kagey-Sobotka, A., Proud, D., and Lichenstein, L. M., 1986, Basophil histamine release induced by a substance from stimulated human platelets, *J. Immunol.* **136:**2240.

Ottaway, C. A., Bernaerts, C., Chan, B., and Greenberg, G. R., 1983, Specific binding of vasoactive intestinal peptide to human circulating mononuclear cells, *Can. J. Physiol. Pharmacol.* **61:**664.

Ottaway, C. A., and Greenberg, G. R., 1984, Interaction of vasoactive intestinal peptide with mouse lymphocytes: Specific binding and the modulation of mitogen response, *J. Immunol.* **132:**417.

Pace, J. L., Russell, S. W., Torres, B. A., Johnson, H. M., and Gray, P. W., 1983, Recombinant mouse gamma-interferon induces the priming step in macrophage activation for tumor cell killing, *J. Immunol.* **130:**2011.

Paetkau, V., Bleackley, R. C., Riendeau, D., Harnish, D. G., and Holowachuk, E. W., 1985, Toward the molecular biology of interleukin 1, *Contemp. Top. Mol. Immunol.* **10:**35.

Page, C. P., Paul, W., and Morley, J., 1984, Platelets and bronchospasm, *Int. Arch. Allergy Appl. Immunol.* **74:**347.

Page, I. H., 1968, *Serotonin,* Year Book Medical Publishers, Chicago.

Palacios, R., 1983, Role of serum thymic factor (FTS) in the development of interleukin 2 producer lymphocytes, *Clin. Immunol. Allergy* **3:**83.

Palaszynski, E. W., Moody, T. W., O'Donohue, T. L., and Goldstein, A. L., 1983, Thymosin alpha₁-like peptides: Localization and biochemical characterization in the rat brain and pituitary gland, *Peptides* **4:**463.

Palkovits, M., 1984, Distribution of neuropeptides in the central nervous system: A review of biochemical mapping studies, *Prog. Neurobiol.* **23:**151.

Palladino, M. A., Welte, K., Ciobanu, N., Mertlesmann, R., and Oettgen, H. F., 1984, Regulation of T-cell proliferation by interleukin 2 in male homosexuals with Acquired Immune Deficiency Syndrome, in: *Thymic Hormones and Lymphokines* (A. L. Goldstein, ed.), pp. 519–524, Plenum, New York.

Papermaster, B. W., Smith, M. E., and McEntire, J. E., 1981, Lymphotoxins: Soluble cytotoxic molecules secreted by lymphocytes, in: *The Lymphokines. Biochemistry and Biological Activity,* (J. W. Hadden and W. E. Stewart II, eds.), pp. 149–180, Humana Press, Clifton, New Jersey.

Papiernik, M., and Homo-Delarche, F., 1983, Thymic reticulum in mice. III. Phagocytic cells of the thymic reticulum in culture secrete both PGE₂ and IL1 which regulate thymocyte proliferation, *Eur. J. Immunol.* **13:**681.

Papiernik, M., and Nabarra, B., 1981, Thymic reticulum in mice. I. Cellular ultrastructure in vitro and functional role, *Thymus* **3:**345.

Papiernik, M., Nabarra, B., Savino, W., Pontous, C., and Barbey, S., 1983, Thymic reticulum in mice. II. Culture and characterization of non-epithelial phagocytic cells of the thymic reticulum: Their role in the syngeneic stimulation of thymic medullary lymphocytes, *Eur. J. Immunol.* **13:** 147.

Parente, L., and Flower, R. J., 1985, Glucocorticoid-induced antiphospholipase proteins, in: *Biochemistry of Arachidonic Acid Metabolism* (W. E., Lands, ed.), pp. 195–201, Martinus Nijhoff, Boston.

Parker, C. W., 1979, Prostaglandins and slow-reacting substance, *J. Allergy Clin. Immunol.* **63**(1): 1.

Parker, C. W., 1987, Lipid mediators produced through the lipoxygenase pathway, *Annu. Rev. Immunol.* **5**:65.

Patterson, R., and Harris, K. E., 1983, The activity of aerosolized and intracutaneous synthetic platelet-activating factor (AGEPC) in rhesus monkeys with IgE-mediated airway responses and normal monkeys, *J. Lab. Clin. Med.* **102**:933.

Pawlikowski, M., Kunert-Radek, J., and Stepien, H., 1978, Somatostatin inhibits mitogenic effect of thyroliberlin, *Experientia* **34**:271.

Pawlikowski, M., Stepien, H., Kunert-Radek, J., and Schally, A. V., 1985, Effect of somatostatin on the proliferation of mouse spleen lymphocytes in vitro, *Biochem. Biophys. Res. Commun.* **129**:52.

Pawlikowski, M., Stepien, H., Kunert-Radek, J., Zelazowski, P., and Schally, A. V., 1987, Immunomodulatory action of somatostatin, in: *Neuroimmune Interactions* (B. D. Jankovic, B. M., Markovic, and N. H. Spector, eds.), *Ann. N.Y. Acad. Sci.* **496**:233.

Payan, D. G., 1985, Receptor-mediated mitogenic effects of substance P on cultured smooth muscle cells, *Biochem. Biophys. Res. Commun.* **130**:104.

Payan, D. G., and Goetzl, E. J., 1985, Modulation of lymphocyte function by sensory neuropeptides, *J. Immunol.* **135**(suppl.):783.

Payan, D. G., Brewster, D. R., and Goetzl, E. J., 1983, Specific stimulation of human T lymphocytes by substance P, *J. Immunol.* **131**:1613.

Payan, D. G., Brewster, D. R., Missirian-Bastian, A., and Goetzl, E. J., 1984a, Substance P recognition by a subset of human T lymphocytes, *J. Clin. Invest.* **74**:1532.

Payan, D. G., Levine, J. D., and Goetzl, E. J., 1984b, Modulation of immunity and hypersensitivity by sensory neuropeptides, *J. Immunol.* **132**:1601.

Payan, D. G., Hess, C. A., and Goetzl, E. J., 1984c, Inhibition by somatostatin of the proliferation of T-lymphocytes and Molt-4 lymphoblasts, *Cell. Immunol.* **84**:433.

Payan, D. G., Missirian-Bastian, A., and Goetzl, E. J., 1984d, Human lymphocyte T subset specificity of the regulatory effects of leukotriene B4, *Proc. Natl. Acad. Sci. U.S.A.* **81**:3501.

Payan, D. G., McGillis, J. P., and Goetzl, E. J., 1986, Neuroimmunology, *Adv. Immunol.* **39**:299.

Payan, D. G., McGillis, J. P., Renold, F. K., Mitsuhashi, M., and Goetzl, E. J., 1987, Neuropeptide modulation of leukocyte function in: *Neuroimmune Interactions* (B. D. Jankovic, B. M. Markovic, and N. H. Spector, eds.), *Ann. N. Y. Acad. Sci.* **496**: 182.

Pazmino, N. H., Ihle, J. N., and Goldstein, A. L., 1978, Induction in vivo and in vitro of terminal deoxynucleotidyl transferase by thymosin in bone marrow cells from athymic mice, *J. Exp. Med.* **147**:708.

Peck, R., 1987, Neuropeptides modulating macrophage functions, in: *Neuroimmune Interactions* (B. D. Jankovic, B. M. Markovic, and N. H. Spector, eds.), *Ann. N.Y. Acad. Sci.* **496**:264.

Peck, R., and Brockhaus, M., 1987, The production and characterization of anti-interleukin 1 monoclonal antibodies, *Lymphokine Res.* **6**:1102 (abst.).

Pernow, B., 1985, Role of tachykinins in neurogenic inflammation, *J. Immunol.* **135**(suppl.):812.

Pernow, B., 1983, Substance P, *Pharmacol. Rev.* **35**:85.

Peroutka, S. J., and Snyder, S. H., 1983, Multiple serotonin receptors and their physiological significance, *Fed. Proc.* **42**:213.

Pert, C. B., Ruff, M. R., Weber, R. J., and Herkenham, M., 1985, Neuropeptides and their receptors: A psychosomatic network, *J. Immunol.* **135**(suppl.):820.

Peters, S. P., MacGlashan, Jr., D. W., Schulman, E. S., Schleimer, R. P., Hayes, E. C., Rokach, J., Adkinson, N. F., Jr., and Lichtenstein, L. M., 1984, Arachidonic acid metabolism in purified human lung mast cells, *J. Immunol.* **132**:1972.

Pichyangkul, S., Hill, N. O., and Khan, A., 1982, Purification of lymphotoxin from RPMI-1788 cell line supernate, in: *Human Lymphokines* (A. Kahn and N. O. Hill, eds.), pp. 173–181, Academic, Orlando, Florida.

Pick, E., (ed.), 1981, *Lymphokines, A Forum for Immunoregulatory Cell Products*, Vol. 3, *Lymphokines in Macrophage Activation*, Academic, Orlando, Florida.

Pinckard, R. N., Farrr, R. S., and Hanahan, D. J., 1979, Physicochemical and functional identify of platelet-activating factor (PAF) release in vivo during IgE anaphylaxis with PAF released in vitro from IgE sensitized basophils, *J. Immunol.* **123**:1847.

Pincus, S. H., Whitcomb, E. A., and Dinarello, C. A., 1987, Interaction of interleukin-1 (IL-1) and PMA in modulation of eosinophil function: Implications for IL-1 mechanism of action, *Lymphokine Res.* **6**:1208 (abst.).

Piotrowski, W. and Foreman, J. C., 1985, On the actions of substance P, somatostatin, and vasoactive intestinal polypeptide on rat peritoneal mast cells and in human skin, *Naunyn-Schmiedebergs Arch. Pharmacol.* **331**:364.

Pirotzky, E., Page, C. P., Roubin, R., Pfister, A., Paul, W., Bonnet, J., and Benveniste, J., 1984, PAF-acether-induced plasma exudation in rat skin is independent of platelets and neutrophils, *Microcirc. Endothelium. Lymphatics* **1**:107.

Pirotzky, E., Page, C., Morley, J., Bidault, J., and Benveniste, J., 1985, Vascular permeability induced by paf-acether (platelet-activating factor) in the isolated perfused rat kidney, *Agents Actions* **16**:17.

Platshon, L. F., and Kaliner, M., 1978, The effects of the immunologic release of histamine upon human lung cyclic nucleotide levels and prostaglandin generation, *J. Clin. Invest.* **62**:1113.

Plaut, M., and Lichtenstein, L. M., 1982, Histamine and immune responses, in: *Pharmacology of Histamine Receptors* (C. R. Ganellin and M. E. Parsons, eds.), pp. 392–435, Wright–PSF, Bristol.

Plotnikoff, N. P. and Miller, G. C., 1983, Enkephalins—endorphins: Immunomodulators in mice, *Int. J. Immunopharmacol.* **5**:437.

Pluznik, D. H., Bickel, M., Tsuda, H., Amstad, P., Mergenhagen, S. E., and S. M. Wahl, 1987, Differential regulation of murine T lymphocyte production of GM-CSF, IL-3, and IL-2, *Lymphokine Res.* **6**:1315 (abst.).

Pollack, S. B., and Hallenback, L. A., 1982, In vivo reduction of NK activity with anti-NK1 serum: Direct evaluation of NK cells in tumor clearance, *Int. J. Cancer* **29**:203.

Poupart, P., Vandenabeele, P., Cayphas, S., Van Snick, J., Haegeman, G., Kruys, V., Fiers, W., and Content, J., 1987, B-cell growth modulating and differentiating activity of recombinant human 26-kDa protein (BSF-2, HuIFN-beta$_2$, HPGF), *EMBO J.* **6**:1219.

Proud, D., MacGlashan, J. W., Jr., Newball, H. H., Schulman, E. S., and Lichtenstein, L. M., 1985, IgE-mediated release of kininogenase from purified human lung mast cells, *Am. Rev. Respir. Dis.* **132**:405.

Proud, D., Togias, A., Naclerio, R., Crush, S. A., Norman, P. S., and Lichtenstein, L. M., 1983, Kinins are generated in vivo following nasal airway challenge of allergic individuals with allergen, *J. Clin. Invest.* **72**:1678.

Radmark, O., Shimizu, T., Jornvall, H., and Samuelsson, B., 1984, Leukotriene A$_4$ hydrolase in human leukocytes: Purification and properties, *J. Biol. Chem.* **259**:12334.

Ralph, P., 1984, Differentiation and functional regulation in macrophage cell lines, in: *The Reticuloendothelial System—A Comprehensive Treatise* (J. A. Bellanti and H. B. Herschowitz, eds.), pp. 43–66, Plenum, New York.

Ramstedt, U., Serhan, C. N., Lundberg, U., Wigzell, H., and Samuelsson, B., 1984, Inhibition of human natural killer cell activity by (14R,15S)-14,15-dihydroxy-5Z,8Z,10E, 12E-icosatetraenoic acid, *Proc. Natl. Acad. Sci. U.S.A.* **81**:6914.

Ranadive, N. S., and Movat, H. Z., 1979, Tissue injury and inflammation induced by immune complexes, in: *Inflammation, Immunity and Hypersensitivity* (H. Z. Movat, ed.), pp. 409–443, Harper & Row, Hagerstown, Maryland.

Raulet, D. H., 1985, Expression and function of interleukin-2 receptor on immature thymocytes, *Nature (Lond.)* **314**:101.

Razin, E., Mencia-Huerta, J. M., Lewis, R. A., Corey, E. J., and Austen, K. F., 1982a, Generation of leukotriene C4 from a subclass of mast cells differentiated in vitro from mouse bone marrow, *Proc. Natl. Acad. Sci. U.S.A.* **79**:4665.

Razin, E., Stevens, R. L., Akiyama, F., Schmid, K., and Austen, K. F., 1982, Culture from mouse bone marrow of a subclass of mast cells possessing a distinct chondroitin sulfate proteoglycan with glycosaminoglycans rich in N-acetylgalactosamine-4,6-disulfate, *J. Biol. Chem.* **257**: 7229.

Rebar, R. W., Miyake, A., Low, T. L. K.,. and Goldstein, A. L., 1981, Thymosin stimulates secretion of luteinizing hormone releasing factor, *Science* **214**:669.

Regoli, D., and Barabe, J., 1980, Pharmacology of bradykinin and related kinins, *Pharmacol. Rev.* **32**:1.

Reid, I. A., 1987, Polypeptides, in: *Basic and Clinical Pharmacology*, 3rd ed. (B. G. Katzung, ed.), pp. 201–210, Appleton & Lange, E. Norwalk, Connecticut.

Renold, F., Chernow, T., Lee, J., Payan, D. G., Furiuchi, R., and Goetzl, E. J., 1985, Somatostatin (SOM) modulation of mediator release by mouse bone marrow derived mast cells (BMMC), rat serosal mast cell (SMC) and rat basophilic cells (RBL-2H3), *Fed. Proc.* **44**:1917.

Rey, A., Klein, B., Zagury, D., Thierry, C., and Serrou, B., 1983, Diminished interleukin 2 activity production in cancer patients bearing solid tumors and its relationship with natural killer cells, *Immunol. Lett.* **6**:175.

Rheinherz, E. L., and Schlossman, S., 1980, Regulation of the immune response-inducer and suppressor T lymphocyte subsets in human beings, *N. Engl. J. Med.* **303**:370.

Rheinherz, E. L., Kung, P., Goldstein, G., and Schlossman, S., 1979, Further characterization of helper/inducer T cell subsets defined by monoclonal antibody, *J. Immunol.* **123**:2894.

Rheinherz, E. L., Morimoto, C., Penta, J. A., and Schlossman, S., 1981, Subpopulations of the T4 positive inducer cell subset in man, *J. Immunol.* **126**:67.

Ribbes, G., Ninio, E., Fontan, P., Record, M., Chap, H., Benveniste, J., and Douste-Blazy, L., 1985, Evidence that biosynthesis of platelet-activating factor (pafacether) by human neutrophils occurs in an intracellular membrane, *FEBS Lett.* **191**:195.

Riccardi, C., Barlozzari, T., Santoni, A., Herberman, R. B., and Cesarini, C., 1981, Transfer to cyclophosphamide-treated mice of natural killer (NK) cells in in vivo natural reactivity against tumors, *J. Immunol.* **126**:1284.

Rimsky, L., Wakasugi, H., Ferrara, P., Robin, P., Capdeville, J., Tursz, T., Fradelizi, D., Bertoglio, J., 1986, Purification to homogeneity and NH_2 terminal amino acid sequence of a novel interleukin-1 species derived from a human B cell line, *J. Immunol.* **136**:3304.

Rinaldi-Garaci, C., 1983, Is Thymosin action mediated by prostaglandin release, *Science* **220**:1163.

Rinaldi-Garaci, C., Garaci, E., DelGobbo, V., Favalli, C., Jezzi, T., and Goldstein, A. L., 1983, Modulation of endogeneous prostaglandins by thymosin alpha$_1$ in lymphocytes, *Cell. Immunol.* **80**:57.

Robb, R. J., Kutney, R. M., and Chowdhry, V., 1983, Purification and partial sequence analysis of human T-cell growth factor, *Proc. Natl. Acad. Sci. U.S.A.* **80**:5990.

Rocha e Silva, M. (ed.), 1978, *Histamine and Antihistamines—Chemistry, Metabolism, and Physiological and Pharmacological Actions, Handbook of Experimental Pharmacology*, Vol. XVIII/2. Springer-Verlag, Berlin.

Rocha e Silva, M., Beraldo, W. T., and Rosenfeld, G., 1949, Bradykinin, a hypotensive and smooth muscle stimulating factor released from plasma globulin by snake venom and by trypsin, *J. Physiol. (Lond.)* **109**:488.

Rocklin, R. E., and Beer, D. J., 1983, Histamine and immune modulation, *Adv. Intern. Med.* **28**: 225.

Roehm, N. W., Leibson, H. J., Zlotnik, A., Kappler, J. W., Marrack, P., and Cambier, J. C., 1984, Interleukin-induced increase in Ia expression by normal mouse B-cells, *J. Exp. Med.* **160**:679.

Rola-Pleszczynski, M., 1985a, Immunoregulation by leukotrienes and other lipoxygenase metabolites, *Immunol. Today* **6**:302.

Rola-Pleszczynski, M., 1985b, Differential effects of leukotriene B4 on T4+ and T8+ lymphocyte phenotype and immunoregulatory functions, *J. Immunol.* **135:**1357.

Rola-Pleszczynski, M., Borgeat, P., and Sirois, P., 1982, Leukotriene B4 induces human suppressor lymphocytes, *Biochem. Biophys. Res. Comun.* **108:**1531.

Rola-Pleszczynski, M., Gagnon, L., and Sirois, P. 1983, Leukotriene B4 augments human natural cytotoxic cell activity, *Biochem. Biophys. Res. Commun.* **113:**531.

Rola-Pleszczynski, M., Gagnon, L., Rudzinski, M., Borgeat, P., and Sirois, P., 1984, Human natural cytotoxic cell activity—enhancement by leukotrienes (LT) A4, B4, and D4, but not by stereoisomers of LTB4 or HETEs, *Prostaglandins Leukotrienes Med.* **13:**113.

Rola-Pleszczynski, M., Chavaillaz, P. A., and Lemaire, I., 1986, Stimulation of interleukin-2 and interferon-gamma production by leukotriene B4 in human lymphocyte cultures, *Prostaglandins Leukotrienes Med.* **23:**207.

Roszman, T. L., Jackson, J. C., Cross, R. J., Titus, M. J., Markesbery, W. R., and Brooks, W. H., 1985, Neuroanatomic and neurotransmitter influences on immune function, *J. Immunol.* **135:** 769.

Roth, R., Leroith, D., Collier, E. S., Weaver, N. R., Watkinson, A., Cleland, C. F., and Glick, S. M., 1985, Evolutionary origins of neuropeptides, hormones, and receptors: Possible applications to immunology, *J. Immunol.* **135**(supp.):816.

Roubin, R., and Benveniste, J., 1985, Release of lipid mediators from macrophages and its pharmacological modulation, in: *The Reticuloendothelial System—A Comprehensive Treatise*, (J. W. Hadden and A. Szentivanyi, eds.), Vol. 8, pp. 73–96, Plenum, New York.

Rouzer, C. A., and Samuelsson, B., 1985, On the nature of the 5-lipoxygenase reaction in human leukocytes: Enzyme purification and requirement for multiple stimulatory factors, *Proc. Natl. Acad. Sci. U.S.A.* **82:**6040.

Rouzer, C. A., Scott, W. A., Hamill, A. L., Liu, F.-T., Katz, D. H., and Cohn, Z. A., 1982, Secretion of leukotriene C and other arachidonic acid metabolites by macrophages challenged with immunoglobulin E immune complexes, *J. Exp. Med.* **156:**1077.

Ruff, M. R., Wahl, S. M., and Pert, C. B., 1985, Substance P receptor-mediated chemotaxis of human monocytes, *Peptides* **6**(Suppl. 2):107.

Ruscetti, F. W., Farrar, W. L., Hill, J. M., and Pert, C. B., 1987, Visualization of the human helper T lymphocyte related antigen (T4) in primate brain, *Lymphokine Res.* **6:**1515 (abst.).

Russell, D. H., Buckley, A. R., Montgomery, D. W., Larson, N. A., Gout, P. W., Beer, C. T., Putnam, C. W., Zukoski, C. F., and Kibler, R., 1987, Prolactin-dependent mitogenesis in Nb 2 node lymphoma cells: Effects of immunosuppressive cyclopeptides, *J. Immunol.* **138**(1):276.

Ryan, J. W., 1982, Processing of the endogenous polypeptides by the lungs, *Annu. Rev. Physiol.* **44:** 241.

Sagi-Eisenberg, R., Ben-Neriah, Z., Pecht, I., Terry, S., and Blumberg, S., 1983, Structure–activity relationship in the mast cell degranulating capacity of neurotensin fragments, *Neuropharmacology* **22:**197.

Said, S. I. (ed), 1982, *Vasoactive Intestinal Peptide,* Raven, New York.

Saito, H., Hirai, A., Tamura, Y., and Yoshida, S., 1985, The 5-lipoxygenase products can modulate the synthesis of platelet-activating factor (alkyl-acetyl GPC) in Ca-ionophore A23187-stimulated rat peritoneal macrophages, *Prostaglandins Leukotriene Med.* **18:**271.

Saklatvala, J., and Sarsfield, S. J., 1985, Purification to homogenicity of two IL-1-like proteins from pig leukocytes, *J. Leukocyte Biol.* **36:**738–739.

Saklatvala, J., Pilsworth, L. M. C., Sarsfield, S. J., Gavrilovic, J., and Heath, J. K., 1984, Pig catabolin is a form of interleukin 1, *Biochem. J.* **224:**461.

Salari, H., Borgeat, P., Fournier, M., Hebert, J., and Pelletier, G., 1985, Studies on the release of leukotrienes and histamine by human lung fragments upon immunologic and nonimmunologic stimulation: Effects of nordihydroguaiaretic acid, aspirin, and sodium cromoglycate, *J. Exp. Med.* **162:**1904.

Samuelsson, B., 1983, Leukotrienes: Mediators of immediate hypersensitivity reactions and inflammation, *Science* **220**:568.

Samuelsson, B., and Hammarstrom, S., 1980, Nomenclature for leukotrienes, *Prostaglandins* **19**: 645.

Sanchez-Crespo, M., Alonso, F., Inarrea, P., and Egido, J., 1981, Nonplatelet mediated vascular actions of 1-*O*-alkyl-2-acetyl-*sn*-3-glycerol phosphorylcholine (a synthetic PAF), *Agents Actions* **11**:566.

Sanchez-Crespo, M., Fernandez-Gallardo, S., Nieto, M.-L., Braanes, J., and Braquet, P., 1985, Inhibition of the vascular actions of IgG aggregates by BN 52021, a highly specific antagonist of PAF-acether, *Immunopharmacology* **10**:69.

Sanderson, C. J., O'Garra, A., Warren, D. J., and Klaus, G. G. B., 1986, Eosinophil differentiation factor also has B-cell growth factor activity: Proposed name interleukin 4, *Proc. Natl. Acad. Sci. U.S.A.* **83**:437.

Sarto, K. T., and Mortensen, R. F., 1985, Enhanced interleukin 1 production mediated by mouse serum amyloid P component, *Cell. Immunol.* **93**:398.

Saunders, R. N., and Handley, D. A., 1987, Platelet-activating factor antagonists, *Annu. Rev. Pharm. Toxicol.* **27**:237.

Saunders, R. N., Handley, D. A., Kowal-DeLillo, A. H., Van Valen, R. G., and Winslow, C. M., 1985, Effects of platelet activating factor in primates, *Thromb. Haemostasis.* **54**:244.

Savino, W., Dardenne, M., Papiernik, M., and Bach, J.-F., 1982, Thymic hormone-containing cells characterization and localization of serum thymic factor in young mouse thymus studies by monoclonal antibodies, *J. Exp. Med.* **156**:628.

Sawchenko, P. E., Swanson, L., and Vale, W. W., 1984, Corticotropin-releasing factor: Coexpression within distinct subsets of oxytocin-, vasopressin- and neurotensin-immunoreactive neurons in the hypothalamus of the male rat, *J. Neurosci.* **4**:1118.

Schachter, M., and Barton, S., 1979, Kallikreins (kininogenases) and kinins. in: *Endocrinology: Metabolic Basis of Clinical Practice* (G. Cahill and L. J. deGroot, eds.), Grune & Stratton, New York.

Schally, A. V., Comaru-Schally, A. M., and Redding, T. W., 1984, Antitumor effects of analogs of hypothalamic hormones in endocrine-dependent cancers, *Proc. Soc. Exp. Biol. Med.* **175**:259.

Schechter, N. M., Choi, J. K., Slavin, D. A., Deresienski, D. T., Sayama, S., Dong, G., Lavker, R. M., Proud, D., and Lazarus, G. S., 1986, Identification of a chymotrypsin-like proteinase in human mast cells, *J. Immunol.* **137**:962.

Schild, H. O., 1936, Histamine release and anaphylactic shock in isolated lungs of guinea pigs, *Q. J. Exp. Physiol.* **26**:165.

Schleimer, R. P., Derse, C., Landy, S., and Lichtenstein, L. M., 1986, Vascular endothelial cell (VEC) supernatants (SUP) cause histamine release (HR) from human basophils, *Fed. Proc.* **45**: 1105.

Schlesinger, D. H., Goldstein, G., and Niall, H. D., 1975, The complete amino acid sequence of ubiquitin: An adenylate cyclase stimulating polypeptide probably universal in living cells, *Biochemistry* **14**:221.

Schlesinger, D. H., Goldstein, G., Scheid, M. P., and Bitensky, M., 1978, Chemical synthesis of a hexadecapeptide segment of ubiquitin that activates adenylatecyclase and induces lymphocytes to differentiate, *Experientia* **34**:703.

Schmitt, D., Monier, J. C., Dardenne, M., Pleau, J. M., DesChaux, P., and Bach, J.-F., 1980, Cytoplasmic localization of FTS (facteur thymique serique) in thymic epithelial cells: An immunoelectronmicroscopical study, *Thymus* **2**:177.

Schrader, J. W., 1981, The in vitro production and cloning of the P-cell, a bone marrow-derived null cell that expresses H2 and Ia antigens, has mast cell-like granules, and is regulated by a factor released by activated T-cells, *J. Immunol.* **126**:452.

Schrader, J. W., and Nossal, G. J. V., 1980, Strategies for the analysis of accessory cell function— The in vitro cloning and characterization of the P-cell, *Immunol. Rev.* **53**:61.

Schrader, J. W., Arnold, B., and Clark-Lewis, I., 1980, Con A-stimulated T-cell hybridoma releases factors affecting hematopoietic colony-forming cells and B-cell antibody responses, *Nature (Lond.)* **283**:197.

Schrader, J. W., Clark-Lewis, I., Crapper, R. M., Wong, G. H. W., and Schrader, S., 1985, P-Cell stimulating factor: Biochemistry, biology and role in oncogenesis, *Contemp. Top. Mol. Immunol.* **10**:121.

Schreier, M. H., Iscove, N. N., Tees, R., Aarden, L., and von Boehmer, H., 1980, Clones of killer and helper T-cells—Growth requirements, specificity and retention of function in long-term culture, *Immunol. Rev.* **51**:315.

Schulman, E. S., Adkinson, N. F., Jr., and Newball, H. H., 1982, Cyclooxygenase metabolites in human lung anaphylaxis—airway vs. parenchyma, *J. Appl. Physiol.* **53**:589.

Schultz, R. M., 1985, The role of macrophage-derived arachidonic acid oxygenation products in the modulation of macrophage and lymphocyte function, in: *The Reticuloendothelial System—A Comprehensive Treatise* (J. W. Hadden and A. Szentivanyi, eds.), Vol. 8, pp. 129–153, Plenum, New York.

Schwartz, J. H., 1981, Chemical basis of synaptic transmission, in: *Principles of Neural Science* (E. R. Kandel and J. H. Schwartz, eds.), pp. 106–131, Elsevier/North-Holland, New York.

Schwartz, L. B., 1985, Monoclonal antibodies against human mast cell tryptase demonstrate shared antigenic sites on subunits of tryptase and selective localization of the enzyme to mast cells, *J. Immunol.* **134**:526.

Schwartz, L. B., 1987, Mediators of human mast cells and human mast cell subsets, *Ann. Allergy* **58**: 226.

Schwartz, L. B., and Austen, K. F., 1984, Structure and function of the chemical mediators of mast cells, *Prog. Allergy* **34**:271.

Schwartz, L. B., and Bradford, T. M., 1986, Regulation of tryptase from human lung mast cells by heparin: Stabilization of the active tetramer, *J. Biol. Chem.* **261**:7372.

Schwartz, L. B., Lewis, R. A., and Austen, K. F., 1981, Tryptase from human pulmonary mast cells: Purification and characterization, *J. Biol. Chem.* **256**:11939.

Schwartz, L. B., Kawahara, M. S., Hugli, T. E., Vik, D., Fearon, D. T., and Austen, K. F., 1983, Generation of C3a anaphylatoxin from human C3 by human mast cell tryptase, *J. Immunol.* **130**:1891.

Schwartz, L. B., Bradford, T. M., Littleman, B. L., and Wintroub, B. U., 1985, The fibronolytic activity of purified tryptase from human lung mast cells, *J. Immunol.* **135**:2762.

Schwartz, L. B., Irani, A.-M. A., Roller, K., Castells, M. C., and Schechter, N. M., 1987, Quantitation of histamine, tryptase, and chymase in dispersed human T and TC mast cells, *J. Immunol.* **138**:2611.

Sehgal, P. B., May, L. T., Tamm, I., and Vilcek, J., 1987, Human beta$_2$ interferon and B-cell differentiation factor BSF-2 are identical, *Science* **235**:731.

Seigel, L. J., 1984, Gene for T-cell growth factor—Location on human chromosome 4Q and feline chromosome B1, *Science* **223**:175.

Seldin, D. C., and Austen, K. F., 1985, Mast cell heterogeneity: The T cell factor-dependent mast cell in vitro and in vivo, in: *The Urticarias* (R. H. Champion, M. W. Greaves, and A. Kobza Black, eds.), Churchill Livingstone, New York.

Seldin, D. C., Austen, K. F., and Stevens, R. L., 1985, Purification and characterization of protease-resistant secretory granule proteoglycans containing chondroitin sulfate di-B and heparin-like glycosaminoglycans from rat basophilic leukemia cells, *J. Biol. Chem.* **260**:11131.

Sen, G. C., 1984, Biochemical pathways in interferon action, *Pharmacol. Ther.* **24**:235.

Serhan, C., 1984, Trihydroxytetraenes: A novel series of compounds formed from arachidonic acid in human leukocytes, *Biochem. Biophys. Res. Commun.* **118**:943.

Serhan, C. N., Hamberg, M., and Samuelsson, B., 1984, Lipoxins—Novel series of biologically active compounds formed from arachidonic acid in human leukocytes, *Proc. Natl. Acad. Sci. U.S.A.* **81**:5335.

Shavit, Y., Terman, G. W., Martin, F. C., Lewis, J. W., Liebeskind, J. C., and Gale, R. P., 1985, Stress, opioid peptides, the immune system and cancer, *J. Immunol.* **135**(Suppl.):834.

Shavit, Y., Lewis, J. W., Terman, G. W., Gale, R. P., and Liebeskind, J. C., 1986, Stress, opioid peptides and immune function, in: *Neuroregulation of Autonomic, Endocrine and Immune Systems* (R. C. A. Frederickson, H. C. Hendrie, J. N. Hingtgen, and M. H. Aprison, eds.), pp. 343–366, Kluwer Academic, Hingham, MA.

Shaw, R. J., Walsh, G. M., Cromwell, O., Moqbel, R., Spry, C. J. F., and Kay, A. B., 1985, Activated human eosinophils generate SRS-A leukotrienes following IgG-dependent stimulation, *Nature (Lond.)* **316**:150.

Shelhamer, J. H., Maron, Z., Sun, F., Bach, M. K., and Kaliner, M., 1982, The effects of arachinoids and leukotrienes on the release of mucous from human airways, *Chest* **81**:36S.

Shepherd, G. M., 1983, *Neurobiology*, Oxford University Press, New York.

Showell, H. J., Naccache, P. H., Borgeat, P., Picard, S., Vallerand, P., Becker, E. L., and Sha'afi, R. I., 1982, Characterization of the secretory activity of leukotriene B4 toward rabbit neutrophils, *J. Immunol.* **128**:811.

Simon, P. L., and Willoughby, W. F., 1981, The role of subcellular factors in pulmonary immune function: Physicochemical characterization of two distinct species of lymphocyte-activating factors produced by rabbit alveolar macrophages, *J. Immunol.* **126**:1534.

Singer, K. H., Harden, E. A., Robertson, A. L., Lobach, D. F., and Haynes, B. F., 1985, In vitro growth and phenotypic characterization of mesodermal-derived and epithelial components of normal and abnormal human thymus, *Hum. Immunol.* **13**:161.

Singer, K. H., Wolf, L. S., Lobach, D. F., Denning, S. M., Tuck, D. T., Robertson, A. L., and Haynes, B. F., 1986, Human thymocytes bind to autologous and allogeneic thymic epithelial cells in vitro, *Proc. Natl. Acad. Sci. U.S.A.* **83**:6588.

Singh, J., 1981, The ultrastructure of epithelial reticular cells, in: *The Thymus Gland* (M. D. Kendall, ed.), pp. 133–150, Academic, Orlando, Florida.

Singh, U., and Goldowitz, D., 1982, Effect of sympathectomy on lymphopoiesis in anterior eye chamber thymic explants, *Int. J. Immunopharmacol.* **4**:301.

Siraganian, R. P., and Osler, A. G., 1971, Destruction of rabbit platelets in the allergic response of sensitized leukocytes. I. Demonstration of a fluid phase intermediate, *J. Immunol.* **106**:1244.

Sirois, P., 1985, Pharmacology of leukotrienes, *Adv. Lipid Res.* **21**:79.

Smith, E. M., and Blalock, J. E., 1981, Human leukocyte production of ACTH and endorphin-like substances: Association with leukocyte interferon, *Proc. Natl. Acad. Sci. U.S.A.* **78**:7530.

Smith, E. M., Meyer, W. J., and Blalock, J. E., 1982, Virus-induced corticosterone in hypothysectomized mice: A possible lymphoid adrenal axis, *Science* **218**:1311.

Smith, E. M., Phan, M., Coppenhaver, D., Kruger, T. E., and Blalock, J. E., 1983, Human leukocyte production of immunorective thyrotropin, *Proc. Natl. Acad. Sci. U.S.A.* **80**:6010.

Smith, E. M., Harbour-McMenamin, D., and Blalock, J. E., 1985, Lymphocyte production of endorphins and endorphin-mediated immunoregulatory activity, *J. Immunol.* **135**(Suppl.):779.

Smith, E. M., Morrill, A. C., Meyer, W. J., III, and Blalock, J. E., 1986, Corticotropin releasing factor induction of leukocyte-derived immunoreactive ACTH and endorphins, *Nature (Lond.)* **324**:884.

Smith, L. J., Greenberger, P. A., Patterson, R., Krell, R. D., Bernstein, P. R., 1985, The effect of inhaled leukotriene D_4 in humans, *Am. Rev. Respir. Dis.* **131**:368.

Smith, M. J. H., Ford-Hutchinson, A. W., and Bray, M. A., 1980, Leukotriene B—A potential mediator of inflammation, *J. Pharmacol.* **32**:517.

Smith, T. J., Hougland, M. W., and Johnson, D. A., 1984, Human lung tryptase, purification and characterization, *J. Biol. Chem.* **259**:11046.

Snapper, C. M., and Paul, W. E., 1987, B cell stimulator factor 1 (interleukin 4) prepares resting murine B cells to secrete IgGl upon subsequent stimulation with bacterial lipopolysaccharide, *J. Immunol.* **139**:10.

Snow, E. C., 1985, Insulin and growth hormone function as minor growth factors that potentiate lymphocyte activation, *J. Immunol.* **135**(Suppl.):776.

Snyder, F., 1985, Chemical and biochemical aspects of platelet activating factor: A novel class of acetylated ether linked choline phospholipids, *Med. Res. Rev.* **5**:107.

Snyder, S. H., 1984, Drug and neurotransmitter receptors in the brain, *Science* **224**:22.

Snyderman, R., and Goetzl, E. J., 1981, Molecular and cellular mechanisms of leukocyte chemotaxis, *Science* **213**:830.

Soter, N. A., Wasserman, S. I., and Austen, K. F., 1976, Cold urticaria—Release into circulation of histamine and eosinophil chemotactic factor of anaphylaxis during cold challenge, *N. Engl. J. Med.* **294**:687.

Soter, N. A., Lewis, R. A., Corey, E. J., and Austen, K. F., 1983, Local effects of synthetic leukotrienes (LTC4, LTD4, LTE4, and LTB4) in human skin, *J. Invest. Dermatol.* **80**:115.

Spangelo, B. L., Hall, N. R., and Goldstein, A. L., 1987, Biology and chemistry of thymosin peptides. Modulators of immunity and neuroendocrine circuits, in: *Neuroimmune Interactions* (B. D. Jankovic, B. M. Markovic, and N. H. Spector, eds.), *Ann. N.Y. Acad. Sci.* **496**:196.

Spector, N. H., 1986, Interactions among the nervous, endocrine and immune systems (NIM), in: *Neuroregulation of Autonomic, Endocrine and Immune Systems* (R. C. A. Frederickson, H. C. Hendrie, J. N. Hingtgen, and M. H. Aprison, eds.), pp. 329–341, Kluwer Academic, Hingham, MA.

Spits, Y., Yssel, H., Arai, K., Takebe, Y., Yokota, T., Lee, F., Arai, N., Banchereau, J., and DeVries, J. E., 1987, The effects of recombinant human IL-4 on T cells, *Lymphokine Res.* **6**: 1815 (abst.).

Stanisz, A. M., Befus, D., and Bienenstock, J., 1986, Differential effects of vasoactive intestinal peptide, substance P, and somatostatin on immunoglobulin synthesis and proliferation by lymphocytes from Peyer's patches, mesenteric lymph nodes, and spleen, *J. Immunol.* **136**:152.

Stanisz, A. M., Scicchitano, R., Payan, D. G., and Bienenstock, J., 1987, In vitro studies of immunoregulation by substance P and somatostatin, in: *Neuroimmune Interactions* (B. D. Jankovic, B. M. Markovic, and N. H. Spector, eds.), *Ann. N.Y. Acad. Sci.* **496**:56.

Stanley, E. R., 1981, Colony stimulating factors, in: *The Lymphokines—Biochemistry and Biological Activity* (J. W. Hadden and W. E. Stewart, II, eds.), pp. 101–132, Humana Press, Clifton, New Jersey.

Stanley, E. R., and Heard, P. M., 1977, Factors regulating macrophage production and growth—Purification and some properties of colony-stiulating factor from medium conditioned by mouse L cells, *J. Biol. Chem.* **252**:4305.

Stavnezer-Nordgren, J., and Sirlin, S., 1986, Specificity of immunoglobulin heavy chain switch correlates with activity of germline heavy chain genes prior to switching, *Eur. Molec. Biol. Org. J.* **5**:95.

Steeg, P. A., Moore, R. N., Johnson, H. M., and Oppenheim, J. J., 1982, Regulation of murine macrophage Ia antigen expression by a lymphokine with immune interferon activity, *J. Exp. Med.* **156**: 1780.

Steel, L. K., and Kaliner, M. A., 1981, Prostaglandin-generating factor of anaphylaxis: identification and isolation, *J. Biol. Chem.* **256**:12692.

Steel, L. K., Bach, D., and Kaliner, M. A., 1982, Prostaglandin-generating factor of anaphylaxis. II. Characterization of activity, *J. Immunol.* **129**:1233.

Stein, M., Keller, St. E., and Schleifer, S. J., 1985, Stress and immunomodulation: The role of depression and neuroendocrine function, *J. Immunol.* **135**(Suppl.):827.

Stenson, W. F., and Parker, C. W., 1979, 12-L-Hydroxy-5,8,10,14-eicosatetraenoic acid, a chemotactic fatty-acid, is incorporated into neutrophil phospholipids and triglyceride, *Prostaglandins* **18**:285.

Stevens, R. L., Razin, E., Austen, K. F., Hein, A., Caulfield, J. P., Seno, N., Schmid, K., and Akiyama, F., 1983, Synthesis of chondroitin SO4 E glycosaminoglycan onto p-nitrophenyl beta-D-xyloside and its localization to secretory granules of rat serosal mast cells and mucosal bone marrow derived mast cells, *J. Biol. Chem.* **258:**5977.

Stevens, R. L., Otsu, K., and Austen, K. F., 1985, Purification and analysis of the protease-resistant intracellular chondroitin sulfate E proteoglycan from the interleukin 3-dependent mouse mast cell, *J. Biol. Chem.* **260:**14194.

Stewart, W. E., II, 1981, *The Interferon System,* 2nd ed., Springer-Verlag, Heidelberg.

Stimler, N. P., Hugli, T. E., and Bloor, C. M., 1980, Pulmonary injury induced by C3a and C5a anaphylatoxins, *Am. J. Pathol.* **100:**327.

Stimler, N. P., Bloor, C. M., Hugli, T. E., Wykle, R. L., McCall, C. E., and O'Flaherty, J. T., 1981, Anaphylactic actions of platelet-activating factor, *Am. J. Pathol.* **105:**64.

Stimler, N. P., Bach, M. K., Bloor, C. M., and Hugli, T. E., 1982, Release of leukotrienes from guinea pig lung stimulated by C5ADES arg anaphylatoxin, *J. Immunol.* **128:**2247.

Stimler, N. P., and O'Flaherty, J. T., 1983, Spasmogenic properties of platelet-activating factor: Evidence for a direct mechanism in the contractile response of pulmonary tissue, *Am. J. Pathol.* **113:**75.

Stites, D. P., Stobo, J. D., and Wells, J. V. (eds.), 1987, *Basic and Clinical Immunology,* Vol. 6, Appleton & Lange, E. Norwalk, Connecticut.

Stjarne, L., Hedqvist, P., Lagercrantz, H., and Wennmalm, A., 1981, *Chemical Neurotransmission,* Academic, London.

Struyker-Boudier, H. A. J., Nievelstein, H. M. N. W., Tijssen, C. M., and Smits, J. F. M., 1985, Regional hemocynamic actions of platelet activating factor (PAF) in conscious spontaneously hypertensive rats (SHR), *Prostaglandins* **30:**726.

Stutman, O., 1983, Role of thymic hormones in T cell differentiation, *Clin. Immunol. Allergy* **3:**9.

Swain, S. L., 1985, Role of BCGFII activity on activated B cells of a purified murine T cell-replacing factor (TRF) from a T cell hybridoma (B151K12), *J. Immunol.* **134:**3944.

Swain, S. L., and Dutton, R. W., 1982, Production of a B cell growth-promoting activity (DL)BCGF, from a cloned T cell line and its assay on the BCLI B cell tumor, *J. Exp. Med.* **156:**1821.

Swain, S. L., Dennert, G., Warner, J. F, and Dutton, R. W., 1981, Culture supernatants of a stimulated T cell line have helper activity that acts synergistically with interleukin 2 in the response of B cells to antigen, *Proc. Natl. Acad. Sci. U.S.A.* **78:**2517.

Swain, S., Howard, M., Kappler, J., Marrack, P., Watson, J., Booth, R., and Dutton, R., 1983, Evidence for two distinct classes of murine B-cell growth factors with activities in different functional assays, *J. Exp. Med.* **158:**822.

Swanson, L. W., and Sawchenko, P. E., 1983, Hypothalamic integration: Organization of the paraventricular and supraoptic nuclei, *Annu. Rev. Neurosci.* **6:**269.

Sykora, K. W., Kolitz, J., Szabo, P. Grzeschik, K. H., Moore, M. A. S., and Mertelsmann, R., 1984, Human interleukin-2 gene is located on chromosome 4, *Cancer Invest.* **2:**261.

Szabo, S., Sandrock, A. W., Nafradi, J., Maull, E. A., Gallagher, G. T., and Blyzniuk, A., 1982, Dopamine and dopamine receptors in the gut: Their possible role in duodenal ulceration, in: *Advances in Dopamine Research,* Vol. 37, *Advances in Bioscience,* (M. Kohsaka, T. Shohmori, Y. Tsukada, and G. N. Woodruff, eds.), pp. 165–170, Pergamon, London.

Szentivanyi, A., 1953, Allergie und zentralnervensystem. Proceedings of Second European Congress of Allergology, *Acta Allergol.* **6:**27.

Szentivanyi, A., 1961, Hypothalamic influences on antibody formation and on bronchial responses to histamine, in: *Proceedings of the Fourth Aspen Conference on Research in Emphysema and Asthma,* p. 78.

Szentivanyi, A., 1968, The beta adrenergic theory of the atopic abnormality in bronchial asthma, *J. Allergy* **42:**203.

Szentivanyi, A., 1971, Effect of bacterial products and adrenergic blocking agents on allergic reactions, in *Textbook of Immunological Diseases,* 2nd ed. (M. Samter, D. W. Talmage, B. Rose, W. B. Sherman, and J. H. Vaughan, eds.), pp. 356–374, Little, Brown, Boston.

Szentivanyi, A., 1988, *The Physiology and Pharmacology of Allergy*, Vol. 81, *Handbook of Experimental Pharmacology*, Springer-Verlag, Heidelberg.

Szentivanyi, A., and Filipp, G., 1956, Experimentelle data zur regulativen rolle des neuroendokriniums in experimenteller anaphylaxie. II. Relazione e communicazione, p. 237, Rome II Pansiero Scientifico.

Szentivanyi, A., and Filipp, G., 1958a, Anaphylaxis and the nervous system. Part II, *Ann. Allergy* 16:143.

Szentivanyi, A., and Fillip, G., 1958b, Anaphylaxis and the nervous system. Part III, *Ann. Allergy* 16:306.

Szentivanyi, A., and Filipp, G., 1958c, Anaphylaxis and the nervous system. Part IV, *Ann. Allergy* 16:389.

Szentivanyi, A., and Fishel, C. W., 1965, Effect of bacterial products on responses to the allergic mediators, in: *Immunological Diseases*, 1st ed. (M. Samter and H. L. Alexander, eds.), pp. 226–241, Little, Brown, Boston.

Szentivanyi, A., and Fishel, C. W., 1966, Die Amin-Mediatorstoffe der Allergishen Reaktion und die Reaktionsfahigkeit ihrer Exfolgszellen. in: *Pathogenese und Therapie Allergischer Reaktionen: Grundlagenforschung und Klinik* (G. Filipp, ed.), pp. 588–683, Ferdinand Enke Verlag, Stuttgart.

Szentivanyi, A., and Fitzpatrick, D. F., 1980, The altered reactivity of the effector cells to antigenic and pharmacologic influences and its relation to cyclic nucleotides. I. Effector reactivities in the efferent loop of the immune response, in: *Allergologie. I. Atiopathogenese* (G. Filipp, ed.), pp. 511–580, Werk-Verlag Dr. Edmund Banaschewski, Munchen-Grafelfing.

Szentivanyi, A., and Szekely, J., 1956, Effect of injury to, and electrical stimulation of, hypothalamic areas on the anaphylactic and histamine shock of the guinea pig, *Ann. Allergy* 14:259.

Szentivanyi, A., and Szekely, J., 1957a, Uber den effekt der schadigung und der elektrischen reizung der hypothalamischen gegenden au den anaphylaktischen und histamin-schock des meerschweinchens, *Allergie Asthmaforsch.* 1:23.

Szentivanyi, A., and Szekely, J., 1957b, Wirkung der konstanten reizung hypothalamischer strukturen durch tiefenelektroden auf den histamin-bedingten und anaphylaktischen schock des meerschweinchens, *Acta Physiol. Hung.* 1141-42(Suppl. V):41.

Szentivanyi, A., and Szentivanyi, J., 1985, Cellular and molecular foundations of immunity, immunologic inflammation and hypersensitivity. Component parts and their relation to neurohumoral control mechanisms, in: *Sodeman's Pathologic Physiology—Mechanisms of Disease* (W. A. Sodeman and T. A. Sodeman, eds.), pp. 113–150, W. B. Saunders, Philadelphia.

Szentivanyi, A., and Williams, J. F., 1980, The constitutional basis of atopic disease, in: *Allergic Diseases of Infancy, Childhood, and Adolescence* (C. W. Bierman and D. S. Pearlman, eds.), pp. 173–210, W. B. Saunders, Philadelphia.

Szentivanyi, A., Filipp, G., and Legeza, I., 1952, Investigations on tobacco sensitivity, *Acta Med. Hung.* 2:175.

Szentivanyi, A., Polson, J. B., and Krzanowski, J. J., 1980, The altered reactivity of the effector cells to antigenic and pharmacological influences and its relation to cyclic nucleotides. I. Effector reactivities in the afferent loop of the immune response, in: *Allergologie. I. Atiopathogenese* (G. Filipp, ed.), pp. 460–510, Werk-Verlag Dr. Edmund Banaschewski, Munchen-Grafelfing.

Szentivanyi, A., Krzanowski, J. J., and Polson, J. B., 1983a, The autonomic nervous system, in: *Allergy—Principles and Practice*, 2nd ed. (E. Middleton, C. E. Reed, and E. F. Ellis, eds.), pp. 303–331, C. V. Mosby, St. Louis.

Szentivanyi, A., Middleton, E., Williams, J. F., and Friedman, H., 1983b, Effect of microbial agents on the immune network and associated pharmacologic reactivities, in: *Allergy—Principles and Practice*, 2nd ed. (E. Middleton, C. E. Reed, and E. F. Ellis, eds.), pp. 211–236, C. V. Mosby, St. Louis.

Szentivanyi, A., Polson, J. B., and Szentivanyi, J., 1985, Adrenergic regulation, in: *Bronchial*

Asthma: Mechanisms and Therapeutics (E. B. Weiss, M. S. Segal, and M. Stein, eds.), pp. 126–150, Little, Brown, Boston.

Szentivanyi, J., Szentivanyi, A., Wiliams, J. F., and Friedman, H., 1986, Virus associated immune and pharmacologic mechanisms in disorders of respiratory and cutaneous atopy, in: *Viruses, Immunity and Immunodeficiency* (A. Szentivanyi and H. Friedman, eds.), pp. 211–244, Plenum, New York.

Szentivanyi, A., Maurer, P., and Janicki, B. W. (eds.), 1987, *Antibodies: Structure, Synthesis, Function, and Immunologic Intervention in Disease,* Plenum, New York.

Szentivanyi, A., Krzanowski, J. J., and Polson, J. B., 1988, The autonomic nervous system and altered effector responses, in: *Allergy—Principles and Practice,* 3rd ed. (E. Middleton, C. E. Reed, and E. F. Ellis, eds.), pp. 461–493, C. V. Mosby, St. Louis.

Takatsu, K., Tanaka, K., Tominaga, A., Kumahara, Y., and Hamaoka, T., 1980a, Antigen-induced T cell-replacing factor (TRF). III. Establishment of T cell hybrid clone continuously producing TRF and functional analysis of released TRF, *J. Immunol.* **125:**2646.

Takatsu, K., Tominaga, A., and Hamaoka, T., 1980b, Antigen-induced T cell-replacing factor (TRF). I. Functional characterization of a TRF-producing helper T cell subset and genetic studies on TRF production, *J. Immunol.* **124:**2414.

Takatsu, K., Harada, N., Hara, Y., Takahama, Y., Yamada, G., Dobashi, K., and Hamaoka, T., 1985, Purification and physicochemical characterization of murine T cell replacing factor (TRF), *J. Immunol.* **134:**382.

Takatsu, K., Kikuchi, Y., Takahashi, T., Honjo, T., Matsumoto, M., Harada, N., Yamaguchi, N., and Tominaga, A., 1987, Interleukin 5, a T-cell-derived B-cell differentiation factor also induces cytotoxic T lymphocytes, *Proc. Natl. Acad. Sci. U.S.A.* **84:**4234.

Takebe, Y., Otsuka, T., Villaret, D., Yokota, T., Lee, F., Arai, K., and Arai, N., 1987, Structural analysis of the mouse and human chromosomal genes encoding interleukin 4 which expresses B cell, T cell, and mast cell stimulating activities, *Lymphokine Res.* **6:**1328 (abst.).

Talbot, S. F., Atkins, P. C., Goetzel, E. J., and Zweiman, B., 1985, Accumulation of leukotriene C4 and histamine in human allergic skin reactions, *J. Clin. Invest.* **76:**650.

Talmage, D. W., 1986, The acceptance and rejection of immunological concepts, *Annu. Rev. Immunol.* **4:**1.

Tanaka, S., Kasuya, Y., Masuda, Y., and Shigenobu, K., 1983, Studies on the hypotensive effects of platelet activating factor (PAF, 1-*O*-alkyl-2-acetyl-*sn*-glyceryl-3-phosphorylcholine) in rats, guinea pigs, rabbits and dogs, *J. Pharmacol. Dyn.* **6:**866.

Taniguichi, T., Matsui, H., Fujita, T., Takaoka, C., Kashima, N., Yoshimoto, R., and Hamuro, J., 1983, Structure and expression of a cloned cDNA for human interleukin 2, *Nature (Lond.)* **302:**305.

Tapia-Arancibia, L., and Reichlin, S., 1985, Vasoactive intestinal polypeptide and PHI stimulate somatostatin release from cat cerebral cortical and diencephalic cells in dispersed cell culture, *Brain Res.* **36:**67.

Terashita, Z., Imura, Y., Nishikawa, K., and Sumida, S., 1985, Is platelet activating factor (PAF) a mediator of endotoxin shock, *Eur. J. Pharmacol.* **109:**257.

Tharp, M. D., Thirlby, R., and Sullivan, T. J., 1984, Gastrin induces histamine release from human cutaneous mast cells, *J. Allergy Clin. Immunol.* **74:**159.

Theoharides, T. C., and Douglas, W. W., 1981, Mast cell histamine secretion in response to somatostatin analogues: Structural considerations, *Eur. J. Pharmacol.* **73:**131.

Thomson, M. A., Seegers, R. M., Keegan, S. C., and Utermohlen, V., 1987, Effect of recombinant interleukin 1 and thymulin on DNFB induced delayed type hypersensitivity in mice, *Lymphokine Res.* **6:**1242 (abst.).

Thueson, D. O., Speck, L. S., Lett-Brown, M. A., and Grant, J. A., 1979, Histamine releasing activity (HRA). II. Interaction with basophils and physiochemical characterization, *J. Immunol.* **123:**633.

Thurman, G. B., Low, T. K. L., Rossio, J. L., and Goldstein, A. L., 1981, Specific and nonspecific macrophage migration inhibition, in: *Lymphokines and Thymic Hormones: Their Potential Utilization in Cancer Therapeutics* (A. L. Goldstein and M. A. Chirigos, eds.), pp. 145–157, Raven, New York.

Timonen, T., Ortaldo, J. R., and Herberman, R. B., 1982, Analysis by a single cell cytotoxicity assay of natural killer (NK) cell frequencies among human large granular lymphocytes and of the effects of interferon on their activity, *J. Immunol.* **128**:2514.

Torres, B. A., Farrar, W. L., and Johnson, H. M., 1982, Interleukin 2 regulates immune interferon (IFN-gamma) production by normal and suppressor cell cultures, *J. Immunol.* **128**:2217.

Tosato, G., Jones, K. D., and Pike, S. E., 1988, Interferon beta-2/B cell stimulatory factor 2/interleukin 6 is a growth factor for Epstein–Barr virus-infected human B cells, *FASEB J.* **2**:A455 (abst. 925).

Touvay, C., Etienne, A., and Braquet, P., 1985, Inhibition of antigen-induced lung anaphylaxis in the guinea-pig by BN 52021, a new specific PAF-acether receptor antagonist isolated from Ginkgo biloba, *Agents Actions* **17**:371.

Touvay, C., Vilain, B., Etienne, A., Clostra, F., and Braquet, P., 1988, Pharmacological control of the contraction of guinea-pig lung strips induced by platelet-activating factor (PAF-acether), *Prostaglandins Leukotrienes Med. Pharmacol. Res. Commun.* **18**:91.

Trainin, N., 1982, Role of thymus humoral factor, a thymic hormone, in the physiology of the thymus, in: *Polypeptide Hormones* (R. F. Beers and E. C. Bassett, eds.), pp. 467–488, Raven, New York.

Tucek, S., 1982, The synthesis of acetylcholine, in: *Handbook of Neurochemistry*, 2nd ed. (A. Lajtha, ed.), Vol. 4, pp. 219–249, Plenum, New York.

Turk, J., Maas, M. L., Brash, A. R., Roberts, L. J., II, and Oates, J. A., 1982, Arachidonic acid 15-lipoxygenase products from human eosinophils, *J. Biol. Chem.* **257**:7068.

Turner, S. R., Tainer, J. A., and Lynn, W. S., 1975, Biogenesis of chemotactic molecules by arachidonate lipoxygenase system of platelets, *Nature (Lond.)* **257**:680.

Twomey, J. J., and Kouttab, N. M., 1982, Selected phenotypic induction of null lymphocytes from mice with thymic and nonthymic agents, *Cell. Immunol.* **72**:186.

Uchiyama, T., Nelson D, Fleisher, T., and Waldmann, T., 1981, A monoclonal antibody (anti-T) reactive with activated and functionally mature human T cells. II. Expression of Tac antigen on activated cytotoxic killer T cells, *J. Immunol.* **126**:1398.

Ullberg, M., Merrill, J., and Tondal, M., 1981, Interferon-induced NK augmentation in humans: an analysis of target recognition, effector cell recruitment and effector cell recycling, *Scand. J. Immunol.* **14**:285.

Umezawa, H., 1972, *Enzyme Inhibitors of Microbial Origin*, University of Toyko Press, Toyko.

Unanue, E. R., and Rosenthal, A. S., 1980, *Macrophage Regulation of Immunity*, Academic, New York.

Uvnas, B., and Tasaka, K. (eds.), 1982, *Advances in Histamine Research*, Vol. 33, *Advances in the Biosciences*, Pergamon, Oxford.

Vahouny, G. V., Kyeyune-Nyombi, E., McGillis, J. P., Tare, N. S., Huang, K. Y., Tombes, R., Goldstein, A. L., and Hall, N. R., 1983, Thymosin peptides and lymphokines do not directly stimulate adrenal corticosteroid production in vitro, *J. Immunol.* **130**:791.

Vale, W., Brazeau, P., Rivier, C., Brown, M., Boss, B., Rivier, J., Burgus, R., Ling, N., and Guillemin, R., 1975, Somatostatin, *Recent Prog. Horm. Res.* **31**:365.

Valone, F. H., Coles, E., Reinhold, V. R., and Goetzl, E. J., 1982, Specific binding of phospholipid platelet-activating factor by human platelets, *J. Immunol.* **129**:1637.

Valone, F. H., and Goetzl, E. J., 1983, Specific binding by human polymorphonuclear leukocytes of the immunological mediator 1-*O*-hexadecyl/octadecyl-2-acetyl-*sn*-glycero-3-phosphorylcholine, *Immunology* **48**:141.

Van Damme, J., DeLey, M., Van Snick, J., Dinarello, C. A., and Billiau, A., 1987, The role of interferon beta$_1$ and the 26-kDa protein (interferon beta$_2$) as mediators of the antiviral effect of interleukin 1 and tumor necrosis factor, *J. Immunol.* **139**:1867.

Vanderhoek, J. Y., Bryant, R. W., and Bailey, J. M., 1980, Inhibition of leukotriene biosynthesis by the leukocyte product 15-hydroxy-5,8,11,13-eicosatetraenoic acid, *J. Biol. Chem.* **255:** 1064.

Van Epps, D. E., and Saland, L., 1984, Beta-endorphin and met-enkephalin stimulate human peripheral blood mononuclear cell chemotaxis, *J. Immunol.* **132:**3046.

van Furth, R. (ed.), 1985, *Mononuclear Phagocytes and Inflammation*, Martinus Nijhoff, Boston.

Vanhoutte, P. M. (ed.), 1985, *Serotonin and the Cardiovascular System*, Raven, New York.

Van Praag, D., and Farber, S. J., 1981, Leukotriene synthesis in rabbit kidney, *Fed. Proc.* **40:**1713.

Vargaftig, B. B., Lefort, J., Chignard, M., and Benveniste, J., 1980, Platelet-activating factor induces a platelet-dependent bronchoconstriction unrelated to the formation of prostaglandin derivatives, *Eur. J. Pharmacol.* **65:**185.

Venter, J. C., Fraser, C. M., Lilly, L., Seeman, P., Eddy, B., and Schaber, J., 1984, The structure of neurotransmitter receptors (adrenergic, dopaminergic and muscarinic cholinergic), in *Catecholamines: Basic and Peripheral Mechanisms* (E. Usdin, A. Carlsson, A. Dahlstrom, and J. Engel, eds.), Alan R. Liss, New York.

Vickroy, T. W., Watson, M., Yamamura, H. I., and Roeske, W. R., 1984, Agonist binding to multiple muscarinic receptors, *Fed. Proc.* **43:**2785.

Vilcek, J., DeMaeyer, E. (eds.), 1984, *Interferon 2: Interferons and the Immune System*, Elsevier/North-Holland, Amsterdam.

Villarreal, H., Canseco, M., Espinoza, L. R., and Zabriskie, J. B., 1983, Post-streptococcal glomerulonephritis. The role of immune complexes, in: *Circulating Immune Complexes. Their Clinical Significance*, (L. R. Espinoza and C. K. Osterland, eds.), pp. 191–218, Futura, Mt. Kisco, New York.

Vitetta, E. S., Brooks, K., Chen, Y.-W., Isakson, P., Jones, S., Layton, J., Mishra, G. C., Pure, E., Weiss, E., Word, C., Yuan, D., Tucker, P., Uhr, J. W., and Krammer, P. H., 1984, T-cell derived lymphokines that induce IgM and IgG secretion in activated murine B-cells, *Immunol. Rev.* **78:**137.

Vitetta, E. S., Ohara, J., Myers, C., Layton, J., Krammer, P. H., and Paul, W. E., 1985, Serological, biochemical, and functional identity of B-cell differentiation factor for IgG1, *J. Exp. Med.* **162:**1726.

Voelkel, N. F., Worthen, N. F., Reeves, J. T., Henson, P. M., and Murphy, R. C., 1982, Nonimmunological production of leukotrienes induced by platelet activating factor, *Science* **218:**286.

Von Euler, U. S. and Gaddum, J. H., 1931, An unidentified depressor substance in certain tissue extracts, *J. Physiol. (Lond.)* **72:**74.

Wagner, F. F. W., Dancygier, H., Fink, R., Hart, R., Berg, J., and Classen, M., 1987, Substance P enhances mitogen-induced interferon gamma production by human peripheral blood mononuclear cells, *Lymphokine Res.* **6:**1459 (abst.).

Wagner-Roos, L., Hauschildt, S., Mock, W., and Bessler, W. G., 1987, Synthetic lipopeptides as B-lymphocyte growth and differentiation factors: Effects on protein kinase C and phosphoinositide metabolism, *Lymphokine Res.* **6:**1821 (abst.).

Waksman, B. H., 1985, Neuroimmunomodulation of homeostasis and host defense, *J. Immunol.* **135** (Suppl.):862.

Wallner, B. P., Mattaliano, R. J., Hession, C., Cate, R. L., Tizard, R., Sinclair, L. K., Foeller, C., Show, E. P., Browning, J. L., Ramachandran, K. L., and Pepinsky, R. B., 1986, Cloning and expression of human lipocortin: A phospholipase A_2 inhibitor with potential anti-inflammatory activity, *Nature (Lond.)* **320:**77.

Walz, A., Vornhagen, R., Bohlen, P., Hirai, K., and Stadler, B. M., 1987, Human IL-3-like activity shows sequence homology with G-CSF, *Lymphokine Res.* **6:**1311 (abst.).

Wang, S. S., Wang, B. S. H., Chang, J. K., Low, T. L. K., and Goldstein, A. L., 1982, Synthesis of thymosin beta-4, *Int. J. Peptide Protein Res.* **18:**413.

Wara, D. W., 1983, Thymic hormones in primary immunodeficiency, *Clin. Immunol. Allergy* **3:** 169.

Warner, J. A., Pienkowski, M. M., Plaut, M., Norman, P. S., and Lichtenstein, L. M., 1986, Identification of a histamine releasing factor in the late phase of cutaneous IgE mediated reactions, *J. Immunol.* **136:**2583.

Wasi, S., Movat, H. Z., Passe, E., and Chan, J. Y. C., 1978, Kinin formation, conversion and inactivation by neutrophil leukocyte proteases, in: *International Symposium on Neutral Proteases of Human Polymorphonuclear Leucocytes: Biochemistry, Physiology and Clinical Significance,* (K. Havemann and A. Janoff, eds.), Urban and Schwarzenberg, Munich.

Webb, D. R., Nowowiejski, I., Healy, C., and Rogers, T. J., 1982, Immunosuppressive properties of leukotriene D-4 and E-4 in vitro, *Biochem. Biophys. Res. Commun.* **104:**1617.

Wedmore, C. V,. and Williams, T. J., 1981, Platelet-activating factor (PAF), a secretory product of polymorphonuclear leukocytes, increases vascular permeability in rabbit skin, *Br. J. Pharmacol.* **74:**916P.

Weinstein, Y., Segal, S., and Melmon, K. L., 1975, Specific mitogenic activity of 8-Br-Guanosine 3′,5′-monophosphate (Br-cyclic GMP) on B lymphocytes, *J. Immunol.* **115:**112.

Weissenbach, J., Chernajovski, Y., Zeevi, M., Shulman, L., Soreq, H., Nir, U., Wallach, D., Perricaudet, M., Toillais, P., and Revel, M., 1980, Two interferon mRNAs in human fibroblasts: In vitro translation and *Escherichia coli* cloning studies, *Proc. Natl. Acad. Sci. U.S.A.* **77:**7152.

Weller, P. F., Lee, C. W., Foster, D. W., Corey, E. J., Austen, K. F., and Lewis, R. A., 1983, Generation and metabolism of 5-lipoxygenase pathway leukotrienes by human eosinophils: Predominant production of leukotriene C4, *Proc. Natl. Acad. Sci. U.S.A.* **80:**7626.

Werle, E., 1937, Uber den aktivitatszustand des kallikreins der bauchspeicheldruse und ihres außeren sekretes beim hund, *Biochem. Z.* **290:**129.

Werle, E., and Berek, U., 1948, Zur kenntnis des kallikreins, *Angew. Chem.* **60:**53.

Westly, H. J., Kleiss, A. J., Kelley, K. W., Wang, P. K. Y., and Yuen, P.-H., 1986, Newcastle disease virus-infected splenocytes express the proopiomelanocortin gene, *J. Exp. Med.* **163:** 1589.

Westly, H. J., Kleiss, A. J., Kelley, K. W., Wang, P. K. Y., and Yuen, P.-H., 1987, The postulated lymphoid-adrenal axis, in: *Neuroimmune Interactions* (B. D. Jankovic, B. M. Markovic, and N. H. Spector, eds.), *Ann. N.Y. Acad. Sci.* **496:**98.

Westmacott, D., Hawkes, J. E., Clarke, L. E., and Wadsworth, J., 1987, Acute phase protein and neutrophilia responses to recombinant human interleukin-1-alpha in mice: Some properties and pharmacological studies, *Lymphokine Res.* **6:**1222 (abst.).

Westmacott, D., Hill, R. P., Nixon, J. S., and Wilkinson, S., 1987, Inhibition of interleukin-1 and phorbol ester-activated synovial cells by inhibitors of protein kinase C, *Lymphokine Res.* **6:**1223 (abst.).

Whittle, B., Jr., and Moncada, S., 1983, Pharmacology of prostacyclin and thromboxanes, *Br. Med. Bull.* **39:**232.

Whittle, B., Jr., Kauffman, G. L., and Moncada, S., 1981, Vasoconstriction with thromboxane A_2 induces ulceration of the gastric mucosa, *Nature (Lond.)* **292:**472.

Wiggins, R. C., and Cochrane, C. C., 1984, Kinins and kinin-forming system, in: *Textbook of Immunopharmacology* (M. M. Dale and J. C. Foreman, eds.), pp. 158–169, Blackwell Scientific Publications, Oxford.

Williams, J. D., Czop, J. K., and Austen, K. F., 1984, Release of leukotrienes by human monocytes on stimulation of their phagocytic receptor for particulate activators, *J. Immunol.* **132:**3034.

Wilson, C. B., and Dixon, F. J., 1983, Immunologic mechanisms in nephritogenesis, in: *The Biology of Immunologic Disease,* (F. J. Dixon and D. W. Fisher, eds.), pp. 209–222, Sinauer, Sunderland, Massachusetts.

Wintroub, B. U., Schechter, N. M., Lazarus, G. S., Kaempfer, C. E., and Schwartz, L. B., 1984,

Angiotensin I conversion by human and rat chymotryptic proteinases, *J. Invest. Dermatol.* **83:** 336.

Wintroub, B. U., Kaempfer, B. S., Schechter, N. M., and Proud, D., 1986, A human lung mast cell chymotrypsin-like proteinase: Identification and partial characterization, *J. Clin. Invest.* **77:** 196.

Wybran, J., Schandene, L., Van Vooren, J.-P., Vandermoten, G., Latinne, D., Sonnet, J., De Bruyere, M., Taelman, H., and Plotnikoff, N. P., 1987, Immunologic properties of methionine-enkephalin and therapeutic implications in AIDS, ARC, and cancer, in: *Neuroimmune Interactions* (B. D. Jankovic, B. M. Markovic, and N. H. Spector, eds.), *Ann. N.Y. Acad. Sci.* **496:** 108.

Xu, G. J., Hannappel, E., Morgan, J., Hempstead, J., and Horecker, B. L., 1982, Synthesis of thymosin beta 4 by peritoneal macrophages and adherent spleen cells, *Proc. Natl. Acad. Sci. U.S.A.* **79:**4006.

Yamamoto, R. S., Harris, P. C., Christensen, C., Orr, S. L., Klostergaard, J., and Granger, G. A., 1982, The identification of two new clases of lymphotoxin released by lectin activated human T lymphocytes that possess Ig-like receptors, in: *Human Lymphokines*, (A. Kahn and N. O. Hill, eds.), pp. 185–198. Academic, Orlando, Florida.

Yokota, T., Otsuka, T., Mosmann, T., Banchereau, J., DeFrance, T., Blanchard, D., DeVries, J. E., Lee, F., and Arai, K.-I., 1986, Isolation and characterization of a human interleukin cDNA clone, homologous to mouse B-cell stimulatory factor 1, that expresses B-cell and T-cell stimulating activities, *Proc. Natl. Acad. Sci. U.S.A.* **83:**5894.

Yokota, T., Otsuka, T., Takebe, Y., Mosmann, T., Banchereau, J., DeVries, J., Arai, N., Miyajima, A., Lee, F., and Arai, K., 1987, Isolation and characterization of mouse and human interleukin (IL-4) genes that express B cell, T cell, and mast cell stimulating activities, *Lymphokine Res.* **6:**1817 (abst.).

Yung, Y.-P., and Moore, M. A. S., 1985, Mast-cell growth factor: Its role in mast cell differentiation, proliferation, and maturation, *Contemp. Top. Mol. Immunol.* **10:**147.

Zweiman, B., 1983, Mast cells in human disease, *Clin. Rev. Allergy* **1:**417.

CHAPTER 5

EARLY BIOCHEMICAL EVENTS IN T-LYMPHOCYTE ACTIVATION BY MITOGENS

JOHN W. HADDEN and RONALD G. COFFEY

1. INTRODUCTION

From the original discovery by Hungerford *et al.* (1959) that extract of kidney bean *Phasiolus vulgaris* caused altered morphology and mitosis in lymphocytes has grown a considerable field of study on the early biochemical events of lymphocyte transformation by plant lectin mitogens. In 1971, the first textbook in the field emerged (Ling, 1971) and was followed in 1975 by a second (Ling and Kay, 1975). Throughout this period, numerous workshops and symposia, including the International Congresses of Immunology (see Progresses in Immunology II–VI), Leukocyte Culture Conferences, and a Cold Spring Harbor Conference on Cell Proliferation (Clarkson and Baserga, 1974), have chronicled the evolution of this field. The list of mitogens has grown from the original phytohemagglutinin (PHA) to include concanavalin A (Con A), and several other plant lectins, phorbol myristate acetate (PMA), calcium ionophore (A23187), and sodium periodate. The relative selectivity of the actions of these mitogens on thymus-dependent (T) lymphocytes has been demonstrated and the general biochemical parameters have been well documented. Central to the study of T-lymphocyte activation by mitogens has been the quest to attach causal significance to early changes and to establish a mitogen signal sequence leading to cellular replication. In some senses this quest has recreated the parable of the blind men and the elephant and to this day there exist schools of adherents to one

JOHN W. HADDEN and RONALD G. COFFEY • Program of Immunopharmacology, Departments of Medicine, Pharmacology, and Medical Microbiology and Immunology, University of South Florida College of Medicine, Tampa, Florida 33612.

causal notion or another. While many different views of the central biochemical mechanisms have evolved, the composite picture clearly establishes the mitogen-activated T lymphocyte as the most extensively studied model for the early biochemical events of cellular activation for proliferation.

The induction of T-lymphocyte proliferation is understood to involve cell–cell interaction and molecular communications. The nature of the intercellular communication on a cell–cell contact basis is not understood, and what evidence is available points to important molecular communications. It is generally accepted that T cells are triggered to proliferate by two signals (see Smith, 1982, for review) (Fig. 1). The mitogen in the relative but not complete absence of accessory cells (Williams *et al.*, 1984) can induce T cells to enter a G_1 phase of the cell cycle from a resting G_0 or ''restricted'' G_1 phase of the cell cycle (Williams *et al.*, 1984; Davis and Lipsky, 1986). This first stage of activation is associated with cellular enlargement or blastogenesis and both RNA and protein synthesis. The lymphocyte does not enter DNA synthesis (S phase) unless a second signal is presented. This second process is thought to be initiated by mitogen interaction directly or indirectly with adherent accessory cells (i.e., monocytes/macrophages), which results in the production of interleukin I (IL-1), previously called lymphocyte activating factor (LAF). The IL-1 thus acts on primed T lymphocytes to induce the production of interleukin II (IL-II, previously called T-cell growth factor (TCGF) and the appearance of cell-surface receptors for IL-2. The cells producing the IL-2 are not known to be the same as or different than the cells expressing IL-2 receptors. In any case, a T cell triggered by mitogen to enter the cell cycle transits a G_1–S boundary as a result of the second signal and completes the cycle. The subsequent divisions do not require re-exposure to the mitogen but do require the presence of IL-2. Relatively little is known about how and precisely when IL-1 is produced by accessory cells like monocytes or macrophages. Its production appears to result from both direct mitogen action and the action of secreted products from activated T lympho-

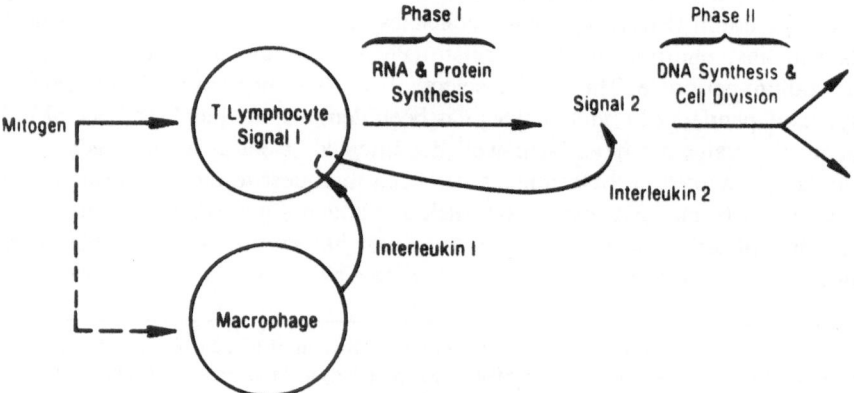

FIGURE 1. Actions of interleukins 1 and 2 (IL-1 and IL-2) in lymphocyte activation.

cytes, such as colony stimulating factor. These accessory cells also down-regulate the process through production of prostaglandins and in turn their effect on lymphocyte cyclic 3',5'adenosine monophosphate (cyclic AMP) level (Folch and Waksman, 1974; Goodwin et al., 1977; Novogrodsky et al., 1979). Little is known of the metabolic events associated with IL-1 action. The vast majority of the studies to date have concentrated on early events following mitogen addition to peripheral blood lymphocytes with the assumptions that the events occur in T cells and are contributive to the replication process.

These studies have also assumed, without proof, that mitogen-induced events are similar or identical to those induced by antigen. These studies have led to hypotheses that a number of different molecules are central to lymphocyte activation, including cyclic AMP (Parker et al., 1974); cyclic 3',5'guanosine monophosphate (cyclic GMP) (Hadden et al., 1979); calcium (Berridge, 1975); cyclic GMP and calcium (Hadden et al., 1975; Hadden, 1977); cyclic AMP, cyclic GMP, and calcium (Whitfield et al., 1976); and others (Resch et al., 1984; Nishizuka, 1984; Berridge, 1984; Kaplan and Owens, 1982). None of these hypotheses has been proved or, for that matter, disproved, and all remain possibilities. In addition to the above, a number of dispassionate reviews have previously appeared (Strom et al., 1977; O'Brien et al., 1978; Hesketh, 1978; Hume and Weidemann, 1980; Robins, 1982). The purpose of the present review is to describe the current status of the information developed on mitogen-induced changes, leading to the initial nuclear activation of T lymphocytes. An attempt is to assess the status of those processes linked to the first signal—the membrane to nuclear signal—to permit evaluation of possible causal events. It may be useful to stress that parallelism between mitogen-induced RNA synthesis and protein (i.e., lymphokine synthesis and/secretion) is a process analogous to the activation for secretion of other cells, such as mast cells and granulocytes. So far, the parallelism of biochemical events is notable. The adaptation of the lymphocyte response to accommodate a second signal, i.e., IL-2, which leads to DNA synthesis, may be unique to the immune system. The processes involved may or may not relate to how other nonlymphoid cells are triggered to divide.

2. SURFACE CHANGES

2.1. Ligand Binding

The first phase of T-lymphocyte transformation is initiated by the binding of the mitogen to cell-surface receptors. It is not necessary for the mitogen to enter the cell, since it has been shown that insolubilized PHA (Greaves and Bauminger, 1972), Con A (Betel and Van den Berg, 1972; Andersson et al., 1972), pokeweed mitogen (W. T. Weber, 1977), and lentil mitogen (Ahmann and Sage, 1974) will induce transformation in the absence of ligand or receptor internalization.

Mitogen responsiveness appears to involve multivalent ligands. Experiments with PHA (Lindahl-Kiessling, 1972), soybean agglutinin (Lotan et al., 1973), and Con A (Wands et al., 1976) suggest that mitogenic ligands must be at least divalent; opinion is divided, however, since two groups (Sawyer et al., 1975; Fraser et al., 1976) have obtained data suggesting that monovalent Con A fragments are capable of stimulating mouse spleen lymphocytes. Reassociation of monovalent Con A dimers into divalent tetramers in the lymphocyte environment was suggested as the explanation by Sawyer et al. (1975); however, Fraser et al. (1976) believed that their freshly prepared monovalent dimers activated lymphocytes before converting to divalent species. In any case, extensive crosslinking and receptor aggregation are not apparently required (McClain et al., 1977).

For both Con A and PHA, ligand binding is virtually complete within 30 min (see Ling and Kay, 1975). It is during this period that the most critical biochemical events are thought to occur. A number of studies have suggested that the mitogen needs to be present for up to 20 hr in order to induce lymphocyte proliferation (see Hadden et al., 1975, for review); however, several works (Soren, 1973; Toyoshima et al., 1976; Milner, 1977) indicate that a single short pulse (3 hr) on either PHA or Con A followed by removal with a competing sugar (N-acetyl galactosamine or α-methyl mannoside, respectively) and washing is sufficient to induce clonal proliferation of lymphocytes. The extent to which proliferation is optimal appears to depend on the mitogen concentration and the time of exposure to the mitogen. Whether all mitogen can be removed under these circumstances is arguable; however, any residual amount would be calculated to be otherwise inactive, on the basis of dose–response relationships. It is clear that a short exposure of mitogen is capable of initiating proliferation in many responsive lymphocytes. This observation indicates a trigger type signal that initiates events that are self sustaining at least long enough to commit the lymphocyte to enter G_1 phase of the cell cycle.

2.2. Membrane Fluidity

Cell-surface proteins can move laterally in the membrane according to the fluid mosaic lipid bilayer model of plasma membranes (Singer and Nicolson, 1972; Bretscher and Raff, 1975). The lipid composition is thought to be crucial in the regulation of the fluidity of the membrane. Using electron paramagnetic resonance of spin-labeled fatty acids to measure fluidity, Barnett et al. (1974) found that PHA or Con A induces rapid increases in fluidity in plasma membranes of mouse and human lymphocytes. The change reached a maximum after 15 or 30 min, respectively and returned to baseline after 60 min. A nonmitogenic lectin, wheat germ agglutinin, had no effect. Similar findings were reported by Toyoshima and Osawa (1975). Inbar and Shinitzky (1975) used fluorescence polarization of the lipophilic 1,6-diphenyl-1,3,5-hexatriene and found no early changes, but rather a slow increase in membrane fluidity that occurred at 24–72 hr in Con A-stimulated rat lymph node cells. Other evidence suggests that these studies may not be conflicting, in that in the latter study the lymph node cells having already been activated by antigen may have different early events. In a recent reinvestigation of membrane fluidity by the fluorescence polarization technique, Tandon et al. (1983) found no changes during the first hour after addition of Con A to rabbit thymocytes.

Other approaches to demonstrate fluidity changes involve direct measurements of membrane lipid composition. Cholesterol content is inversely related to lipid fluidity while the degree of unsaturation of fatty acids in phospholipids is directly related. The decreased cholesterol content of proliferative leukemic cells has been related to increased fluidity in their membranes (Inbar and Shinitzky, 1974a,b); however, normal lymphocytes apparently do not undergo a change in cholesterol when stimulated by mitogens (Resch and Ferber, 1972). Gradual changes in fluidity may also result from changes in phospholipid composition, as shown first in mitogen-activated lymphocytes by Fisher and Mueller (1969). They showed that PHA stimulates accumulation of phosphatidylethanolamine and phosphatidylserine during the first 24 hr and phosphatidylcholine and phosphatidylinositol at 24–48 hr. Detailed studies of changes in fatty acid moieties of activated lymphocyte membranes (Rode et al., 1982) have confirmed the notion that mitogens induce early increases in fluidity due to increasing unsaturation of fatty acids (Ferber et al., 1974, 1975). The changes contributing to the increased unsaturation of fatty acids are discussed further in Section 2.4.

2.3. Microtubule and Microfilament-Associated Events

Lymphocyte shape and motility are functions of the cytoskeletal contractile structures, which include microfilaments (diameter 50–700 Å) and microtubules ($d = 240$ Å). Microfilaments consist largely of actin, which constitutes 6% of the total protein of resting peripheral blood lymphocytes (Stark et al., 1982). Myosin interacts with actin under certain conditions requiring calcium and ATP; the ATPase of myosin complexed with actin provides the contractile force for microfilament-regulated shape change and cell motility.

Several actin-related changes are induced in lymphocytes by activation with mitogens. These include (1) conversion from the monomeric G form to the polymerized F form within 10 min; (2) reorganization of actin at about 30 min, associated with a rapid flattening of the cell, followed by the development of a prominent fibrous process termed the uropod (Sundquist et al., 1980); and (3) the appearance of actin-containing microvilli and ridges or ruffles on the cell surface at 1–2 days after mitogen stimulation, followed by the loss of microvilli and the development of an actin-containing protuberance at 3 days in cells that had undergone blast transformation (Otteskog et al., 1983). Each of the described changes is inhibited by the actin-specific fungal metabolite cytochalasin B and not by the microtubule-specific drugs colchicine or vinblastine.

Proof of a role for microfilaments in lymphocyte activation is dependent on showing that the effects of inhibitors are specific. If one accepts the actions of cytochalasins as restricted to inhibition of microfilament functions, it seems clear from several studies that these structures play more than one role in activation: Potentiation of mitogen stimulation of DNA synthesis was reported at low doses and inhibition at high doses of cytochalasin B (Yoshinaga et al., 1972; Bernard et al., 1975; Greene et al., 1976b; Gery and Eidinger, 1977; Hoffman et al., 1977). This is also true of the other cytochalasins (Greene et al., 1976b). Hume et al. (1978a) carefully titrated the dose of cytochalasin B against the glucose requirement for Con A stimulation of rat thymocytes and attributed the inhibition of DNA synthesis by cytochalasin B to its inhibition of early glucose uptake and not to its effect on microfilaments. Hume and co-workers proposed that this could even account for the inhibition by the drug of phospholipid synthesis reported by Resch et al. (1976). Belmont and Rich (1981) showed that cytochalasin B, like colchicine, had little effect during the first 4 hr after Con A but had to be present during the entire incubation period to inhibit effectively. Curiously, cytochalasins B, E, and A augment mitogen-induced calcium uptake and increase cyclic AMP levels and AIB uptake (Greene and Parker, 1975). It is quite possible that cytochalasins act at more than one site, since they were shown to bind to three types of receptors (Mookerjee and Jung, 1982). Cytosolic actin represents the site thought to participate in the inhibition of PHA activation of human peripheral blood lymphocytes by cytochalasin B, but two membrane-binding sites might be important in other functions related to glucose uptake and possibly unrelated to actin. It is also entirely possible that cell-surface actin of unknown function (Owen et al., 1978) represents one of these binding sites.

Microtubules consist largely of tubulin, and they participate in cell motility and form part of the cytoskeleton. Assembly and disassembly are controlled by both phosphorylation and calcium. Colchicine blocks the polymerization of tubulin, thereby inhibiting movement mediated by microtubules. Only a small percentage of quiescent lymphocytes have parallel tubular structures, most of which are T lymphocytes (Smit et al., 1983). Murine spleen cells responding to Con A stimulation exhibit a more extensive microtubule network after several hours, as measured by immunofluorescence with fluoresceinated antitubular antibody (Waterhouse et al., 1983). Tubulin is increased in activated cells by 24 hr (0.8–1.3% of total protein); this increase is maintained through 48 hr, by which time a fivefold increase has occurred in the number of microtubule fibers radiating from the centrosome (Kecskemethy and Schafer, 1982).

The early increases (prior to 6 hr) in both actin and tubulin are achieved by post-transcriptional processing steps such as polyadenylation and methylation of RNA, both of which double during the first 2 hr, whereas later increases, nearly fourfold in 10 hr (Degen et al., 1983), are probably due to increases in the rate of RNA synthesis, which begins after 6 hr (Kecskemethy and Schafer, 1982).

The importance of microtubules in mitosis in unquestioned, but they appear to be unrelated to questions of early signal transmission. Edelman and co-workers (Yahara and Edelman, 1972, 1973, 1975; Gunther et al. 1973, 1976; Edelman et al., 1973; McClain and Edelman, 1976; Wang et al., 1975a,b) observed that ligand-bound antibody or Con A receptors form patches and caps on the lymphocyte surface. High doses of Con A inhibited cap formation by interfering with receptor mobility in the plasma membrane. Colchicine relieved the inhibition by Con A or immunoglobulin (Ig) capping in B lymphocytes and promoted Con A capping on mouse splenic T lymphocytes. The effects of colchicine were assumed to be correlated with disassembly of microtubules, which were thought to restrict the mobility of surface receptors. The many elegant experiments described in the cited publications prompted Edelman (1976) to formulate the surface-modulating assembly (SMA) hypothesis. This assembly consisted of submembranous arrays of microtubules, microfilaments, and associated contractile and membrane proteins. It was thought to control the mobility of cell-surface receptors and to regulate signals from the cell surface to the interior. An important aspect of the hypothesis was the notion that microtubules were involved in the initiation of lymphocyte transformation by mitogens. Specifically, a role in commitment was suggested by inhibition with colchicine added during the first 20 hr (Gunther et al., 1976).

Data collected from several laboratories in the ensuing years have confirmed Edelman's notions of microtubule restriction of receptor mobility and colchicine augmentation of receptor capping (e.g., Schreiner and Unanue, 1975; Oliver et al., 1980). The capping phenomenon, however, has turned out to be irrelevant to mitogenesis.

The consensus on a role for microtubules in the early events of proliferation initiation is negative (Medrano et al., 1974; Betel and Martijnse, 1976; Greene et al., 1976a; Resch et al., 1977, 1981; Sherline and Mundy, 1977; Rudd et al., 1979; Belmont and Rich, 1981; Hall et al., 1982; Cuthbert and Shay, 1983). Definitions of initiation are important; early processes found to be unaffected by colchicine in mitogen activated lymphocytes include phospholipid turnover, lymphotoxin synthesis, RNA synthesis (Resch et al., 1977, 1981), cell volume increase at 24 hr (Cuthbert et al., 1983), and calcium uptake (Greene et al., 1976a). Parker (1982) observed modest reduction by colchicine of PHA-induced AA release; however, relatively high concentrations of colchicine (10 μM) were required to exceed 50% inhibition. Schellenberg and Gillespie (1980) reported inhibition by colchicine of phosphatidylinositol labeling but not breakdown. They also saw inhibition of phosphatidylinositol labeling by D_2O, which has the opposite effect of colchicine on microtubule formation; they appropriately concluded that the reported inhibitory effects of colchicine might be on some other system in addition to microtubules. The most definitive study of thymidine uptake and DNA synthesis kinetics (Hall et al., 1982) showed convincingly that colchicine does not inhibit commitment of stimulated lymphocytes to enter the cell cycle, but it decreases the rate of entry into S phase. The biochemical steps involved are not known. Finally, colchicine was found not to inhibit activation by neuraminidase and galactose oxidase (Rasmussen and Davis 1977) and to potentiate periodate stimulation of lymphocyte proliferation (Stenzel *et al.*, 1978).

In conclusion, the experiments to date do not support direct roles for either microtubules or microfilaments in the initiating events of lectin-induced lympho-cyte proliferation. It is now clear that patch and cap formation and the surface-modulating assembly are not essential to initiation of T-lymphocyte proliferation by Con A, since succinylated dimeric Con A and other mitogens induce pro-liferation without their involvement (Gunther *et al.*, 1976). Their involvement can more realistically be related to the mechanism by which Con A at high doses inhibits its own mitogenic action (high-dose inhibition) (Hadden *et al.*, 1976; McClain and Edelman, 1978).

In that regard, high doses of native Con A have been demonstrated to induce receptor aggregation and (in the presence of further crosslinking) a process of capping by which the receptors are moved to one extreme of the cell and re-moved. Under these circumstances, both actin (Toh and Hard, 1977) and mem-brane-bound adenylate cyclase (Earp *et al.*, 1977) co-cap with Con A receptors. In the case of adenylate cyclase, both membrane localized increases in cyclic AMP (Bloom *et al.*, 1973) and increases in cellular levels of cyclic AMP have been observed under capping circumstances. A relationship of these cyclic AMP changes to the capping process (Bourguignon and Hsing, 1983; Butman *et al.*, 1981; Hadden *et al.*, 1976) and to high-dose mitogen inhibition of proliferation (Hadden *et al.*, 1976) has been suggested.

2.4. Membrane Lipid Changes

The earliest experiments providing information on mitogen-induced lipid changes were those of Fisher and Mueller (1968) and of Kay (1968). These represented, respectfully, the fields of phosphatidylinositol (PI) and phos-phatidylcholine (PC) metabolism. Each field has acquired a considerable and separate following in the ensuing years, with only a few attempts to interrelate them. In this review, we discuss each field separately, followed by a review of the actions of the products of the phospholipid changes, with a final attempt to synthesize the various findings.

2.4.1. The PI Response

Fisher and Mueller (1968) observed that PHA induces a 10-fold stimulation of ^{32}P-labeled inorganic phosphate incorporation into membrane PI of human blood lymphocytes within 10 min. No large changes occurred in other lipids. Further studies (Fisher and Mueller, 1971b) demonstrated that PHA induces an 18-fold increase in [^{3}H]inositol labeling of PI. At the same time a fourfold increase in [^{32}P]phosphate labeling of plasma membrane phosphatidic acid occurred. A comprehensive analysis of phospholipid changes within 3 min of PHA addition showed that the earliest changes in phosphate labeling of phosphatidic acid were in fact greater than PI, with PC and major phospholipids showing minor changes. Combined with data derived from glycerol incorporation, which was slight, the results indicated that PA was synthesized by phosphorylation of 1,2-diglyceride rather than acylation of glycerol phosphate. The collected data provided strong evidence for mitogen-induced stimulation of the PI–diglyceride–phosphatidic acid–PI cycle (Fig. 2) as originally proposed for hormone responses by Hokin and Hokin (1953). In support of the importance of these reactions, an inhibitor of inositol reactions (γ-hexachlorocyclohexane) prevented the mitogen-stimulated cycle as well as RNA and DNA synthesis (Fisher and Mueller, 1971a). Lucas et al. (1971) also showed PHA stimulation of phosphate incorporation into PI. By separating stimulated cells on gradients, they showed that the cells with enhanced PI labeling were the same cells that went on to make DNA after 3 days. Further confirmation of the specificity of the response came from Masuzawa et al. (1973), who found that a host of T-cell mitogens stimulated inositol labeling of PI in human T lymphocytes. In these studies, PHA increased phosphate-labeled PI up to 10-fold within 30 min, while PC and other phospholipids were not appreciably labeled until after 3 hr. Neither T- nor B-cell mitogens (e.g., PWM) stimulated labeling in B cells in the studies of Masuzawa et al. (1973) or of Betel et al. (1974). Maino et al. (1975) also found that only transforming lectins stimulated PI labeling of pig lymph node lymphocytes. These workers observed good correspondence between the ascending limbs of the mitogen dose for both the phosphate uptake response and the thymidine response; however, the phosphate uptake showed no high-dose inhibition. Hasegawa-Sasaki and Sasaki (1982) confirmed the latter finding with rat lymphoid cells. Several other laboratories subsequently confirmed all the essential PI labeling findings discussed above (Betel et al., 1974; Schumm et al., 1974; Maino et al., 1975; Schellenberg and Gillespie, 1977, 1980; Miller, 1979; Hui and Harmony, 1980c; Hasegawa-Sasaki and Sasaki, 1981; Sasaki and Hasegawa-Sasaki, 1981; Kaibuchi et al., 1982; Rode et al., 1982; Sugiura and Waku, 1984; Taylor et al., 1984). The response is apparently limited to T-cell mitogens (Betel et al., 1974). Hui and Harmony (1980a,b) demonstrated a remarkably specific effect of low-density lipoproteins (LDL), which inhibit lymphocyte proliferation, to inhibit the early changes in PHA-induced PI labeling, cyclic GMP increases, and calcium uptake coordinately. Slightly lower ID_{50} values were obtained for PI labeling compared with the cyclic GMP and calcium increases, suggesting that the latter may be consequences of the former. A mutual dependency of PI turnover and calcium uptake is suggested by the data of Crumpton et al. (1976), who found that inositol labeling of PI was inhibited by calcium chelating agents.

A major alteration in thinking about the phosphoinositide cycle was prompted by findings in a variety of cells, stimulated by a variety of calcium-linked but

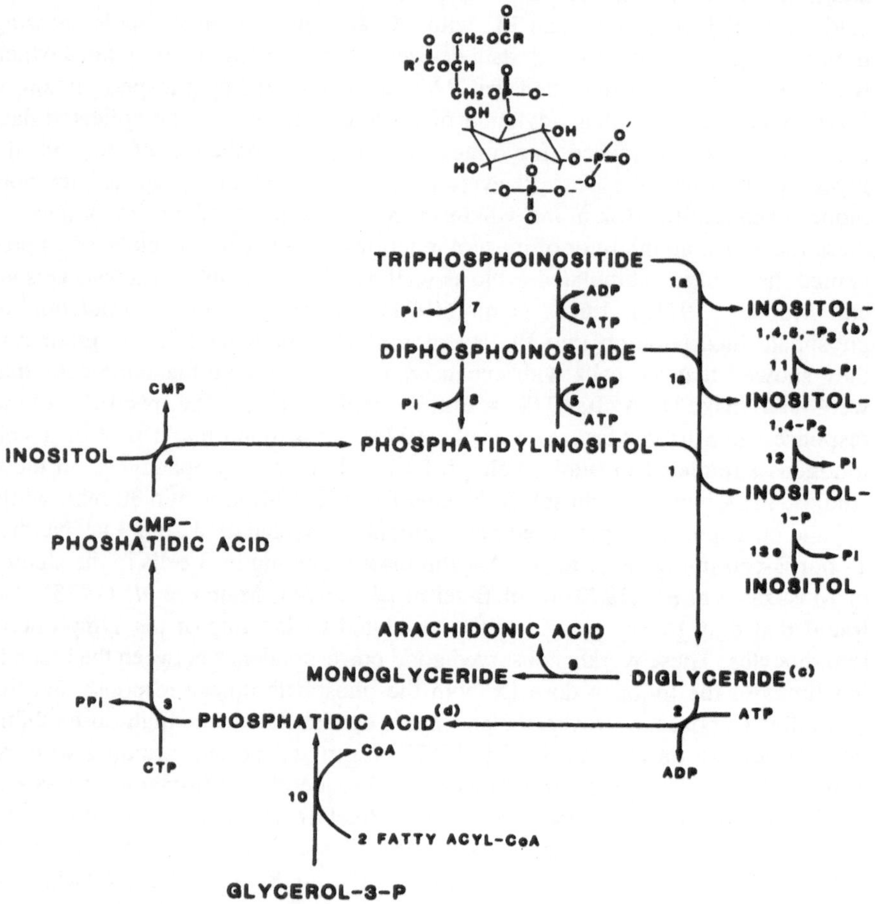

FIGURE 2. The phosphoinositide cycle. Enzymes catalyzing the indicated reactions are as follows: 1, phospholipases C (or phosphoinositide phosphodiesterases); 2, diglyceride kinase (or 1,2-diacylglycerol kinase); 3, phosphatidic acid: CTP cytidyltransferase; 4, CMP-phosphatidic acid inositol phosphatidyltransferase; 5, phosphatidylinositol kinase; 6, phosphatidylinositol-4-P kinase; 7, phosphatidylinositol-4,5-diP phosphatase (or trisphosphoinositide phosphomonoesterase); 8, phosphatidylinositol-4-P phosphatase (or diphosphoinositide phosphomonoesterase; 9, diglyceride lipase; 10, *de novo* pathway; 11, inositol triphosphatase; 12, inositol bisphosphatase; 13, inositol 1-phosphatase. *Notes:* a, Phospholipases C acting on polyphosphoinositides—may be confined to the plasma membrane to a greater extent than enzymes acting on PI; b, mobilizes calcium from intracellular stores; c, activates protein kinase C (with calcium and phosphatidylserine); d, acts as a calcium ionophore; e, Inhibited by Li^+.

cyclic AMP-independent agents, that PI breakdown occurred earlier in time than PI synthesis. The findings prompted Michell (1975) to elaborate the hypothesis now known as the PI response, in which stimulation of phospholipase C and its hydrolysis of PI to form diglyceride and inositol-1-P represents the first event following cell activation. In many (but not all) cases, this is coupled to, or followed by, calcium influx and cyclic GMP increases (Michell, 1975, 1982; Michell *et al.*, 1981). The diglyceride formed by this reaction can be phosphory-lated by a specific kinase to form phosphatidic acid or deacylated by a di-glyceride lipase to form arachidonic acid and monoglyceride (see Fig. 2). To form a cycle, phosphatidic acid must interact with CTP to form CMP-phos-phatidic acid, which then reacts with inositol to produce PI and CMP. Each step of this cycle is catalyzed by a specific enzyme. The rapidity of the PI breakdown response (Michell, 1982; Farese, 1983) is measured by the appearance of labeled diglyceride (or, less directly, of phosphatidic acid), of labeled inositol-1-P, or by the disappearance of labeled PI in cells preincubated with the appropriate precur-sor (e.g., [^{14}C]-fatty acid, [^{3}H]inositol, [^{32}P]phosphate). Since a major fraction of cell membrane PI is often hydrolyzed in the early minutes of cell activation, chemical analysis of unlabeled membrane lipids is often employed as well.

Analysis of the PI cycle demonstrates that the most direct route of phosphate labeling of PI occurs following ATP formation, its interaction with diglyceride to form phosphatidic acid, and two more enzymatic steps. However, an analysis of phosphate-labeling patterns showed that PHA induced greater labeling of PI than of phosphatidic acid (Allan and Michell, 1977). This finding suggests that PI can be labeled by reactions other than shown in Fig. 2; other publications reviewed by Farese (1983) offer some possibilities. It seems difficult to compare the Fisher and Mueller hypothesis directly with the Michell hypothesis merely on the basis of kinetics of labeling of two components of the cycle.

By comparing the kinetics of labeling of several lipids simultaneously, important inferences can be drawn. Such a study was conducted by Hasegawa-Sasaki and Sasaki (1982) using rat lymph node cells preincubated with labeled arachidonate to label all lipids containing this fatty acid. The proportion of label appearing in PI and PC resembled the mole percent of these phospholipids reported earlier (Fisher and Mueller, 1971b), and the percentage change in each of eight lipid moieties was followed from 15 sec to 15 min after addition of Con A. Phosphatidic acid increases and PI decreases were evident at 0.5–1 min; diglyceride increased only 10% but significantly so at 2 min, at which time phosphatidic acid was twice the control. A major portion of diglyceride may have been converted to monoglyceride and arachidonate, but this was not dem-onstrated. PI decreased from 1 to 5 min (90% of control) and then increased. No changes were found in PC, phosphatidylethanolamine, phosphatidylserine, tri-glycerides, or fatty acids during the first 15 min. Fisher and Mueller interpreted the data to indicate that PI breakdown precedes PI synthesis and may be the initial step in the lymphocyte PI response to Con A. They remarked at the relatively small change in PI compared with other cell types stimulated with various agents, although this could reflect the small percent of cells responding to Con A, and were reluctant to conclude that the PI response is an essential event for lymphocyte activation.

For reasons discussed in relationship to Fisher and Mueller's work, and discussed below, we are inclined to believe that the PI response is essential. Human blood contains a higher percentage of Con A-responding T cells than does rat lymph node. It is therefore of considerable interest to examine the data of Hasegawa-Sasaki and Sasaki (1981) concerning glycerol and [^{32}P]phosphate incorporation in peripheral blood lymphocytes. Although both Con A and PHA stimulated PI synthesis from both precursors, the comparisons suggested that Con A acts primarily by stimulating the cycle and PHA the *de novo* pathway. It is important to compare the data of Parker *et al.* (1979a) with those just reviewed. After allowing human blood lymphocytes to incorporate [^{14}C]arachidonic acid (AA), Parker *et al.* added PHA and followed labeled AA release. It occurred in 1 min, peaked at 10 min, and accounted for 40% of the cellular PI stores. Whereas most of the AA is incorporated into PC of resting lymphocyte membranes, most of the AA appearing after stimulation is derived from PI, not PC (Parker *et al.*, 1979a; Homa *et al.*, 1984). Parker *et al.* (1979a) suggested that phospholipase C and diglyceride lipase were closely coupled in producing the AA.

Before proceeding to other areas of phospholipid changes, it would be useful to examine the relevance of Michell's hypothesis that the PI response is somehow liked to, or even responsible for, calcium uptake. First, lymphocyte phospholipase C has been shown to be present in lymphocytes; it is calcium dependent and inhibited by chlorpromazine (Allan and Michell, 1974). Second, inhibition of PI breakdown also prevented calcium ion uptake (Hui and Harmony, 1980a). Using the calcium ionophore A23187, Maino *et al.* (1974) obtained data suggesting that a rise in cellular calcium triggered PI turnover. In a comparison of PHA and A23187, Allan and Michell (1977) found that the ionophore stimulated a greater production of phosphatidic acid that was abolished by the removal of calcium from the medium. Interestingly, the stimulation of PI labeling was not so inhibited. Since glycerol uptake into phosphatidic acid was unexpectedly reduced by A23187, a calcium-dependent effect on *de novo* synthesis was discounted. Other data suggested that the ionophore has an additional effect to stimulate triglyceride lipase, thereby increasing diglyceride, phosphatidic acid, and, ultimately, PI label. The principal effect of PHA, however, was the breakdown of PI, a response that was only modestly reduced by eliminating most of the extracellular calcium. Confirming this relatively calcium-independent effect, Hui and Harmony (1980c) reported that PHA stimulates PI hydrolysis in a calcium-free medium. It thus seems clear that extracellular calcium is not required for the lectin mitogen-stimulated PI response, whereas the PI response may be essential for calcium uptake.

Several findings suggest how the latter might occur. Phosphatidic acid is thought to regulate the calcium channel in the surface membrane (Michell, 1975;

Rittenhouse-Simmons, 1980) and has been found, among several phospholipids, to be an effective calcium ionophore (Serhan et al., 1982).

More recently, interest has been renewed in inositol 1,4,5-trisphosphate (IP_3) as a calcium mobilizer. It arises from PI-4,5-bisphosphate, a minor component of cell membranes, by the action of a phospholipase C (see Berridge, 1984, for review). In a cultured human T-lymphoblastoid cell line, inositol trisphosphate was released in less than 10 sec after stimulation with PHA (Hasegawa-Sasaki and Sasaki, 1983). At 1 min, 28% of PI-4,5-bisphosphate has broken down, and this decrease precedes the breakdown of PI and the appearance of phosphatidic acid. One suspects that the relevant phospholipase C differs in both substrate preference and in subcellular location from the primarily soluble enzyme described by Allan and Michell (1974). EGTA or quinacrine inhibit about one half the phosphatidic acid formation from prelabeled cells, suggesting again that two enzymes, of differing calcium requirements, are involved. The results extend the findings of Hui and Harmony (1980a) that inositol bis- and trisphosphates are released along with inositol-1-P after stimulation of human peripheral blood lymphocytes with PHA. These data can be interpreted in light of a rapidly growing body of evidence that inositol trisphosphate acts within seconds to mobilize intracellular calcium ion (Joseph et al., 1984; Dawson and Irvine, 1984; Berridge, 1984; Burgess et al., 1984). This has been demonstrated in liver and several other tissues and represents an early response to a variety of cell activators that act in a calcium-dependent manner but do not require extracellular calcium ion. The membrane sources of calcium appear to be microsomal (e.g., plasma membrane and/or endoplasmic reticulum, cytoskeleton), and not mitochondrial. If this system is verified as a very early response of lymphocytes to mitogens it will serve to connect the phospholipid response to calcium-dependent effects.

If calcium mobilization is due to one product of phospholipase C action, calcium effects are probably dependent in large part on the other product, diglyceride. This lipid stimulates a recently described protein kinase that requires phosphatidylserine and calcium ion (reviewed by Nishizuka, 1984; Kuo et al., 1984). Once stimulated, this kinase C translocates from the cytoplasm to the plasma membrane, where it catalyzes phosphorylation of specific membrane protein substrates. The phosphorylated forms of these are characteristic of transformed cells. In lymphocytes, Ogawa et al. (1981) and Ku et al. (1981) demonstrated the existence of this kinase and verified that it is stimulated by mitogens acting on intact cells. The kinase has also been found to be stimulated directly by phorbol myristate acetate (PMA) (Castagna et al., 1982), a tumor promoter and mitogen for a subset of human T lymphocytes (Touraine et al., 1977). Diglyceride can substitute for PMA as a co-mitogen in human lymphocytes completely freed of macrophages (Kaibuchi et al., 1985), further supporting a role for protein kinase C in mitogenesis (see Section 2.4.3).

It has not yet been shown in lymphocytes how the PI-diglyceride–phosphatidic acid response, when activated, results in enhanced uptake of calcium ion from the medium. The effect of phosphorylation of membrane proteins or the ionophoretic influence of phosphatidic acid appear to be good candidates for research. In any event, the inhibition studies of Fisher and Mueller (1971a) strongly suggest that a compound capable of competitive antagonism of inositol or inositol phosphates could be of considerable use in exploring these possibilities.

2.4.2. The Phosphatidylcholine Response

Leaving PI metabolism, we shall briefly discuss the other area of phospholipid changes that has received considerable attention. PC synthesis by different routes (Fig. 3) is stimulated by T-cell mitogens as measured by enhanced incorporation of choline (Kay, 1968; Fisher and Mueller, 1969; Resch and Ferber, 1972, Wertz and Mueller, 1978, 1980; Chen, 1979; Nathaniel et al., 1983), of unsaturated fatty acids (Resch et al., 1971, 1972, 1976, 1978, 1981; Northoff et al., 1978), and by methylation of phosphatidylethanolamine (Fisher and Mueller, 1969, Hirata and Axelrod 1980b; Toyoshima et al., 1982a,b; Bougnoux et al., 1983). Incorporation of choline into lymphocytes appears to be a late event; incorporation into T cells is not noticeable until 1 hr after mitogen stimulation (Resch and Ferber, 1972; Chen 1979), and B-cell incorporation does not begin until 16 hr (Chien and Ashman, 1983; Ashman et al., 1984). Apparently the stimulation of choline incorporation by PMA in T cells requires prior arachidonate release and metabolism by lipoxygenase (Wertz and Mueller, 1980). By contrast, mitogen stimulation of fatty acid incorporation has been seen as early as 10 min (Resch et al., 1972; Ferber and Resch, 1973) but is usually not measured until after 1–3 hr (Resch et al., 1971, 1978). Oleic acid labels PC to a greater extent than phosphatidylethanolamine, and position 1 is preferred (Resch et al., 1971). AA, found almost exclusively in position 2 of PC, is not incorporated into human lymphocytes at enhanced rates following PHA according to Parker et al. (1979a). By contrast, Rode et al. (1982) found enhanced incorporation of AA into PC, phosphatidylethanolamine, and PI within minutes of adding Con A to rabbit thymocytes. The preference of AA compared with other fatty acids became absolute at 4 hr, contributing to a new membrane of greater fluidity. The relative importance in mitogen action of PC synthesis by either choline or fatty acid incorporation is questionable, since both can be inhibited (by dapsone) without preventing subsequent DNA synthesis (Nathaniel and Mellors, 1983).

Perhaps more relevant is the conversion of PE to PC by a sequence of three transmethylation reactions in response to mitogens. This change is much more rapid than the PC synthesis schemes discussed above. Hirata et al. (1980a) and Toyoshima et al. (1982a,b) found that Con A and PHA stimulate phosphatidylethanolamine (PE) methylation in mouse spleen T cells within 2 min, and the increase peaked at 10 min—a time when AA release was just beginning. The

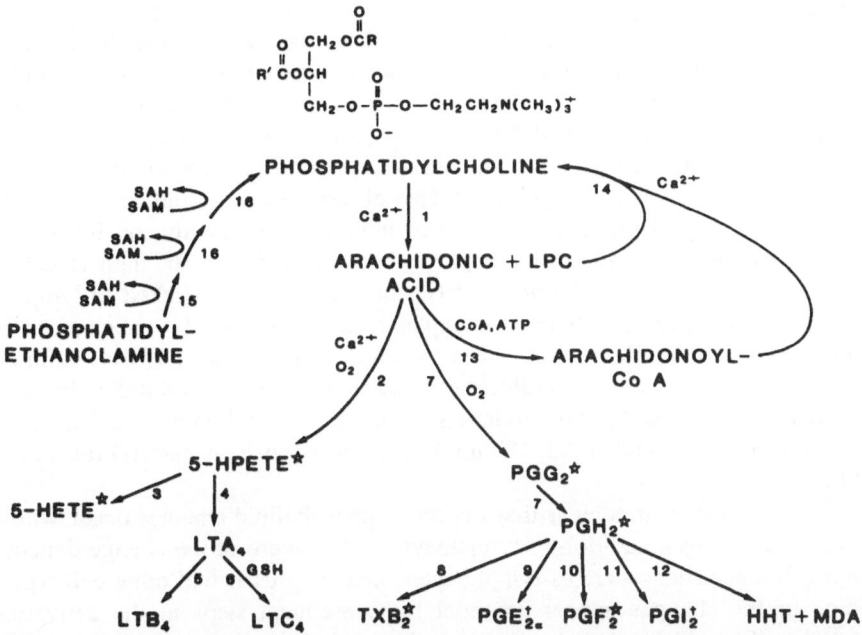

FIGURE 3. Arachidonic acid formation and metabolism. Enzymes catalyzing the indicated reactions are as follows: 1, phospholipase A_2; 2, 5-lipoxygenase (other lipoxygenases produce other HPETEs); 3, HPETE peroxidase (or nonenzymatic); 4, HPETE dehydrase; 5, leukotriene A_4 hydrolase (this enzyme produces 5S, 12R-diHETE; nonenzymatic reactions produce biologically inactive epimers); 6, glutathione S-transferase (the product, LTC_4, may be converted sequentially to LTD_4 and LTE_4 by other enzymes in other tissues); 7, cyclooxygenase; 8, thromboxane synthetase; 9, endoperoxide isomerase; 10, endoperoxide reductase; 11, prostacyclin synthetase; 12, nonenzymatic; 13, acyl-CoA synthetase; 14, acyl-CoA:lysolecithin acyltransferase; 15, phospholipid methyltransferase I; 16, phospholipid methyltransferase II. CoA, coenzyme A; GSH, glutathione; HETE, hydroxyeicosate-trienoic acid; HPETE, hydroperoxyeicosatetraenoic acid; HHT, 12-hydroxyheptadecatrienoic acid; LPC, lysophosphatidylcholine; LT, leukotriene; MDA, malondialdehyde; PG, prostaglandin; SAH, S-adenosylhomocysteine; SAM, S-adenosylmethionine; TX, thromboxane. *Stimulates cyclic GMP accumulation. † Stimulates cyclic AMP accumulation.

magnitude of methylation was proportional to that of eventual thymidine uptake. Like DNA synthesis, methylation was inhibited by high Con A concentrations and both were prevented by specific S-adenosyl methionine antagonists of trans-methylation reactions. In lymphocytes (Toyoshima et al., 1982a) and in other systems (Ishizaka et al., 1980) phospholipid methylation precedes activation of calcium ion influx by a variety of appropriate cell stimuli. In fact, methylations are catalyzed by two calcium-independent enzymes. It was suggested that mono-methyl PE, the product of the first transmethylation, may function as a calcium ionophore (Waxdal, 1980), possibly mediating calcium ion influx and AA re-lease. The importance of the transmethylation reactions may lie in the area of calcium or other trigger signals rather than as a source of PC, since the primary source of AA released by mitogen action is PI, not PC. The early enthusiasm for the critical nature of phospholipid methylation (reviewed by Hirata and Axelrod, 1980; Pike and Snyderman, 1981; Ishizaka *et al.*, 1980) has possibly been dampened by the report of J. P. Moore *et al.* (1982) that Con A did not stimulate methylation of PE during the first 60 min in spite of the positive demonstration of enhanced PI turnover and glycolysis. This observation was confirmed by Ashman (1984). No adequate explanation of inhibition of calcium ion influx and mitogenesis by methylation inhibitors has been offered; perhaps their effect on key protein carboxymethylations or RNA base methylations linked to lymphocyte activation provide alternative explanations. Interestingly, when used in combination, the inhibitors have been shown to increase cyclic AMP (Zimmerman *et al.*, 1980), a known inhibitor of early events as discussed in Section 2.7. In any event, phospholipid methylation is not a general link in the mechanism of all mitogens, since neither A23187 nor PMA induces such changes (Hirata *et al.*, 1980a).

In conclusion, it is clear that important phospholipid changes occur within minutes of mitogen addition to lymphocytes. The nature of the change depends on the mitogen, the source of lymphocytes, and the presence of other cell types. Some of the changes appear essential for subsequent steps in the activation sequence (PI or PI-bisphosphate hydrolysis and diglyceride formation); some do not appear essential (PI and PC synthesis), and some remain controversial (phosphatidylethanolamine methylation). Some products of phospholipid metabolism may function as second messengers (diglyceride, phosphatidic acid, inositol trisphosphate), and calcium is involved in some of these steps. Diglyceride (together with phosphatidylserine) activates protein kinase C by increasing the affinity of the enzyme for calcium; phosphatidic acid may bring calcium into the cell or translocate calcium from membrane stores to other sites; inositol trisphosphate may serve a similar function. The requirement for extracellular calcium in the actions of lectin mitogens is documented, but its role in the initiation of phospholipid metabolism remains controversial. Since Kay (1968) and Fisher and Mueller (1968) showed that early increases in PC and PI metabolism do not require protein synthesis, and since the mass of PI does not increase concomitantly with the mass of phosphatidic acid, *de novo* phospholipid synthesis is probably not involved in lymphocyte responses to mitogens. Conflicting results from labeled glycerol incorporation (cf. Fisher and Mueller (1971a) and of Allan and Michell (1977) with Hasegawa-Sasaki and Sasaki (1981)) are relevant to this discussion and remain to be explained.

2.4.3. Protein Kinase C

Protein kinase C has been shown to be both activated and translocated from the cytoplasm to the plasma membrane in lymphocytes by various mitogens, including PHA, OKT3, and PMA (Kaibuchi et al., 1985; Farrar and Ruscetti, 1986; Mire et al., 1986). While the membrane substrates it phosphorylates can be considered to be many, examples in lymphocytes include tyrosine protein kinase (56 kda), the IL-2 receptor, and adenylate cyclase (with down regulation) (Casnellie and Lamberts, 1986; Gaulton and Eardley, 1986; Farrar and Ruscetti, 1986; Beckner and Farrar, 1986). Another likely candidate in lymphocytes is guanylate cyclase, since inhibition of protein kinase C blocks guanylate cyclase activation by PMA (Coffey, 1986). Similarly, a link between protein kinase C and the *de novo* RNA-dependent induction of IL-2 receptor gene expression has been suggested (Depper et al., 1985; Farrar and Ruscetti, 1986); however, the mechanism of the latter can only be speculated on. It has been presumed that because PMA mimics many of the effects of IL-1, IL-1 will activate protein kinase C; this remains to be demonstrated. It is notable that PMA induces IL-2 receptors, but does not imply important differences in their mechanism of action (Malek et al., 1985). The activation of protein kinase C has been suggested to be independent of calcium influx or increased $[Ca^{2+}]$; since PMA as a lymphocyte mitogen does not induce these calcium changes (Gelfand et al., 1985; Oettgen et al., 1985). Its relationship to phosphorylation events previously observed in mitogen-stimulated lymphocytes (see Section 2.7 and 2.8) and to the other initiation processes (Section 2.5.2) remains to be clarified. On the basis of its hypothesized role in the activation of other cells, including tumor cells (see Nishizuka, 1984), studies to pursue these relationships are timely.

2.4.4. Arachidonic Acid Release

The third and most tangled web of lipid reactions involves AA and its metabolism as an early response to mitogens. As depicted in Figs. 2 and 3, AA may derive from PC or PI (or other phospholipids) by the action of phospholipase A_2 or the sequential action of phospholipase C and diglyceride lipase. Parker et al. (1979a) reported that most of the AA released from HPBL in response to PHA came from PI, not PC. This was confirmed in rat spleen lymphocytes by Homa et al. (1984) and is in agreement with the positive demonstration of phospholipase C (Allan and Michell, 1974) and the failure to measure a phospholipase A_2 (Trotter and Ferber, 1981; Resch et al., 1984) in lymphocytes carefully freed of macrophages. [Parenthetically, phospholipase A_2 activity does occur in chronic lymphocytic leukemia B cells (Suzuki et al., 1980), macrophages (Resch et al., 1984), and natural killer (NK) cells (Hoffman et al., 1981).]

Despite the absence of lymphocyte phospholipase A, Trotter and Ferber (1981), Trotter et al. (1982), and Resch et al. (1984) believe that in mitogen-activated lymphocytes, AA can derive from PC by the action of an acyl CoA : lysophosphatide acyltransferase, operating in reverse. In mouse thymocytes, Trotter and Ferber (1981) showed that when Con A was added to PC, lysophosphatidylcholine and acyl CoA appear. PI did not function as acyl donor in this first step. In the second reaction, lysophosphatidylethanolamine plus acyl CoA yielded PE and CoA. Lysophosphatidylcholine or lysophosphatidyinositol did not substitute for lysophosphatidylethanolamine. In an alternative second reaction (not definitively demonstrated), an acyl CoA hydrolase would cleave acyl CoA to yield free fatty acid (FFA). Combining PC with CoA and acyltransferase plus the hydrolase, AA would thus be derived from PC, and evidence for release of AA in both lymphocytes and macrophages by this mechanism was reported by Trotter et al. (1982). Evidence for mitogen activation of the entire pathway is lacking. However, Resch et al. (1984) summarized extensive evidence accumulated over several years (Ferber and Resch, 1973, Ferber et al., 1974, 1975, 1976; Reilly and Ferber, 1976; Szamel and Resch, 1981a,b, Szamel et al., 1981, Trotter and Ferber, 1981; Trotter et al., 1982; Resch et al., 1983) that the acyltransferase is activated three- to fourfold very soon after the exposure of intact cells to Con A. The acyltransferase is enriched in a Con A-binding fraction of plasma membranes. Na^+, K^+-ATPase is also enriched in the same fraction and is also activated indirectly by Con A. Both enzymes were shown to be activated in membranes isolated from cells incubated with Con A at 0° or 37°C, ruling out an energy or metabolic requirement. In membranes isolated from untreated cells, both enzymes were activated by polyunsaturated fatty acids such as AA, mimicking the action of the mitogen in intact cells. The source of the stimulatory fatty acids is thought to be triglycerides.

These data form the core of a new proposal for the activation of lymphocytes, involving a supramolecular complex of the two enzymes and their lipid matrix (Resch et al., 1984). In support of one aspect of the proposal, Szamel and Resch (1981b) showed that ouabain inhibited mitogen activation of acyltransferase, lipid turnover, and lymphocyte transformation. The effective concentrations of ouabain (5×10^{-8} M) were said to be much lower than required to inhibit monovalent cation transport. It is perhaps too early to comment decisively on this proposal, except to point out five reasons for caution: (1) it requires free AA to be already present in lymphocytes, even at 0°C, to initiate the release of more AA after Con A binds, a fact not well supported by the literature; (2) most of the mitogen-stimulated free AA is derived from PI, which Trotter and Ferber (1981) found was not a donor of acyltransferase-mediated AA release; (3) triglycerides were not found to be significantly altered following the addition of mitogen (Hasegawa-Sasaki and Sasaki, 1982); (4) some workers observed inhibition rather than stimulation of acyltransferase by Con A (Dobson and Mellors, 1980); and (5) the effects of ouabain have not been shown to be independent of Na^+/K^+, transport; for example, Quastel and Kaplan (1968) showed inhibition of uridine uptake by exactly the same concentration of ouabain, and this was reversed by K^+, suggesting that the effects of ouabain were primarily on the K^+-binding site of the monovalent cation pump. Nevertheless, mitogens induce a small amount of AA release from PC (Parker et al., 1979a) and the normal functioning of acyltransferase, to build PC, could well account for a portion of the increase in the percent of polyenoic fatty acids found in lipids of mitogenically stimulated cells (Ferber *et al.*, 1975; Rode *et al.*, 1982).

We favor the view that most of the AA derives from PI, but that some portion of AA may also be hydrolyzed from PC, possibly by an acyltransferase-mediated step. In any event, AA release occurs soon after mitogen addition (Parker *et al.*, 1979a; Parker, 1982; Hirata *et al.*, 1980; Homa *et al.*, 1984), and inhibition of its release results in inhibition of guanylate cyclase activation (Coffey *et al.*, 1981; Coffey and Hadden, 1981a,b, 1983a,b), IL-2 production (Namiuchi *et al.*, 1984), and ultimately of DNA synthesis (Hirata *et al.*, 1980; Parker, 1982; Coffey and Hadden, 1981b; Coffey *et al.*, 1981; Namiuchi *et al.*, 1984). Some of the inhibitors used have been considered specific for phospholipase A_2 (mepacrine or quinacrine, tetracaine, p-bromophenacylbromide), while others (e.g., cyclic AMP) have been shown to inhibit both phospholipase A_2 and C (Lapetina, 1982). Recently, mepacrine (Best *et al.*, 1984) and p-bromophenacylbromide (Kyger and Franson, 1984) were also found to inhibit phospholipase C.

2.4.5. Arachidonic Acid Metabilities

The liberated AA may serve as an energy source or may be quickly metabolized by one of three routes: the acyltransferase discussed above, cyclooxygenase, or the lipoxygenases (see Fig. 3). Cyclooxygenase (with its associated peroxidase) produces the endoperoxides PGG_2 and PGH_2, which are quickly converted to prostaglandins (PG), thromboxanes, or prostacyclin; the products vary, depending on the cell (Samuelsson *et al.*, 1978). Lipoxygenases form hydroperoxy derivatives of AA (HPETE), which are converted by peroxidases or nonenzymatically to hydroxy counterparts (HETE). In the case of 5-lipoxygenase, uniquely sensitive to calcium activation and possibly to diglyceride stimulation as well, the product 5-HPETE may also be converted, via the 5,6-epoxide intermediate (leukotriene A_4) to leukotrienes B_4 or C_4 (Lands, 1984; Samuelsson, 1982).

Evidence has accumulated to implicate lipoxygenase but not cyclooxygenase activity in lymphocyte activation. In several studies, (Goodwin *et al.*, 1977; Tomar *et al.*, 1981), the specific cyclooxygenase inhibitor indomethacin did not prevent lymphocyte activation at concentrations adequate to inhibit cyclooxygenase. High indomethacin concentrations may block due to other mechanisms (Wang *et al.*, 1978). In many cases, indomethacin augmented DNA synthesis, possibly by preventing inhibition by prostaglandin E_2 (PGE_2) produced by macrophages (Goodwin *et al.*, 1977; Coffey and Hadden, 1981b). Many workers (Bray *et al.*, 1981; Goldyne and Stobo, 1982) found no PGs in either resting or activated lymphocytes, while others found a small PG production in stimulated cells (C. A. Phillips *et al.*, 1978; Tomar *et al.*, 1981). PG synthesis seems to be required for the generation of suppressor T cells from precursors (Orme and Shand, 1981); glass wool-adherent T-suppressor cells apparently manufacture PGs in a way that may depend on macrophages (Webb and Nowowiejski, 1981). Thromboxanes A_2 and B_2 were reported to be synthesized in significant amounts in lymphocytes following mitogen stimulation (Parker et al., 1979b) and some evidence exists for attenuation of DNA synthesis by relatively nonspecific inhibitors of thromboxane synthesis (Kelly and Parker, 1979b; Udey and Parker, 1982). Overall, a comparison of several chemically unrelated and highly potent inhibitors of thromboxane synthesis showed no correlation between the latter and DNA synthesis in human peripheral blood lymphocytes stimulated by four different mitogens (Gordon et al., 1981). This is in agreement with the fact that indomethacin, which blocks completely the formation of the thromboxane precursor PGG_2, does not inhibit transformation. It seems safe to presume that while the data concerning whether T cells make prostaglandins is controversial, there are no data to convince one that any cyclooxygenase product is critical for mitogen activation.

By contrast, lipoxygenase inhibitors do prevent mitogen action. Kelly and Parker (1979) observed inhibition of human peripheral blood lymphocyte stimulation by PHA, A23187, or PWM by the early addition of low concentrations of either nordihydroguaiaretic acid, which inhibits lipoxygenase but not cyclooxygenase, or of 5,8,11,14-eicosatetraynoic acid (ETYA), which inhibits both. High concentrations of indomethacin, found by others (Rittenhouse-Simmons, 1980) to prevent AA release, were partially inhibitory to mitogenesis. Nordihydroguaiaretic acid and ETYA, but not indomethacin, were also shown to inhibit PHA activation of guanylate cyclase at concentrations inhibitory to thymidine incorporation (Coffey and Hadden, 1981b; E. M. Hadden, unpublished observations). Since lipoxygenase depends on free radicals to sustain its chain reaction (Lands, 1984), free radical absorbing compounds also inhibit lipoxygenase and guanylate cyclase activation and, relatedly, mitogenesis (Novogrodsky et al., 1982).

At least five lipoxygenase products have been identified in mitogen-activated human blood lymphocytes within minutes of stimulation. Parker et al. (1979b) reported the rapid PHA stimulation by 4- to 12-fold of both 5-HETE and 12-HETE in lymphocytes freed of platelet contamination. Goetzl (1981) and Atluru et al. (1986) observed large increases in 5-,11-,12-,15-mono-HETES and 5,12-diHETE (leukotriene B_4) in PHA-, Con A-, or A23187-stimulated human T lymphocytes freed of monocytes. It remains uncertain whether all the products listed above are formed in the same cells. Goldyne (1984) maintains that T lymphocytes do not make any of them; however, the high concentration of AA used has been shown to inhibit their production by T lymphocytes (Atluru et al., 1986). It is possible that some HETEs are formed by macrophages from AA liberated by activated lymphocytes. The levels of all lipoxygenase products, each of which depends on a separate enzymatic activity, increased after addition of

PHA, Con A, or A23187. Activation of lipoxygenase(s) is therefore a common step in the mechanism of three disparate mitogens, one of which (A23187) does not share the property of activating phospholipid methylation. The 5-lipoxygenase may be stimulated by the direct, calcium-independent action of diglyceride, as reported by Parker (1984) to occur in leukemia cells.

Many effects of lipoxygenase products in promoting lymphocyte activation are implicated: 5-HETE and leukotriene B_4, added to intact lymphocytes, promote chemokinesis (Payan and Goetzl, 1981); and 5-HETE stimulates lymphocyte guanylate cyclase when added to intact cells (Coffey and Hadden, 1981b, 1985). Like PHA, 5-HETE activates primarily the membrane-bound form of guanylate cyclase. The effects of 5-HETE, like those of PHA, are blocked by inhibitors of phospholipases and of lipoxygenases, suggesting that 5-HETE promotes further AA release and metabolism by cellular lipoxygenases. Other mono-HETES, such as 11-HETE and 12-HETE, mimic to a lesser extent the guanylate cyclase-stimulating effects of 5-HETE. These observations indicate that lipoxygenase products, particularly 5-HETE, provide the link between the various membrane-related events discussed, as well as cyclic GMP production.

The activation of guanylate cyclase is a result of the lipoxygenation of AA (presumably released by phospholipase A) and represents a critical step in several aspects of the activation sequence. It occurs in the relative absence of adherent accessory cells (Coffey et al., 1981), indicating that it may result from direct actions of the mitogen on T lymphocytes. It has been shown that the action of IL-1 to induce IL-2 is dependent on the lipoxygenase pathway and associated with 5- and 15-HETE production (Bailey et al., 1986; Farrar and Humes, 1985; Dinarello et al., 1983). Although the link to cyclic GMP production is only tentative (preliminary data of J. W. Hadden, R. G. Coffey, and J. J. Oppenheim), it seems likely that IL-1 action will involve this pathway in T lymphocytes. It is also now apparent that IL-2 action involves this pathway; IL-2 promotes the lipoxygenation of arachidonate to form 5- and 15-HETE (Farrar and Humes, 1985), inhibitors of 5-lipoxygenase block IL-2 action or its target cells (Farrar and Humes, 1985; Bailey et al., 1986), and IL-2 increases cellular lymphocyte levels or cyclic GMP in mitogen-primed T cells freed of adherent cells (Hadden et al., 1987).

The extent that products of the lipoxygenase pathway of cyclic GMP will mimic the effects of IL-1 or IL-2 or restore their actions following inhibition of the pathway has not yet been determined. It has been noted that cyclic GMP will replace the effect of IL-2 to induce gamma IFN production in activated T lymphocytes (Johnson et al., 1982). It appears likely that cyclic GMP is an intracellular messenger for indirect mitogens actions via IL-1 and IL-2 as well as direct effects (see Section 2.8.1).

In contrast to the stimulatory effects of 5-HETE, 15-HETE and its precursor 15-HPETE do not augment, but rather inhibit, lymphocyte activation by mitogens (Goodman, et al., 1981; Payan and Goetzl, 1981, 1983; Bailey et al.,

1982a,b; Gualde *et al.*, 1982, 1983, 1985b; Mexmain *et al.*, 1984). This may result from two mechanisms. One mechanism results from the inhibition by 15-HETE of the 5-lipoxygenase pathway (Vanderhoek and Bailey, 1980; Payan and Goetzl, 1981). 15-HETE also inhibits activation of guanylate cyclase by mitogens or by 5-HETE (Coffey and Hadden, 1985). By this mechanism, 15-HPETE and/or HETE operate as a negative feedback within the same cells or closely related cells to prevent the production of other 5-lipoxygenase products necessary for the activation sequence. The second mechanism involves action of LTB_4 and/or 15-HPETE to activate, in a positive way, suppressor/cytotoxic T lymphocytes, in turn surpressing the proliferative response (Rola-Pleszczynski *et al.*, 1982; Gualde *et al.*, 1985a; Rola-Pleszczynski, 1985). This latter mechanism has both cyclic GMP production and proliferation as part of the process (Payan *et al.*, 1984, Mexmain *et al.*, 1985; Gualde *et al.*, 1985a).

The relative importance of the various lipoxygenases in mixed leukocyte systems depends on their affinities for AA. At physiological AA levels, the affinity of 5-lipoxygenase for substrate is much greater than that of 15-lipoxygenase, while at high (10-μM) levels, the 15-lipoxygenase is enhanced and the 5-lipoxygenase is inhibited (DeLaclos *et al.*, 1984). Inhibitor studies also demonstrate discordance in the lipoxygenases. The capacity of nordihydroguaiaretic acid to inhibit 5-lipoxygenase exceeds that of 15-lipoxygenase by a factor of 100 (Salari *et al.*, 1984). Considering these observations, a reasonable sequel to mitogen activation of phospholipase C would be the stimulation, by calcium and/or diglyceride released from PI, of 5-lipoxygenase to form 5-HPETE and 5-HETE, which promote many aspects of lymphocyte activation. As AA levels rise, 5-lipoxygenase products decline and 15-HPETE and LTB_4 increase, attenuating further activation.

As a final comment, AA itself may, without further metabolism, activate certain processes. Kelly and Parker (1979) showed that it augmented PHA stimulation of HPBL transformation at 0.5–1 μM (but inhibited at higher doses). Homa *et al.* (1984) observed stimulation of membrane AA conversion to several products by extracellular AA. Coffey and Hadden (1981b) showed that 1 μM AA stimulates guanylate cyclase activation in intact cells by a mechanism not dissimilar to that of mitogens acting on the cell surface, i.e., by conversion to eicosanoids. A possible mechanism for some of the actions of AA is the stimulation of the phospholipid-dependent calcium-requiring protein kinase C, as shown in human neutrophils (McPhail *et al.*, 1984). AA accomplishes this in a manner that can be further augmented by diglyceride but not by phosphatidylserine. AA thus seems to replace phosphatidylserine in the protein kinase C activation mechanism, as PMA replaces diglyceride.

2.5. Membrane Transport and Monovalent Cation Changes

Among the earliest changes observed after stimulation of lymphocytes are increased fluxes of ions and substrates across the plasma membrane. Several different membrane carriers or mediators of transport are involved; enzyme activities have been identified with some. In this section, the transport of K^+, amino acids, glucose, and nucleosides is reviewed. Roles of iron, pH, and membrane potential are also discussed. Uptake of fatty acids, phosphate, choline, and calcium are considered in other sections.

2.5.1. Potassium Transport

The plasma membrane Na^+/K^+ pump has been unequivocally identified with the Na^+,K^+-ATPase that spans the plasma membranes of animal cells. This enzyme transports K^+ inward and Na^+ outward against chemical gradients, using the energy derived from the hydrolysis of ATP. Ouabain binds in a highly selective way to sites on the cell surface and inhibits the pump. K^+ reverses the ouabain inhibition. At least 16 laboratories have contributed nearly 50 papers to document the stimulation of K^+ influx and the increase in the Na^+,K^+-ATPase by T-cell mitogens or the effects of ouabain to inhibit various aspects of lymphocyte mitogens.

The first report involving the system was that of Quastel and Kaplan (1968), who showed that ouabain inhibited PHA stimulation of uridine uptake into RNA, as well as DNA synthesis, with an IC_{50} of 50 nM. K^+ reversed the effect, providing strong evidence for the importance of the Na^+/K^+ pump and/or intracellular K^+ for uridine incorporation. Quastel and Kaplan (1970) later found that PHA stimulated both $^{42}K^+$ uptake and efflux; ouabain inhibited only the uptake. The rapidity of the response was demonstrated by Averdunk (1972), who saw an increase in the uptake of $^{86}Rb^+$, a K^+ analogue, within 30 sec of PHA addition. Kinetic analysis indicated that the V_{max} was increased, while the K_{nm} remained unchanged by PHA. The same year, Kay (1972) published evidence that the early increase in K^+ influx might be a homeostatic response of the lymphocyte to a mitogen-induced increase in membrane permeability, which causes K^+ depletion. The importance of maintaining K^+ levels was reflected by the inhibition of protein synthesis and, later (26 hr), of RNA synthesis by ouabain. Since ouabain did not affect uridine incorporation at 1 hr, Kay (1972) concluded that the early stimulation of uridine uptake by PHA was not dependent on activation of the pump.

2.5.2. Potassium Permeability, Membrane Potential, and Intracellular pH

The mitogen-induced K^+ permeability or leak flux has been confirmed by several laboratories to occur in minutes after mitogen addition (Averdunk and Lauf, 1975; Segel et al., 1975; Negendank and Collier, 1976; Matteson and Deutsch, 1984). Some consequences of this increased K^+ permeability include increased intracellular levels of Na^+ and calcium in addition to decreased Mg^{2+} and K^+ (Averdunk et al., 1976). Segel et al. (1976) and Segel and Lichtman

(1976) measured K^+ in human lymphocytes for 24 hr after PHA. These investigators found no net change in K^+ levels, as the PHA-induced increase in influx (from 20 to 38 nmoles/liter cell water) was almost exactly balanced by the efflux (from 19 to 38 nmoles/liter cell water). In confirmation of Kay's suggestion, they concluded that the enhanced influx was a homeostatic response to the primary alteration in permeability. Interestingly, the mitogen dose–K^+ flux response paralleled the mitogen dose–DNA synthetic response. The stimulation of the active transport system was calculated to be a cellular response to a small increase (from 15 to 21 mM) of intracellular Na^+ resulting from the leak (Segel et al., 1979a). Hamilton and Kaplan (1977) and Negendank and Shaller (1979) confirmed the findings of Segel and co-workers regarding the balanced K^+ influx and leak. When K^+ levels appeared to be reduced by mitogen, this was determined to be an artifact of cell washing and resuspension (Negendank and Shaller, 1979). The only question remaining is one of priority. If the increased leak precedes increased transport, it should be possible to determine this experimentally. However, Averdunk (1972) showed that increased K^+ transport occurred as early as 30 sec. More recently, it was determined that Con A caused slightly greater active transport than efflux of K^+ (or Rb^+) (Owens and Kaplan, 1980; Kaplan and Owens, 1982). The difference caused a net intracellular K^+ increase, from 14 to 16 fmole/cell (Kaplan and Owens, 1980). If cell water volume expands proportionately, there would be no change in K^+ concentration (Owens and Kaplan, 1980).

Potassium ions are now understood to be exported from cells by several quite specific types of ion channels, and the nomenclature for these will probably replace the terms "permeability" and "leak flux." Two types of calcium-activated K^+ channels were discovered recently in smooth muscle and other cells (reviewed by Walsh and Singer, 1983; Peterson and Maruyama, 1984). Rink and Deutsch (1983) obtained evidence for calcium-activated K^+ channels in mouse thymocytes, as well as indirect evidence for activation of such channels by hyperpolarization resulting from A23187-induced increases in cellular calcium. However, they stated that membrane potential plays no critical role in the response to lectin mitogens for the first 2–3 hr. Rink and Deutsch (1983) also discussed a new patch-clamp technique that has revealed the presence of voltage-gated K^+ channels in lymphocytes.

DeCoursey et al. (1984) and Chandy et al. (1984) used patch-clamp techniques to determine that a voltage-gated K^+ channel was the predominant ion channel in human T lymphocytes. The channels open with sigmoid kinetics during depolarizing voltage steps, distinguishing them from calcium-gated K^+ channels. PHA altered K^+ channel gating within 1 min, causing channels to open more rapidly and at more negative membrane potentials. By using inhibitors (4-aminopyridine, tetraethylammonium), some correspondence was found between inhibition of K^+ current and of PHA-stimulated leucine incorporation and DNA synthesis. Calcium channel blockers (verapamil, diltiazem) and a calcium-activated K^+ channel blocker (quinine) were also effective, but Chandy et al. (1984) suggested that these agents can also act on the voltage-gated K^+ channels. Gupta and co-workers interpret their data as indicating that the calcium-independent K^+ channels may participate in early events and may be necessary for protein and DNA synthesis. Gelfand et al. (1986a,b) excluded a role for these channels in mitogen-induced calcium permeability. The ability of the inhibitors to block DNA synthesis even when added 20 hr after mitogen, as well as their inability to block the new expression of IL-2 receptors on T cells, suggests that these channels are necessary for proliferation but are not involved in initial signal transmission.

Membrane potential changes accompanying ion fluxes in innervated tissues and might be expected to occur immediately upon activation of other types of cells. Several studies indicate that potential changes do occur in mitogen activated lymphocytes, but the effects are variable and slow to develop. Shapiro et al. (1979), Kiefer et al. (1980), and Felber and Brand (1983) observed that mitogens such as PHA and Con A induce a depolarization of transmembrane potential in spleen and peripheral blood lymphocytes, using a variety of techniques ranging from micropuncture to cationic dyes. Kiefer et al. (1980) found that mouse spleen T cells have a normal surface charge of -65 mV and became depolarized at 2–3 hr after addition of Con A. Repolarization occurred over the next 7 hr, and hyperpolarization characterized the final 24–48 hr before mitosis. Similar changes were observed using splenic B lymphocytes stimulated by LPS. The specificity of the mitogens for lymphocyte types supported the notion that depolarization relates to mitogen action.

By contrast, others (Tsien et al., 1982; Felber and Brand, 1983; Tatham and Delves, 1984; June et al., 1986) observed that T-cell mitogens, including the calcium ionophore A23187, do not induce depolarization or instead induce hyperpolarization of blood and lymph node lymphocytes and thymocytes. This effect was calcium ion dependent and, based on the action of inhibitors, it was concluded that it resulted from effects on calcium-gated K^+ channels. Felber and Brand attributed the difference in the mitogen-induced responses of peripheral T lymphocytes and of murine thymocytes to the fact that calcium-dependent K^+ channels are already maximally activated in peripheral lymphocytes; therefore, only the thymocytes could show the calcium-dependent hyperpolarization effect.

The collected observations do not make it likely that K^+ efflux via either calcium dependent or calcium independent, voltage-regulated K^+ channels is essential to the initial activation process, and that since both hyperpolarization and depolarization result from mitogen stimulation of various T cells, changes in transmembrane potential are not crucial early processes.

The work of Quastel and Kaplan (1968, 1970) suggested that the Na^+,K^+-ATPase enzymatic activity would be elevated by mitogens. Such measurements require careful isolation of plasma membranes, in order to detect activity of the

Na^+,K^+-ATPase (which also requires Mg^{2+}) in the presence of other Mg^{2+}-dependent ATPases found throughout the cell. Lichtman and Weed (1969) measured an elevated activity in leukemic lymphocytes (CLL) compared with normal peripheral blood lymphocytes. Early attempts to measure an increase in the enzyme by direct addition of PHA (Averdunk, 1972) or Con A (Novogrodsky, 1972) to crude lymphocyte membrane preparations were not successful. However, Averdunk and Lauf (1975) and Pommier et al. (1975) detected mitogen-induced increases in Na^+,K^+-ATPases of human, sheep, and mouse lymphocytes. The increases were seen only after preincubating intact cells with mitogen.

In a more detailed study, Averdunk et al. (1976) found that preincubation with Con A stimulated the Mg^{2+}-ATPase (twofold) as well as the Na^+,K^+-ATPase (fivefold) in intact human blood lymphocytes. Curiously, they also reported an increase in the Na^+,K^+-ATPase after adding Con A directly to membranes. The fact that lectins can stimulate an isolated membrane Na^+,K^+-ATPase was confirmed in MOPC cells (Aubry et al., 1979) and liver (Riordan et al., 1977), but whether mitogenic lectins do so in lymphocytes has not been confirmed (Dornand et al., 1978; Segel et al., 1979b). The effects of mitogens acting on intact cells to stimulate the Na^+,K^+-ATPase have been abundantly documented in calf thymocytes by Resch and colleagues (Szamel and Resch, 1981a,b; Szamel et al., 1981; Resch et al., 1983, 1984) and in rabbit thymocytes (Tandon et al., 1983).

Whereas Resch et al. (1983) observed a Con A-induced decrease in Mg^{2+}-ATPase, several others (Novogrodsky, 1972; Ellegard and Dimitrov, 1973; Krishnaraj and Talwar, 1973; Averdunk and Lauf, 1975; Pommier et al., 1975; Tandon et al., 1983) measured an increase in this activity after mitogen addition to lymphocytes. This increase is smaller than the increase in Na^+,K^+-ATPase, but since the total activity of Mg^{2+}-ATPase far exceeds that of Na^+,K^+-ATPase, Tandon et al. (1983) concluded that the net effect of Con A was greater on Mg^{2+}-ATPase. No physiological significance has yet been associated with plasma membrane Mg^{2+}-ATPase, and the effects of mitogens on this activity cannot be interpreted at this time. Ellegard and Dimitrov (1973) attributed part of the increased activity to a mitochondrial origin, and therefore represented the disorganized ATP synthesis system operating in reverse. By contrast, Pommier et al. (1975) stated that their Mg^{2+}-ATPase measurements represented a cell-surface ectoenzyme. It is of interest to note, however, that the Mg^{2+}-ATPase activity (and not the Na^+,K^+-ATPase) is considerably elevated in mouse spleen after immunization with antigen (Friedman and Kateley, 1974).

In addition to the above activities, mitogen-induced increases of calcium-ATPase have been observed (Dornand et al., 1974; Averdunk and Gunther, 1980). This activity has been identified with calcium transport (efflux) of plasma membranes and is stimulated by calmodulin in lymphocytes (Lichtman et al., 1981) as in other cells. Its stimulation by mitogens would account for the increased calcium efflux observed by Mikkelson and Schmidt-Ulrich (1980).

Specific inhibition of several consequences of mitogen action by ouabain may be interpreted as presumptive evidence for a requirement of the Na^+, K^+ pump in these events, although actions disassociated from those on the pump have been described in macrophages (Leu et al., 1973). Among such events are the late increases in uridine uptake (Quastel and Kaplan, 1968; Kay, 1972; Szamel et al., 1981), acyltransferase activation, and oleate incorporation, IL-2 production and response to IL-2 (Stoeck et al., 1983), and ultimately, DNA synthesis (Quastel and Kaplan, 1968; Wright et al., 1973). Inhibition of the mitogen-induced changes is reversed by washing, indicating the above are not merely toxic effects (Wright et al., 1973).

Ouabain binds to specific high-affinity sites on Na^+, K^+-ATPase facing the external surface of cells, and PHA-induced increases in ouabain binding to human blood lymphocytes have been observed (Quastel et al., 1974; Quastel and Kaplan, 1975). The effect is due to increased V_{max}, representing an increased number rather than affinity of binding sites. It occurs within minutes after PHA addition to lymphocytes, in parallel with PHA-induced increases in active K^+ transport (Quastel and Kaplan, 1975). K^+ reverses ouabain binding and also its inhibition of transport and uridine uptake. K^+ reversal studies of the other ouabain-inhibited events have not been performed to our knowledge. Resch and co-workers (Szamel and Resch, 1981b; Stoeck et al., 1983; Resch et al., 1984) believe that ouabain acts at some point in addition to the ATPase since its potency for inhibiting activation of acyl transferase and other early events (0.1–2 mM) exceeds the potency usually found for inhibiting Na^+, K^+-ATPase (1–10 μM), and the concentration required for inhibiting IL-2 production is much greater (1 mM). Conclusions based on the assumed selectivity of a drug can be misleading. In this case, ouabain inhibition of the Na^+, K^+-pump may occur at a lower concentration than measurable for inhibition of membrane ATPase because binding sites of intact cells may be more accessible. Zachowski et al. (1977) found that ouabain effectively inhibits Na^+, K^+-ATPase in "inside-out" vesicles at 10^{-7} M, but not in "right-side-out" vesicles in which 10^{-4} M was required. These workers suggested that the inhibition in right-side-out vesicles was impeded by a protein (30-kDa) that could be removed by EDTA. Since EDTA is often used in the purification of Na^+, K^+-ATPase, such an effect would not be seen in studies of the purified enzymes. Other modulatory effects, including Na^+, K^+-ATPase, inhibition by cyclic AMP may be mediated by a kinase, present in membrane systems but not in the more purified Na^+, K^+-ATPase preparations.

In conclusion, it appears that mitogen activation of lymphocytes results in early permeability changes and ion fluxes and that compensatory mechanisms involving ATPase are activated to restore normal balances. The regulatory rule of these processes has not been established; further evidence is needed to determine the dependency or independence of early nuclear activation processes on these events. Normal function of ATPase, as demonstrated by ouabain inhibition studies, is essential for lymphocyte proliferation, as it probably is ultimately for viability.

Intracellular pH measurements have recently been made possible by three new technologies:

1. A new application of nuclear magnetic resonance (NMR) was employed by Deutsch *et al.* (1982) to measure the pH value of human lymphocytes without the possible discrepancies of equilibrium distribution of weak acids and bases used in other methods. A pH value of 7.17 was found in human peripheral blood lymphocyte by the NMR method. These workers determined that lymphocytes regulate closely their pH at the expense of energy, showing only minor changes within the external pH range of 6.8–7.4; they reported that mitogenesis proceeds best when cells are within this pH range.

2. Gerson and Kiefer (1982) employed the pH-dependent fluorochrome, 4-methyl-umbelliferone, to show that activation of mouse splenic lymphocytes by Con A or LPS is accompanied by a gradual increase in intracellular pH from 7.15 to 7.45. Furthermore, they found that these virus-transformed cell lines with high mitotic activity were about 0.5 pH units higher than normal cells. The quene 1 fluorescence technique also gave a pH value of 7.15 for thymocytes (Rogers *et al.*, 1983a). The pH value was found to be insensitive to calcium or Mg^{2+} but declined if the medium pH was lowered. In contrast to the results of Deutsch *et al.* (1982), Rogers *et al.* (1983b) observed no change in intracellular pH with quene 1 upon increasing the medium pH to 8.0, and they saw no change during the first 30 min after mitogen addition.

3. Gerson *et al.* (1982) measured a resting cell pH of 7.18 in mouse spleen cells with $[^{14}C]$-5,5-dimethyl oxazoline-2,4-dione. This value is remarkably similar to the one obtained by Deutsch *et al.* (1982). With this labeled substance, they observed two increases in pH following mitogen addition: pH increased by about 0.2 units at 1–6 hr, declined to control levels at 20 hr, then increased gradually to 7.5 over the next 50 hr. The second increase was proportional to DNA synthesis, and the final decline in pH was coincident with mitosis.

Doubts concerning the interpretation of the data of Gerson *et al.* (1982) have been raised by Grinstein *et al.* (1984), who found that apparent increases in the pH of actively cycling thymocytes were actually due to increases in the number of mitochondria per unit cell volume. In agreement with Deutsch *et al.* (1982), they found that certain pH indicators distribute preferentially in these organelles, which are more basic than lymphocyte cytoplasm. By contrast, Hesketh *et al.* (1985) found that a wide variety of mitogenic substances increased the pH of mouse thymocytes as well as 3T3 fibroblasts within 30 min and that this change was dependent on a transient (5 min) increase in intracellular ionized calcium (see Section 2.6).

It is interesting to note that one mechanism for simultaneously increasing intracellular pH and Na^+ content, the membrane Na^+/H^+ antiport, has now been described in human peripheral blood lymphocytes (Grinstein *et al.*, 1984). This system may be activated by protein kinase C (Besterman *et al.*, 1985), which is activated by mitogens (as described in Section 2.4.1). This system is inhibited by amiloride analogues; recent data (Mills *et al.*, 1986b) using such analogues indicate that the Na^+/H^+ antiport is not an obligatory requirement for lymphocyte activation or proliferation. The alterations in pH like those of surface potential cannot, therefore, be considered as primary activation signals. They may contribute to late cycle events, but it is unlikely that they are critical events.

2.5.3. Amino Acid Uptake

In basic studies of nonstimulated human peripheral blood lymphocytes, Yunis *et al.* (1963) found that the active transport of 2-aminoisobutyric acid (AIB), glycine, proline, alanine, and glutamic acid requires Na^+. Transport of these amino acids is stimulated by calcium and inhibited by ouabain. Amino acids whose uptake is independent of these influences include arginine, lysine, leucine, histidine, and methionine. In lymphocytes the transport of several amino acids is enhanced by mitogens, as attested by more than 20 papers from at least 14 laboratories.

The earliest reports of mitogen-stimulated amino acid transport involve leucine (Na^+-independent): Kay (1968) and Hausen *et al.* (1969) found that rates of uptake of this amino acid doubled by 4–6 hr after addition of mitogen to lymphocytes. Activation of uptake of the nonmetabolizable AIB (Na^+-dependent) was measured at 30 min (Mendelsohn *et al.*, 1971) and may begin at 5 min (Van den Berg and Betel, 1971, 1973a,b; Averdunk, 1972). Ouabain inhibited the mitogen-stimulated transport of AIB in rat lymph node cells (Van den Berg and Betel, 1973a), as did a host of inhibitors of oxidative phosphorylation, glycolysis, and protein synthesis, whereas RNA and DNA synthesis inhibitors did not (Van den Berg and Betel, 1974b). Only amino acids whose transport is Na^+-dependent were found to be stimulated in rat lymph node cells by Con A (Van den Berg and Betel, 1974b). However, detailed analysis of three transport systems in pig blood lymphocytes by Borghetti *et al.* (1979) and human blood lymphocytes by Segel *et al.* (1981) produced different conclusions. The A transport system of these cells is Na^+ dependent and uniquely increases as an adaptive response to a period of amino acid deprivation. It is responsible for AIB uptake and, of the three systems, it is the most dramatically increased by PHA (Borghetti *et al.*, 1979). The ASC system is also Na^+ dependent, has a broader substrate specificity than the A system (including proline and alanine), and was enhanced by PHA to a similar degree as the A system in human lymphocytes (Segel and Lichtman, 1981). The third system, the L system, is Na^+ independent, transports leucine and several other amino acids, and is also increased by PHA (Borghetti *et al.*, 1979; Segel and Lichtman, 1981). The increases occur much later than with AIB (16–20 hr in these studies, 6–8 hr in the studies of Kay, 1968, and Hausen *et al.* 1969), and to a much lesser extent than with the A and ASC systems.

Kinetic studies (Mendelsohn *et al.*, 1971; Greene *et al.*, 1976a) indicated that AIB transport (A system) increases as a result of increased V_{max}, rather than an effect on K_m, reaching a sixfold elevation of AIB compared with control at 9 hr. The greatly increased intracellular amino acid concentration reflects not only the increased rate of uptake but also the relatively insignificant increase in efflux (Averdunk, 1972). Mitogen-induced increase in AIB transport was found to be inhibited by colchicine (Greene *et al.*, 1976d; Resch *et al.*, 1981) but augmented by the cytochalasins (Greene *et al.*, 1976b). It was not affected by protein synthesis inhibitors in HPBL (Mendelsohn *et al.*, 1971) but was inhibited by cycloheximide in leukemic cells and rat lymph node cells (Baran *et al.*, 1972; Van den Berg and Betel, 1974b). Actinomycin D and mitocycin D did not inhibit AIB, asparagine, or glycine transport increases induced by Con A in rat lymph node cells (Van den Berg and Betel, 1974b). It may be concluded that mitogen stimulation of the amino acid transport systems does not require DNA or RNA synthesis but may require protein synthesis and energy, depending on the species.

Van den Berg and Betel (1973a, 1974a) found a good correlation between AIB uptake stimulation and lectin mitogenicity in mouse and rat lymphocytes, but Udey *et al.* (1980) found that the nonmitogenic wheat germ agglutinin (WGA) stimulated uptake in human peripheral blood lymphocytes. Since WGA also inhibited AIB uptake stimulated by Con A (Greene *et al.*, 1976c), the essentiality of the early stimulation of the A transport system to lymphocyte activation is doubtful. Resch *et al.* (1981) reached similar conclusions based on the findings that colchicine suppressed early Con A-stimulated AIB uptake but suppressed DNA synthesis even if added 20 hr after Con A—a time when the presence of the mitogen is no longer required. Later events do require amino acid transport, since cysteine and glutamine are essential for DNA synthesis (Van den Berg and Betel, 1974a,b). It is possible that stimulation of the L system is the only essential feature of mitogen action on amino acid uptake.

2.5.4. Glucose Uptake

Lymphocytes treated with PHA incorporate glucose or its nonmetabolizable analogues, 3-*O*-methyl glucose and 2-deoxyglucose, at a greatly accelerated rate within minutes (Hadden *et al.*, 1971a,b; Peters and Hausen, 1971b; Yasmeen *et al.*, 1977; Averdunk, 1972). Experiments with Con A and A23187 have confirmed that this response is a general one for mitogens (Reeves, 1975; Whitesell *et al.*, 1977; Hume *et al.*, 1978a). Glucose is transported by facilitated diffusion in mitogen stimulated as well as control lymphocytes. The effect of PHA in increasing transport is due entirely to increased V_{max} and is not inhibited by cycloheximide, actinomycin D, or puromycin; it may therefore represent a direct effect on the cell membrane to increase the availability of carrier sites (Peters and Hausen, 1971b).

Energy-linked processes in mitogen action are suggested by the inhibitory effects of oligomycin and dinitrophenol on A23187-stimulated (but not on control) glucose uptake (Reeves, 1975). Calcium was also necessary for the stimulation, but not for the maintenance, of mitogen-stimulated glucose transport rate. Cyclic AMP, agents that increase cyclic AMP, and hydrocortisone inhibit glucose transport (Hadden et al., 1971a,c; Munck, 1971, Boyett and Hoffert, 1972). The inhibitory effects of cyclic AMP and agents that increase its intracellular level, on both Con A and A23187 stimulation of glucose uptake in rat thymocytes, were interpreted with reference to inhibition of calcium uptake (Whitesell et al., 1977). Calcium ion was also found necessary for Con A stimulation of glucose uptake in these cells (Yasmeen et al., 1977; Nordenberg et al., 1983). Activation by Con A, but not PMA, of glucose uptake could be inhibited by p-bromophenacyl bromide in addition to dibuturyl cyclic AMP and 1-methyl-3-isobutylxanthine. Nordenberg et al. (1983) suggested that all the agents act at a common point, inhibiting calcium-dependent phospholipase. More specific inhibitors of mitogen-activated glucose uptake include cytochalasin B, which is thought to bind to glucose carriers (Hume et al., 1978a), and quercetin, which closely resembles phloretin (Hume et al., 1979). Mookerjee and Jung (1982) showed that six different cytochalasins inhibit PHA stimulation of glucose uptake and proliferation. They found three binding sites for cytochalasin B; site M was specifically displaced by glucose.

All the experiments reviewed above have produced important information basic to understanding lymphocyte physiology. Again, the relevance to early events of lymphocyte activation is not definitively proven, since work reviewed in the microfilament section suggests that inhibition of glucose transport by cytochalasin B has little effect on lymphocyte activation if it occurs only during the first few hours.

2.5.5. Nucleoside Uptake

Stimulation of nucleoside transport by mitogens has not received as much experimental attention as the other transport topics. Increased uptake of uridine occurs almost immediately after addition of PHA to human blood lymphocytes (Z. J. Lucas, 1967; Hausen and Stein, 1968; Kay, 1968; Quastel and Kaplan, 1968). Like transport of K^+, glucose, and amino acids, the effect of PHA on uridine transport involves increased V_{max}, with no effect of K_m. The increase reaches a maximum rate at about 8 hr after PHA and, since uridine kinase rises accordingly, Hausen and Stein (1968) suggested that the kinase was rate limiting. However, Z. J. Lucas (1967) first observed uridine and cytidine kinase increases at 16 hr and claimed that uridine kinase was induced by uridine in a

RNA- and protein synthesis-dependent fashion. Kay and Handmaker (1970) measured enhanced uridine uptake prior to increased kinase activity and stated that uridine uptake and even its incorporation into RNA was not limited by uridine kinase.

Inhibitor studies have been useful in two aspects of nucleoside uptake. First, Kay (1972) observed that the early (1-hr) increase induced by PHA in human peripheral blood lymphocytes was insensitive to ouabain, while the later (26-hr) increase was inhibited by it. The later effect was thought to be secondary to an effect of ouabain on protein synthesis. Second, the most definitive study involved dipyridamole, which inhibits uptake of several nucleosides. Peters and Hausen (1971a) found this agent to prevent uridine uptake but not the stimulation by PHA or uridine and cytidine kinases. Most importantly, dipyridamole did not limit lymphocyte transformation, ruling out any further debate concerning the role of nucleoside uptake in the early events of lymphocyte activation. The metabolism of nucleosides and nucleic acid synthesis are reviewed in Section 3.

The roles of iron and transferrin in lymphocyte activation have recently come under scrutiny. The collected data (reviewed by Brock and Mainou-Fowler, 1983; Pelosi et al., 1986) suggest that activated lymphocytes have an increased need for iron, for its transport protein transferrin, or both. Iron is an indispensable part of heme, which is found in many proteins, including the cytochromes, cyclooxygenase, and guanylate cyclase. Iron is also required for ribonucleotide reductase, a key enzyme in DNA synthesis. Using serum free media, Brock (1981) showed markedly enhanced responses of mouse lymph node cells to Con A or LPS with transferrin which was partly saturated with iron. Larrick and Creswell (1979) first showed increases in the binding of transferrin to transferrin receptors of human blood lymphocytes after addition of PHA or Con A. Weiel and Hamilton (1984) established that transferrin receptors are present intracellularly in resting lymphocytes but increase fivefold and appear partly on the surface of activated lymphocytes. The increase in receptors occurs only after the appearance of IL-2 receptors and the addition of IL-2 (>6 hr) (Hamilton, 1982, 1983; Neckers and Crossman, 1983), in agreement with the data of Brock and Rankin (1981), which indicate that significant iron uptake occurs at about 20 hr after addition of mitogen. Iron is made available to the cell only after the transferrin–transferrin receptor complex is internalized. Recycling of the receptors to the cell surface is associated with a phosphorylation–dephosphorylation cycle, which may be regulated by protein kinase C (May et al., 1984).

Mendelsohn et al. (1983) found that DNA synthesis in human blood lymphocytes, cultured in serum-free medium, could be blocked by a monoclonal antibody against the transferrin receptor. These investigators concluded that transferrin is needed throughout the cell cycle. However, inhibition could be reversed by removing the antibody after 48 hr of incubation, suggesting that either transferrin is needed only in the latter stages of the cell cycle or the inhibition is nonspecific. The fact that inhibition could also be partially reversed by an iron containing compound (ferric nitrilotriacetate) suggests that the transferrin receptor may be important to increase cellular levels of iron or other ions. In this regard, Phillips and Azair (1974) have observed that transferrin complexed with zinc rather than iron could augment mitogen action in association with zinc uptake by lymphocytes and several observations support an important role for zinc in mitogen-induced lymphocyte transformation (R. O. Williams and Loeb, 1973; Berger and Skinner, 1974; Chesters, 1975; Phillips, 1976).

2.6. Calcium

During the late 1960s, data derived from other cell biology systems placed calcium in a central role in stimulus-coupling mechanisms. It was natural to think of lymphocytes within this context, as two seminal observations focused attention on these cells. Whitfield *et al.* (1969) observed that concentrations of calcium in excess of 1.2 mM (i.e., approximately four times normal serum levels) would induce rat thymocytes to enter DNA synthesis and to undergo mitosis. While this was not the case for resting lymphocytes in the blood or other lymphoid tissues, this observation was initially taken to mean that calcium was mitogenic for lymphocytes in general. Only in subsequent years was it realized that the effect of calcium in this system was to induce immature thymocytes to move from a G_1–S restriction point to enter S phase (Whitfield *et al.*, 1976), an action, as it turns out, that is more relevant to how second signals, such as IL-2, or T-cell growth factor (TCGF), might act rather than how mitogens might initiate proliferation in resting lymphocytes in G_0 or a restricted G_1 phase of the cell cycle. The second observation (Alford, 1970) was that calcium chelators such as disodium(ethylenedinitrilo)tetracetate (EDTA) and citrate blocked PHA-induced lymphocyte proliferation, and this effect was reversed by calcium. While a great variety of nutritive and ionic constituents might be envisioned to be necessary for cell growth, these observations placed calcium in center stage for lymphocytes and led to the findings of Allwood *et al.*, (1971) showing that PHA induces calcium influx.

During the past 15 years, more than 60 papers have probed the requirements for calcium in lymphocyte activation and its participation in the initiation process. Considerable controversy has clouded the area during this period; however, a sizable amount of data has been derived to support the participation of calcium in lymphocyte activation. While earlier reviews (see Berridge 1975; Hesketh, 1978; Hume and Wiedemann, 1980) tended to emphasize technical discrepancies and the controversial aspects, it appears to us that a consensus has emerged and it is our intent to summarize its salient features here.

The strategies that have been employed to evaluate the role of calcium in mitogen-induced lymphocyte activation include the study of:

1. The effect of deletion of calcium from the medium and its further chelation with relatively specific chelators, such as ethylene glycol-bis(diaminoethyl ether) N,N'-tetra acetic acid (EGTA)
2. The effect of mitogens to induce calcium influx
3. The actions of the calcium ionophore A23187 to mimic lectin mitogens
4. The calcium dependence of enzymatic processes thought to be central in the triggering process

2.6.1. Extracellular Calcium

The first of these strategies has been revealing in its insights, but not devoid of pitfalls. Although a number of studies employing calcium-free medium, in fact, failed to consider the presence of calcium in the small amounts (generally 10%) of serum present, it did become apparent that lymphocyte proliferation, in general, required more than trace amounts of calcium and 0.1–1 mM was found to be optimal (Ling and Kay, 1975). Chelation of calcium with EGTA blocked both RNA and DNA synthesis induced by PHA and allogeneic cells and addition of excess calcium reversed the block (Alford, 1970; Kay, 1971; Whitney and Sutherland, 1972a,b; Diamantstein and Ulmer, 1975a). The addition of EGTA was suspected to modify PHA binding; however, Whitney and Sutherland (1973b) found that addition of EGTA 1–2 hr after PHA addition, and therefore after PHA binding, effectively inhibited the effects of PHA; they concluded that the effect was not on binding. Brewer *et al.* (1974) concluded that calcium is not necessary for Con A binding as long as another transitional metal is present. Lindahl-Kiessling (1976) observed that EGTA (1.5 mM) prevented PHA binding by 90% at 37°C but not at 4°C and had no effect on binding if added 1 hr after PHA, under which circumstance it still blocked proliferation (see also Bard *et al.*, 1978). These observations pointed to a metabolically dependent EGTA-affected step in PHA binding and placed in some doubt conclusions made on the basis of EGTA additions with PHA. More recently, Resch (1976) stated that concentrations of EGTA sufficient to block Con A-induced proliferation do not inhibit binding; Ananthakrishnan *et al.* (1981) showed that EGTA (2 mM) in calcium-free media reduced PHA binding by approximately 50%. In the latter study, it was concluded that 1 mM EGTA allowed sufficient PHA to bind to produce a half-maximal proliferative response; therefore, early metabolic events induced by PHA that are completely blocked by EGTA at this concentration can be concluded to be dependent on calcium. The use of EGTA in calcium-free and serum-free media in this study inhibited early events to a greater degree than deletion of calcium in the medium, implying that cell-associated, even intracellular, calcium is thus chelated and that intracellular processes dependent on this calcium source are thus blocked. Experiments employing the calcium ionophore A23187 carry less liability of interpretation, since binding of A23187 is unaffected by calcium and the mitogenic effects of the ionophore seem to depend entirely on extracellular calcium. A number of conclusions made as a result of the use of EGTA have been independently corroborated by calcium ionophore experiments.

Several experiments have attempted to show a restricted period of calcium requirement by adding EGTA at various times after PHA addition to culture (Whitney and Sutherland, 1972c, 1973a,b; Diamantstein and Ulmer, 1975a; Bard et al., 1978). Addition of EGTA 48 hr after PHA does not affect PHA proliferation, while addition of EGTA for the first 12 hr completely blocks PHA action. Addition of EGTA at times after 12 hr results in progressively diminished effects of EGTA to block. While Diamantstein and Ulmer (1975a) emphasized, in contrast to their data, the prolonged requirement for calcium, it is apparent that calcium is required principally for the first 12–24 hr of PHA action. Since this time period precedes measurable DNA synthesis, extracellular calcium is thought necessary only for the initial activation events.

The interpretation has been further corroborated by experiments using blockers of the action of calcium, which presumably have no effect on mitogen binding. Luckasen et al. (1974) showed that lanthanum that competes for calcium binding but is otherwise inactive blocks PHA-induced lymphocyte proliferation. Ferguson et al. (1975, 1976) showed that chlorpromazine and lidocaine, two calcium-blocking agents, block Con A-induced proliferation during the first 3–4 hr and had no effect after 24 hr. Blitstein-Willinger and Diamantstein, (1978) further showed that verapamil, a calcium-channel blocker, prevented PHA- and Con A-induced lymphocyte proliferation principally at early times (<8 hr) but had little or no effect later. These observations were recently confirmed by Birx et al. (1984) with several calcium-channel blockers.

Several laboratories (Lichtman et al., 1982; Kimoto et al., 1983; Cheung et al., 1983; Bachvaroff et al., 1984) showed that trifluoperazine (TFP) and chlorpromazine, which inhibit calmodulin-stimulated enzymes and protein kinase C, block mitogen and MLC-induced proliferation. Metcalfe et al., (1980) showed that delayed addition of calcium to lymphocytes stimulated by mitogen in calcium-free media results in corresponding delays of the increase in thymidine incorporation into DNA. These observations suggest that the cells entered the proliferative cycle only when calcium influx was allowed to occur.

These collected observations offer strong argument that extracellular and cell-associated calcium is critical in the initiation process and that influx and calmodulin- or protein kinase C-linked processes are involved. Of the other early metabolic events, calcium deletion and calcium-blocker studies show that medium- or cell-associated calcium is necessary for lectin mitogen-induced leucine and uridine incorporation (2 hr) (Kay, 1971), cell aggregation (3 hr) (Ferguson et al., 1975, Neely et al., 1976), amino acid transport (Whitney and Sutherland, 1973a; Betel and Van den Berg, 1975), cyclic GMP increases and guanylate cyclase activation (5–10 min) (Hadden, 1977; Coffey et al., 1977; Coffey and Hadden, 1978), nuclear RNA synthesis (1 hr) (Ananthakrishnan et al., 1981), glucose uptake (Reeves, 1975; Yasmeen *et al.*, 1977), pyruvate oxidation (Hume *et al.*, 1978b), increases of ornithine decarboxylase (Otani *et al.*, 1980, 1982) and IL-2 production (Mills *et al.*, 1985a). Similar studies indicate that the following processes are not dependent on calcium: AIB transport, cyclic AMP increases, and phosphatidylinositol turnover (Greene *et al.*, 1976a) and IL-2 receptor display and IL-2 action (Mills *et al.*, 1985b).

Before turning to a discussion of calcium influx, it is important to evaluate whether calcium is specific in triggering the initial events (Alford, 1970; Allwood *et al.*, 1971). Kay (1971) reported that the effects of EDTA were partially reversed by Mg (20 mM); however, others (Whitney and Sutherland, 1972a,b) showed that the effects of EGTA were reversed by calcium, but not by magnesium. Alford (1970) observed the effects of iron and zinc to promote proliferation of lymphocytes in the presence of EDTA and calcium; it was not clear, however, whether these metals merely displaced calcium for the chelator. Subsequent experiments have indicated that zinc itself is a T-cell mitogen that is perhaps dependent on the macrophage (Ruhl and Kirchner, 1978) and that iron transferrin and/or lactoferrin is a cofactor in lymphocyte proliferation (Neckers and Crossman, 1983). Resch *et al.* (1978) further suggested that magnesium and manganese may compete with calcium for influx, but these observations probably relate to B cells. Another trace metal, mercury, at high concentrations has also been shown to be a T-lymphocyte mitogen. In none of these studies has it been suggested that the requirement of calcium for mitogen-induced proliferation is not highly specific and biologically relevant.

2.6.2. Calcium Influx

Since Allwood *et al.* (1971) first showed that PHA induced calcium influx, no less than 18 studies have been performed to confirm this observation with mitogens (Table I). The following T-cell mitogens have been confirmed to induce calcium influx by one or another technique: PHA, Con A, succinylated Con A, periodate, zinc, mercury, and an anti T-cell mitogenic monoclonal antibody. Lymphocytes used in these studies include human blood lymphocytes, mouse splenocytes, rat thymocytes, and rabbit and guinea pig lymph node cells. The calcium influxes have been observed with a variety of T-cell mitogens in T cells (Freedman, 1979; O'Flynn *et al.*, 1984) but not with B-cell mitogens in T cells (Freedman, 1979) or with nonmitogens (Parker, 1974). Similarly B-cell mitogens, but not T-cell mitogens, induce calcium influx in B lymphocytes (Freedman, 1979). Additional evidence supporting the interpretation that, for T-cell mitogens, these changes are T-cell specific is that the effects do not occur in athymic nude mice spleen cells. The effects correlate with dose–response curves for the mitogens where tested (Freedman *et al.*, 1975; Freedman, 1979).

While 21 studies are positive, one failed to show a Con A effect in pig lymph node cells and mouse splenocytes (Hesketh *et al.*, 1977). The impact of

TABLE I
Calcium Influx Studies with T-Cell Mitogens[a,b]

Investigators	Mitogen	Lymphocyte source	Cell collection	Results
Allwood et al. (1971)	PHA	Human blood	Filter	↑ 40 to 80 min
Whitney and Sutherland (1972c)	PHA	Human blood	Filter	↑ 60 min
Whitney and Sutherland (1973b)	PHA	Human blood	Cell pellet	Progressive increase ↑ 5–90 min
Parker (1974)	PHA Con A Periodate ZN and HG	Human blood	Filter	↑ at 60 min
Freedman et al. (1975)	PHA Con A	Mouse spleen	Water-impermeable barrier	↑ 60 sec
Hadden et al. (1975)	PHA	Human blood	Filter	Progressive ↑ 10–60 min
Greene et al. (1976a)	PHA Con A	Human blood	Filter	Peak at 2 min ↑ to 10 min, 10–60 min
Hesketh et al. (1977)	Con A	Pig lymph node Mouse spleen	Filter	No effect to 30 min
Ozato et al. (1977)	Con A	Mouse spleen	Cell pellet	Progressive ↑ to 0–60 min
Whitesell et al. (1977)	Con A	Rat thymus	Cell pellet	Progressive ↑ 2–40 min
Freedman (1979)	Con A	Mouse spleen	Water barrier	↑ 6–45 min, then decline
	PHA	Mouse spleen		↑ 6 min–5 hr, then decline
Hui and Harmony (1977)	PHA	Human blood	Water	Progressive to 60 min
Otani et al. (1980)	PHA	Guinea pig lymph node	Filter	↑ to 30–60 min
Tsien et al. (1982)	Con A	Guinea pig lymph node	Quin 2	↑ to 2–3 min
	PHA	Mouse spleen		
Toyoshima et al. (1982a)	Con A	Mouse spleen	Filter	↑ 5 min
Deutsch and Price (1982)	S-Con A	Human blood	Filter	Progressive ↑ to 40 min
Hesketh et al. (1983a,b)	Con A S-Con A	Mouse thymus Guinea pig lymph node	Quin 2	↑ 1 min
O'Flynn et al. (1984)	PHA	Human blood	Quin 2	↑ 2 min

[a]Con A, concanavalin A; PHA, phytohemagglutinin.
[b]Excludes calcium ionophore.

this negative observation on the field and the challenges it produced have been great; however, it is of note that Hesketh and co-workers have since presented an hypothesis that calcium influx is nevertheless central to lymphocyte activation (Metcalfe et al., 1980). In the controversy that ensued, it was soon clear that different techniques used to measure calcium (^{45}Ca) uptake could produce somewhat different results. Most of the earlier studies involved washing, centrifugation, and trapping of lymphocytes on filters (Table I). It was legitimately pointed out by Resch (1976) that the trauma involved in the collection procedure is sufficient to induce erythrocytes preloaded with chromium (^{51}Cr) to lose most of their label. To a varying degree, depending on the specifics of the experimental procedure, lymphocytes collected in this manner must also be affected, leading one to conclude that mitogen-induced calcium uptake by this procedure may underestimate influx and reflect to a greater degree than the other techniques cell-bound versus free cytosol calcium.

Techniques using cell pellet counting without trapping on filters and separation of cells from the water-soluble isotope using a silicone oil or similar barrier represent theoretically more reliable ways to assess total calcium uptake. These studies (Whitney and Sutherland, 1972c, 1973b; Freedman et al., 1975; Ozato et al., 1977; Whitesell et al., 1977; Freedman, 1979; Hui et al., 1979; Hui and Harmony, 1980a; Toyoshima et al., 1982a,b; and Kimoto et al., 1983) generally describe progressive influx of calcium following PHA or Con A stimulation over the first 30–60 min. These increases are first detectable at 30 sec (Freedman et al., 1975). Notable are the data of Freedman (1979) describing progressive uptake of calcium for 45 min after Con A stimulation but flat uptake after 6 min with PHA. The latter observation is unexplainably discrepant to those of others (Whitney and Sutherland, 1973; Hui et al., 1979).

After 60–90 min, the levels peak and decline to near control levels at 6–20 hr and remain low in two studies with Con A (Freedman, 1979; Kimoto et al., 1983) and in one study with PHA (Freedman, 1979) but progressively increase to 68 hr in another experiment with PHA (Whitney and Sutherland, 1972c).

A study of the calcium efflux pump in lymphocytes (Hadden et al., 1975) showed that it functioned in an ATP-dependent manner very similar to the one described in erythocytes. These observations were subsequently confirmed and extended by Hesketh et al. (1977), Metcalfe et al. (1980), and Lichtmann et al. (1981). It seems likely that mitogen-induced influx would be matched to a great extent by efflux; therefore, a critical test of the hypothesis that calcium is essential for lymphocyte activation (Berridge, 1975; Metcalfe et al., 1980) depends on the demonstration that net cytosolic calcium concentrations are increased. The inference from indirect data is that they are increased (Metcalfe et al., 1980; Tsien et al., 1982; Hesketh et al., 1983a).

Much has been said about calcium channels to account for calcium influx; however, several observations may be applicable in casting doubt on selective uptake. It is apparent that within minutes of lectin mitogen action, there is a rapid intracellular increase of various substrates studied (e.g., glucose, amino acids, and nucleotides) (see Sections 2.5.3–2.5.5 on transport). Also apparent, following PHA, is a rapid exchange of monovalent cations that is compensated for by an equally rapid activation of ion-exchange ATPase-dependent pump mechanisms (see Section 2.5.2). In unpublished studies, we observed that PHA-stimulated lymphocytes take up trypan blue dye within minutes and subsequently extrude it by 30–60 min. Taken collectively, these observations suggest that lectin mitogen stimulation may entail, in the initial phase (first 15 min), a rather massive but transient change in plasma membrane permeability. Such a speculation would account for the appearance of cyclic nucleotides (e.g., cyclic GMP) in relatively large amounts extracellularly (Hadden *et al.*, 1975). This permeability process is probably transient (i.e., 20 min), on the basis of the trypan blue dye and chromium uptake data and may explain the early transient uptake of calcium observed by Greene *et al.* (1976a). This interpretation implies that the initial phases would not appear to result from so-called gated channels.

With this logic in mind, it is interesting to note the results of Greene *et al.* (1976a), who showed peaks in mitogen-induced calcium influx at 2 min with PHA and Con A, which declined by 10 min. This type of observation differs from the progressive increases seen by employing pelleting or flotation methods. Hadden *et al.* (1975) reported using a filter technique that the first observable influx of calcium occurred at 20 min following PHA addition and that the intersection with control appeared to be at 10 min. Not reported in the data presented at that time was an observation that was considered an artifact. In each of 10 experiments, a brisk peak of calcium influx was observed that disappeared at some point during the first 10 min. While significantly different than that of control, the effect could not be described as influx. In retrospect, these data might indicate that a portion of the calcium possibly taken up by transient binding is subsequently dissociated or extruded by active efflux. Mikkelson and Schmidt-Ulrich (1980) recently presented evidence for mitogen-induced efflux of calcium from intracellular stores.

Several groups further confirmed the mitogen-induced calcium influxes using a fluorescent probe Quin 2 (Tsien *et al.*, 1982; Hesketh *et al.*, 1983a,b; O'Flynn *et al.*, 1984). These studies indicate significant increases in calcium influx within 1–2 min with PHA, Con A, succinylated Con A, and a mitogenic monoclonal antibody.

A kinetic analysis of calcium transport performed by Whitney and Sutherland (1973b) indicated that PHA lowers the K_m value of the carrier for calcium without altering its V_{max}. By contrast, in similar studies, Ozato *et al.* (1977) found that Con A induces an increase in V_{max} with no change in K_m. Using metabolic inhibitors, Whitney and Sutherland (1972b, 1973b) found no energy requirements for influx, while Ozato *et al.* (1977) and Landry *et al.* (1978) concluded that the process is energy dependent. Gelfand *et al.* (1984) demonstrated that lectin-induced calcium permeability changes are dependent on the maintenance of the transmembrane potential and independent of depolarization, extracellular sodium, and monovalent cation fluxes. Furthermore, changes in calcium permeability have been attributed to changes in phospholipid methylation, inositol trisphosphate (IP_3), and phosphatidic acid formation (see Section 2.4). Because of the difference in techniques and the other variables mentioned, it is not clear what the active carrier is and whether it is dependent on energy; further work is required.

In the studies conducted by Freedman et al. (1975) and Freedman (1979), cyclic GMP promoted mitogen-induced calcium influx, while cyclic AMP inhibited it. Whitney and Sutherland (1973b) and Parker (1974) showed small increases of calcium influx with cyclic AMP or cyclic AMP-raising agents in control lymphocytes but no effect on PHA-induced influx. Tsien et al. (1982) further confirmed the effect of cyclic AMP to inhibit mitogen induced calcium influx as sensitively measured by the fluorescent probe Quin 2. Whether this effect of the cyclic nucleotide is related to the calcium carrier or other mechanisms remains to be determined.

2.6.3. Calcium Ionophore

Maino et al. (1974) and Luckasen et al. (1974) were the first to observe that the calcium ionophore A23187, a carboxylic antibiotic from *Streptomyces chartreusensis,* induces lymphocyte proliferation in a calcium-dependent manner blocked by lanthanum, which inhibits calcium ion transport. Freedman et al. (1975, 1981) and Reeves (1975) confirmed the action of A23187 to induce calcium ion influx in lymphocytes (Table II). Greene et al. (1976a) showed that the effects of A23187 only roughly paralleled its characteristic dose response of proliferation; i.e., while optimal concentration of 0.6 μg/ml gave optimal proliferation and calcium influx, concentrations that were mitogenic (0.2–0.4 μg/ml) did not induce significant calcium influx, and toxic levels 0.8 μg/ml gave high values for influx. Hesketh et al. (1977) were unable to correlate the effects of A23187 on calcium influx in lymphocytes with proliferation and raised serious questions about the validity of this probe. A number of studies have confirmed and extended the original findings and have shown using various cell collection techniques that A23187 at a mitogenic concentration induces calcium uptake as measured by ^{45}Ca uptake (Hovi et al., 1976; Resch, 1976; Jensen and Rasmussen, 1977; Freedman, 1979; Otani et al., 1982), DPH fluorometry (Freedman et al., 1981), graphite furnace atomic absorption spectrometry (Jensen and Rasmussen, 1977; Lichtman et al., 1979), and Quin 2 fluoresence spectroscopy (Whitesell et al., 1977). For suboptimal and optimal concentrations, a reasonable correlation of calcium influx and proliferation exists; however, for high concentrations, greater influx (Freedman et al., 1981) correlates with the toxicity of the ionophore (Kaiser and Edelman, 1978). The toxic effect of high concentrations has been attributed to excessive influx (Jensen and Rasmussen, 1977;

TABLE II
Calcium Influx Studies with Calcium Ionophore A23187

Investigators	Lymphocyte source	Cell collection	Results
Freedman *et al.* (1975)	Mouse spleen	Water barrier	15 min
Reeves (1975)	Rat thymocyte	Filter	0–15 min
Greene *et al.* (1976a)	Human blood	Filter	To 30 min
Hovi *et al.* (1976)	Human blood	Water barrier	To 30 min
Hesketh *et al.* (1977)	Guinea pig lymph node	Filter	At 30 min only at superoptimal dose
	Mouse spleen	Pellet	To 30–60 min
Whitsell *et al.* (1977)	Rat thymus	Cell pellet	2–40 min
Lichtman *et al.* (1979)	Human blood	Atomic spectrometry	At 30 min
Resch *et al.* (1978)	Rabbit lymph node	Filter	At 90 min
Freedman, (1979)	Mouse spleen	Water barrier	At 30 min
Freedman *et al.* (1981)	Mouse spleen	DPH fluorometry	Progressive to 60 min
Otani *et al.* (1980, 1982)	Guinea pig lymph node	Filters	To 30–60 min
Tsien *et al.* (1982)	Guinea pig lymph node	Quin 2	1 min
	Mouse spleen		

Metcalfe *et al.*, 1980; Lichtman *et al.*, 1983). The initial discrepancies concerning a lack of correlation of low doses of ionophore to induce proliferation may be accounted for by the effects of the ionophore to liberate intracellular sources of calcium (e.g., mitochondria) (Mikkelsen and Schmidt-Ullrich, 1980). Such would be the case for transformed lymphocytes that contain numerous mitochondria as would be found in spleen and lymph node as used by Hesketh *et al.* (1977).

The uptake of calcium induced by A23187 would appear to be progressive for the first hour, followed by a decline to near-control levels at 7 hr (Jensen and Rasmussen, 1977; Freedman, 1979; Freedman *et al.*, 1981). As was apparent for mitogen dependency on calcium influx, the ionophore needs to be present for approximately a 5-hr calcium-sensitive phase (Cheung *et al.*, 1983). The effect of the ionophore appears to be relatively specific for mouse T cells (Freedman, 1979; Freedman *et al.*, 1981); however, differing results have been reported for rabbit lymphocytes (Resch, 1976), which may be explained by the fact that lymphocytes of this species bear characteristics of both B and T cells (Sell and Linthicum, 1975) and that the role of calcium influx in B lymphocyte activation is less clear (Resch, 1976; Freedman, 1979).

The action of the ionophore to mimic, in a calcium-dependent manner, the initial events induced by lectin mitogens has been demonstrated for PI turnover, cyclic AMP increase and AIB transport (Greene *et al.*, 1976a), cyclic GMP increases (Coffey *et al.*, 1977), and glucose transport (Reeves, 1975).

Several investigators have attempted to assess quantitatively the influxes with the presumption that a single process of mitogen-induced calcium influx is involved. Since active efflux is an unquantitated factor, these calculations share the liability that cellular isotope increases may grossly overestimate unbound cellular concentration.

2.6.4. Actions of Calcium

The fourth strategy to implicate calcium in activation events by showing its direct effect on enzymatic processes known to be stimulated by mitogens will be detailed in other sections. The processes and enzymes may be summarized as follows:

Membrane: phospholipases, guanylate cyclase, acyl transferase, calcium ATPase, calcium-gated potassium channels

Cytoplasm: cyclic GMP-dependent and calmodulin-dependent protein kinases, protein kinase C activation and translocation to membrane, lipoxygenase

Nucleus: DNA-dependent RNA polymerases in intact nuclei

2.6.5. Intracellular Calcium

Estimates of total lymphocyte calcium, on the basis of atomic absorption measurements, are within the range of $2-3 \times 10^{-3}$ M (Jensen and Rasmussen, 1977; Lichtman *et al.*, 1979). Free cytosolic calcium levels ($[Ca^{2+}]_i$) have been estimated using Quin 2 as a fluorescent probe at $1.1-1.2 \times 10^{-7}$ M (Tsien *et al.*, 1982; Hesketh *et al.*, 1983a; O'Flynn *et al.*, 1984). On this basis, approximately 0.005% of total calcium is free. Levels of intracellular free calcium induced by mitogens range from $2-4 \times 10^{-7}$ M using Quin 2 (Tsien *et al.*, 1982; O'Flynn *et al.*, 1984; Hesketh *et al.*, 1983b) to $0.2-1.9 \times 10^{-3}$ M using ^{45}Ca measurements (Freedman, 1979; Deutsch and Price, 1982; Metcalfe *et al.*, 1980) to $4-6 \times 10^{-3}$ M using atomic absorption measurements (Lichtman *et al.*, 1979). The wide discrepancy between measurements with Quin 2 and the other methods indicates that, if the measurements can be considered reliable estimates, the vast majority (99.99%) of the calcium influx induced by mitogens appears to exist as bound rather than as free calcium. Hesketh *et al.* (1983a) placed an upper limit on free calcium concentration of 1×10^{-5} M based on intracellular concentrations, which would be inhibitory. It seems reasonable to conclude that on mitogen stimulation total calcium is increased anywhere from 2- to 100-fold, that free calcium increases perhaps 1.5-fold, and that, quantitatively, the major increase is in cell bound calcium (99%). In light of these estimates, it would seem that the technical problems in accurately measuring changes in free calcium concentrations are significant and that new methods are needed. The large changes in total calcium can be measured by conventional methods (such as atomic absorption) and need confirmation. If confirmed, the emphasis should shift from thinking about free cytosol concentrations to analysis of where and to what structures (e.g., mitochondria, calmodulin, nucleus) calcium is bound or sequestered. Such changes in free and bound calcium are consistent with a central role for calcium in lymphocyte activation, based on consideration of other systems; however, the fact that mere increases in extracellular calcium levels can effect intracellular changes equivalent to those of mitogen (Hesketh *et al.*, 1983a) without inducing proliferation and that PMA is mitogenic for T lymphocytes without apparently increasing intracellular free calcium (Gelfand *et al.*, 1985) suggests that the nature of the signal and other factors also need to be considered. The localization of intracellular calcium in lymphocytes is not clear. The cell-surface glycocalix is thought to be one major site of calcium binding. Mitochondrial sequestration of calcium also has been shown in studies of rat and rabbit lymphocytes (Ozato *et al.*, 1977; Landry *et al.*, 1978). Cytoplasmic calmodulin is another important site of calcium binding. On the basis of nuclear activation studies (Ananthakrishnan *et al.*, 1981; Williams *et al.*, 1986), the nucleus is also a probable site of binding following mitogen stimulation. Clearly, the potential exists for tracking the location of the influxed calcium using autoradiography and/or fractionation of subcellular components. The localization following calcium influx due to mitogen action will be important in determining sequential aspects of mitogen action.

The accumulated data are inferentially strong in implicating calcium in mitogen-induced lymphocyte activation; recent data also suggest that antigen receptor activation yields similar events (see Section 3). Substantial data support (1) a calcium dependence of the activation process, which is restricted to probably 3–5 hr but perhaps as long as 20 hr after mitogen addition (this phase corresponds to the estimates for the length of the G_1 phase of the cell cycle in mitogen-stimulated lymphocytes); (2) a short but as yet uncharacterized influx process (1–2 hr) partially balanced by active efflux but probably sufficient to yield transient levels of free calcium of 2–4×10^{-7} M; and (3) a close correlation of calcium influx with calcium-dependent and, in some cases, calcium influx-dependent processes thought to be critical for lymphocyte activation.

2.7. Cyclic AMP

During the late 1970s, the lymphocyte represented a "black box" being probed by a growing legion of workers initiated into the field as a result of the discovery that lectin mitogens induced lymphocyte proliferation. The concomitant discovery of the mechanism of hormone action via the second messenger cyclic 3′,5′-adenosine monophosphate (cyclic AMP) by Earl Sutherland and co-workers led a number of investigators, including ourselves, to examine the possible role played by cyclic AMP in lectin-activated lymphocyte proliferation. A series of studies (see Hadden, 1977; Strom *et al.*, 1977; Robins, 1982, for reviews) indicated that cyclic AMP, its dibutyryl analogue, and agents that increased cellular levels of cyclic AMP (e.g., isoproterenol and theophylline) could inhibit PHA-induced lymphocyte proliferation even when introduced as a short 10-min pulse exposure with PHA (Hadden *et al.*, 1970). These studies suggested that cyclic AMP played an antiproliferative role in lymphocyte activation, a notion shared by investigators in other areas of the study of the control of cellular proliferation (see Clarkson and Baserga, 1974).

Novogrodsky and Katchalski (1970) were the first to report that PHA had no effect over a broad range of concentrations on the cyclic AMP levels of rat lymph node cells. Working independently with other cells, J. W. Smith *et al.* (1971) produced opposite results. They found that PHA, particularly at higher concentrations, raised cyclic AMP levels in human peripheral blood lymphocytes from 25% to 300% in 1–2 min and the levels declined by 6 hr. These observations prompted the hypothesis that cyclic AMP, perhaps in a localized compartment, participated in the signal mechanism induced by PHA (see Wedner and Parker, 1976, for review). A series of investigations ensued to confirm or disprove this hypothesis (see Table III). Over a period of 14 years, 23 laboratories have taken one side or the other of the controversy.

Concerning early (0–15 min) changes in cyclic AMP levels, a series of reports confirm the observations of J. W. Smith *et al.* (1971) (see Table III). It is notable that virtually all the studies reporting positive data with PHA or Con A at optimal mitogenic doses employed centrifugation prior to extraction and assay of cyclic AMP levels (see + on right-hand column of Table III). We have observed that centrifugation of cells with Con A, but not with succinylated Con A, artifactually increases lymphocyte levels of cyclic AMP (unpublished and confirmed by T. R. Hesketh, personal communication); thus, this artifact may contribute to the experimental findings.

Evident in these early studies were several points. The first observation was that nonmitogenic lectins such as WGA also increased cyclic AMP levels (Greene *et al.*, 1976b; Hadden and Coffey; unpublished observations) and that a highly agglutinating impure preparation of PHA (PHA-M) (Hadden *et al.*, 1972) increased cyclic AMP levels, whether centrifugation was used or not, indicating an association between agglutination and the cyclic AMP increases. The second observation was that nonlectin mitogens such as periodate (Hadden *et al.*, 1976) and A23187 (Hadden, 1977; Coffey *et al.*, 1978; Rochette-Egly and Kempf, 1981) did not induce early increases in cyclic AMP levels, suggesting that cyclic AMP increases were not a consistent feature of T-lymphocyte mitogen action. The third, a consistent finding from all laboratories, was that supraoptimal concentrations of purified PHA and purified native (tetrameric) Con A increased cyclic AMP levels, whether centrifugation was used or not. A notable exception to this observation was that with succinylated Con A (Con A-S) (Hadden *et al.*,

TABLE III

Cyclic AMP in Mitogen Action[a]

Investigators	Sources	Mitogen	Optimal mitogen			Supraoptimal			Centrifugation[b]
			0–15	15–60	Late	0–15	15–60	Late	
Novogrodsky and Katchalski (1970)	Rat LN	PHA	0	0					0
Parker and co-workers (1971)[c]	HPBL	PHA	↑	↑	→	↑↑	↑↑		+
		Con A	↑	→					
		A23187	↑						
Hadden and co-workers (1972)[d]	HPBL	PHA-M	↑	↑		↑↑	↑↑		0
		PHA-P	0	0					
		Con A-N	0	0		↑↑			
		Con A-S	0	0		0		0	
		A23187	0			↑			
		PMA	0	0					
Webb et al. (1973, 1975)	HPBL	PHA-M	↑	→	→	↑↑	→	→	+
	Con A			→	→				
Krishnaraj and Talwar (1973)	HPBL	PHA	↑			↑↑			+
		Con A	↑						
DeRubertis et al. (1974)	HPBL	PHA	0						
		Con A	0						
Whitfield et al. (1974)	Rat thymocyte	Con A	↑						+
Monahan et al. (1975)	HPBL	PHA	↑		↑ 4 hr				+
Watson (1976)	Mouse spleen	PHA	↑			↑			0
		Con A	↑			↑			

(continued)

TABLE III (Continued)

Investigators	Sources	Mitogen	Optimal mitogen			Supraoptimal			Centrifugation[b]
			0–15	15–60	Late	0–15	15–60	late	
Weber and Goldberg (1975)	HPBL	PHA	0			↑			0
Jegasothy et al. (1976)	Rat LN	PHA	↑						+
Burleson and Sage (1976)	Guinea pig LN	PHA		←					
		LcL	←	←			0		
Haddox et al. (1976)	Mouse spleen	Perio-date	0						+
Wang et al. (1978)	Mouse	Con A		0	↑↑				
Tam and Walford (1978, 1980)	Young mouse spleen	PHA	→	→					0
	Old mouse spleen	Con A	→	←					
		PHA	←	←					
		Con A	0	←					
Stolc (1980)	HPBL	A23187	↑						+

Reference	Cell	Mitogen					
Domand et al. (1980)	Mouse thymocyte	Con A					+
Carpentieri et al. (1980a,b)	HPBL	PHA	0	↕24L	↑		+
Hui and Harmony (1980b)	HPBL	PHA	0				+
Rochette-Egly and Kempf (1981)	HPBL	PHA / Con A / PMA	0 0 0	↑ ↑ ↑			
Takigawa and Waksman (1980)	Mouse spleen	Con A / Con A-S	↑ 0	↑ ↑ ↑	↑ 0	↑ ↑	+
Goodman and Weigle (1983)	Mouse spleen	Con A	0				+
Chisari and Curtis (1981)	HPBL	PHA	↑				+
Largen and Votta (1983)	Mouse	Con A	0				

[a]LN, lymph node; HPBL, human peripheral blood lymphocyte; PHA-M, phytohemagglutinin-M (crude); PHA-P, phytohemagglutinin-P (purified); Con A, concanavalin A; Con A-N, concanavalin A–native; Con A-S, concanavalin A–succinylated; LcL, *Lensularis* lectin.
[b]Employed centrifugation of cells prior to cyclic AMP assay.
[c]Smith et al. (1971); Parker (1974); Lyle and Parker (1974); Wedner et al. (1975); Greene et al. (1976a–d); Atkinson et al. (1978).
[d]Hadden et al. (1972, 1975, 1976, 1977); Coffey et al. (1978); Coffey and Hadden (1983a,b).

1976; Takigawa and Waksman, 1980) did not increase cyclic AMP at any concentration. Elaboration on this exception is important. Both PHA and Con A have bell-shaped dose–response curves in which supraoptimal doses progressively lose activity. Succinylated Con A (Con A-S), composed of dimers and monomers of native Con A, has a flat dose–response curve above optimal concentrations and does not, up to 200 μg/ml, induce high-dose inhibition characteristic of Con A. The lack of effect of Con A-S at either low dose or high dose to increase cyclic AMP further indicates that the observable increases in cyclic AMP are not a necessary part of the mitogen signal. More importantly, it implies a role for cyclic AMP in the mechanism by which high doses of mitogens inhibit lymphocyte proliferation. Also, throughout these studies, the only correlation of the magnitude of observed cyclic AMP increases is with progressive suppression of proliferation by Con A (Hadden et al., 1976).

Another important distinction about the Con A-S data is that Con A-S does not induce cap formation and microtubular-based freezing of the lymphocyte plasma membrane. Both processes were initially thought to be intrinsic to the mitogen activation signal (see Section 2.3); however, work with Con A-S has indicated that these were not necessary events and, in fact, were associated with the mechanism of high dose inhibition (McClain and Edelman, 1976) and linked to cyclic AMP (Hadden et al., 1976; Butman et al., 1981). PG produced by accessory cells is not involved as indicated by the observation that indomethacin, a PG synthesis inhibitor, does not block high-dose Con A inhibition (Hadden, unpublished observations). It is not known whether T-cell suppressor factors might contribute to this process. It is clear that when lectin-induced cyclic AMP changes occur, they do so in adherent cell-free (Hadden et al., 1977) and virtually pure T-cell populations (Atkinson et al., 1978).

When the cation dependence of early cyclic AMP increases with lectin mitogen have been examined they have been shown to be calcium dependent for Con A in human peripheral blood cells (Greene et al., 1976a) and mouse thymocytes (Whitfield et al., 1976) and calcium dependent for one but not all preparations of A23187 (Greene et al., 1976a; Coffey et al., 1977). Thus, the cyclic AMP involvement appears to relate to the particular preparation of ionophore used.

A large literature has accumulated to indicate that a variety of agents that increase cyclic AMP levels inhibit mitogen-induced lymphocyte proliferation (see Strom et al., 1977; Hadden et al., 1979; Hadden and Coffey, 1982; Coffey and Hadden, 1984, for review). These include β-adrenergics, adenosine, Bordatella pertussis, cholera toxin, inhibitor of DNA synthesis (IDS), prostaglandins, theophylline, and cyclic AMP itself. On the basis of their addition with mitogen and, in some cases, their presumed rapid metabolism, their actions are envisioned to be on the early phases of lymphocyte activation. Demonstrated actions by which cyclic AMP may inhibit early activation events include possible inhibitory effects on phospholipase (Lapetina, 1982), Na^+/K^+ ATPase (Coffey et al., 1975), glucose uptake and glycogen accumulation (Hadden et al.,

1971a,b), guanylate cyclase activation and cyclic GMP production (Coffey *et al.*, 1981; Hadden *et al.*, 1976), and IL-2 production and IL-2 action (Gilmore and Weiner, 1986; Beckner and Farrar, 1986; M. Wiranowska and J. W. Hadden, unpublished observations, 1985; Farrar *et al.*, 1987).

Using a novel microinjection technique, Ohara and Watanabe (1982) showed that anticyclic AMP antibodies delivered intracellularly enhance Con A-induced lymphocyte proliferation. These observations further support the notion that cyclic AMP is not needed for early stages of mitogen-induced proliferation and antagonizes it. While these collected observations provided an explanation for thinking that cyclic AMP played only an inhibitory role in lymphocyte activation, they did not rule out the possibility that small, perhaps localized cyclic AMP increases were part of the signal process.

In general, hormone-action studies have employed phosphodiesterase inhibitors to demonstrate not only that the hormone acts via adenylate cyclase but also to accentuate the cyclic AMP increases, which in many tissues may be brief and marginal in magnitude. The lectin-induced increases in cyclic AMP levels are observed in the presence of phosphodiesterase inhibitors (Hui and Harmony, 1980b), indicating that lectins stimulate adenylate cyclase to increase the production of cyclic AMP either directly or indirectly. Con A or PHA have not been shown to activate adenylate cyclase in broken cell preparations, and the evidence as to whether PHA increases adenylate cyclase activity of cells stimulated intact and then broken is controversial (Novogrodsky and Katchalski, 1971; Makman, 1971; Smith *et al.*, 1971; Krishnaraj and Talwar, 1973; DeRubertis *et al.*, 1974). Nevertheless, the potentiation of mitogen-induced cyclic AMP increases by phosphodiesterase inhibitors makes it likely that cyclic AMP increases derive from increased production rather than from inhibited catabolism. Parker and co-workers employed fluorescent anticyclic AMP antibody to show that PHA increases cyclic AMP detectable in micropatches along the plasma membrane (Bloom *et al.*, 1973). Whether the membrane-associated cyclic AMP is bound to adenylate cyclase, phosphodiesterase, or protein kinase is speculative; however, this localization of cyclic AMP is such that the protein that binds the cyclic AMP appears to be part of a mobile lectin receptor-linked enzyme complex. Since early transient cyclic AMP increases have been observed in neutrophil and mast cell activation by a variety of stimuli, they cannot be totally excluded in the process of lymphocyte activation. The magnitude of lectin-induced cyclic AMP increases observed in the absence of phosphodiesterases is not an important issue, since cyclic AMP turnover and compartmentalized production may well occur undetectable by current methodology.

2.7.1. Cyclic AMP Actions in Early Events

Cyclic AMP is thought to act exclusively through activation of cyclic AMP-dependent protein kinases, termed I and II according to the order of recovery from columns. The data to support changes in total and type I or II cyclic AMP-dependent protein kinases during the first hours of mitogen action are controversial. Wedner and Parker (1975) showed that PHA induces the phosphorylation of nonnuclear proteins parallel to the effect produced by cyclic AMP itself and presumed that a cyclic AMP-dependent protein kinase was involved. Later studies (Chaplin et al., 1980) failed to show that cyclic AMP could mimic protein phosphorylation induced by PHA, Con A, or the calcium ionophore. They also found that activation of adenylate cyclase by PG abolished mitogen-induced effects on protein phosphorylation. These data suggested that cyclic AMP-dependent kinase is not involved in early events. Cyclic AMP-dependent kinase activation and membrane phosphorylation have not been detected in other studies of lymphocyte activation within the first hour (Klimpel et al., 1979; Carpentieri et al., 1981). Recent observations using immunofluorescence detection of cyclic AMP and protein kinase I and II subunits during the first hour showed no change in protein kinases and a decrease in the number of cells staining for cyclic AMP at 5 min after Con A addition (Largen and Votta, 1983).

In marked contrast, several reports indicate that PHA and Con A induce early increases in type I cyclic AMP-dependent protein kinase within the first hour; no increase was observed in type II-dependent protein kinase (Byus et al., 1977, 1978). Somewhat paradoxically, these investigators noted that cellular increases in cyclic AMP levels, provoked by the addition of cyclic AMP, activated both kinase I and II associated with inhibition of proliferation. Subsequent studies by these investigators (Klimpel et al., 1979) emphasized later changes in cyclic AMP-dependent protein kinases. Medniecks and Jungmann (1982) elaborated on these studies and found that Con A induced a small early increase (20–90 min) in total cytoplasmic kinase associated with a decrease in kinase II and an increase in kinase I. They also observed the converse in nuclear fractions (i.e., a decrease in total kinase and kinase I and an increase in kinase II) and suggested that translocation of cyclic AMP-dependent protein kinase, particularly kinase I, from nucleus to cytoplasm occurred and represented a molecular basis for changes in nuclear regulation. The nature of events associated with cyclic AMP-dependent protein kinases in the first hour remains to be clarified; in any case, these are transient events not sufficiently explored to determine their relevance.

Several investigators observed late increases in cyclic AMP levels after 1 hr and before 6 hr (see Table III). In this time frame, Klimpel et al. (1979) observed overall increases in cyclic AMP-dependent protein kinase that parallel the induction of ornithine decarboxylase (ODC). Cyclic AMP added with mitogen blocks mitogen induction of ODC, while cyclic GMP stimulates it (Klimpel et al., 1979; Mizoguchi et al., 1975). Klimpel et al. (1979) postulated that type I cyclic AMP-dependent protein kinase stimulates and type II inhibits ODC induction. In the absence of data showing that other nonmitogenic agents that increase cyclic AMP induce ODC by activating type I kinase, it is difficult to evaluate this apparent paradox. Another possibility is that the column-purified kinase catalytic activity that increases is not derived from type I kinase holoenzyme but from a cyclic GMP-dependent or calcium-dependent kinase C. In any case, the inability of most laboratories to show cyclic AMP-dependent protein kinase activation during the first hour and the promoting effects of cyclic GMP and inhibiting effects of cyclic AMP leaves the regulation of ODC induction by cyclic nucleotides and their kinases in lymphocytes an open question to be resolved.

2.8. Cyclic GMP in T-lymphocyte Activation

In 1972, we observed that PHA and Con A induced early increases in lymphocyte levels of cyclic GMP (Hadden et al., 1972). The levels peaked at 20 min and declined to control levels by 30 min. They conformed to what appeared to be a trigger type of signal indicated by the other, then concomitant, studies of mitogen action. On the basis of these data, a lack of effect of relatively nonagglutinating lectin preparation on lymphocyte cyclic AMP levels, and the known effect of cyclic AMP active agents to inhibit mitogen-induced proliferation, it was suggested that cyclic GMP acted as an active signal in promoting lymphocyte proliferation and that cyclic AMP acted as a limiting regulatory influence. Much controversy ensued (Table IV).

The major issue concerned the reproducibility of the cyclic GMP measurements. The original assay was an enzyme cycling assay following extensive purification of the extracted cyclic GMP. The 10- to 50-fold increases observed under these circumstances have never been reproduced using the generally employed radioimmunoassay (RIA) for cyclic GMP. Since 1973, an average of 3- to 6-fold increases have been observed with a variety of mitogens, including PHA, Con A, succinylated Con A, phorbol myristate acetate (PMA), and A23187. These increases have peaked within the first 2–15 min. Over the years, the methodological nuances of measuring cyclic GMP have been studied in the femtomole amounts existing in lymphocytes and the pitfalls have been reviewed (Coffey, 1977; Coffey and Hadden, 1983a). Our major conclusion is that successful and reliable detection of cyclic GMP levels in lymphocytes requires rigorous efforts involving three column-purification procedures. Conditions of cell concentration, sample size, recovery of cells from the cyclic AMP-raising effect of Ficoll hypaque (Patrick et al., 1975), and purification all play a role. For example, the positive studies confirming mitogen-induced cyclic GMP increases have usually employed significantly lower cell concentrations than the negative studies (5×10^6/sample versus 5×10^7/sample) and lower basal levels (0.12 pm/10^7 cells versus 0.35 pm/10^7 cells). Nevertheless, there are exceptions to these averages and to conditions in which individual laboratories have reported positive results without purification, with large samples, or with higher basal levels, so that to this day no satisfactory explanation can be offered as to why certain laboratories after extensive effort have been unsuccessful.

To date 17 laboratories (22 reports) have reported effects of PHA, Con A, succinylated Con A, periodate, A23187, and PMA to increase lymphocyte levels of cyclic GMP. The levels of increase range from 1.2- to >10-fold with most in the range of 2- to 4-fold (see Table IV). The peaks have occurred within the first 30 min and in each case decline to control levels by 10–60 min. Cell sources include rat and human peripheral blood and mouse spleen and thymus. The mitogen-induced increases have been confirmed to occur in T-cell-enriched preparations, free of adherent cells (Coffey *et al.*, 1978) and in highly purified T cells (Carpentieri *et al.*, 1980c). The increases induced by PHA, Con A, and A23187 closely parallel their dose–response curves for proliferation (Coffey *et al.*, 1978; Hui and Harmony, 1980b). The increases in cyclic GMP have been shown to be dependent in part or totally on extracellular calcium for Con A, PHA, and A23187 (Whitfield *et al.*, 1974, Hadden *et al.*, 1975; Coffey *et al.*, 1978; Hui and Harmony, 1980b; Rochette-Egly and Kempf, 1981), but not periodate (Haddox *et al.*, 1976). Effects of PMA appear to involve intracellular calcium (Coffey and Hadden, 1981b). Only a few studies have employed phosphodiesterase inhibitors, and the cyclic GMP increases have been augmented by the use of imidazole at 10^{-4} M (Hadden *et al.*, 1975) but not 10^{-3} M, which blocks the increase (Whitfield *et al.*, 1974) indicating that mitogen action is to increase production and not to decrease metabolism.

The earliest increase recorded is 2 min with PMA, Con A, and PHA (Whitfield *et al.*, 1974; Coffey *et al.*, 1978; Coffey and Hadden, 1983a). Cyclic GMP is detected in the media in significant amounts following stimulation. The changes in lymphocyte levels of cyclic GMP are thought to represent a small fraction of the turnover of cyclic GMP based on the duration and extent of guanylate cyclase activation (Coffey *et al.*, 1981a,b) and on ^{18}O-GTP turnover (N. D. Goldberg, personal communication).

Deviller *et al.* (1975) first showed that PHA will activate guanylate cyclase of intact lymphocytes within 2 min after stimulation through an effect on V_{max} rather than K_m. Neither PHA nor Con A stimulated the enzyme in broken cells. Katagiri *et al.* (1976) showed that calcium activated lymphocyte guanylate cyclase; they suggested that the action of lectin mitogens might be indirect via this mechanism. Coffey *et al.* (1978, 1981) showed that PHA activates both membrane and soluble forms of lymphocyte guanylate cyclase from lymphocytes stimulated intact. The effect of PHA was dependent in great part on the presence of calcium in the external media and addition of EGTA completely ablated the response. Furthermore, the increases in guanylate cyclase were observed in the presence of magnesium, manganese, or calcium in the guanylate cyclase assay, yet the effect of calcium in the assay was insufficient to explain the action of PHA on the intact cell. The earliest change (1 min) occurred in plasma membrane-associated guanylate cyclase, followed by increases in cytosolic enzyme, both of which increases were present up to 1 hr. The effects appear to be on V_{max}, not K_m. The dose–response curve for a PHA effect on guanylate cyclase also paralleled that on DNA synthesis. Coffey and Hadden (1981, 1983a) also showed that PMA activates membrane and soluble guanylate cyclase of intact

TABLE IV
Cyclic GMP in T-Cell Activation[a]

Investigators	Cell source	Mitogen	Cyclic GMP increase 0-60'
Hadden and co-workers (1982–1983)[b]	HPBL	PHA-M	↑ >10 × peak 20' ↓ by 30'
		PHA-P	↑
		Con A	↑
		Con A	↑ 3 × peak 5–10'
		Con A-S	↑ 6 × peak 10'
		A23187	↑ 4 × peak 10'
		PHA	↑ 3 × peak 15'
		PMA	↑ 3 × peaks 2' and 40'
Webb et al. (1973, 1975)	HPBL	PHA	↑ 2 × 0–5'
	Con A		↑ 1.5 ×
Schumm et al. (1974)	Rat PBL	PHA	↑ >10 × peak 20' ↓ by 50'
Whitfield et al. (1974)	Rat thymus	Con A	↑ 2.5 × peak 2' ↓ by 4'
Parker and co-workers (1975–1978)[c]	HPBL	Con A	0 varying times and doses
		PHA	0 varying times and doses
Weber and Goldberg (1975)	Human adenoids	PHA	0 (2 experiments)
DeRubertis and Zenser (1976)	Mouse spleen	Con A	0 varying time and doses
		PHA	0 varying time and doses
Burleson and Sage (1976)	Guinea pig lymph node	PHA	0 varying time and doses
Katagiri et al. (1976)	Mouse spleen	Con A	↑ 3 × peak at 20'
Haddox et al. (1976)	Mouse and guinea pig spleen	Periodate	↑ 5 × 2' ↓ by 10'
Watson (1976)	Mouse spleen	PHA	↑ 1.7 ×
		Con A	↑ 1.7 ×
Tam and Walford (1978)	Mouse spleen	PHA	↑ 2 × peak at 25'
		Con A	↑ 5 × peak at 15'
Carpentieri et al. (1980a,b)	HPBL	PHA	↑ 5 × peak at 30' ↓ by 60'
Hui and Harmony (1980b)	HPBL	PHA	↑ 2 × peak at 30' ↓ by 60'
Rochette-Egly and Kempf (1981)	HPBL	PHA	↑ 3 × peak 10' ↓ by 30'
		Con A	↑ 4 × peak 5' ↓ by 30'
		PMA	↑ 4 × peak 5' ↓ by 30'
		A23187	↑ 4 × peak 5' ↓ by 30'
Goodman et al. (1981)	Mouse	Con A	0 at 15'
Largen and Votta (1983)	Mouse	Con A	↑ 3 × 20'–60'
Takemoto et al. (1979)	HPBL	Con A	↑ 2.5 × 20'

[a]See Table III for abbreviations.
[b]Hadden et al. (1972, 1975, 1976); Coffey et al. (1977, 1978); Coffey and Hadden (1983a,b).
[c]Wedner et al. (1975, 1976); Greene et al. (1976b); Atkinson et al. (1978).

cells in a calcium-dependent manner. Inhibitor studies (Coffey and Hadden, 1983b) implicate products of AA in the activation of guanylate cyclase by both PHA and PMA (see Section 2.4.3 for further discussion). Inhibitors of phospholipase and lipoxygenase, but not cyclooxygenase, inhibit mitogen-induced activation of membrane and soluble guanylate cyclase isolated from cells stimulated while intact. They do so in a manner directly parallel to their effects to inhibit mitogen-induced lymphocyte proliferation. Arachidonic acid added to lymphocyte homogenates activates guanylate cyclase, and the effect is blocked by inhibition of the lipoxygenase but not the cyclooxygenase pathway. The observations underscore the critical nature of the lipoxygenase pathway in guanylate cyclase activation. Notably the enzymes involved in both arachidonic acid release and the lipoxygenase pathway are calcium dependent.

Several products of the lipoxygenase pathway have been implicated in the direct activation of guanylate cyclase. Goldberg *et al.* (1978) and Graff *et al.* (1978) showed that a variety of HPETEs will stimulate guanylate cyclase of mouse spleen cells. Coffey and Hadden (1981b) showed that 5-, 11-, and 12-hydroxyeicosatetraenoic acid (HETEs), all reported to be possible products of arachidonic acid oxidation in mitogen-activated lymphocytes will stimulate human lymphocyte guanylate cyclase. Notably 15-HETE, an inhibitor of mitogen-induced lymphocyte proliferation (Bailey *et al.*, 1982a,b), inhibits 5-HETE activation of guanylate cyclase (Coffey and Hadden, 1985). These observations implicate several lipoxygenase products in the mitogen activation of lymphocyte guanylate cyclase. The specific mechanisms remain to be determined; however, oxidative processes are implicated by indirect evidence. A nonoxidative system also exists for activiting guanylate cyclase, i.e., through protein kinase C-mediated phosphorylation (Zwiller *et al.*, 1985).

Cyclic GMP in Early Events

Cyclic GMP-dependent protein kinase activity increases three- to fourfold following the cyclic GMP increases, peaking at 2–4 hr and declining to control levels by 8 hr (Carpentieri *et al.*, 1980a,b) confirmed by S. Kamiserenko and J. W. Hadden (presented at the Kyoto International Congress of Immunology, 1983). The phosphorylated substrates for the cyclic GMP-dependent protein kinase in lymphocytes are not known; however, phosphorylation of nonhistone acidic nuclear proteins closely parallels the increase in kinase activity (E. M. Johnson *et al.*, 1974). Cyclic GMP has been reported to reverse certain inhibitory effects of cyclic AMP on lymphocytes (Watson *et al.*, 1973; Watson, 1976) and to promote calcium influx (Freedman, 1979). H. M. Johnson *et al.* (1982) implicated cyclic GMP as the messenger in the action of IL-2 to produce γ interferon, independent of effects on proliferation. We have implicated cyclic GMP in the actions of IL-2 (see Section 5). Gupta (1979) linked cyclic GMP to

T-helper cell receptor display also independent of proliferation. These observations underscore the need for studies of cyclic nucleotide involvement in T-cell subset function unrelated to proliferation. Other actions of cyclic GMP have been related to nuclear events (see Section 4). Using fluorescent immunoperoxidase-labeled antisera to cyclic GMP and cyclic GMP-dependent protein kinase, Largen and Votta (1983) showed a Con A-induced increase in the number of cells staining positively for cyclic GMP at 30–60 min and for cyclic GMP-dependent protein kinase at 5–60 min. These observations support the close association of kinase activation and/or synthesis with early changes in cellular and nuclear levels of cyclic GMP and imply, as do the biochemical data with cyclic GMP-dependent protein kinase (Carpentieri *et al.*, 1980a,b) that cyclic GMP-dependent processes are involved throughout the approximately 8-hr period considered essential for the initiation process.

A large body of supporting evidence indicates that agents that increase cyclic GMP promote mitogen-induced lymphocyte proliferation, including levamisole, thymosin, thymopoietin, and lymphocyte activating factor (LAF) (see Hadden and Coffey, 1982, for review). Cyclic GMP itself induces B-cell proliferation (Weinstein *et al.*, 1974, 1975); the effect has been attributed to the induction of IL-1 (LAF) production by macrophages (Diamantstein and Ulmer, 1975b–d). Certain other guanosine analogues are also active to induce B-cell proliferation apparently by substituting for helper T-cell influences (Goodman and Weigle, 1983). While these data on effects of added cyclic GMP are interesting, it is important to note that a variety of agents that increase lymphocyte cyclic GMP levels, including those listed above, do not induce T-lymphocyte proliferation by themselves, so that the notion that cyclic GMP is the only effector of the membrane-mediated signal is inadequate and other concommitant processes must also be taken into account in the interaction process.

2.9. Other Early Cytoplasmic Events

The membrane events described that give direct rise to cytoplasmic events, including increased free Ca^{2+} from influx and intracellular mobilization, protein kinase C activation, AA metabolism to thromboxane and other eicosonoids, and soluble guanylate cyclase activation and increased levels of cyclic nucleotides and protein kinases, have been discussed in direct relation to the membrane events thought to contribute to them. They can be viewed as potentially localized events in close proximity to the plasma membrane but may also be more dispersed in the cytoplasm. Certainly cyclic nucleotide and calcium actions are envisioned to occur in multiple cellular compartments. A number of other cytoplasmic processes occur early following mitogen stimulation that not only may reflect the mitogen signal but may contribute as well.

Within minutes of mitogen addition, the generation of oxygen radicals (e.g., superoxide, singlet oxygen, hydroxyl ion, and H_2O_2) as expressed by chemiluminescence has been observed (Mookerjee et al., 1980; Weidemann and Kolbuck-Braddon, 1982). These events are inhibited by catalase, calmodulin/protein kinase inhibitors, and are partially dependent on extracellular calcium. They may reflect the products of oxidases involved, on the one hand, in AA metabolism or, on the other, in glucose metabolism and H_2O_2 generation via the hexose monophosphate (HMP) shunt. Certainly glucose uptake and utilization to form glycogen and to be metabolized to pentose by the HMP shunt and the Embden–Meyerhoff pathway to lactate occur early following mitogen addition and persist through much of the early cycle (Roos et al., 1970, 1972; Hadden et al., 1971a,b). Increased phosphofructokinase and other glycolytic enzymes are apparently involved in the latter process (Wang et al., 1980; Hume and Weidemann, 1980; Diaz-Espada and Lopez-Alarcon, 1982). Protein synthesis begins measurably within 4 hr and is generally considered essential, but not regulatory, for subsequent events (Ling and Kay, 1975; Cooper and Braverman, 1980; Varesio and Holden, 1980; Varesio et al., 1980). Naturally, lipid synthesis also occurs (Sternholm and Falor, 1970), as do all other processes essential to the metabolism in cell replication.

Protease increase, in part from lysosomal degranulation, has been considered an important event, but little recent evidence supports its role in activation. Speculation about a role for calcium-activated neutral protease is justifiable (Nishizuka, 1984), yet the levels of calcium required may be higher than those thought obtainable. Early changes in transglutaminase following mitogen have been reported (Novogrodsky et al., 1978); however the relevance and function of this enzyme in lymphocyte activation remain to be determined.

Several reports have suggested that mitogens activate cytoplasmic ornithine decarboxylase (ODC), which converts ornithine to putrescine and regulates the production of spermine and spermidine. This effect on ODC is observed at 4–14 hr (Kay and Cooke, 1971), with increases in polyamine synthesis by 12 hr. Inhibitors of ODC block DNA but not RNA synthesis (Fillingame and Morris, 1973; Fillingame et al., 1975; Otani et al., 1977; Byus et al., 1977; Morris et al., 1977; Knutson and Morris, 1978). These observations may implicate ODC in the initiation of DNA synthesis. The regulation of ODC by cyclic nucleotides is discussed in Section 2.7.1. It remains to be determined how polyamine metabolism signals or modulates mitogen activation processes (see Holta et al., 1981; Patt et al., 1982, for further discussion).

3. EARLY EVENTS IN ACTIVATION BY MONOCLONAL ANTIBODIES TO T-CELL RECEPTOR MOLECULES

It is clear from the foregoing sections that the actions of mitogens involve a series of biochemical events that may involve several different pathways, including both direct actions and indirect actions involving IL-1 and IL-2. The recent development of monoclonal antibodies to discrete epitopes of T-lymphocyte surface receptors has provided useful tools to dissect these direct and indirect pathways (see Walls et al., 1984; Davis et al., 1986; Huet et al., 1986; Kroozck et al., 1986; Yang et al., 1986; Weiss et al., 1986; Nel et al., 1987; Oettgen and Terhorst, 1987, for review).

The T-cell membrane antigen receptor (Ti) is thought to be composed of two disulfide-linked heterodimer glycoproteins, termed α- and β-chains, in close association with a third, termed the γ-chain. The cell-surface α- and β-chains provide the variable regions necessary for antigen recognition and binding. The T-cell antigen receptor exists in close physical association with the T_3 receptor complex, which also is made up of three peptide chains. The two complexes (T_3/Ti) together are thought to represent the receptor–transmembrane signaling unit. Antibodies directed against either the Ti or the T_3 receptor complex provide an initial first pathway that, in the presence of an activating signal for a second pathway, will trigger T-lymphocyte proliferation. The second of these two pathways is activated by accessory cells, IL-1, PMA, or IL-2 (Meuer et al., 1984, 1986; Ledbetter et al., 1986a,b).

The first pathway activated by T_3/Ti receptor modulation using monoclonal antibodies is associated with PI turnover, transient protein kinase C activation (Galbraith et al., 1985; Manger et al., 1987), increases in inositol triphosphate and $[Ca^{2+}]_i$ (independent of extracellular calcium), increases in calcium influx (dependent on extracellular calcium) (Oettgen et al., 1985; Rabinovitch et al., 1986), a brief cycle AMP increase (1 min) (Ledbetter et al,. 1986b), and IL-2 receptor induction (Weiss et al., 1986). This signal is not associated with IL-2 production, unless the anti-T_3/Ti monoclonal antibody is crosslinked by Sepharose, indicating that the antigen receptor is linked to mechanisms of IL-2 production, but increased $[Ca^{2+}]_i$ alone is not sufficient for IL-2 production. Activation of the first pathway is mimicked by the calcium ionophore and depends on transmembrane potential in that both depolarization or hyperpolarization inhibit; a voltage-gated calcium channel would thus appear to be excluded (Oettgen et al., 1985). IL-1, PMA, and IL-2 will activate the second pathway.

The action of IL-1 in this regard is unknown; however, dependence on the integrity of the lipoxygenase pathway has been demonstrated (Dinarello et al., 1983; Kato et al., 1986). Its intracellular messenger remains to be determined. The demonstrated actions of PMA include prolonged protein kinase C activation (Farrar and Ruscetti, 1986; Manger et al., 1987), phosphorylation and downregulation of the T_3 receptor (Cantrell et al., 1985), and lipoxygenase and guanylate cyclase activation with cyclic GMP production (Coffey and Hadden, 1981b; Coffey et al., 1981). PMA does not increase $[Ca^{2+}]_i$ in T lymphocytes (Gelfand et al., 1985; Oettgen et al., 1985).

Interleukin-2 actions are discussed in Section 4 and presumably relate more to the second signal than to the first signal. In any case, insufficient uniformity of information exists on these three agents activating the second pathway to determine whether they all share the same biochemical mechanisms.

Recent work by Ledbetter et al. (1986a,b) using monoclonals to non T_3/Ti receptors (CD5 and Tp44) indicates that their activation will mimic the actions of accessory cells, IL-1, and PMA; i.e., they will, with T_3/Ti-receptor complex modulation, induce IL-2 production and subsequent proliferation. Activation of both these non T_3/Ti receptors leads to increases in cellular levels of cyclic GMP, but not of cyclic AMP. Interestingly, the activation of only one receptor (CD5) leads to increased $[Ca^{2+}]_i$, suggesting a disassociation, in this case, of calcium mobilization and guanylate cyclase activation.

These observations suggest a coordinate association of inositol trisphosphate formation, transient protein kinase C activation, calcium mobilization, cyclic AMP increase, and IL-2 receptor induction with the first pathway and prolonged protein kinase C activation, cyclic GMP increase, and IL-2 production with the second pathway. The role of PI turnover and diacylglyceride production in these two pathways is unclear. The use of antireceptor monoclonal antibodies and of new mitogenic agents such as teleocidin (Isakov et al., 1985) offer excellent probes to dissect the various pathways of activation by mitogens and should lead to discriminating studies on how these cell-surface signals are transduced in the nucleus into specific gene activation. The use of these new probes cannot, however, be assumed to avoid the pitfalls of prior mitogens and may introduce new complexities (see Feister and Sage, 1986).

4. EARLY EVENTS IN LYMPHOCYTE NUCLEAR ACTIVATION

A central question in the study of the biochemistry of T-lymphocyte activation is how do cell-surface-derived signals give rise to early nuclear events. A number of studies have attempted to relate intracellular cytoplasmic signals, such as cyclic nucleotides, calcium, polyamines, and proteases, to nuclear activation. To provide a background for understanding these efforts, a brief summary of those studies that have probed the events that occur sequentially in nuclei of mitogen-activated lymphocytes is presented.

Within 15 min of activation of lymphocytes by PHA or Con A, initiation of a number of metabolic events related to nuclei occurs: (1) RNA synthesis in isolated nuclei (Pogo et al., 1966) followed by increases in total cellular RNA detectable at 12 hr (Forsdyke, 1968; Mitchell et al., 1978); and (2) protein synthesis (Pogo et al., 1966), including the synthesis and translocation to the nucleus of nonhistone acidic nuclear proteins (Rosenberg and Levy, 1972; Levy et al., 1973; E. M. Johnson et al., 1974). Early events associated with the initiation of nuclear RNA synthesis at 15–30 min are the acetylation of arginine-rich histones (Pogo et al., 1966), the phosphorylation of nonhistone acidic nuclear proteins (Kleinsmith et al., 1966; E. M. Johnson et al., 1974), an increase in histone kinase (Cross and Ord, 1971) an increase in RNA initiation sites (Ananthakrishan et al., 1981, and increases in actinomycin D and acridine orange binding to DNA (Darzynkewicz *et al.*, 1969). During this early period, nuclear transcription assays indicate that genes for the IL-2 receptor and the proto-oncogenes c-myc and c-fos are activated, followed later (4 hr) by those for IL-2, interferon (IFN), and the transferrin receptor (Kronke *et al.*, 1985; Reed *et al.*, 1987). These events occur in association with an increase in chromatin dispersion and a decrease in nuclear refringency (Pompidou *et al.*, 1984). A number of these early events are sensitive to actinomycin D and cycloheximide, indicating an interdependence of both RNA and protein synthesis.

The initial increases in RNA synthesis by PHA are associated with an activation of DNA-dependent RNA polymerase I (RNA associated) that increases progressively over the first 2 hr (Pogo, 1972), a small increase in RNA polymerase III (RNA associated) that occurs during the first hour), and a decline in RNA polymerase II (mRNA associated) during the first hour, followed by progressive increases after 1 hr. The RNA synthesized during the first hour is magnesium dependent and is insensitive to α-amanatin (Kay *et al.*, 1969; Pogo, 1972; Anathakrishnan *et al.*, 1981). It is 4–5 S in size, G-C rich, poly A poor, and mostly methylated (Pogo, 1972; Howard, 1972; Cooper and Rubin, 1965; Mitchell *et al.*, 1978).

The initial RNA synthesis is characteristic of transfer RNA (tRNA) products of RNA polymerase III and incomplete ribosomal RNA (rRNA) products of polymerase I. An initial increase in ribonuclease activity is evident (Anathakrishnan *et al.*, 1981), which may explain the lack of early 45S rRNA precursor.

Only after the first 12 hr is there an increased production of 28 and 18S rRNA (Cooper, 1968, 1972; Purtell and Anthony, 1975) and of poly A-rich in mRNA (Mitchell *et al.*, 1978). In lymph node cells, poly A-rich RNA is observed within 2 hr of Con A stimulation (Hauser *et al.*, 1978), perhaps because these cells are preactivated and have a short G_1 phase.

Within 2–10 hr following mitogen stimulation, an increased flow of ribosomes occurs from an inactive pool of 80S single ribosomes through the active subunit to form functioning ribosomes (Cooper, 1974; Jagus and Kay, 1979; Cooper and Braverman, 1980, 1981; Cooper and Lester, 1982). Cooper and Lester (1982) recently presented evidence indicating that the early tRNA synthesis may play an important initiator role in lymphocyte protein synthesis. In mitogen-activated lymphocytes, the G_1 phase of the cycle involving RNA and protein synthesis is thought to vary, depending on the lymphocyte. Progression to the S phase and DNA synthesis occur only after 12–24 hr, depending on the type of lymphocyte and the presence of T-cell growth factor (IL-2) and its receptors. At this time, activation of DNA polymerases is evident (Loeb and Agarwal, 1971).

It is important to remember that T-cell mitogens such as PHA and Con A activate 25–40% of the cells that are usually present in such experiments (Darzynkewicz *et al.*, 1969); the metabolic events described may be relevant to T cells induced to proliferate, but they may also be relevant to helper and suppressor cell activation or to interleukin production by T cells and accessory cells independent of proliferation. They may also relate to the recruitment of B cells via B-cell growth factor (Duncan and Hadden, 1982). Clearly, work with isolated interleukins and subpopulations will be necessary to clarify the picture fully; however, for the present, it can be safely concluded that the T lymphocyte, as other cell populations, requires rRNA and messenger RNA (mRNA) synthesis and protein synthesis in order to move from early G_1 into DNA synthesis.

4.1. Membrane to Nuclear Signals

A major question is how these nuclear events are regulated and orchestrated to occur. One crude but insightful approach is to mix cytoplasm of activated lymphocytes with nuclei of resting lymphocytes. This type of approach has been taken late in G_1 by Jazwinski et al. (1976), Wang et al. (1981), and Gutowski et al. (1984), and cytoplasmic phosphoproteins have been detected that will initiate DNA synthesis in isolated nuclei. Evidence indicates that at least one is a T-cell growth factor-induced protein. No such studies have been performed in the first hours of mitogen activation.

4.1.1. Calcium in Nuclear Signals

Ananthakrishnan et al. (1981) showed that deletion of extracellular calcium markedly reduces α-amanatin, RNAase-sensitive RNA synthesis in nuclei isolated at 1 hr after PHA and that further addition of EGTA completely prevents the initiation of RNA synthesis in isolated nuclei. Under these circumstances of calcium restriction, cellular cyclic GMP increases and guanylate cyclase activation were blocked. Early Con A-induced changes in nuclear refringence are also dependent on the presence of extracellular calcium as well as an intact lipoxygenase pathway (Pompidou et al., 1980, 1984, 1986). Cross and Ord (1971) found that chlorpromazine, a calmodulin inhibitor, among other actions, blocks early uridine incorporation in RNA. These studies point to a central role of calcium influx and calcium presence in the early nuclear activation process.

In experiments adding calcium to isolated lymphocyte nuclei, Burgoyne et al. (1970) attributed the increased DNA synthesis to DNA nicking and to increased endonuclease activity. In similar experiments, Johnson and Hadden (1975) observed that calcium increases magnesium-dependent RNA polymerase I-mediated RNA synthesis to a small but consistent degree. Ananthakrishnan et al. (1981) extended this approach using high salt conditions to restrict reinitiation and presented evidence to show that calcium (10^{-4} M) would induce in isolated nuclei increased RNA synthesis attributable to an increase in initiation sites. The mechanisms of such calcium-induced events can only be speculated on at this time; however, they support the evidence that calcium influx and/or mobilization is critical for nuclear activation. Recent data indicate a leak between nuclear calcium influx into the nucleus and IL-2 gene expression (White and Morris, 1986; Williams *et al.*, 1986).

Calcium influx has been implicated in the labilization of lysosomes; Hirschhorn *et al.* (1969) suggested that PHA might act through a redistribution of cytoplasmic acid hydrolases to the nucleus. In support, they showed that PHA increases lymphocyte nuclear template activity for exogenous RNA polymerase within minutes, its effects are blocked by EDTA and reproduced when trypsin is added to isolated lymphocyte nuclei. Little more has been written about this notion.

4.1.2. Cyclic AMP in Nuclear Signals

A number of experiments have probed a possible role of cyclic AMP in nuclear activation. Cross and Ord (1971) showed that cyclic AMP added to pig lymphocytes, without mitogen, increased uridine incorporation associated with increases in the phosphate pool and ATP concentration. The effects of PHA to increase histone kinase activity and phophorylation of histones were attributed to cyclic AMP, since it would stimulate the isolated kinase. Similar effects of cyclic AMP (without mitogen) to increase RNA synthesis were reported by Averner *et al.* (1972). The interaction of PHA and cyclic AMP was not studied. Johnson and Hadden (1975) showed that cyclic AMP and agents that increase cyclic AMP inhibit the overall phosphorylation of nonhistone acidic nuclear protein; however, several specific proteins were increased in their phosphorylation. Cyclic AMP added to isolated lymphocyte nuclei inhibits RNA synthesis (Ananthakrishnan *et al.*, 1981). Rosenfield *et al.* (1972) found that cyclic AMP by itself would simulate the effects of PHA on the late production of poly A-rich mRNA synthesis. By contrast, cyclic AMP blocked the effect of PHA to induce mRNA. In studies with fluorescent anticyclic AMP antibodies, Bloom *et al.* (1973) did not observe nuclear localization following PHA stimulation, nor has this been reported in other studies (E. M. Rosenberg *et al.*, 1980). Bloom *et al.* (1973) noted that a nuclear increase in cyclic AMP occurred with isoproterenol, and a nuclear membrane adenylate cyclase and phosphodiesterase have been described (Wedner and Parker, 1975; Coulson and Kennedy, 1971). Dobson and Mellors (1980) and Dornand *et al.* (1980) failed to confirm the presence of a nuclear adenylate cyclase in lymphocytes. It would be necessary to study the effects of cyclic AMP in combination with mitogen on other early events to prove the point, but it seems likely from the evidence presented so far that cyclic AMP cannot reproduce the effects of mitogens on early RNA synthesis-related events in lymphocyte nuclei. It is important to note that histamine and adenosine will activate suppressor T cells via a cyclic AMP mechanism (Rocklin, 1976; Birch and Polmar, 1982) and that while the induction of T-cell suppressor factor has not been shown to depend on RNA synthesis, it is very possible that it is and that there is an effect of cyclic AMP, in the absence of mitogen, on RNA mechanisms related to suppressor cell activation.

A better case can be made for the correlation of mitogen-induced increases in cyclic AMP and cyclic AMP-dependent protein kinase occurring after 1 hr with the increases in DNA-dependent RNA polymerase II activation and mRNA synthesis. Kranias et al. (1977) showed that cyclic AMP would stimulate lymphocyte nuclear cyclic AMP-dependent protein kinase and would induce the phosphorylation of, and an increase in, the activity of RNA polymerase II. Regulation by cyclic AMP of other processes also seems likely, particularly since lymphocyte nuclei contain cyclic AMP-dependent protein kinase(s) (Johnson, 1977; Medniecks and Jungmann, 1982). This kinase(s) is thought to function as a histone kinase (Farago et al., 1978), in the phosphorylation of a 22kDa nuclear protein (Hashizume et al., 1983) and perhaps in nuclear pore formation (Schumm and Webb, 1978). In addition to phosphorylation of protein substrates in nuclei by the catalytic subunit, the observation by Johnson et al. (1975a) that the cyclic AMP-bound regulatory 4S subunit binds tightly to DNA suggests that an inductive action by the subunit, like that of the steroid bound 4S receptor seems possible and deserves testing.

4.1.3. Ornithine Decarboxylase

Another process thought to be cyclic AMP dependent in other tissues is the induction of ODC (see Russell, 1973, for review). Recent data suggest that protein kinase C and increased $[Ca^{2+}]_i$ may also or alternatively be involved in ODC induction (Buckley et al., 1986). ODC is a cytoplasmic enzyme that converts ornithine to putrescine, thereby regulating the production of the two polyamines spermine and sperimidine. It has also been suggested to bind to and stimulate RNA polymerase I (Manen and Russell, 1977). Both PHA and Con A increase ODC and polyamine synthesis after 6–12 hr (Kay and Cooke, 1971). Inhibition of ODC blocks DNA but not RNA synthesis (Fillingame and Morris, 1973; Fillingame et al., 1975; Otani et al., 1977; Byus et al., 1977). These observations implicate ODC and polyamines in late events in the lymphocyte cycle and may relate more to T-cell growth factor action than to initial mitogen effects.

4.1.4. Cyclic GMP

A possible role for cyclic GMP in lymphocyte nuclear activation has been studied by several groups. Preliminary experiments with isolated lymphocyte nuclei indicated that low levels of cyclic GMP can stimulate RNA synthesis (Hadden et al., 1972; Goldberg et al., 1974). In intact cells, cyclic GMP in the presence, but not the absence, of PHA was shown to increase uridine incorporation into RNA (Averner et al., 1972), and acetylcholine (ACh), which increases cyclic GMP in lymphocytes, was shown to augment RNA and protein synthesis (Hadden *et al.*, 1975). In none of these cases was cyclic GMP shown to induce DNA synthesis. Furthermore, cyclic GMP and agents that increase cyclic GMP levels in lymphocytes induce transient increases in the phosphorylation of non-histone acidic nuclear protein parallel to the pattern of phosphorylation induced by Con A (Johnson and Hadden, 1975). These observations suggested a unique association of cyclic GMP with nuclear RNA synthesis; however, the relationship of this effect to DNA synthesis remained to be established.

The dependence on calcium of cyclic GMP production by mitogens has been discussed. On the basis of this evidence, it seemed likely that cyclic GMP and calcium represent co-partners in mitogen-induced nuclear activation (Hadden *et al.*, 1975; Coffey *et al.*, 1977). A number of observations using isolated nuclei and nuclear constitutients support this hypothesis. Johnson and Hadden (1975, 1977) showed that cyclic GMP at low concentrations stimulated the incorporation of nucleoside triphosphates into RNase-sensitive RNA of isolated nuclei. The effect was observed maximally at 10^{-8} M cyclic GMP, required calcium, and was α-amanatin resistant, consistent with stimulation of DNA-dependent RNA polymerase I (rRNA-associated) or III (tRNA-associated). Cyclic GMP inhibited RNA polymerase II activity. In both cases, cyclic GMP in the presence of calcium reproduced in the nucleus those effects that occur in the nucleus when the intact lymphocyte is stimulated by PHA. When lymphocyte nuclear RNA polymerases were isolated and partially purified, it was shown that all the polymerases bind cyclic GMP and that low levels of cyclic GMP, in the absence of calcium, stimulate RNA polymerase I and III and inhibit polymerase II. Cyclic AMP was not active in these studies insofar as tested. These studies have been confirmed and extended by Ananthakrishnan *et al.* (1981). Using high salt conditions to restrict reinitiation in isolated lymphocyte nuclei, cyclic GMP at low concentrations, but no cyclic AMP, increases α-amanatin-resistant RNA synthesis principally through chain elongation. This effect was shown in the absence of calcium and was consistent with RNA polymerase I or III activation. The effect of calcium under these conditions, as mentioned, was consistent with increased initiation. The combination of cyclic GMP and calcium was additive and paralleled in nature and magnitude the effects induced in the nucleus of the cell stimulated intact by PHA. In each case, the RNA products of the isolated nuclei were small (4-5S) and therefore may relate to early RNA synthesis by either RNA polymerase I or III. These observations are consistent with the hypothesis that cyclic GMP and calcium act in a complementary manner to initiate RNA synthesis in lymphocytes stimulated by mitogens.

Cyclic GMP at low concentrations has also been shown to bind specifically to a number of nuclear proteins having high affinity for DNA (E. M. Johnson *et al.*, 1975b; Allfrey *et al.*, 1975; E. M. Johnson and Hadden, 1977; Farago *et al.*, 1978). The regulatory function of these proteins remains to be determined, however, as they include both histones and acidic nuclear proteins. Their role in regulating transcription can be surmised. To date, a nuclear cyclic GMP-dependent protein kinase has not been studied, nor has its possible role in the phosphorylation of histones or acidic nuclear proteins.

The binding of cyclic GMP in the intact nucleus of lymphocytes using a fluorescein-labeled anticyclic GMP antibody has not been specifically studied. It has been studied, however, in other tissues (Earp et al., 1977; Rosenberg et al., 1980); cyclic GMP, but not cyclic AMP, is found in aggregates associated with DNA condensation and in nucleoli in which RNA polymerase I is also localized. These latter observations have prompted the investigators to suggest, independently, a role of cyclic GMP in regulating nuclear function. Cyclic GMP has also been implicated in late cycle nuclear events. Chambers et al. (1974) reported that cyclic GMP stimulates and cyclic AMP inhibits the activity of phosphoribosyl pyrophosphate (PRPP) synthetase induced in lymphocytes by 20-hr exposure to Con A. This enzyme is critical for both the purine salvage pathway and the de novo pathway of nucleic acid synthesis. It has also been suggested that cyclic GMP may function in nuclear pore formation and the translation of RNA (Schumm and Webb, 1978).

Collectively, these observations are compelling for thinking that cyclic GMP and calcium are important in the initial events of nuclear activation; however, the relationship of these events to DNA synthesis and to T-cell growth factor production and action remains to be determined. As previously mentioned, subpopulations need to be specifically analyzed and the action of accessory cells and molecules probed. The mechanisms by which these and other surface and cytoplasmic nuclear signals operate have only been hinted at. The growth of molecular biology in recent years has created the technologies to probe the relevant mechanisms in molecular depth and, it is hoped, will be applied to these important biological problems in the future.

5. LATE EVENTS ASSOCIATED WITH IL-2 ACTION

Cyclic GMP was first implicated in late cycle events by Waksman and co-workers, who described effects of lymphocyte activating factor (LAF or IL-1) to increase cyclic GMP levels after 12 hr in lymph node cells following PHA priming (Katz et al., 1978; Waksman et al., 1980). Cyclic GMP-active agents mimic the LAF effect on proliferation of these cells, and EGTA blocked it. These investigators suggest that LAF acts via cyclic GMP changes at a G_1–S boundary restriction point. T-cell growth factor (IL-2) is induced by LAF (IL-1) and is thought to act at the G_1–S boundary. Thus, the effect of LAF described by Waksman may be mediated by IL-2 and its effects on cyclic GMP.

Toyoshima et al. (1976) suggested that the second signal provided by IL-2 would be independent of calcium influx, in contrast to the first signal, which clearly involves calcium influx. Only recently have studies of IL-2 action been reported (see Farrar et al., 1986). Three laboratories have reported that IL-2 induces calcium influx and increased $[Ca^{2+}]_i$ in its target cells and that the effects of IL-2 are prevented by calcium-channel blockers (H. M. Johnson et al., 1985; Fleisher and Birx, 1985; Nakanishi and Utsunomiya, 1986). By contrast, Mills et al. (1985b), LeGrue (1987), and Harris et al. (1987) were unable to show that IL-2 increases $[Ca^{2+}]_i$ influx. Thus, the role of calcium in IL-2 action remains unclear.

Mills et al. (1986b) were unable to show that IL-2 induces membrane phospholipid changes, including PI turnover, diacylglycerol production, or AA release. Other events known to be involved in the mechanism of IL-2 action include activation and translocation of protein kinase C (Farrar and Anderson, 1985; Farrar and Ruscetti, 1986), phosphorylation of membrane proteins including the IL-2 receptor (Gaulton and Eardley, 1986), and phosphorylation and down-regulation of adenylate cyclase (Beckner and Farrar, 1986). Farrar and Humes (1985) showed that IL-2 activates the lipoxygenase pathway in its target cells with production of 5- and 15-HETEs and that inhibitors of the pathway block IL-2 action as well as lymphocyte proliferation (confirmed by M. Wiranowska and J. W. Hadden, unpublished observations). The source of the arachidonic acid used in this pathway remains to be determined.

We recently showed that IL-2 increases cyclic GMP but not cyclic AMP levels in mitogen-primed T cells without accessory cells (Hadden et al., 1987). There may be several mechanisms by which IL-2 acts to increase cyclic GMP levels. Calcium influx and/or increased $[Ca^{2+}]_i$ may be involved in the activation of guanylate cyclase. These effects also presumably derive from the actions of hydroxy and hydroperoxy eicosatetraenoic acids and/or leukotrienes to activate guanylate cyclase. Finally, it is also possible that one of the substrates phosphorylated and activated by protein kinase C is guanylate cyclase (see Zwiller et al., 1985).

The actions of cyclic GMP that might relate to an IL-2 intracellular signal can only be speculated on. Johnson et al. (1985) implicated cyclic GMP in IFN$_\gamma$ induction by IL-2, and a gene-activation mechanism may be involved. Cyclic GMP has been linked to a number of nuclear events, including DNA-dependent RNA polymerases, phosphorylation of chromatin-binding, acidic nuclear proteins, and nuclear RNA synthesis (see Section 4). The ultimate actions of IL-2 that translate into DNA synthesis are unclear; they may include the induction of phosphoproteins, including a protease linked to the initiation of DNA synthesis (Gutowski et al., 1984; Cohen et al., 1986). Neckers and Crossman (1983) suggested an obligatory intermediary role of IL-2-induced transferrin receptor in this process.

Cyclic Nucleotides in Other Late-Cycle Events

Late changes in cyclic AMP generally have been observed (see Table I) with peaks at 30–36 hr (Wang et al., 1978; Chisari and Curtis, 1981; Rochette-Egly and Kempf, 1981) and decline to control levels by 48 hr. Wang et al.

(1978) showed that indomethacin, at a concentration sufficient to inhibit PG synthesis, blocks both the cyclic AMP increase and DNA synthesis; if removed, the return of both responses is coordinate. These investigators also observed a discrete increase in cyclic AMP-dependent protein kinase activity at the cyclic AMP peak at 30–36 hr. Carpentieri *et al.* (1978) failed to show increases in cyclic AMP-dependent protein kinase activity at 24 or 48 hr; however, as with several of the studies of cyclic AMP levels at these times, these investigators may have missed a discrete peak at 30–36 hr. Evidence supporting a positive role for cyclic AMP in later cycle events has been extensively reviewed by Whitfield and co-workers (1976). A body of evidence (Whitfield *et al.*, 1969, 1974, 1976; Morgan *et al.*, 1975) indicates that agents that increase cyclic AMP and others, such as parathormone (PTH), antidiuretic hormone (ADH), calcitonin, vasopressin (also linked to cyclic AMP) promote in a magnesium-dependent, calcium-independent manner the traversement by thymocytes of a G_1–S boundary restriction. These actions of these agents, hence cyclic AMP itself, may, under these circumstances, be as much involved in differentiation of thymocytes to one or another subset as in simply allowing them to enter DNA synthesis and complete their cycle.

To the contrary, Waksman and co-workers have implicated a cyclic AMP-mediated inhibitory event during this period based on work with a lymphocyte-produced inhibitor of DNA synthesis (IDS) (Jegasothy *et al.*, 1976, 1978; Wagshal *et al.*, 1978; Wagshal and Waksman, 1978). Since cyclic AMP-deficient mutant lymphoid cells have no difficulty traversing the cell cycle, it remains to be determined what these midcycle events mean. In any case, the ultimate decline of mitogen-induced DNA synthesis after 72 hr is associated with progressive elevations of cyclic AMP levels (Monahan *et al.*, 1975; Carpentieri *et al.*, 1981) that may result from either nutritional deprivation or suppressor cell activation.

On balance, it is clear that both early and late changes in cyclic AMP levels occur in lymphocytes under certain circumstances. Their meaning in relationship to triggering events and cell-cycle traversement (G_1–S binding) remains to be unequivocally established. The distinct possibility exists that the induction and regulation, as well as the expression, of T-suppressor cells (Rocklin, 1976) or T-helper cells (Ohara *et al.*, 1978) by mitogens may involve cyclic AMP-related mechanisms. Analyses of the mechanism of T-cell subset function independent of the induction of the proliferation are needed to better define these issues.

Whitfield *et al.* (1976), Whitfield and MacManus (1972), and Morgan *et al.* (1975) presented evidence that cyclic GMP and cyclic GMP-related hormonal influences (e.g., PTH, insulin, ACh, and histamine) promote, in a calcium-dependent manner, rat thymocytes to enter DNA synthesis from a G_1–S restriction point. In this regard, thymocytes may have regulatory events different from those of peripheral T cells. A late peak of cyclic GMP and cyclic GMP-dependent protein kinase activity was observed by Carpentieri *et al.* (1981) at 72 hr during maximum DNA synthesis in PHA-stimulated cultures and may correspond to mitosis-associated changes. These data imply that cyclic GMP-related processes may be important in late events of the T-lymphocyte cycle in addition to IL-2 action and may be related to differentiation, proliferation, or both; however, appropriate studies in models employing discrete synchronized subpopulations are needed to clarify these issues.

6. BIOLOGICAL CORRELATES OF CYCLIC NUCLEOTIDES AND CALCIUM IN LYMPHOCYTE ACTIVATION

The foregoing predicts several possible biological correlates. The first is that there will be described defects of the early mitogen events critical to activation in disease states in which T lymphocytes and/or accessory cells are absent or are present but hyporesponsive. Few studies of cyclic nucleotides have been reported for these disease states. The second is that defects will be described under circumstances of uncontrolled lymphocyte proliferation. Several published studies relate to cyclic nucleotides in lymphocyte malignancies.

Schumm et al. (1974) and Tam et al. (1979) showed that PHA-induced increases in cyclic GMP are defective in blood lymphocytes of mice and rats bearing tumors, as are their mitogen responses. Spach and Aschkenasy (1979) showed that protein-deprived rats show defects in in vivo cyclic nucleotide responses compared with normal mice in association with depressed T-dependent B-cell antibody responses. Wess and Archer (1981, 1982) showed that butylated hydroxyanisole, an antioxidant and inhibitor of thymus-dependent antibody responses, blocks splenic mitogen-induced cyclic GMP responses and that the depressed immune response can be reversed by addition of exogenous cyclic GMP or calcium. Tam et al. (1979) and Tam and Walford (1980) showed that the defects of lymphocyte mitogen responses in aged humans and mice are associated with elevated basal cyclic GMP and lowered basal cyclic AMP levels and with impaired PHA-induced early increase in cyclic GMP. Krall et al. (1981, 1983) and Abrass and Scarpace (1982) presented evidence to indicate that the cyclic AMP-related defect in lymphocytes of the aged reflects an impairment of adenylate cyclase. Kennes et al. (1981) suggested that the age-related defect in lymphocyte responsiveness to PHA stimulation reflects an impairment in calcium-dependent processes.

A number of reports have appeared and indicate that cyclic nucleotide abnormalities are present in various leukemias. Reported cellular levels of cyclic AMP in leukemia cells have been variable in the same type of leukemia and in different leukemias (Monahan et al., 1975; Kemp et al., 1975; Coffey, 1977; Peracchi et al., 1980; W. Weber et al., 1981; Takemoto et al., 1982). The most frequent observation has been a lowered level of cyclic AMP. This has been associated with depressed adenylate cyclase activity and response to stimulants

(Polgar *et al.*, 1973, 1977; Carpentieri *et al.*, 1981) and an increase in cyclic AMP-dependent phosphodiesterase (Hait and Weiss, 1975, 1977; Scher *et al.*, 1976; Weiss and Winchurch, 1978). Cyclic AMP binding and protein kinase have also been described as depressed in leukemic cells (Weber *et al.*, 1981).

By contrast, cellular levels of cyclic GMP have been reported to be elevated in various leukemic cell populations (Coffey, 1977; Scavennec *et al.*, 1981; Takemoto *et al.*, 1982; Peracchi *et al.*, 1980). Elevated levels of cyclic GMP in plasma and urine during leukemogenesis have also been reported (Chauwla *et al.*, 1980; Scavennec *et al.*, 1981; Wood *et al.*, 1984). This disturbance in cyclic GMP metabolism has been associated with increased or variable levels of guanylate cyclase (Carpentieri *et al.*, 1981; Takemoto *et al.*, 1982) and with increased levels of cyclic GMP phosphodiesterase (Hait and Weiss, 1977; Epstein *et al.*, 1977). The processes contributing to these cyclic nucleotide changes have not been elucidated.

Alterations in T-Cell Leukemias

A number of reports have examined acute lymphocyte leukemia (ALL) for alterations in membrane enzymes and cyclic nucleotide levels. The lymphocyte of ALL is perhaps comparable to T lymphocytes activated by mitogens; however, comparison of an actively cycling population with a recently activated resting T-cell population has intrinsic limitations.

We are among the first to record cellular increases in cyclic GMP in ALL (Coffey, 1977). This observation was confirmed by some (Scavennec *et al.*, 1981; Takemoto *et al.*, 1982) but not by others (Peracchi *et al.*, 1980). Conversely, most, but not all (Carpentieri *et al.*, 1980c; Peracchi *et al.*, 1980; Scavennec *et al.*, 1981; Liangxu *et al.*, 1981) studies have reported low levels of cyclic AMP. All studies showed increased cyclic GMP/cyclic AMP ratios and concluded significance of the cyclic nucleotide alterations. A number of studies showed elevated plasma and urinary cyclic GMP levels in acute leukemia (Scavennec *et al.*, 1981; Peracchi *et al.*, 1983, 1985) with low plasma and variable urinary cyclic AMP levels. In parallel with these findings, elevated guanylate cyclase levels (Carpentieri *et al.*, 1981) and cyclic GMP-dependent protein kinase and low levels of cyclic AMP-dependent protein kinase (Carpentieri *et al.*, 1980a,b) have been observed. Elevated levels of casein kinase and low histone kinase have also been observed (Pena *et al.*, 1983). The status of adenylate cyclase and cyclic nucleotide phosphodiesterases has not been reported for ALL.

Other studies hint at meaningful alterations in plasma membrane structure and function that may contribute to these cyclic nucleotide disturbances; however, an integrated view is not possible at this time. Carpentieri *et al.* (1980a) reported increased levels of PGE_1 and PGE_2 in ALL, an observation that may reflect more on enhanced AA release from membrane phospholipids rather than any action of these PGs on cyclic nucleotide metabolism. Several studies (Ben-Bassat *et al.*, 1977; Tsuda *et al.*, 1981; Liebes *et al.*, 1981; Spiegel *et al.*, 1981; Van Blitterswijk *et al.*, 1982; Humphries and Lovejoy, 1983) show increased fluorescence polarization of ALL cells, using several membrane probes; these studies suggest an increased membrane fluidity. No structural basis involving phospholipid or cholesterol content or ratio has been shown to account for these changes (Koizumi *et al.*, 1980; Spiegel *et al.*, 1981; Liebes *et al.*, 1981). Other changes include increased Na^+/K^+-ATPase activity and increased permeability to Na^+ and Ca^{2+} of ALL cells (Logan and Newland, 1982). All the findings are consistent with early changes observed in mitogen-activated lymphocytes; however, a more meaningful comparison to detect malignancy-associated changes would be with mitogen-activated lymphoblasts in cycle. Nevertheless, the foregoing summary of changes in mitogen-activated T lymphocytes offers a wealth of possibilities for probing membrane-associated pathways in search for clues to the malignancy-related changes. It would be important to know the status of IL-2 production, receptors, and responsiveness in ALL and in T-cell malignancies.

Increased understanding of the biochemical events associated with lymphocyte activation by mitogens will ultimately translate into some interesting new approaches to manipulating leukemic cell proliferation. One example is provided by the observations of Takemoto *et al.* (1982) and Claflin *et al.* (1977), who have shown that the balsam pear-derived inhibitor of guanylate cyclase preferentially inhibits leukemic cell guanylate cyclase; these workers have suggested that it may be useful to inhibit leukemia cell proliferation, as it does mitogen-induced lymphocyte proliferation.

While the biological correlates of early events of lymphocyte activation have centered almost exclusively on cyclic nucleotide-related events in immunodeficiency or leukemia, it seems reasonable to extend them to a variety of other mechanisms discussed in this review and that may be involved in these disorders. For example, a basic defect in membrane lipids could underlie defects in fluidity, in permeability, and in responses to lymphocyte-triggering agents, if indeed the earliest of these responses involves lipid metabolism.

7. CONCLUSIONS AND FUTURE CONSIDERATIONS

At the risk of oversimplification, we conclude with a synopsis of our current view on the central biochemical events involved in the initial activation of T lymphocytes by mitogens. Mitogens bind to the surface receptors of T cells and accessory cells by distinct receptors. They initiate two series of events without apparently entering the cells. In the accessory cells, they initiate IL-1 production and secretion, which alone or in conjunction with mitogen induces responder T cells to synthesize IL-2 and their receptors. Accessory cells may also contribute products of AA, such as PGs and eicosanoids, which modulate the subsequent T-cell response. In the absence of accessory cell function, the T cell responds directly to the mitogen with a series of events over a period of perhaps 3 hr that commit the cell to RNA and protein synthesis and blastogenesis. Once this first phase is completed, a second phase initiated by IL-2 and its interaction with appropriate receptors leads to DNA synthesis and clonal replication.

The events of the first phase initiated by the mitogen in the T lymphocyte are the subject of this review. Following interaction of the mitogen with its receptors there occurs a clustering of receptors and probably also associated enzymes. As a result, a transmembrane trigger-type signal is propagated that has both positive and negative correlates. The negative signal is exemplified with high mitogen concentrations and is associated with membrane freezing, microtubular aggregation, microfilament-based receptor capping, adenylate cyclase activation, and large cellular cyclic AMP increases. These events are not associated with subsequent DNA synthesis; however, they may occur concomitant with one or several manifestations of the positive signal. The polymerization and aggregation of microtubules and the microfilament-related changes are clearly not essential for lymphocyte activation.

For reasons that are not yet clear, the mitogen induces an early change in membrane permeability and transport with flux of cations, including calcium and potassium ion influxes, as well as sodium efflux. It is difficult to discern whether the earliest permeability change reflects organized biochemical events involving one or another "channel" or merely reflects indiscriminant uptake of molecules from the surrounding medium. In any case, activation of several membrane transport ATPases occurs, and a balance is re-established such that Na^+/K^+ levels are maintained and no consistent change in transmembrane potential occurs that can be considered essential to the positive signal. A variety of transport processes are stimulated (e.g., glucose, amino acids, and nucleosides) and pH increases occur; these events are associated with, but may not be essential for, triggering.

A collected series of early membrane lipid changes occur that can be considered essential for the positive signal. These include the uptake from both intra- and extracellular sources of AA and other fatty acids, choline, phosphate, and other molecules. These substances are incorporated into membrane phospholipids, particularly PI. The methylation of PE may occur following the action of some mitogens, but not others and is therefore not seen as a critical event. The mitogen induces a turnover of PI with the production of diglyceride and inositol phosphates. A series of enzymes are activated in this process including phospholipase C, acyl CoA transferase, inositol phosphatases, and phosphoinositide kinases. It is possible, but it has not been conclusively shown, that the initial event involves phospholipase C. The turnover of PI and the associated fatty acid changes are correlated with an increase in membrane fluidity that may or may not contribute to signal propagation.

The major products of these reactions involving PI that contribute to signal formation include (1) inositol trisphosphate itself, which has been shown to give rise to calcium mobilization; and (2) diacylglycerol, which activates a cytoplasmic protein kinase C, another possible participant in the signal, yet without well-established actions (tentatively linked to the phosphorylation of guanylate cyclase, the IL-2 receptor, and adenylate cyclase). Diacylglycerol also gives rise, by way of mitogen-activated diglyceride kinase, to phosphatidic acid, which has also been suggested to contribute to calcium influx and/or mobilization. Diacylglycerol also gives rise to AA release by way of a mitogen-activated diglyceride kinase.

Perhaps the two most completely documented events associated with mitogen action are calcium influx/mobilization and AA release. These two products of the transmembrane signal have been clearly demonstrated to be essential for activation and to contribute to reactions that lead to nuclear activation. Arachidonic acid may give rise to PGs and thromboxanes; however, these metabolites apparently do not contribute to a positive signal and may play a role in negative components of the signal through effects on the adenylate cyclase/cyclic AMP system. Arachidonic acid may be reincorporated into other phospholipids of the membrane by the acyltransferase reaction and contribute to later changes in fluidity and transport. Finally, and most importantly, AA gives rise to eicosanoids such as 5-, 11-, 12-, and 15-hydroxyperoxy- and hydroxyeicosatetraenoic acids and leukotriene B_4 and C_4. At this point, it appears that this pathway is essential for activation through the production of 5- and perhaps 11- and 12-HPETEs and HETEs. It also appears that 15-HETE and LTB_4 may act as either negative feedback signals or inducers of suppressor T cells, or both.

The activation of the 5-lipoxygenase, a critical calcium-dependent step, leads via the production of 5-HPETE and 5-HETE and possibly other products to the activation of membrane and soluble guanylate cyclase and the production of increased cellular levels and turnover of cyclic GMP. Cyclic GMP production appears to be essential for mitogen activation. It facilitates mitogen-induced calcium influx.

Calcium influx/mobilization is clearly central to mitogen action. Lectin mitogens are ionophoretic for calcium. The calcium ionophore mimics most, but not all, of the actions of lectin mitogens. Only PMA does not induce calcium influx, yet its actions appear to be dependent on intracellular calcium. Much of the calcium that enters the cell appears to be bound; however, free calcium concentration increases markedly. The prevention of mitogen-induced calcium entry, mobilization, and action with various experimental manipulations made it clear that calcium ion is central and essential to the trigger signal.

Through its influx and mobilization from cellular stores, calcium is thought to contribute directly and indirectly through the action of calmodulin, protein kinase C, and perhaps other systems to the activation of a number of enzymatic processes involved in the positive signal. These include phospholipase C, diglyceride kinase and lipase, 5-lipoxygenase, and guanylate cyclase. Calcium has also been shown to cooperate with cyclic GMP in the initiation of nuclear RNA synthesis, perhaps through an effect on regulating initiation site frequency.

It seems reasonable to consider cyclic GMP and calcium ion as the best-documented candidates for membrane to nuclear signal mechanisms leading to early RNA and protein synthesis. The adenylate cyclase–cyclic AMP system plays a complex role in lymphocyte activation. Clearly, potent activation of the system in the very early phases by high doses of mitogen or by accessory cell-produced PG blocks positive signal transmission, perhaps through protein kinase A activation and inhibition of phospholipase, calcium influx, and IL-2 production and action. Small, perhaps localized, early increases of cyclic AMP may play a role in a positive signal formation through protein kinase A activation and membrane protein phosphorylation; however, this remains to be conclusively demonstrated. Late increases in cyclic AMP and cyclic AMP-dependent protein kinases and in ornithine decarboxylase and polyamine metabolism are probably events essential to the latter part of the first phase essential for ultimate entry into DNA synthesis upon reception of the second IL-2 signal. The significance of other events remains to be determined.

Recent studies employing the differential actions of monoclonal antibodies to the T_3/Ti receptor complex or calcium ionophores in conjunction with PMA have begun to unravel components of the first signal discussed in this review into two pathways. The first involves T-cell receptor activation, inositol trisphosphate production, and calcium mobilization, and the second involves protein kinase C activation, lipoxygenation of AA, and cyclic GMP production. The actions of IL-1 to yield IL-2 production remain to be clarified; however, appear to involve the second pathway. The second signal for proliferation involving IL-2 action is incompletely understood but may involve components of both pathways, particularly the second. It remains to dissect the signal pathways further with these differential probes.

The foregoing represents a simplified version of the common denominators and cause–effect relationships following mitogen action in the T lymphocyte. While it represents a great accumulation of information since the first experiments were performed almost 20 years ago, it produces many more new questions to be asked than we possibly could have envisioned at that time. To conclude this review, we would like to highlight some of the general questions and directions that might be approached in the future.

Purified mitogens and recombinant IL-1 and IL-2 are now available, and the techniques exist to separate individual T-cell and accessory cell populations to explore their interactions. It remains to explore the biochemical mechanisms involved in IL-1 production and action, particularly the involvement of protein kinase C.

The possibility has been raised that arachidonate metabolites, including both PGs and eicosanoids, participate in intercellular communication; it may well be that many of the events described herein are not occurring in T cells destined to enter DNA synthesis, but in regulatory accessory cells. It has also been suggested that lymphokine interactions (e.g., production of CSF-1 by T cells) induce IL-1 (R. N. Moore *et al.*, 1981) and may contribute to positive feedback loops. The role of cell–cell contact and intercellular functions remains to be explored in the activation process.

While receptors have been identified for mitogen, they need to be characterized and particularly in association with what appear to be macromolecular intramembranous complexes containing enzymes involved in signal formation. New approaches to submembrane biology and biochemistry using immobilized lectins and/or monoclonal antibodies in conjunction with membrane fractionation procedures should lead to dissection of the membrane and the elucidation of such complexes. Ultimately, when the transmembrane signal sequence is sufficiently clarified, it should be possible to be reconstructed in its simplest form. Mitogen activation of key enzymes in broken cells and membrane preparations should be a first step in this process.

Comparison of the actions of lectin mitogens with the processes induced by mitogenic probes (e.g., PMA and calcium ionophore) by hormones acting on related pathways and by nonmitogenic lectins will be important. As first steps, it seems crucial to dissect early, perhaps nonspecific, leak events from discrete channel regulated fluxes and transports. The experimental work with so-called "channels" may not reflect meaningful events critical to activation. Such studies could well benefit from comparisons with nonmitogenic lectins and mitogeneic probes. It seems possible that discrete signals may be propagated in the absence of all but calcium flux and in the absence of the compensatory ion transport changes. It seems important to document further any importance of Na^+/H^+ carrier transport in mitogen action, since it has been advanced by Berridge (1984) and others as being critical in cell division in general. If one assumes, as we have, that calcium mobilization is central to lymphocyte activation, the mechanism should be clarified and the role of phosphatidic acid and inositol trisphosphate as ionophores further probed.

Clearly, further elucidation of phospholipid turnover will yield profitable insights. Key questions include the following: Does the same phospholipase C hydrolyze PI and PI-4,5-bisphosphate? Is there a phospholipase D that converts PI directly to phosphatidic acid, bypassing the formation of diglyceride? Is there a mechanism in lymphocytes, as in platelets (Lapetina, 1982), for phosphatidic acid (derived from PI) to stimulate a phospholipase A_2-mediated breakdown of PC? Or, as an alternative to diglyceride lipase, is there in lymphocytes, as in platelets (Billah *et al.*, 1981), a phospholipase A_2 with specificity for phosphatidic acid? Is there an acyltransferase with a specificity for PI?

It remains to be determined whether the activation of protein kinase C is critical, particularly in IL-1 action, and what its phosphorylated substrates are and whether there are critical interactions with calcium influx and/or cyclic nucleotide-related mechanisms. The roles of membrane G proteins, ADP ribosylation, and tyrosine kinase need to be examined. The proximal stimulants and regulators in the eicosanoid/guanylate cyclase sequence remain to be clarified, and the mechanisms for stable and persistent activation of both particulate and soluble guanylate cyclase need elucidation.

The role of proton generation in guanylate cyclase activation, as advanced by Goldberg, needs investigating as it relates to mitogen actions. The substrates and products of all putative messengers (Cyclic nucleotides, calcium, inositol trisphosphate, diglyceride, protein kinase AI and AII, C, and G) need to be elucidated and linked to the signal sequence or shown to be noncritical. In turn, there is a great need for the linking of component signal sequence pathways with activation of specific genes required for proliferation.

For the most part, cytoplasmic events do not seem critical in initiation; however, the activation of ornithine decarboxylase and its direct or indirect action through its polyamine products to initiation events critical to proliferation and/or differentiation needs to be unraveled. Other critical events will also be uncovered.

Two approaches to the nuclear activation issue seem very relevant. The first is the biological one reviewed herein, where the nucleus is isolated soon after cellular activation and some parameter of early RNA synthesis is measured in order to ask whether a cell surface event is critical, if stimulated or inhibited, for nuclear activation and whether membrane or cytoplasmically derived messengers act in the nucleus to recreate the activation. The second approach is a molecular biological one to piece together the sequence critical to new RNA synthesis, like histone phosphorylation and acetylation, acidic nuclear protein phosphorylation, DNA-dependent RNA polymerase activation, nuclease activation, and so forth, and those critical to specific gene activation. On the basis of two-dimensional gel analysis, several new proteins are synthesized, and a large variety are increased in their synthesis. The specific genes encoding proteins associated with and leading to activation (e.g., IL-2 receptor, c-fos, c-myc), those secreted as lymphokines (e.g., IL-2 and IFN), as well as those associated with activation surface receptors (Cotner et al., 1982; Newman et al., 1986), will ultimately be detected and their regulation determined with great benefit to our understanding of the processes involved.

Particularly interesting will be the clarification of late receptor activation events and nuclear induction of phosphoproteins implicated in the entry of the primed T cell into DNA synthesis (See Gutowski et al., 1984).

Finally, it is clear that T-lymphocyte activation by mitogens leads to proliferation of helper, suppressor, and other subsets having different functions. It is very possible that the mechanisms will differ. Both cyclic AMP-related mechanisms, including histamine and PG (Webb and Jamieson, 1976) and 15-HETE and LTB_4 (Goodwin, 1986), have been implicated in the activation of suppressor cells both with and without proliferation. It may be that these signals, if imposed on the positive signals, may contribute to activation of suppressor mechanisms in cells that ultimately proliferate. In any case, such possibilities need to be explored. The ultimate goal of all these endeavors will be to relate the mechanisms of induction of proliferation by mitogens to those by antigen and growth factors, like IL-2, and also to the events associated with the concomitant induction of differentiation in these cells and their progeny.

REFERENCES

Abraham, R. T., Steffan, N., and McKean, D. J., 1986, Signal requirements for the activation of an interleukin-1 responsive T cell lymphoma, *Sixth International Congress of Immunology, Toronto Canada*, p. 230 (abst.).

Abrass, I., and Scarpace, P., 1982, Catalytic unit of adenylate cyclase: Reduced activity in aged-human lymphocytes, *J. Clin. Endocrinol. Metabol.* **55**:1026–1028.

Ahmann, G. B., and Sage, H. J., 1974, Stimulation of guinea pig lymphocytes by lenz culinaris lectin-A, *Cell. Immunol.* **10**:183–195.

Alford, R. H., 1970, Metal cation requirements for phytohemagglutinin-induced transformation of human peripheral blood lymphocytes, *J. Immunol.* **104**:698–703.

Allan, D., and Michell, R. H., 1974, Phosphatidylinositol cleavage catalyzed by the soluble fraction from lymphocytes, *Biochem. J.* **142**:591–597.

Allan, D., and Michell, R. H., 1977, A comparison of the effects of PHA and of calcium ionophore A23187 on the metabolism of glycerolipids in small lymphocytes, *Biochem. J.* **164**:389–397.

Allfrey, V. G., Inoue, A., Karn, J., Johnson, E. M., Good, R. A., and Hadden, J. W., 1975, Sequence-specific DNA-binding by non-histone proteins of the lymphocyte nucleus and evidence for their migration from cytoplasm to nucleus at times of gene activation, in: *The Structure and Function of Chromatin*, Ciba Foundation Symposium, **28**:199–228.

Allwood, G., Asherson, G. L., Davey, M. J., and Goodford, P. J., 1971, The early uptake of radioactive calcium by human lymphocytes treated with phytohaemagglutinin, *Immunology* **21**:509–516.

Ananthakrishnan, R., Coffey, R. G., and Hadden, J. W., 1981, Cyclic GMP and calcium in lymphocyte activation by phytohemagglutinin, *Lymphocyte Diff.* **1**:183–196.

Andersson, J., Edelman, G. M., Moller, G., and Sjoberg, O., 1972, Activation of B lymphocytes by locally concentrated concanavalin A, *Eur. J. Immunol.* **2**:233–235.

Ashman, R. F., 1984, The influence of cell interactions on early biochemical activation events in human mononuclear cells, *Prog. Immunol.* **5**:339–359.

Atkinson, J. P., Kelly, J. P., Weiss, A., Wedner, J. H., and Parker, C. W., 1978, Enhanced intracellular cGMP concentrations and lectin-induced lymphocyte transformation, *J. Immunol.* **121**:2282–2291.

Atluru, D., Lianos, E. A., and Goodwin, J. S., 1986, Arachidonic acid inhibits 5-lipoxygenase in human T cells, *Biochem. Biophys. Res. Commun.* **135**:670–676.

Aubry, J., Zachowski, A., Paraf, A., and Colombani, J., 1979, Modulation of membrane-bound enzyme activity by binding of antibodies to major histocompatability complex antigens, *Ann. Immunol.* **130C**:17–27.

Averdunk, R., 1972, Uber die wirking von phytohemagglutinin und antilymphozytenserum auf den kalium-, glucose- und aminosaure-transport bei menschlichen lymphozyten, *Hoppe Seylers Z. Physiol. Chem.* **353**:79–87.

Averdunk, R., and Lauf, P. K., 1975, Effects of mitogens on sodium–potassium transport, ^{3}H-ouabain binding and adenosine triphosphatase activity in lymphocytes, *Exp. Cell. Res.* **93**:331–342.

Averdunk, A., and Gunther, T., 1980, Effect of concanavalin A on Ca^{2+} binding, Ca^{2+} uptake and the Ca^{2+} ATPase of lymphocyte plasma membranes, *Biochem. Biophys. Res. Commun.* **97:** 1146–1153.

Averdunk, R., Mueller, J., and Wenzel, B., 1976, Studies on the mechanism of activation of lymphocyte membrane ATPase by concanavalin A, *J. Clin. Chem. and Clin. Biochem.* **14:**339–344.

Averner, M. J., Brock, M. L., and Jost, J. P., 1972, Stimulation of ribonucleic acid synthesis in horse lymphocytes by exogenous cyclic adenosine 3′,5′-monophosphate, *J. Biol. Chem.* **247:** 413–417.

Bachvaroff, R. J., Miller, F., and Rapoport, F. T., 1984, The role of calmodulin in the regulation of human lymphocyte activation, *Cell Immunol.* **85:**135–153.

Bailey, J. M., Bryant, R. W., Low, C.-E., Pupillo, M. B., and Vanderhoek, J. Y., 1982a, Regulation of T-lymphocyte mitogenesis by the leukocyte product 15-hydroxy-eicosatetraenoic acid (15-HETE), *Cell. Immunol.* **67:**112–120.

Bailey, J. M., Bryant, R. W., Low, E. C., Pupillo, M. B., and Vanderhoek, J. Y., 1982b, Role of lipoxygenases in regulation of PHA and phorbol ester-induced mitogenesis, *Adv. Prostaglandins Thromboxanes Leukotrienes Res.* **9:**341–353.

Bailey, J. M., Coffey, R., Merrit, W. D., and Hadden, J. W., 1986, Role of licosanoids in lymphocyte activation: A review, in: *Advances in Immunopharmacology.* Vol. 3 (L. Chedid, J. W. Hadden, F. Spreafice, P. Dukor, and D. Willoughby, eds.), pp. 177–188, Pergamon, Oxford.

Baran, D. T., Lichtman, M. A., and Peck, W. A., 1972, Alpha-aminoisobutyric acid transport in human leukemic lymphocytes: In vitro characteristics and inhibition by cortisol and cyclohexi-mide, *J. Clin. Invest.* **51:**2181–2189.

Bard, E., Colwill, R., L'Anglais, R., and Kaplan, J. G., 1978, Response of human lymphocytes to mitogen: At what stage is there a requirement for Ca^{2+}?, *Can. J. Biochem.* **56:**900–904.

Barnett, R. E., Scott, R. E., Furcht, L. T., and Kersey, J. H., 1974, Evidence that mitogenic lectins induce changes in lymphocyte membrane fluidity, *Nature (Lond.)* **249:**465–466.

Beckner, S. K., and Farrar, W. L., 1985, Generation of lymphokine activated killer (LAK) cells and stimulation of proliferation by interleukin 2 (IL-2) are both modulated by cAMP; regulation of growth factor mediated differentiation and proliferation by common mechanism. *Fed. Proc.* **44:** 1792.

Beckner, S. K., and Farrar, W. L., 1986, Interleukin 2 modulation of adenylate Cyclase, *J. Biol. Chem.* **261:**3043–3047.

Belmont, J. W., and Rich, R. R., 1981, Role of calcium and magnesium and of cytochalasin-sensitive processes in lectin-stimulated lymphocyte activation, *Cell. Immunol.* **59:**276–288.

Ben-Bassat, H., Poliak, A., Rosenbaum, S., Naparstek, E., Shouval, D., and Inbar, M., 1977, Fluidity of membrane lipids and lateral mobility of concanavalin A receptors in the cell surface of normal lymphocytes and lymphocytes from patients with malignant lymphomas and leuke-mias, *Cancer Res.* **37:**1307–1312.

Berger, N. A., and Skinner, A. M., 1974, Characterization of lymphocyte transformation induced by zinc ions, *J. Cell. Biol.* **61:**45–55.

Bernard, D. P., Carboni, J. M., and Waksman, B. H., 1975, Regulation of lymphocyte responses in vitro. VI. Potentiation of the response to phytohemagglutinin by cytochalasin B, *Ann. Immunol.* **126:**107–120.

Berridge, M. J., 1975, The interaction of cyclic nucleotides and calcium in the control of cellular activity, *Adv. Cyclic Nucleotide Res.* **6:**1–98.

Berridge, M. J., 1984, Inositol triphosphate and diacylglycerol as second messengers, *Biochem. J.* **220:**345–360.

Best, K., Sever, A., Mathias, P. C. F., and Malaisse, W. J., 1984, Inhibition by mepacrine and p-bromophenacyl bromide of phosphoinositide hydrolysis, glucose oxidation, calcium uptake and insulin release in rat pancreatic islets, *Biochem. Pharmacol.* **33:**2657–2662.

Besterman, J. M., May, W. S., Levine, H., Cragoe, E. J., and Cuatrecases, P., 1985, Amiloride inhibits phorbol ester-stimulated Na$^+$/H$^+$ exchange and protein kinase C, *J. Biol. Chem.* **260:** 1155–1159.

Betel, I., and Martijnse, J., 1976, Drugs that disrupt microtubuli do not inhibit lymphocyte activation, *Nature (Lond.)* **261:**318–319.

Betel, I., and Van den Berg, K. J., 1972, Interaction of concanavalin A with rat lymphocytes, *Eur. J. Biochem.* **30:**571–578.

Betel, I., and Van den Berg, K. J., 1975, The relationship between "early events" and DNA synthesis in mitogen stimulated lymphocytes, in: *Immune Recognition,* Proceedings of the Ninth Leukocyte Culture Conference (A. S. Rosenthal, ed.), pp. 505–509, Academic, New York.

Betel, I., Martijnse, J., and Van den Berg, K. J., 1974, Absence of an early increase of phospholipid-phosphate turnover in mitogen stimulated B lymphocytes, *Cell. Immunol.* **14:**429–434.

Billah, M. M., Lapetina, E. G., and Cautrecasas, P., 1981, Activity specific for phosphatidic acid. A possible mechanism for the production of arachidonic acid in platelets, *J. Biol. Chem.* **256:** 5399–5403.

Birch, R. E., and Polmar, S. H., 1982, Pharmacological modification of immunoregulatory T lymphocytes. I. Effect of adenosine, H$_1$ and H$_2$ histamine agonists upon T lymphocyte regulation of B lymphocyte differentiation *in vitro, Clin. Exp. Immunol.* **48:**218–230.

Birx, D. L., Berger, M., and Fleisher, T. A., 1984, The interference of T cell activation by calcium channel blocking agents, *J. Immunol.* **133:**2904–2909.

Blitstein-Willinger, E., and Diamantstein, T., 1978, Inhibition by isoptin (a calcium antagonist) of the mitogenic stimulation of lymphocytes prior to the S-phase, *Immunology* **34:**303–308.

Bloom, F. E., Wedner, H., and Parker, C. W., 1973, The use of antibodies to study cell structure and metabolism, *Pharmacol. Rev.* **25:**343–358.

Borghetti, A. F., Kay, J. E., and Wheeler, K. P., 1979, Enhanced transport of natural amino acids after activation of pig lymphocytes, *Biochem. J.* **182:**27–32.

Bougnoux, P., Bonvini, E., Chang, Z. L., and Hoffman, T., 1983, Effect of interferon on phospholipid methylation by peripheral blood mononuclear cells, *J. Cell. Biochem.* **20:**215–224.

Bourguignon, L. Y. W., and Hsing, Y-C., 1983, The participation of adenylate cyclase in lymphocyte capping, *Biochim. Biophys. Acta* **728:**186–190.

Boyett, J. D., and Hofert, J. F., 1972, Stimulatory effect of insulin on glucose metabolism of thymus lymphocytes, *Horm. Metab. Res.* **4:**163–167.

Bray, M. A., Powell, R. G., and Lydyard, P. M., 1981, Prostaglandin generation by separated human blood mononuclear cell fractions, *Int. J. Immunopharmacol.* **3:**377–381.

Bretscher, M. S., and Raff, M. C., 1975, Mammalian plasma membranes, *Nature (Lond.)* **258:**43–49.

Brewer, C. F., Marcus, D. N., Grollman, A. P., 1974, Interactions of saccharides with concanavalin A, *J. Biol. Chem.* **249:**4614–4616.

Brock, J. H., 1981, The effect of iron and transferrin on the response of serum-free cultures of mouse lymphocytes to concanavalin A and LPS, *Immunology* **43:**387–392.

Brock, J. H., and Mainou-Fowler, T., 1983. The role of iron and transferrin in lymphocyte transformation, *Immunol. Today* **4:**347–351.

Brock, J. H., and Rankin, C., 1981, Transferrin binding and iron uptake by mouse lymph node cells during transformation in response to concanavalin A, *Immunology* **43:**393–398.

Buckley, A. R., Montgomery, D. W., Kibler, R., Putnam, C. W., Zukoski, C. F., Gout, P. W., Beer, C. T., and Russell, D. H., 1986, Prolactin stimulation of ornithine decarboxylase and mitogenesis in Nb$_2$ node lymphoma cells: The role of protein kinase C and calcium mobilization. *Immunopharmacology* **12:**37–51.

Burgess, G. M., Godfrey, P. P., McKinney, J. S., Berridge, M. J., Irvine, R. F., and Putney, J. W., Jr., 1984, The second messenger linking receptor activation to internal Ca release in liver, *Nature (Lond.)* **309:**63–65.

Burgoyne, L. A., Wagar, M. A., and Atkinson, M. R., 1970, Initiation of DNA synthesis in rat thymus: Correlation of calcium-dependent initiation in thymocytes and in isolated thymus nuclei, *Biochem. Biophys. Res. Commun.* **39:**918–922.

Burleson, D. G., and Sage, H. J., 1976, Effect of lectins on the levels of cAMP and cGMP in guinea pig lymphocytes: Early responses of lymph node cells to mitogenic and non-mitogenic lectins, *J. Immunol.* **116:**696–703.

Butman, B. T., Jacobsen, T., Cabatu, O. G., and Bourguignon, L. Y. W., 1981, The involvement of cAMP in lymphocyte capping, *Cell. Immunol.* **61:**397–403.

Byus, C. V., Klimpel, G. R., Lucas, D. O., and Russell, D. H., 1977, Type I and type II cyclic AMP-dependent protein kinase as opposite effectors of lymphocyte mitogenesis, *Nature (Lond.)* **268:**63–64.

Byus, C. V., Klimpel, G. R., Lucas, D. O., and Russell, D. H., 1978, Ornithine decarboxylase induction in mitogen-stimulated lymphocytes is related to the specific activation of type I adenosine cyclic 3′,5′-monophosphate-dependent protein kinase, *Mol. Pharmacol.* **14:**431–441.

Cantrell, D. A., Davies, A. A., and Crumpton, M. J., 1985, Activators of protein kinase C down-regulate and phosphorylate the T3/T-cell antigen receptor complex of human T lymphocytes. *Proc. Natl. Acad. Sci. USA* **82:**8158–8162.

Carpentieri, U., Brouhard, B. H., LaGrone, L., and Lockhart, L. H., 1980a, Observations on prostaglandins in normal and leukemic human lymphocytes, *Prostaglandins* **20:**1117–1129.

Carpentieri, U., Minguell, J. J., and Haggard, M. E., 1980b, Variation of activity of protein kinase in unstimulated and phytohemagglutinin-stimulated normal and leukemic human lymphocytes, *Cancer Res.* **40:**2714–2718.

Carpentieri, U., Monahan, T. M., and Gustavson, L. P., 1980c, Observations on the level of cyclic nucleotides in three populations of human lymphocytes in culture, *J. Cyclic Nucleotide Res.* **6:**253–259.

Carpentieri, U., Minguell, J. J., and Gardner, F. H., 1981, Adenylate cyclase and guanylate cyclase activity in normal and leukemic human lymphocytes, *Blood* **57:**975–978.

Casnellie, J. E., and Lamberts, R. J., 1986, Tumor promoters cause changes in the state of phosphorylation and apparent molecular weight of a tyrosine protein kinase in T lymphocytes. *J. Biol. Chem.* **261:**4921–4925.

Castagna, M., Takai, Y., Kaibuchi, K., Sano, K., Kikkawa, U., and Nishizuka, Y., 1982, Direct activation of calcium-activated, phospholipid-dependent protein kinase by tumor-promoting phorbol esters, *J. Biol. Chem.* **257:**7847–7851.

Chambers, D. A., Martin, D. W., Jr., and Weinstein, Y., 1974, The effect of cyclic nucleotides on purine biosynthesis and the induction of PRPP synthetase during lymphocyte activation, *Cell* **3:**375–380.

Chandy, K. G., DeCoursey, T. E., Cahalan, M. D., McLaugulin, C., and Gupta, S., 1984, Voltage-gated potassium channels are required for human T lymphocyte activation, *J. Exp. Med.* **160:**369–385.

Chaplin, D. D., Wedner, H. J., and Parker, C. W., 1980, Protein phosphorylation in human peripheral blood lymphocytes: Mitogen-induced increases in protein phosphorylation in intact lymphocytes, *J. Immunol.* **124:**2390–2398.

Chauwla, R. K., Shlaer, M., Laurson, D. H., Murray, T., Schmidt, F., Shoji, M., Nixon, D., Richmond, A., Rudman, D., 1980, Elevated plasma and urinary guanosine 3′,5′-monophosphate and increased production rate in patients with neoplastic disease, *Cancer Res.* **40:**3915–3920.

Chen, S-H. S., 1979, Relationship between phosphatidylcholine biosynthesis and cellular commitment in concanavalin A-stimulated lymphocytes, *Exp. Cell. Res.* **121:**283–290.

Chesters, J. K., 1975, Comparison of the effects of zinc deprivation and actinomycin D on ribonucleic acid synthesis by stimulated lymphocytes, *Biochem. J.* **150:**211–218.

Cheung, R. K., Grinstein, S., Gelfand, E. W., 1983, Permissive role of calcium in the inhibition of T cell mitogenesis by calmodulin antagonists, *J. Immunol.* **131:**2291–2294.

Chien, M. M., and Ashman, R. F., 1983, Phospholipid synthesis by activated human B lymphocytes, *J. Immunol.* **130:**2568–2573.

Chisari, F. V., and Curtis, L. K., 1981, Modulation of peripheral blood mononuclear cell cyclic adenosine monophosphate levels of human very low density lipoprotein, *Cell. Immunol.* **65:** 325–336.

Claflin, A., Vesely, D., Hudson, J., Bagwell, C., Lekotay, D., Lo, T., Fletcher, M., Block, N., and Levey, G., 1977, Inhibition of growth and guanylate cyclase activity of an undifferentiated prostate adenocarcinoma by an extract of the balsam pear (*Momordica charantia abbreviata*), *Proc. Natl. Acad. Sci. USA* **75:**989–993.

Clarkson, B., and Baserga, R., 1974, *Control of Proliferation in Animal Cells*, Cold Spring Harbor Conferences on Cell Proliferation, Vol. 1, Cold Spring Harbor Laboratory, Cold Spring Harbor, New York.

Coffey, R. G., 1977, Assays for cyclic nucleotides including clinical applications, in: *Immunopharmacology* (J. Hadden, R. Coffey, and F. Spreafico, eds.), pp. 389–412, Plenum, New York.

Coffey, R. G., 1986, Phosphatidylserine and phorbol myristate acetate stimulation of human lymphocyte guanylate cyclase, *Int. J. Biochem.* **18:**665–670.

Coffey, R. G., and Hadden, J. W., 1981a, Phorbol myristate acetate stimulation of lymphocyte guanylate cyclase, *Biochem. Biophys. Res. Commun.* **101:**584–590.

Coffey, R. G., and Hadden, J. W., 1981b, Arachidonate and metabolites in mitogen activation of lymphocyte guanylate cyclase, in: *Advances in Immunopharmacology* (J. Hadden, L. Chedid, R. Spreafico, and P. Mullen, eds.), pp. 365–373, Pergamon, Oxford.

Coffey, R. G., and Hadden, J. W., 1983a, Phorbol myristate acetate stimulation of lymphocyte guanylate cyclase and cyclic guanosine 3′,5′-monophosphate phosphodiesterase and reduction of adenylate cyclase, *Cancer Res.* **43:**150–158.

Coffey, R. G., and Hadden, J. W., 1983b, Calcium and guanylate cyclase in lymphocyte activation, in: *Advances in Immunopharmacology*. Vol. 2 (L. Chedid, J. Hadden, and A. Willoughby, eds.), pp. 87–94, Pergamon, Oxford.

Coffey, R. G., and Hadden, J. W., 1984, Cyclic nucleotides in neurohumoral and hormonal regulation of cells of the immune system, in: *Stress, Immunity, and Aging* (E. L. Cooper, ed.), pp. 225–247, Dekker, New York.

Coffey, R. G., and Hadden, J. W., 1985, Stimulation of lymphocyte guanylate cyclase by HETEs, in: *Prostaglandins, Leukotrienes, and Lipoxins: Biochemistry, Mechanism of Action, and Clinical Applications* (J. M. Bailey, ed.), pp. 501–509, Plenum, New York.

Coffey, R. G., Hadden, E. M., and Hadden, J. W., 1975, Norepinephrine stimulation of membrane ·ATPase in human lymphocytes, *Endocrinol. Res. Commun.* **12:**179–198.

Coffey, R. G., Hadden, E. M., and Hadden, J. W., 1977, Evidence for cyclic GMP and calcium mediation of lymphocyte activation by mitogens, *J. Immunol.* **119:**1387–1394.

Coffey, R. G., Hadden, E. M., Lopez, C., and Hadden, J. W., 1978, Cyclic GMP and calcium in the initiation of cellular proliferation, *Adv. Cyclic Nucleotide Res.* **9:**661–676.

Coffey, R. G., Hadden, E. M., and Hadden, J. W., 1981, Phytohemagglutinin stimulation of guanylate cyclase in human lymphocytes, *J. Biol. Chem.* **256:**4418–4424.

Cohen, S., Wong, R., Gutowski, J., and Goldfarb, R. H., 1986, The cytoplasmic protein (ADR) that triggers DNA synthesis in interleukin 2-stimulated lymphocytes appears to be a protease, *Sixth International Congress of Immunology, Toronto, Canada*, p. 236 (abst.).

Cooper, H. L., 1968, Ribonucleic acid metabolism in lymphocytes stimulated by phytohemagglutinin. II. Rapidly synthesized ribonucleic acid and the production of ribosomal ribonucleic acid, *J. Biol. Chem.* **243:**34–43.

Cooper, H. L., 1972, Studies on RNA metabolism during lymphocyte activation, *Transplant Rev.* **11:**3–38.

Cooper, H. L., 1974, Studies of poly(A)-bearing RNA in resting and growing human lymphocytes, in: *Control of Proliferation in Animal Cells* (B. Clarkson and R. Baserga, eds.), Vol. 4, pp. 769–800, Cold Spring Harbor Laboratory, Cold Spring Harbor, New York.

Cooper, H. L., and Braverman, R., 1980, Protein synthesis in resting and growth-stimulated human peripheral lymphocytes, *Exp. Cell. Res.* **127**:351–359.

Cooper, H. L., and Braverman, R., 1981, Close correlation between initiator methionyl-tRNA level and rate of protein synthesis during human lymphocyte growth cycle, *J. Biol. Chem.* **256**:7461–7467.

Cooper, H. L., and Lester, E. P., 1982, Nuclear activation and regulation of lymphocyte protein synthesis, in: *Advances in Immunopharmacology*, Vol. 2, (J. Hadden, L. Chedid, P. Dukor, and D. Willoughby, eds.), pp. 95–100, Pergamon, New York.

Cooper, H. L., and Rubin, A. D., 1965, RNA metabolism in lymphocytes stimulated by phytohemagglutinin: Initial response to phytohemagglutinin, *Blood* **25**:1014–1027.

Cotner, T., Williams, J. M., Strom, T. B., and Strominger, J. L., 1982, The relationship between early T cell activation antigens and T cell proliferation, in: *Advances in Immunopharmacology*, Vol. 2 (J. Hadden, L. Chedid, P. Dukor, F. Spreafico, and D. Willoughby, eds.), pp. 63–68, Pergamon, Oxford.

Coulson, A. S., and Kennedy, L. A., 1971, Lymphocyte membrane enzymes, *Blood* **38**:485–490.

Cross, M. E., and Ord, M. G., 1971, Changes in histone phosphorylation and associated early metabolic events in pig lymphocyte cultures transformed by phytohaemagglutinin or 6-N,2'-O-dibutyryladenosine 3',5'-cyclic monophosphate, *Biochem. J.* **124**:241–248.

Crumpton, M. J., Auger, J., Green, N. M., and Maino, V. C., 1976, Surface membrane events following activation by lectins and calcium ionophore, in: *Mitogens in Immunobiology* (J. J. Oppenheim and D. L. Rosenstreich, eds.), pp. 85–101, Academic, New York.

Cuthbert, J. A., and Shay, J. W., 1983, Microtubules and lymphocyte responses: Effects of colchicine and taxol on mitogen-induced human lymphocyte activation and proliferation, *J. Cell. Physiol.* **116**:127–134.

Darzynkiewicz, A., Bolund, L., and Ringertz, N. R., 1969, Nucleoprotein changes and initiation of RNA synthesis in PHA stimulated lymphocytes, *Exp. Cell. Res.* **56**:418–424.

Davis, L., and Lipsky, P. E., 1986, Signals involved in T cell activation, *J. Immunol.* **136**:3588–3596.

Davis, L., Vida, R., and Lipsky, P. E., 1986, Regulation of human T lymphocyte mitogenesis by antibodies to CD3, *J. Immunol.* **137**:3758–3767.

Dawson, A. P., and Irvine, R. F., 1984, Inositol (1,4,5)-triphosphate-promoted Ca^{2+} release from microsomal fractions of rat liver, *Biochem. Biophys. Res. Commun.* **120**:858–864.

DeCoursey, T. E., Chandy, K. G., Gupta, S., and Cahalan, M. D., 1984, Voltage gated K^+ channels in human T lymphocytes: A role in mitogenesis?, *Nature (Lond.)* **307**:465–468.

Degen, J. L., Neubauer, M. G., Degen, S. J. F., Seyfried, C. E., and Morris, D. R., 1983, Regulation of protein synthesis in mitogen-activated bovine lymphocytes. Analysis of active-specific and total mRNA accumulation and utilization, *J. Biol. Chem.* **258**:12153–12162.

DeLaclos, B. F., and Braquet, P., and Borgeat, P., 1984, Characteristics of leukotriene and HETE synthesis in human leukocytes in vitro. Effect of arachidonic acid concentration, *Prostaglandins Leukotrienes Med.* **13**:47–52.

Depper, J. M., Leonard, W. J., Drogula, C. L., Kronke, M., Waldmann, T. A., and Greene, W. C., 1985, *J. Cell. Biochem.* **27**:267–276.

DeRubertis, F. R., and Zenser, T., 1976, Activation of murine lymphocytes by cyclic guanosine 3',5'-monophosphate: Specificity and role in mitogen action, *Biochim. Biophys. Acta* **428**:91–103.

DeRubertis, F. R., Zenser, T. V., Adler, W. H., and Hudson, T., 1974, Role of cyclic adenosine 3',5'-monophosphate in lymphocyte mitogenesis, *J. Immunol.* **113**:151–161.

Deutsch, C., and Price, M. A., 1982, Cell calcium in human peripheral blood lymphocytes and the effect of mitogen, *Biochim. Biophys. Acta* **687**:211–218.

Deutsch, C., Taylor, J. S., and Wilson, D. F., 1982, Regulation of intracellular pH by human peripheral blood lymphocytes as measured by ^{19}F NMR, *Proc. Natl. Acad. Sci. USA* **79**:7944–7948.

Deviller, P., Cille, Y., and Betuel, H., 1975, Guanyl cyclase activity of human blood lymphocytes, *Enzyme* **19**:300–313.

Diamantstein, T., and Odenwald, M. V., 1974, Control of the immune response in vitro by calcium ions, *Immunology* **27**:531–541.

Diamantstein, T., and Ulmer, A., 1975a, The control of immune response in vitro by Ca^{2+}. II. The Ca^{2+}-dependent period during mitogenic stimulation, *Immunology* **28**:121–126.

Diamantstein, T., and Ulmer, A., 1975b, Effect of cyclic nucleotides on DNA synthesis in mouse lymphoid cells, *Immunol. Commun.* **4**:51–62.

Diamantstein, T., and Ulmer, A., 1975c, Regulation of DNA synthesis by guanosine-5'-diphosphate, cyclic guanosine-3',5'-monophosphate, and cyclic adenosine-3',5'-monophosphate in mouse lymphoid cells, *Exp. Cell. Res.* **93**:309–314.

Diamantstein, T., and Ulmer, A., 1975d, Stimulation by cyclic GMP of lymphocytes mediated by soluble factor released from adherent cells, *Nature (Lond.)* **256**:418–419.

Diaz-Espada, F., and Lopez-Alarcon, L., 1982, Mitogen-induced changes in glycolytic enzymes of mouse lymphocytes: Influence of insulin on cell activation in vitro, *Immunology* **46**:705–712.

Dinarello, C. A., Marnoy, S. O., and Rosenwasser, L. J., 1983, Role of arachidonate metabolism in the immunoregulatory function of human leukocyte pyrogen/lymphocyte-activating factor in interleukin 1, *J. Immunol.* **130**:890–895.

Dobson, P., and Mellors, A., 1980, Inhibition of acyltransferase in lymphocytes by concanavalin A, *Biochim. Biophys. Acta* **629**:305–316.

Dornand, J., Mani, J-C., Mousseron-Canet, M., and Pau, B., 1974, Properties of a Ca^{2+} and Mg^{2+} dependent ATPase from plasmic membranes of lymphocytes. Effects of concanavalin A upon membrane ATPases, *Biochimie* **56**:1425–1432.

Dornand, J., Reminiac, C., and Mani, J-C., 1978, Studies of $(Na^+ + K^+)$ sensitive ATPase activity in pig lymphocytes. Effects of concanavalin A, *Biochim. Biophys. Acta* **509**:194–200.

Dornand, J., Bonnafous, J-C., Mani, J-C., 1980, 5'-Nucleotidase-adenylate cyclase relationships in mouse thymocytes, *FEBS Lett.* **110**:30–34.

Duncan, M. R., and Hadden, J. W., 1982, Concanavalin-induced human lymphocyte mitogenic factor: Activity distinct from interleukin 1 and 2, *J. Immunol.* **129**:56–62.

Earp, H. S., Utsinger, P. D., Yount, W. J., Logue, M., and Steiner, A. L., 1977, Lymphocyte surface modulation and cyclic nucleotides, *J. Exp. Med.* **145**:1087–1092.

Edelman, G. M., 1976, Surface modulation in cell recognition and cell growth, *Science* **194**:218–226.

Edelman, G. M., Yahara, I., and Wang, J. L., 1973, Receptor mobility and receptor–cytoplasmic interactions in lymphocytes, *Proc. Natl. Acad. Sci. USA* **70**:1442–1446.

Ellegaard, J., and Dimitrov, N. V., 1973, Ouabain-sensitive and oligomycin-sensitive adenosine triphosphatase activities of normal human lymphocytes, *Br. J. Haematol.* **25**:309–320.

Epstein, P., Mills, J., Ross, C., Strada, S., Hersh, E., and Thompson, W., 1977, Increased cyclic nucleotide phosphodiesterase activity associated with proliferation and cancer in human and murine lymphoid cells, *Cancer Res.* **37**:4016–4023.

Farago, A., Hasznos, P., Antoni, F., and Romhanji, T., 1978, Two types of cyclic GMP binding site associated with the cyclic AMP-dependent protein kinase from lymphocytes, *Biochim. Biophys. Acta* **538**:493–504.

Farese, R. V., 1983, The phosphatidate-phosphoinositide cycle: An intracellular messenger system in the action of hormones and neurotransmitters, *Metabolism* **32**:628–641.

Farrar, W. L., Evans, S. W., Rapp, U. R., and Cleveland, J. J., 1987, Effects of anti-proliferative cyclic AMP on interleukin 2-stimulated gene expression, *J. Immunol.* **139**:2075–2080.

Farrar, W. L., and Anderson, W. B., 1985, Interleukin-2 stimulates association of protein kinase C with plasma membrane, *Nature (Lond.)* **315**:233–235.

Farrar, W. L., and Humes, J. L., 1985, The role of arachidonic acid metabolism in the activities of interleukin 1 and 2, *J. Immunol.* **135**:1153–1159.

Farrar, W. L., and Ruscetti, F. W., 1986, Association of protein kinase C activation of IL-2 receptor expression, *J. Immunol.* **136**:1266–1273.

Farrar, W. L., Cleveland, J. L., Beckner, S. K., Bonvini, E., and Evans, S. W., 1986, Biochemical and molecular events associated with interleukin 2 regulation of lymphocyte proliferation. *Immunol. Rev.* **92**:49–65.

Feister, A. J., and Sage, H. J., 1986, Stimulation of phosphatidylinosital turnover by concanavalin A is not sufficient to activate mouse thymocytes, *Biochem Biophys. Res. Commun.* **141**:657–664.

Felber, S. M., and Brand, M. D., 1983, Early plasma-membrane potential changes during stimulation of lymphocytes by concanavalin A, *Biochem. J.* **210**:885–891.

Ferber, E., and Resch, K., 1973, Phospholipid metabolism of stimulated lymphocytes: Activation of acyl-CoA: Lysolecithin acyl transferases in microsomal membranes, *Biochim. Biophys. Acta* **296**:335–349.

Ferber, R., Reilly, C. E., DePasquale, G., and Resch, K., 1974, Lymphocyte stimulation by mitogens: Increase in membrane fluidity caused by changes of fatty acid moieties of phospholipids, in: *Lymphocyte Recognition and Effector Mechanisms* (K. Lindahl-Kiessling and D. Osoba, eds.), pp. 529–534, Academic, New York.

Ferber, E., DePasquale, G. G., and Resch, K., 1975, Phospholipid metabolism of stimulated lymphocytes: Composition of phospholipid fatty acids, *Biochim. Biophys. Acta* **398**:364–376.

Ferber, E., Reilly, C. E., and Resch, K., 1976, Phospholipid metabolism of stimulated lymphocytes. Comparison of the activation of acyl-CoA: Lysolecithin acyltransferase with the binding of concanavalin A to thymocytes, *Biochim. Biophys. Acta* **448**:143–154.

Ferguson, R. M., Schmidtke, J. R., and Simmons, R. L., 1975, Concurrent inhibition by chlorpromazine of concanavalin A-induced lymphocyte aggregation and mitogenesis, *Nature (Lond.)* **256**:744–745.

Ferguson, R., Schmidtke, J. R., and Simmons, R. L., 1976, Inhibition of mitogen-induced lymphocyte transformation by local anesthetics, *J. Immunol.* **116**:627–634.

Fillingame, R. H., and Morris, D. R., 1973, Accumulation of polyamines and its inhibition by methyl glyoxol bis-(guanylhydrazone) during lymphocyte transformation, In: *Polyamines in Normal and Neoplastic Growth* (D. H. Russell, ed.), pp. 249–260, Raven, New York.

Fillingame, R. H., Jorstad, C. M., and Morris, D. R., 1975, Increased cellular levels of spermidine or spermine are required for optimal DNA synthesis in lymphocytes activated by concanavalin A, *Proc. Natl. Acad. Sci. USA* **72**:4042–4045.

Fisher, D. B., and Mueller, G. C., 1968, An early alteration in the phospholipid metabolism of lymphocytes by PHA, *Proc. Nat. Acad. Sci. USA* **60**:1396–1402.

Fisher, D. B., and Mueller, G. C., 1969, The stepwise acceleration of phosphatidylcholine synthesis in PHA-treated lymphocytes, *Biochim. Biophys. Acta* **176**:316–323.

Fisher, D. B., and Mueller, G. C., 1971a, Gamma-hexachlorocyclohexane inhibits the initiation of lymphocyte growth by phytohaemagglutinin, *Biochem. Pharmacol.* **20**:2515–2518.

Fisher, D. B., and Mueller, G. C., 1971b, Studies on the mechanism by which phytohemagglutinin rapidly stimulates phospholipid metabolism of human lymphocytes, *Biochim. Biophys. Acta* **248**:434–448.

Fleisher, T. A., and Birx, D. L., 1985, The role of calcium in IL-2 dependent proliferation, *Fed. Proc.* **44**:1309 (abst.).

Folch, H., and Waksman, B., 1974, Regulation of lymphocyte responses in vitro. V. Suppression activity of adherent and non-adherent rat lymphoid cells, *Cell. Immunol.* **9**:12–24.

Forsdyke, D. R., 1968, Studies of the incorporation of [5-³H]uridine during activation and transformation of lymphocytes induced by phytohemagglutinin, *Biochem. J.* **107**:197–205.

Fraser, A. R., Hemperly, J. J., Wang, J. L., and Edelman, G. M., 1976, Monovalent derivatives of concanavalin A, *Proc. Natl. Acad. Sci. USA* **73**:790–794.

Freedman, M. H., 1979, Early biochemical events in lymphocyte activation, *Cell Immunol.* **44:**290–313.

Freedman, M. H., Raff, M. C., and Gomperts, B., 1975, Induction of increased calcium uptake in mouse T-lymphocytes by concanavalin-A and its modulation by cyclic nucleotides, *Nature (Lond.)* **255:**378–382.

Freedman, M. H., Khan, N. R., Frew-Marshall, B. J., Cupples, C. G., and Mely-Goubert, B., 1981, Early biochemical events in lymphocyte activation, *Cell. Immunol.* **58:**134–146.

Friedman, H., and Kateley, J. R., 1974, Enhanced splenic ATPase activity in immunized mice, *Proc. Soc. Exp. Biol. Med.* **147:**460–463.

Galbraith, R. M., Nel, A. E., Dirienzo, W., Canonica, W., and Goldschmidt-Clermont, P. J., 1985, T_3-mediated activation of human T cells involves translocation of Ca^{2+}/phospholipid-dependent C-kinase, *Fed. Proc.* **44:**1132.

Gaulton, G. N., and Eardley, D. D., 1986, Interleukin 2-dependent phosphorylation of interleukin-2 receptors and other T cell membrane proteins, *J. Immunol.* **136:**2470–2477.

Gelfand, E. W., Cheung, R. K., and Grinstein, S., 1984, Role of membrane potential in the regulation of lectin-induced calcium uptake, *J. Cell. Physiol.* **121:**533–539.

Gelfand, E. W., Cheung, R. K., Mills, G. B., and Grinstein, S., 1985, Mitogens trigger a calcium-independent signal for proliferation in phorbol ester-treated lymphocytes, *Nature (Lond.)* **315:**419–424.

Gelfand, E. W., Cheung, R. K., and Grinstein, S., 1986a, Mitogen-induced changes in Ca^{2+} permeability are not mediated by voltage-gated K^+ channels, *J. Biol. Chem.* **261:**11520–11525.

Gelfand, E. W., Cheung, R. K., Grinstein, S., and Mills, G. B., 1986b, Characterization of the role for calcium influx in mitogen-induced triggering of human T cells. Identification of calcium-dependent and calcium-independent signals. *Eur. J. Immunol.* **16:**907–912.

Gerson, D. F., and Kiefer, H., 1982, High intracellular pH accompanies mitotic activity in murine lymphocytes, in *J. Cell. Physiol.* **112:**1–4.

Gerson, D. F., Kiefer, H., and Eufe, W., 1982, Intracellular pH of mitogen-stimulated lymphocytes, *Science* **216:**1009–1010.

Gery, I., and Eidinger, D., 1977, Selective opposing effects of cytochalisn B and other drugs on lymphocyte responses to different doses of mitogens, *Cell. Immunol.* **30:**147–155.

Gilmore, W., and Weiner, L. P., 1985, The role of cyclic nucleotides and guanine nucleotide binding proteins in interleukin-2 production. *Fed. Proc.* **44:**505.

Goetzl, E. J., 1981, Selective feed-back inhibition of the 5-lipoxygenation of arachidonic acid in human T-lymphocytes, *Biochem. Biophys. Res. Commun.* **101:**344–350.

Goldberg, N. D., Haddox, M. K., Dunham, E., Lopez, C., and Hadden, J. W., 1974, The Yin Yang hypothesis of biological control: Opposing influences of cyclic GMP and cyclic AMP in the regulation of cell proliferation and other biological processes, in: *Control of Proliferation in Animal Cells* (B. Clarkson and R. Baserga, eds.), *Cold Spring Harbor Conf. Cell Prolif.* **1:**609–626.

Goldberg, N. D., Graff, G., Haddox, M. K., Stephenson, J. H., Glass, D. B., and Moser, M. E., 1978, Redox modulation of splenic cell soluble guanylate cyclase activity: Activation by hydrophilic and hydrophobic oxidants represented by ascorbic and dehydroascorbic acids, fatty acid hydroperoxides and prostaglandin endoperoxides, *Adv. Cyclic Nucleotide Res.* **9:**101–130.

Goldyne, M. E., 1984, The generation of 5-lipoxygenase-derived arachidonic acid metabolites among human lymphocytes and monocytes, *Prostaglandins and Leukotrienes '84—Fourth Int. Washington Spring Symposium.*

Goldyne, M. E., and Stobo, J. D., 1982, Human monocytes synthesize eicosanoids from T lymphocyte-derived arachidonic acid, *Prostaglandins* **24:**623–630.

Goodman, M. G., and Weigle, W. O., 1983, T cell-replacing activity of C8-derivatized guanine ribonucleosides, *J. Immunol.* **130:**2042–2044.

Goodman, M. G., Brunton, L. L., and Weigle, W. O., 1981, Modulation of lymphocyte activation, *Cell. Immunol.* **58**:85–96.

Goodwin, J. S., 1986, Regulation of T cell activation of leukotriene B4, *Immunol. Res.* **5**:233–248.

Goodwin, J. S., Baukhurst, A. D., and Messner, R. P., 1977, Suppression of human T-cell mitogenesis by prostaglandin. Existence of a prostaglandin-producing suppressor cell, *J. Exp. Med.* **146**:1719–1734.

Gordon, D., Nouri, A. M. E., and Thomas, R. U., 1981, Selective inhibition of thromboxane biosynthesis in human blood mononuclear cells and the effects on mitogen-stimulated lymphocyte proliferation, *Eur. J. Pharmacol.* **74**:469–476.

Graff, G., Stephenson, J. H., Glass, D. B., Haddox, M. K., and Goldberg, N. D., 1978, Activation of soluble splenic cell guanylate cyclase by prostaglandin endoperoxides and fatty acid hydroperoxides, *J. Biol. Chem.* **253**:7662–7676.

Greaves, M. F., and Bauminger, S., 1972, Activation of T and B lymphocytes by insoluble phytomitogens, *Nature New Biol.* **235**:67–70.

Greene, W., and Parker, C. W., 1975, A role for cytochalasin-sensitive proteins in the regulation of calcium transport in activated human lymphocytes, *Biochem. Biophys. Res. Commun.* **65**:456–463.

Greene, W. C., Parker, C. M., and Parker, C. W., 1976a, Calcium and lymphocyte activation, *Cell. Immunol.* **25**:74–89.

Greene, W. C., Parker, C. M., and Parker, C. W., 1976b, Opposing effects of mitogenic and nonmitogenic lectins on lymphocyte activation, *J. Biol Chem.* **251**:4017–4025.

Greene, W. C., Parker, C. M., and Parker, C. W., 1976c, Cytochalasin sensitive structures and lymphocyte activation, *Exp. Cell. Res.* **103**:109–118.

Greene, W. C., Parker, C. M., and Parker, C. W., 1976d, Colchicine-sensitive structures and lymphocyte activation, *J. Immunol.* **117**:1015–1022.

Grinstein, S., Cohen, S., Lederman, H. M., and Gelfand, E. W., 1984, The intracellular pH of quiescent and proliferating human and rat thymic lymphocytes, *J. Cell. Physiol.* **121**:87–95.

Gualde, N., Rabinovitch, H., Fredon, M., and Rigaud, M., 1982, Effects of 15-hydroperoxyeicosatetraenoic acid on human lymphocyte sheep erythrocyte rosette formation and response to concanavalin A associated with HLA system, *Eur. J. Immunol.* **12**:773–777.

Gualde, N., Chabel-Rabinovitch, H., Motta, C., Durand, J., Beneytout, J. L., and Rigaud, M., 1983, Hydroperoxyeicosatetraenoic acids: Potent inhibitors of lymphocyte responses, *Biochim. Biophys. Acta* **750**:429–433.

Gualde, N., Atluru, D., and Goodwin, J., 1985a, Effect of lipoxygenase metabolites of arachidonic acid on proliferation of human T cells and T cell subsets, *J. Immunol.* **134**:1125–1128.

Gualde, N., Rigaud, M., and Goodwin, J. S., 1985b, Induction of suppressor cells from peripheral blood T cells by 15-hydroperoxyeicosatetraenoic acid (15-HPETE), *J. Immunol.* **135**:3424–3429.

Gunther, G. R., Wang, J. L., Yahara, I., Cunningham, B., and Edelman, G. M., 1973, Concanavalin A derivatives with altered biological activities, *Proc. Natl. Acad. Sci. USA* **70**:1012–1016.

Gunther, G. R., Wang, J. L., and Edelman, G. M., 1976, Kinetics of colchicine inhibition of mitogenesis in individual lymphocytes, *Exp. Cell. Res.* **98**:15–22.

Gupta, S., 1979, Subpopulations of human T lymphocytes. XII. In vitro effects of agents modifying intracellular levels of cyclic nucleotides on T cells with receptors for IgM (Tu), IgG (Ty), or IgA (Ta), *J. Immunol.* **123**:2664–2668.

Gutowski, J. K., Mukherji, B., and Cohen, S., 1984, The role of cytoplasmic intermediates in IL-2-induced T cell growth, *J. Immunol.* **133**:3068–3074.

Hadden, J. W., 1977, Cyclic nucleotides in lymphocyte proliferation and differentiation, in: *Immunopharmacology* (J. W. Hadden, R. G. Coffey, and F. Spreafico, eds.), pp. 1–28, Plenum, New York.

Hadden, J. W., and Coffey, R. C., 1982, Cyclic nucleotides in mitogen induced lymphocyte proliferation, *Immunology Today* **3**:299–304.

Hadden, J. W., Hadden, E. M., and Middleton, E., Jr., 1970, Lymphocyte blast transformation. I. Demonstration of adrenergic receptors in human peripheral lymphocytes, *J. Cell. Immunol.* **1:** 583–595.

Hadden, J. W., Hadden, E. M., and Good, R. A., 1971a, Adrenergic mechanisms in human lymphocyte metabolism, *Biochim. Biophys. Acta* **237:**339–347.

Hadden, J. W., Hadden, E. M., and Good, R. A., 1971b, Alpha adrenergic stimulation of glucose uptake in the human erythrocyte, lymphocyte, and lymphoblast, *Exp. Cell. Res.* **68:**217–219.

Hadden, J. W., Hadden, E. M., and Good, R. A., 1971c, Lymphocyte blast transformation. II. The mechanism of action of alpha-adrenergic receptor effects, *Int. Arch. Allergy Appl. Immunol.* **40:** 526–539.

Hadden, J. W., Hadden, E. M., Haddox, M. K., and Goldberg, N. D., 1972, Guanosine 3′,5′-cyclic monophosphate: A possible intracellular mediator of mitogen influences in lymphocytes, *Proc. Natl. Acad. Sci. USA* **69:**3024–3027.

Hadden, J. W., Johnson, E. M., Hadden, E. M., Coffey, R. G., and Johnson, L. D., 1975, Cyclic GMP and lymphocyte activation, in: *Immune Recognition* (A. Rosenthal, ed.), pp. 359–389, Academic, New York.

Hadden, J. W., Hadden, E. M., Sadlik, J. R., and Coffey, R. G., 1976, Effects of concanavalin A and a succinylated derivative on lymphocyte proliferation and cyclic nucleotide levels, *Proc. Natl. Acad. Sci. USA* **73:**1717–1721.

Hadden, J. W., Coffey, R. G., Ananthakrishnan, R., and Hadden, E. M., 1979, Part V. Role of intracellular factors in immunity: Cyclic nucleotides and calcium in lymphocyte regulation and activation, *Ann. NY Acad. Sci.* **332:**241–254.

Hadden, J. W., Hadden, E. M., and Coffey, R. G., 1987, IL-2 increases cyclic GMP levels in immature thymocytes and mitogen primed lymphocytes, *Int. J. Immunopharmacol.* **10:**851– 858.

Haddox, M. K., Furcht, L. T., Gentry, S. R., Moser, M. E., Stephenson, J. H., and Goldberg, N. D., 1976, Periodate-induced increase in cyclic GMP in mouse and guinea pig splenic cells in association with mitogenesis, *Nature (Lond.)* **262:**146–148.

Hait, W., and Weiss, B., 1975, Increased cyclic nucleotide phosphodiesterase activity in leukemic lymphocytes, *Nature (Lond.)* **259:**321–323.

Hait, W., and Weiss, B., 1977, Characteristics of the cyclic nucleotide phosphodiesterases of normal and leukemic lymphocytes, *Biochim. Biophys. Acta* **497:**86–100.

Hall, D. J., O'Leary, J. J., and Rosenberg, A., 1982, Commitment and proliferation kinetics of human lymphocytes stimulated in vitro: Effects of colchicine on mitogen response, *J. Cell. Physiol.* **112:**157–161.

Hamilton, T. A., 1982, Regulation of transferrin receptor expression in concanavalin A stimulated and gross virus transformed rat lymphoblasts, *J. Cell. Physiol.* **113:**40–46.

Hamilton, T. A., 1983, Receptor-mediated endocytosis and exocytosis of transferrin in concanavalin A-stimulated rat lymphocytes, *J. Cell. Physiol.* **114:**222–228.

Hamilton, L. J., and Kaplan, J. G., 1977, Flux of ^{86}Rb in activated human lymphocytes, *Can. J. Biochem.* **55:**774–778.

Hasegawa-Sasaki, H., and Sasaki, T., 1981, Phytomitogen-induced stimulation of synthesis do novo of PtdIns, phosphatidic acid and diacylglycerol in rat and human lymphocytes, *Biochim. Biophys. Acta* **666:**252–258.

Hasegawa-Sasaki, H., and Sasaki, T., 1982, Rapid breakdown of PtdIns accompanied by accumulation of phosphatidic acid and diacylglycerol in rat lymphocytes, *J. Biochem.* **91:**463–468.

Hasegawa-Sasaki, H., and Sasaki, T., 1983, Phytohemagglutinin induces rapid degradation of phosphatidyl-inositol-4,5-bis-phosphate and transient accumulation of phosphatidic acid and diacylglycerol in a human T-lymphoblastoid cell line, CCRF-CEM, *Biochim. Biophys. Acta* **754:**305–314.

Hashizume, H., Yoneda, M., and Kanemoto, K., 1983, Phosphorylation of specific polypeptides in isolated murine splenocyte nuclei which is controlled by cyclic nucleotides, *J. Biochem.* **94:** 961–966.

Hausen, P., and Stein, H., 1968, On the synthesis of RNA in lymphocytes stimulated by phytohemagglutinin, *Eur. J. Biochem.* **4:**401–406.

Hausen, P., Stein, H., and Peters, H., 1969, On the synthesis of RNA in lymphocytes stimulated by phytohemagglutinin, *Eur. J. Biochem.* **9:**542–549.

Hauser, H., Knippers, R., and Schafer, K. P., 1978, Increased rate of RNA-polyadenylation, *Exp. Cell. Res.* **111:**175–184.

Hesketh, R., 1978, Cation fluxes and lymphocyte transformation, in: *The Molecular Basis of Immune Cell Function*, (J. Gordin Kaplin, ed.), pp. 39–56, Elsevier/North-Holland Biomedical Press, Amsterdam.

Hesketh, T. R., Smith, G. A., Housley, M. D., Warren, G. B., and Metcalf, J. C., 1977, Is an early calcium flux necessary to stimulate lymphocytes?, *Nature (Lond.)* **267:**490–494.

Hesketh, T. R., Smith, G. A., Moore, J. P., Taylor, M. V., and Metcalfe, J. C., 1983a, Limits to the early increase in free cytoplasmic calcium concentrations during the mitogenic stimulation of lymphocytes, *Biochem. J.* **212:**685–690.

Hesketh, T. R., Smith, G. A., Moore, J. P., Taylor, M. V., and Melcalfe, J. C., 1983b, Free cytoplasmic calcium concentration and the mitogenic stimulation of lymphocytes, *J. Biol. Chem.* **258:**4876–4882.

Hesketh, T. R., Moore, J. P., Morris, J. D. H., Taylor, M. V., Rogers, J., Smith, G. A., and Metcalfe, T. C., 1985, A common sequence of calcium and pH signals in the mitogenic stimulation of eukaryotic cells, *Nature (Lond.)* **313:**481–484.

Hirata, F., and Axelrod, J., 1980, Phospholipid methylation and biological signal transmission, *Science* **209:**1082–1090.

Hirata, F., Toyoshima, S., Axelrod, J., and Waxdal, M. J., 1980, Phospholipid methylation: A biochemical signal modulating lymphocyte mitogenesis, *Proc. Natl. Acad. Sci. USA* **77:**862–865.

Hirschhorn, R., Troll, W., Brittinger, G., Weissman, G., 1969, Template activity of nuclei from stimulated lymphocytes, *Nature (Lond.)* **222:**1247–1250.

Hoffman, R., Ferguson, R., and Simmons, R. L., 1977, Effect of cytochalasin B on human lymphocyte responses to mitogens. Time and concentration dependence, *J. Immunol.* **118:**1472–1479.

Hoffman, T., Hirata, F., Bougnoux, P., Fraser, B. A., Goldfarb, R. H., Haberman, R. B., and Axelrod, J., 1981, Phospholipid methylation and phospholipase A_2 activation in cytotoxicity by human natural killer cells, *Proc. Natl. Acad. Sci. USA* **78:**3839–3843.

Holta, E., Korpela, H., and Hovi, T., 1981, Several inhibitors of ornithine and adenosylmethionine decarboxylases may also have antiproliferative effects unrelated to polyamine depletion, *Biochim. Biophys. Acta* **677:**90–102.

Hokin, M. R., and Hokin, L. E., 1953, Enzyme secretion and the incorporation of P^{32} into phospholipids of pancreas slices, *J. Biol. Chem.* **203:**967–977.

Homa, S. T., Conroy, D. M., and Smith, A. D., 1984, Unsaturated fatty acids stimulate the formation of lipoxygenase and cyclooxygenase products in rat spleen lymphocytes, *Prostaglandins Leukotrienes Med.* **14:**417–427.

Hovi, T., Allison, A. C., and Williams, S. C., 1976, Proliferation of human peripheral blood lymphocytes induced by A23187, a streptomyces antibiotic, *Exp. Cell. Res.* **97:**92–100.

Howard, E. F., 1972, Low molecular weight nuclear RNA in human lymphocytes, *Exp. Cell. Res.* **82:**280–286.

Huet, S., Wakasugi, H., Sterkers, G., Gilmour, J., Fursz, F., Boumsell, L., and Bernard, A., 1986, T cell activation via CD 2 [T, gp50]: The role of accessory cells in activating resting T cells via CD 2. *J. Immunol.* **137:**1420–1428.

Hui, D. Y., and Harmony, J. A. K., 1980a, Inhibition of Ca^{2+} accumulation in mitogen-activated lymphocytes: Role of membrane-bound plasma lipoproteins, *Proc. Nat. Acad. Sci. USA* **77:**4764–4768.

Hui, D. Y., and Harmony, J. A. K., 1980b, Inhibition by low density lipoproteins of mitogen-stimulated cyclic nucleotide production by lymphocytes, *J. Biol. Chem.* **255**:1413–1419.

Hui, D. Y., and Harmony, J. A. K., 1980c, Phosphatidylinositol turnover in mitogen-activated lymphocytes, *Biochem. J.* **192**:91–98.

Hui, D. Y., Berebisky, G. L., and Harmony, J. A. K., 1979, Mitogen-stimulated calcium ion accumulation by lymphocytes, *J. Biol. Chem.* **254**:4666–4673.

Hume, D. A., and Wiedemann, M. J., 1980, Intracellular second messengers in Mitogenic Lymphocyte Transformation, *Res. Monog. Immunol.* **2**:183–225.

Hume, D. A., Hansen, K., Weidemann, M. J., and Ferber, E., 1978a, Cytochalasin B inhibits lymphocyte transformation through its effects on glucose transport, *Nature (Lond.)* **272**:359–362.

Hume, D. A., Vijayakumar, E. K., Schweinberger, F., Russell, L. M., Weidemann, M. J., 1978b, The role of ions in the regulation of rat thymocyte pyruvate oxidation by mitogens, *Biochem. J.* **174**:711–716.

Hume, D. A., Weidemann, M. J., and Ferber, E., 1979, Preferential inhibition by quercetin of mitogen-stimulated thymocyte glucose transport, *J. Natl. Cancer Inst.* **62**:1243–1246.

Humphries, G. M. K., and Lovejoy, J. P., 1983, Cholesterol-free phospholipid domains may be the membrane feature selected by *N*-dansyl-1-lysine and merocyanine 540, *Biochem. Biophys. Res. Commun.* **111**:768–774.

Hungerford, D. A., Donnelly, A. J., Nowell, P. C., and Beck, S., 1959, The chromosome constitution of a human phenotype intersex, *Am. J. Hum. Genet.* **11**:215–236.

Imboden, J. B., and Stobo, J. D., 1985, Transmembrane signalling by the T cell antigen receptor, *J. Exp. Med.* **161**:446–456.

Imboden, J., Weiss, A., and Stobo, J., 1985, The antigen receptor on a human T cell line initiates activation by increasing cytoplasmic free calcium, *J. Immunol.* **134**:663–665.

Inbar, M., and Shinitzky, M., 1974a, Increase of cholesterol level in the surface membrane of lymphoma cells and its inhibitory effect on ascites tumor development, *Proc. Natl. Acad. Sci. USA* **71**:2128–2130.

Inbar, M., and Shinitzky, M., 1974b, Cholesterol as bioregulator in the developmental inhibition of leukemia, *Proc. Natl. Acad. Sci. USA* **71**:4229–4231.

Inbar, M., and Shinitzky, M., 1975, Decrease in microviscosity in lymphocyte surface membrane associated with stimulation induced by concanavalin A, *Eur. J. Immunol.* **5**:166–170.

Isakov, N., Bleackley, R. C., Shaw, J., and Altman, A., 1985, The tumor promoter teleocidin induces IL-2 receptor expression and IL-2-independent proliferation of human peripheral blood T cells, *J. Immunol.* **135**:2343–2350.

Ishizaka, T., Hirata, F., Ishizaka, K., and Axelrod, J., 1980, Stimulation of phospholipid methylation, Ca^{2+} influx, and histamine release by bridging of IgE receptors on rat mast cells, *Proc. Natl. Acad. Sci. USA* **77**:1903–1906.

Jagus, R., and Kay, J., 1979, Distribution of lymphocyte messenger RNA during stimulation by phytohaemagglutinin, *Eur. J. Biochem.* **100**:503–510.

Jazwinski, S. M., Wang, J. L., and Edelman, G. M., 1976, Initiation of replication in chromosomal DNA induced by extracts from proliferating cells, *Proc. Natl. Acad. Sci. USA* **73**:2231–2235.

Jensen, P., and Rasmussen, H., 1977, The effect of A23187 upon calcium metabolism in the human lymphocyte, *Biochim. Biophys. Acta* **468**:146–156.

Jegasothy, B. V., Pachner, A. R., Waksman, B. H., 1976, Cytokine inhibition of DNA synthesis: Effect on cyclic adenosine monophosphate in lymphocytes, *Science* **193**:1260–1262.

Jegasothy, B. V., Namba, Y., and Waksman, B. H., 1978, Regulatory substances produced by lymphocytes. VII. IDS (inhibitor of DNA synthesis) inhibits stimulated lymphocyte proliferation by activation of membrane adenylate cyclase at a restriction point in late G, *Immunochemistry* **15**:551–555.

Johnson, E. M., 1977, Cyclic AMP-dependent protein kinase and its nuclear substrate proteins, in:

Advances in Cyclic Nucleotides Research, Vol. 8 (P. Greengard, and G. A. Robison, eds.), pp. 267–309, Raven, New York.

Johnson, E. M., and Hadden, J. W., 1975, Phosphorylation of lymphocyte nuclear acidic proteins: Regulation by cyclic nucleotides, *Science* **1807:**1198–1200.

Johnson, E. M., Karn, J., and Allfrey, V. G., 1974, Early nuclear events in the induction of lymphocyte proliferation by mitogens, *J. Biol. Chem.* **249:**4990–4999.

Johnson, E. M., Hadden, J. W., Inoue, A., Allfrey, V. G., 1975a, DNA binding by cyclic adenosine 3′,5′-monophosphate dependent protein kinase from calf thymus nuclei, *Biochemistry,* **14:** 3873–3884.

Johnson, E. M., Inoue, A., Crouse, L. J., Allfrey, V. G., and Hadden, J. W., 1975b, Effects of cyclic GMP upon DNA binding by a calf thymus nuclear protein fraction, *Biochem. Biophys. Res. Commun.* **65:**714–721.

Johnson, H. M., Archer, D. L., and Torres, B. A., 1982, Cyclic GMP as the second messenger on helper cell requirement for gamma-interferon production, *J. Immunol.* **129:**2570–2572.

Johnson, H. M., Vallaso, T., and Torres, B. A., 1985, Interleukin 2-mediated events in γ-interferon production are calcium dependent at more than one site, *J. Immunol.* **134:**967–970.

Johnson, L. D., and Hadden, J. W., 1975, Cyclic GMP and lymphocyte proliferation: Effects on DNA-dependent RNA polymerase I and II activities, *Biochem. Biophys. Res. Commun.* **66:** 1498–1505.

Johnson, L. D., and Hadden, J. W., 1977, Modification of human DNA-dependent RNA polymerase activity by cyclic GMP, *Nucleic Acids Res.* **4:**4007–4014.

Joseph, S. K., Thomas, A. P., Williams, R. J., Irvine, R. F., and Williamson, J. R., 1984, Myo-inositol 1,4,5-triphosphate, a second messenger for the hormonal mobilization of intracellular Ca^{2+} in liver, *J. Biol. Chem.* **259:**3077–3081.

June, C. H., Ledbetter, J. A., Rabinovitch, P. S., Beatty, P. G., Martin, P. J., and Hansen, J. H., 1986, in: *Sixth International Congress of Immunology, Toronto, Canada,* p. 232 (abst.).

Kaibuchi, K., Takai, Y., Ogawa, Y., Kimura, S., Nishizuka, Y., Nakamura, T., Tonomura, A., and Ichihara, A., 1982, Inhibitory action of adenosine 3′,5′-monophosphate on phosphatidylinositol turnover, *Biochem. Biophys. Res. Commun.* **104:**105–112.

Kaibuchi, K., Takai, Y., and Nishizuka, Y., 1985, Protein kinase C and calcium ion in mitogenic response of macrophage-depleted human peripheral lymphocytes, *J. Biol. Chem.* **260:**1366– 1369.

Kaiser, N., and Edelman, I. S., 1978, Calcium dependence of ionophore A23187-induced lymphocyte cytotoxicity, *Cancer Res.* **38:**3599–3603.

Kaplan, J. G., and Owens, T., 1980, Activation of lymphocytes of man and mouse: Monovalent cation fluxes, *Ann. NY Acad. Sci.* **339:**191–200.

Kaplan, J. G., and Owens, T., 1982, The cation pump as a switch mechanism controlling proliferation and differentiation in lymphocytes, *Biosci. Rep.* **2:**577–581.

Katagiri, T., Terao, T., and Osawa, T., 1976, Activation of mouse splenic lymphocyte guanylate cyclase by calcium ion, *J. Biochem.* **79:**849–852.

Kato, K., Koshihara, Y., and Murota, S., 1986, Contribution of lipoxygenase metabolites to IL-2 production in the early phase of lymphocyte activation, *Prosta, Leuk. Med.* **22:**301–311.

Katz, S. P., Kierszenbaum, F., and Waksman, B. H., 1978, Mechanisms of action of ''lymphocyte-activating factor'' (LAF), *J. Immunol.* **121:**2386–2391.

Kay, J. E., 1968, Early effects of phytohemagglutinin on lymphocyte RNA synthesis, *Eur. J. Biochem.* **4:**225–232.

Kay, J. E., 1971, Interaction of lymphocytes and phytohaemagglutinin: Inhibition by chelating agents, *Exp. Cell. Res.* **68:**11–16.

Kay, J. E., 1972, Lymphocyte stimulation by phytohaemagglutinin: Role of the early stimulation of potassium uptake, *Exp. Cell. Res.* **71:**245–247.

Kay, J. E., and Cooke, A., 1971, Ornithine decarboxylase and ribosomal RNA synthesis during the stimulation of lymphocytes by phytohaemagglutinin, *FEBS. Lett.* **16:**9–12.

Kay, J. E., and Handmaker, S. D., 1970, Uridine incorporation and RNA in normal and phytohaemagglutinin-stimulated human lymphocytes, *Biochim. Biophys. Acta* **186**:62–84.

Kay, J. E., Leventhal, B. G., and Cooper, H. L., 1969, Effects of inhibition of ribosomal RNA synthesis on the stimulation of lymphocytes by phytohaemagglutinin, *Exp. Cell. Res.* **54**:94–100.

Kecskemethy, N., and Schafer, K. P., 1982, Lectin induced changes among polyadenylated and non-polyadenylated mRNA in lymphocytes, *Eur. J. Biochem.* **126**:573–582.

Kelly, J. P., and Parker, C. W., 1979, Effects of arachidonic acid and other unsaturated fatty acids on mitogenesis in human lymphocytes, *J. Immunol.* **122**:1556–1562.

Kelly, J. P., Johnson, M. C., and Parker, C. W., 1979, Effect of inhibitors of arachidonic acid metabolism on mitogenesis in human lymphocytes: Possible role of thromboxanes and products of the lipoxygenase pathway, *J. Immunol.* **122**:1563–1571.

Kemp, R. G., Hsu, P-Y., and Duquesnoy, R. J., 1975, Changes in lymphoid cyclic adenosine 3':5'-monophosphate metabolism during murine leukemogenesis, *Cancer Res.* **35**:2440–2445.

Kennes, B., Hubert, C. L., Brohee, D., and Neve, P., 1981, Early biochemical events associated with lymphocyte activation in aging, *Immunology* **42**:119–126.

Kiefer, M., Blume, A. J., and Kaback, H. R., 1980, Membrane potential changes during mitogenic stimulation of mouse spleen lymphocytes, *Proc. Natl. Acad. Sci. USA* **77**:2200–2204.

Kimoto, H., Nakao, Y., Kobayashi, N., Baba, Y., Sobue, K., Kabuichi, S., and Fujita, T., 1983, Heterogeneous pathways of Ca^{2+} metabolism in the triggering of the proliferative process in rat thymocytes, *Biochim. Biophys. Acta* **762**:25–30.

Kleinsmith, L., Allfrey, V., and Mirsky, A., 1966, Phosphorylation of nuclear protein early in the course of gene activation in lymphocytes, *Science* **154**:780–781.

Klimpel, G. R., Byers, C. V., Russell, D. H., and Lucas, D. O., 1979, Cyclic AMP-dependent protein kinase activation and the induction of ornithine decarboxylase during lymphocyte mitogenesis, *J. Immunol.* **123**:817–824.

Knutson, J. C., and Morris, D. R., 1978, Cellular polyamine depletion reduces DNA synthesis in isolated lymphocyte nuclei, *Biochim. Biophys. Acta* **520**:291–301.

Koizumi, K., Kano-Tanaka, K., Shimizu, S., Nishida, K., Yamanaka, N., and Ota, K., 1980, Lipids of plasma membranes from rat thymic lymphoid cell: Deficiency of sphingomyelin, *Biochim. Biophys. Acta* **619**:344–352.

Krall, J. F., Connelly, M., Tuck, M. L., 1981, Evidence for reversibility of age-related decrease in human lymphocyte adenylate cyclase activity, *Biochem. Biophys. Res. Commun.* **99**:1028–1034.

Krall, J. F., Connelly-Fittingoff, M., and Tuck, M. L., 1983, Lymphocyte adenylate cyclase and human aging, *Proc. Soc. Exp. Biol. Med.* **173**:475–480.

Kranias, E. G., Schweppe, J. S., and Jungmann, R. A., 1977, Phosphorylative and functional modifications of nucleoplasmic RNA polymerase II by homologous adenosine 3':5'-monophosphate-dependent protein kinase from calf thymus and by heterologous phosphate, *J. Biol. Chem.* **252**:6750–6758.

Krishnaraj, R., and Talwar, G. P., 1973, Role of cyclic AMP in mitogen induced transformation of human peripheral leukocytes, *J. Immunol.* **111**:1010–1017.

Kroczek, R. A., Gunter, K. C., Seligmann, B., and Shevach, E. M., 1986, Induction of T cell activation by monoclonal anti-thy-1 antibodies, *J. Immunol.* **136**:4379–4384.

Kronke, M., Leonard, W. J., Depper, J. M., and Greene, W. C., 1985, Sequential expression of genes involved in human T lymphocyte growth and differentiation, *J. Exp. Med.* **161**:1593–1598.

Ku, Y., Kishimoto, A., Takai, Y., Ogawa, Y., Kimura, S., and Nishizuka, Y., 1981, A new possible regulatory system for protein phosphorylation in human peripheral lymphocytes. II. Possible relation to phosphatidylinositol turnover induced by mitogens, *J. Immunol.* **127**:1375–1379.

Kuo, J. F., Schatzman, R. C., Turner, R. S., and Mazzei, G. J., 1984, Phospholipid sensitive Ca^{2+}-dependent protein kinase: A major protein phosphorylation system, *Mol. Cell. Endocrinol.* **35**:65–73.

Kyger, E. M., and Franson, R. C., 1984, Nonspecific inhibition of enzymes by p-bromophenacylbromide. Inhibition of human platelet phospholipase C and modification of sulfhydryl groups, *Biochim. Biophys. Acta* **794:**96–103.

Landry, Y., Vincent-Viry, M., and Jodin, C., 1978, Energy requirement for calcium uptake by thymus lymphocytes, *FEBS Lett.* **88:**305–308.

Lands, W., 1984, Biological consequences of fatty acid oxygenase reaction mechanisms, *Prostaglandins Leukotrienes Med.* **13:**35–46.

Lapetina, E. G., 1982, Regulation of arachidonic acid production: Role of phospholipase C and A_2, *Trends Pharmacol. Sci.* **3:**115–118.

Largen, M. T., and Votta, B., 1983, Immunocytochemical evidence for 3′,5′-cGMP and 3′,5′-cGMP-dependent protein kinase involvement in lymphocyte proliferation, *J. Cyclic Nucleotide Prot. Phosphor. Res.* **9:**231–244.

Larrick, J. W., and Creswell, P., 1979, Modulation of cell surface iron transferrin receptors by cellular density and state of activation, *J. Supramol. Struct.* **11:**579–586.

Ledbetter, J. A., June, C. H., Martin, P. J., Spooner, C. E., Hansen, J. A., and Meier, K. E., 1986a, Valency of CD3 binding and internalization of the CD_3 cell-surface complex control T cell responses to second signals: Distinction between effects on protein kinase C, cytoplasmic free calcium, and proliferation, *J. Immunol.* **136:**3945–3952.

Ledbetter, J. A., Parsons, M., Martin, P. J., Hansen, J. A., Rabinovitch, P. S., and June, C. H., 1986b, Antibody binding to CD5 (Tp67) and Tp44 T cell surface molecules: Effects on cyclic nucleotides, cytoplasmic free calcium, and cAMP mediated suppression, *J. Immunol.* **137:**3299–3305.

LeGrue, S. J., 1987, Interleukin-2 stimulus–response coupling is calcium independent, *Lymph. Res.* **6:**1–11.

Leu, R. W., Eddleston, A. W., Good, R. W., and Hadden, J. W., 1973, Paradoxical effects of ouabain on the migration of peritoneal and alveolar macrophages, *Exp. Cell. Res.* **76:**458–461.

Levy, R., Levy, S., Rosenberg, S. A., and Simpson, R. T., 1973, Selective stimulation of nonhistone chromatin protein synthesis in lymphoid cells by phytohemagglutinin, *Biochemistry* **12:**224–228.

Liangxu, W., Shipeng, H., Sunxi, Z., Yunqin, G., Zhongmin, L., and Chenjiang, L., 1981, Peripheral leukemic cell cAMP level changes in acute leukemic and clinical observations, *Chinese Med. J.* **94:**47–50.

Lichtman, M. A., and Weed, R. I., 1969, Monovalent cation content and adenosine triphosphatase activity of human normal and leukemic granulocytes and lymphocytes: Relation to cell volume and morphologic age, *Blood* **34:**645–660.

Lichtman, A., Segal, G. B., and Lichtman, M. A., 1979, Total and exchangeable calcium in mitogen-treated lymphocytes, in: *The Molecular Basis of Immune Cell Function* (J. G. Kaplan, ed.), pp. 417–419, Elsevier North-Holland Biomedical Press, Amsterdam.

Lichtman, A. H., Segel, G. B., and Lichtman, M. A., 1981, Calcium transport and calcium-ATPase activity in human lymphocyte plasma membrane vesicles, *J. Biol. Chem.* **256:**6148–6154.

Lichtman, A. H., Segel, G. B., and Lichtman, M. A., 1982, Effects of trifluoperazine and mitogenic lectins on calcium ATPase activity and calcium transport by human lymphocyte plasma membrane vesicles, *J. Cell. Physiol.* **111:**213–217.

Lichtman, A. H., Segel, G. B., and Lichtman, M. A., 1983, The role of calcium in lymphocyte proliferation, *Blood* **61:**413–422.

Liebes, L. F., Pelle, F., Zucker-Franklin, D., and Silber, R., 1981, Comparison of lipid composition and 1, 6-dephenyl-1,3,5-Lexatriene fluorescence polarization measurements of hairy cells with monocytes and lymphocytes from normal subjects and patients with chronic lymphocytic leukemia, *Cancer Res.* **41:**4050–4056.

Lindahl-Kiessling, K., 1972, Mechanism of phytohemagglutinin (PHA) action. V. PHA compared with concanavalin A (Con A), *Exp. Cell. Res.* **70:**17–26.

Lindahl-Kiessling, K. M., 1976, Calcium dependency of the binding and mitogenicity of phytohemagglutinin. Differentiation between calcium-dependent and independent events, *Exp. Cell. Res.* **103**:151–158.

Ling, N. R., 1971, *Lymphocyte Stimulation*, North-Holland, Amsterdam.

Ling, N. R., and Kay, J. E., 1975, *Lymphocyte Stimulation*, North-Holland, Amsterdam.

Loeb, L. A., and Agarwal, S. S., 1971, DNA polymerase, *Exp. Cell. Res.* **66**:299–304.

Logan, J. C., and Newland, A. C., 1982, Leukocyte sodium–potassium adenosine triphosphate and leukemia, *Clin. Chim. Acta* **123**:39–43.

Lotan, R., Lis, H., Rosenwasser, A., Novogrodsky, A., and Sharon, N., 1973, Enhancement of the biological activities of soybean agglutinin by cross-linking with glutaraldehyde, *Biochem. Biophys. Res. Commun.* **55**:1347–1355.

Lucas, D. O., Shohet, S. B., and Merler, E., 1971, Changes in phospholipid metabolism which occur as a consequence of mitogenic stimulation of lymphocytes, *J. Immunol.* **106**:768–772.

Lucas, Z. J., 1967, Pryimidine nucleotide synthesis: Regulatory control during transformation of lymphocytes *in vitro, Science* **156**:1237–1240.

Luckasen, J. R., White, J. G., and Kersey, J. H., 1974, Mitogenic properties of a calcium ionophore, A23187, *Proc. Natl. Acad. Sci. USA* **71**:5088–5090.

Lyle, L. R., and Parker, C. W., 1974, Cyclic adenosine 3',5'-monophosphate responses to concanavalin A in human lymphocytes. Evidence that the response involves specific carbohydrate receptors on the cell surface, *Biochem.* **13**:5416–5420.

Maino, V. C., Green, N. M., and Crumpton, M. J., 1974, The role of calcium ions in initiating transformation of lymphocytes, *Nature (Lond.)* **251**:324–327.

Maino, V. C., Hayman, M. J., and Crumpton, M. J., 1975, Relationship between enhanced turnover of phosphatidylinositol and lymphocyte activation by mitogens, *Biochem. J.* **146**:247–252.

Makman, M. H., 1971, Properties of adenylate cyclase of lymphoid cells, *Proc. Natl Acad. Sci. USA* **68**:885–889.

Malek, T. R., Schmidt, J. A., and Shevack, E. M., 1985, The murine IL-2 receptor, *J. Immunol.* **134**:2405–2412.

Manen, C-A., and Russell, D. H., 1977, Ornithine decarboxylase may function as an initiation factor for RNA polymerase I, *Science* **195**:505–506.

Manger, B., Weiss, A., Imboden, J., Laing, T., and Stobo, J., 1987, The role of protein kinase C in transmembrane signaling by the T cell antigen receptor complex. *J. Immunol.* **139**:2755–2760.

Masuzawa, Y., Osawa, T., Inoue, K., and Nojima, S., 1973, Effects of various mitogens on the phospholipid metabolism of human peripheral lymphocytes, *Biochim. Biophys. Acta* **326**:339–344.

Matteson, D. R., and Deutsch, C., 1984, K Channels in T lymphocytes: A patch clamp study using monoclonal antibody adhesion, *Nature (Lond.)* **307**:468–471.

May, W. S., Jacobs, S., and Cuatrecasas, P., 1984, Association of phorbol ester-induced hyperphosphorylation and reversible regulation of transferrin membrane receptors in HL60 cells, *Proc. Natl. Acad. Sci. USA* **81**:2016–2020.

McClain, D. A., and Edelman, G. M., 1976, Analysis of the stimulation–inhibition paradox exhibited by lymphocytes, *J. Exp. Med.* **144**:1494–1508.

McClain, D. A., and Edelman, G. M., 1978, Surface modulation and transmembrane control, *Birth Defects* **14**:1–28.

McClain, D. A., D'Eustachio, P., and Edelman, G. M., 1977, Role of surface modulating assemblies in growth control of normal and transformed fibroblasts, *Proc. Natl. Acad. Sci. USA* **74**:666–670.

McPhail, L. C., Clayton, C. C., and Snyderman, R., 1984, A potential second messenger role for unsaturated fatty acids: Activation of Ca^{2+}-dependent protein kinase, *Science* **224**:622–625.

Mednieks, M. I., and Jungmann, R. A., 1982, Selective expression of type I and type II cyclic AMP-dependent protein kinases in subcellular fractions of concanavalin A-stimulated rat thymocytes, *Arch. Biochem. Biophys.* **213**:127–138.

Medrano, E., Piras, R., and Mordoh, J., 1974, Effect of colchicine, vinblastine, and cytochalasin B on human lymphocyte transformation by phytohemagglutinin, *Exp. Cell. Res.* **86**:295–300.

Mendelsohn, J., Skinner, A., and Kornfeld, S., 1971, The rapid induction by phytohemagglutinin of increased alpha-aminoisobutyric acid uptake by lymphocytes, *J. Clin. Invest.* **50**:818–826.

Mendelsohn, J., Trowbridge, I., Castagnola, J., 1983, Inhibition of human lymphocyte proliferation by monoclonal antibody to transferrin receptor, *Blood* **62**:821–826.

Metcalfe, J. C., Pozzan, T., Smith, G. A., and Hesketh, T. R., 1980, A calcium hypothesis for control of cell growth, *Biochem. Soc. Symp.* **45**:1–26.

Meuer, S. C., Hussey, R. E., Cantrell, D. A., Hodgolon, J. C., Schlossman, S. F., Smith, K. A., and Reinherz, E. L., 1984, Triggering of the T3-T: Antigen–receptor complex results in clonal T-cell proliferation through an interleukin 2-dependent autocrine pathway. *Proc. Natl. Acad. Sci. USA* **81**:1509–1513.

Meuer, S. C., and Meyer zum Buschenfelde, K-H., 1986, T cell receptor triggering induces responsiveness to interleukin 1 and interleukin 2 but does not lead to T cell proliferation, *J. Immunol.* **136**:4106–4112.

Mexmain, S., Gualde, N., Aldigier, J. C., Motta, C., Chable-Rabinovitch, H., and Rigaud, M., 1984, Specific binding of 15 HETE to lymphocytes. Effects on the fluidity of plasmatic membranes, *Prostaglandin Leuktrienes Med.* **13**:93–97.

Mexmain, S., Cook, J., Aldigier, J. C., Gualde, N., and Riguad, M., 1985, Thymocyte cyclic AMP and cyclic GMP response to treatment with metabolites issued from the lipoxygenase pathway, *J. Immunol.* **135**:1361–1365.

Michell, R. H., 1975, Inositol phospholipids and cell surface receptor function, *Biochim. Biophys. Acta* **415**:81–147.

Michell, R. H., 1982, Inositol lipid metabolism in dividing and differentiating cells, *Cell Calcium* **3**:429–440.

Michell, R. H., Kirk, C. J., Jones, L. M., Downes, C. P., and Creba, J. A., 1981, The stimulation of inositol lipid metabolism that accompanies calcium mobilization in stimulated cells: Defined characteristics and unanswered questions, *Phil. Trans. R. Soc. Lond. B.* **296**:123–137.

Mikkelsen, R. B., and Schmidt-Ullrich, R., 1980, Concanavalin A induces the release of intracellular Ca^{2+} in intact rabbit thymocytes, *J. Biol. Chem.* **255**:5177–5183.

Miller, J., 1979, Oncodazole (R 17934) an inhibitor of the turnover of phosphatidyl inositol in concanavalin A induced lymphocytes, *Biochem. Pharmacol.* **28**:2967–2968.

Mills, G. B., Cheung, R. K., Grinstein, S., and Gelfand, E. W., 1985a, Increase in cytosolic free calcium concentration is an intracellular messenger for the production of interleukin 2 but not for expression of the interleukin 2 receptor. *J. Immunol.* **134**:1640–1645.

Mills, G. B., Cheung, R. K., Grinstein, S., and Gelfand, E. W., 1985b, Interleukin 2-induced lymphocyte proliferation is independent of increases in cytosolic-free calcium concentrations, *J. Immunol.* **134**:2431–2435.

Mills, G. B., Stewart, D. J., Mellors, A., and Gelfand, E. W., 1986a, Interleukin 2 does not induce phosphatidylinositol hydrolysis in activated T cells, *J. Immunol.* **136**:3019–3024.

Mills, G. B., Cheung, R. K., Cracol, E. J., Jr., Grinstein, S., and Gelfand, E. W., 1986b, Activation of the Na^+/H^+ antiport is not required for lectin-induced proliferation of human T lymphocytes, *J. Immunol.* **136**:1150–1154.

Milner, S., 1977, Activation of mouse spleen cells by a single short pulse of mitogen, *Nature (Lond.)* **268**:441–442.

Mire, A. R., Wickremasinghe, G., and Hoffbrand, A. V., 1986, Phytohemagglutinin treatment of T lymphocytes stimulates rapid increases in activity of both particulate and cytosolic protein kinase C, *Biochem. Biophys. Res. Commun.* **137**:128–134.

Mitchell, M., Bard, E., L'Anglais, R., and Kaplan, J. G., 1978, Transport of RNA from nucleus to cytoplasm following mitogenic stimulation of human lymphocytes, *Can. J. Biochem.* **56**:659–666.

Mizoguchi, Y., Otani, S., Matsui, I., and Morisawa, S., 1975, Control of ornithine decarboxylase activity by cyclic nucleotides in the phytohemagglutinin induced lymphocyte transformation, *Biochem. Biophys. Res. Commun.* **66**:328–335.

Monahan, T. M., Marchand, N. W., Fritz, R. R., and Abell, C. W., 1975, Cyclic adenosine 3':5'-monophosphate levels and activities of related enzymes in normal and leukemic lymphocytes, *Cancer Res.* **35**:2540–2547.

Mookerjee, B. K., and Jung, C. Y., 1982, The effects of cytochalasins on lymphocytes: Mechanism of action of cytochalasin A on responses to phytomitogens, *J. Immunol.* **128**:2153–2159.

Mookerjee, B. K., Ferber, E., Ernst, M., Sharon, N., and Fischer, H., 1980, Chemiluminescence and immune cell activation: General features of the thymocyte chemiluminescence responses to plant lectins, *Immunol. Commun.* **9**:653–676.

Moore, J. P., Smith, G. A., Hesketh, T. R., and Metcalfe, J. C., 1982, Early increases in phospholipid methylation are not necessary for the mitogenic stimulation of lymphocytes, *J. Biol. Chem.* **257**:8183–8189.

Moore, R. N., Oppenheim, J., Farrar, J., Carter, C. G., Waheed, J., and Shadduck, R., 1981, Production of lymphocyte-activating factor (interleukin I) by macrophages activated with colony-stimulating factors, *J. Immunol.* **125**;1302–1305.

Morgan, J. I., Hall, A. K., and Perris, A. D., 1975, Requirements for divalent cations by hormonal mitogens and their interactions with sex steroids, *Biochem. Biophys. Res. Commun.* **66**:188–194.

Morris, D. R., Jorstad, C. M., Seyfried, C. E., 1977, Inhibition of the synthesis of polyamines and DNA in activated lymphocytes by a combination of alpha-methylornithine and methylglyoxal bis (guanylhydrazone), *Cancer Res.* **37**:3169–3172.

Munck, A., 1971, Glucocorticoid inhibition of glucose uptake by peripheral tissues: Old and new evidence, molecular mechanisms, and physiological significance, *Perspect. Biol. Med.* **14**:265–289.

Nakanishi, M., and Ulsunomiya, N., 1986, Early transmembrane events in cytotoxic T lymphocyte activation as revealed by stopped-flow fluorometry, in *Sixth International Congress of Immunology, Toronto, Canada,* p. 231 (abst.).

Namiuchi, S., Kumagai, S., Imura, H., Suginoshita, T., Hattori, T., and Hirata, F., 1984, Quinacrine inhibits the primary but not secondary proliferative response of human cytotoxic T cells to allogeneic non-T cell antigens, *J. Immunol.* **132**:1456–1461.

Nathaniel, D., and Mellors, A., 1983, Mitogen effects on lipid metabolism during lymphocyte activation, *Mol. Immunol.* **20**:1259–1266.

Neckers, L. M., and Crossman, J., 1983, Transferrin receptor induction in mitogen-stimulated human T lymphocytes is required for DNA synthesis and cell division and is regulated by interleukin 2, *Proc. Natl. Acad. Sci. USA* **80**:3494–3498.

Neely, A., Sitzmann, J. V., and Kersey, J. H., 1976, EGTA and proteinase reversal of cellular aggregation of activated lymphocytes, *Nature (Lond.)* **264**:770–771.

Negendank, W. G., and Collier, C. R., 1976, Ion contents of human lymphocytes, *Exp. Cell. Res.* **101**:31–40.

Negendank, W., and Shaller, C., 1979, Potassium-sodium distribution in human lymphocytes: Description by the association-induction hypothesis, *J. Cell. Physiol.* **98**:95–105.

Nel, A. E., Bouic, P., Lattanze, G. R., Stevenson, H. C., Miller, P., Dirienzo, W., Stefanini, F., and Galbraith, R. M., 1987, Reaction of T lymphocytes with anti-T3 induces translocation of C-kinase activity to the membrane and specific substrate phosphorylation, *J. Immunol.* **138**:3519–3524.

Newman, W., Fanning, V. A., Rao, P. E., Westberg, E. F., and Patten, E., 1986, Early events in lymphocyte activation as defined by three new monoclonal antibodies, *J. Immunol.* **137**:3702–3708.

Nishizuka, Y., 1984, The role of protein kinase C in cell surface transduction and tumor promotion, *Nature (Lond.)* **308**:693–698.

Nordenberg, J., Stenzel, K. H., and Novogrodsky, A., 1983, 12-O-tetradecanoyl-phorbol-13-acetate and concanavalin A enhanced glucose uptake in thymocytes by different mechanisms, *J. Cell Physiol.* **117**:183–188.

Northoff, H., Dorken, B., and Resch, K., 1978, Ligand-dependent modulation of membrane phospholipid metabolism in Con A-stimulated lymphocytes, *Exp. Cell. Res.* **113**:189–196.

Novogrodsky, A., 1972, Concanavalin A stimulation of rat lymphocyte ATPase, *Biochim. Biophys. Acta* **266**:343–349.

Novogrodsky, A., and Katchalski, E., 1970, Effect of phytohemagglutinin and prostaglandins on cyclic AMP synthesis on rat lymphnode lymphocytes, *Biochim. Biophys. Acta* **215**:291–296.

Novogrodsky, A., and Katchalski, E., 1971, Lymphocyte transformation induced by concanavalin A and its reversion by methyl-alpha-D-mannopyranoside, *Biochim. Biophys. Acta* **228**:579–583.

Novogrodsky, A., Quittner, S., Rubin, A. L., and Stenzel, K., 1978, Transglutaminase activation in human lymphocytes: Early activation by phytomitogens, *Proc. Natl. Acad. Sci. USA* **75**:1157–1161.

Novogrodsky, A., Rubin, A., and Stenzel, K., 1979, Selective suppression by adherent cells, prostaglandin and cyclic AMP analogues of blastogenesis induced by different mitogens, *J. Immunol.* **122**:1–7.

Novogrodsky, A., Ravid, A., Rubin, A. L., and Stenzel, K. H., 1982, Hydroxyl radical scavengers inhibit lymphocyte mitogenesis, *Proc. Natl. Acad. Sci. USA* **79**:1171–1174.

O'Brien, R. L., Parker, J. W., and Dixon, J. F. P., 1978, Mechanisms of lymphocyte transformation, *Prog. Mol. Subcell. Biol.* **6**:201–270.

Oettgen, H. C., and Terhorst, C., 1987, The T-cell receptor–T3 complex and T-lymphocyte activation, *Hum. Immunol.* **18**:187–204.

Oettgen, H. C., Terhorst, C., Cantley, L. C., and Rosoff, P. M., 1985, Stimulation of the T3–T cell receptor complex induces a membrane-potential-sensitive calcium influx, *Cell* **40**:583–590.

O'Flynn, K., Linch, D. C., and Tatham, P. E. R., 1984, The effect of mitogenic lectins and monoclonal antibodies on intracellular free calcium concentration in human T-lymphocytes, *Biochem. J.* **219**:661–666.

Ogawa, Y., Takai, Y., Kawahara, Y., Kimura, S., and Nishizuka, Y., 1981, A new possible regulatory system for protein phosphorylation in human peripheral lymphocytes. I. Characterization of a calcium-activated, phospholipid-dependent protein kinase, *J. Immunol.* **127**:1369–1374.

Ohara, J., and Watanabe, T., 1982, Microinjection of macromolecules into normal murine lymphocytes by cell fusion technique. I. Quantitative microinjection of antibodies into normal splenic lymphocytes, *J. Immunol.* **128**:1090–1096.

Ohara, J., Kishimoto, T., and Yamomura, Y., 1978, *In vitro* immune response of human peripheral lymphocytes, *J. Immunol.* **121**:2088–2096.

Oliver, J. M., Gelfand, E. W., Pearson, C. B., Pfeiffer, J. R., and Dosch, H-M., 1980, Microtubule assembly and concanavalin A capping in lymphocytes: Reappraisal using normal and abnormal human peripheral blood cells, *Proc. Natl. Acad. Sci. USA* **77**:3499–3503.

Orme, I. M., and Shand, F. L., 1981, Inhibitors of prostaglandin synthetase block the generation of suppressor T cells induced by concanavalin A, *Int. J. Immunopharmacol.* **3**:15–19.

Otani, S., Matsui, I., and Morisawa, S., 1977, Suppression of phytohemagglutinin-induction of thymidine uptake in guinea pig lymphocytes by methylglyoxal bis(guanylhydrazone) treatment, *Biochim. Biophys. Acta* **478**:417–427.

Otani, S., Matsui, I., and Morisawa, S., Masutani, M., Mizoguchi, Y., and Morisawa, S., 1980, Induction of ornithine decarboxylase in guinea pig lymphocytes by the divalent cation ionophore A23187 and phytohemagglutinin, *J. Biochem.* **88**:77–85.

Otani, S, Kuramoto, A., Matsui, I., and Morisawa, S., 1982, Induction of ornithine decarboxylase in guinea pig lymphocytes by the divalent cation ionophore A23187, *Eur. J. Biochem.* **125**:35–40.

Otteskog, P., Wanger, L., and Sundquist, K. G., 1983, Cytochalasins distinguish by their action resting human T lymphocytes from activated T cell blast, *Eur. Cell Res.* **144**:443–454.

Owen, M. J., Auzer, J., Barber, B. H., Edwards, A. J., Walsh, F. S., and Crumpton, M. J., 1978, Actin may be present on the lymphocyte surface, *Proc. Natl. Acad. Sci. USA* **75**:4484-4488.

Owens, T., and Kaplan, J. G., 1980, Increased cationic fluxes in stimulated lymphocytes of the mouse: Response of enriched B- and T-cell subpopulations to B- and T-cell mitogens, *Can. J. Biochem.* **58**:831-839.

Ozato, K., Huang, L., and Ebert, J. D., 1977, Accelerated calcium ion uptake in murine thymocytes induced by concanavalin-A, *J. Cell. Physiol.* **93**:153-160.

Parker, C. W., 1974, Correlations between mitogenicity and stimulation of calcium uptake in human lymphocytes, *Biochem. Biophys. Res. Commun.* **61**:1180-1186.

Parker, C. W., 1982, Pharmacologic modulation of release of arachidonic acid from human mononuclear cells and lymphocytes by mitogenic lectins, *J. Immunol.* **128**:393-397.

Parker, C. W., 1984, Intracellular activation in mast cells and lymphocytes, *Prog. Immunol.* **5**:327-337.

Parker, C. W., Smith, J. W., and Steiner, A. L., 1971, Early effects of phytohemagglutinin (PHA) on lymphocyte cyclic AMP levels, *Int. Arch. Allergy Appl. Immunol.* **41**:40-46.

Parker, C. W., Sullivan, T. J., and Wedner, H. J., 1974, Cyclic AMP and the immune response, *Adv. Cyclic Nucleotide Res.* **4**:1-80.

Parker, C. W., Kelly, J. P., Falkinhein, S. F., and Huber, M. G., 1979a, Release of arachidonic acid from human lymphocytes in response to mitogenic lectins, *J. Exp. Med.* **149**:1487-1503.

Parker, C. W., Stenson, W. F., Huber, M. G., and Kelly, J. P., 1979b, Formation of thromboxane B$_2$ and hydroxy arachidonic acids in purified human lymphocytes in the presence and absence of PHA, *J. Immunol.* **122**:1572-1577.

Patrick, J. C., Rengachary, S., and Melnykovych, G., 1975, Elevation of adenosine 3′,5′-cyclic monophosphate in established mammalian cell strains by hypaque (sodium diatrizoate), *In Vitro* **11**:404-408.

Patt, L., Barrantes, D. M., and Houck, J., 1982, Inhibition of lymphocyte DNA-synthetic responses by spermine-derived polycations, *Biochem. Pharmacol.* **31**:2353-2360.

Payan, D. G., and Goetzl, E. J., 1981, The dependence of human T-lymphocyte migration on the 5-lipoxygenation of endogenous arachidonic acid, *J. Clin. Immunol.* **1**:266-270.

Payan, D. G., and Goetzl, E., 1983, Specific suppression of human T lymphocyte function by leukotriene B$_4$, *J. Immunol.* **131**:551-553.

Payan, D. G., Missirian-Bastian, A., and Goetzl, E. J., 1984, Human T-lymphocyte subset specificity of the regulatory effects of leukotriene B$_4$, *Immunology* **81**:3501-3505.

Pelosi, E., Testa, U., Louache, F., Thomopoulos, P., Salvo, G., Samoggia, P., and Peschle, C., 1986, Expression of transferrin receptors in phytohemagglutinin-stimulated human T-lymphocytes, *J. Immunol.* **261**:3036-3042.

Pena, J. M., Itarte, E., Domingo, A., and Cusso, R., 1983, Cyclic adenosine 3′:5′-monophosphate-dependent and -independent protein kinases in human leukemic cells, *Cancer Res.* **43**:1172-1175.

Peracchi, M., Maiolo, A., Lombardi, L., Catena, F., and Polli, E., 1980, Patterns of cyclic nucleotides in normal and leukaemic human leucocytes, *Br. J. Cancer* **41**:360-371.

Peracchi, M., Lombardi, A. T., Maiolo, F., Bamonti-Catena, V., Toschi, O., Chiorboli, O., Mozzana, R., and Polli, E. E., 1983, Plasma and urine cyclic nucleotide levels in patients with acute and chronic leukemia, *Blood* **61**:429-434.

Peracchi, M., Lombardi, L., Bareggi, B., Maiolo, A. T., Bamonti-Catena, F., Toschi, V., Cortelezzi, A., and Polli E. E., 1985, Plasma cyclic nucleotide levels in monitoring acute leukemia patients, *Cancer Detect. Prev.* **8**:291-295.

Peters, J. H., and Hausen, P., 1971a, Effect of PHA on lymphocyte membrane transport, I. Stimulation of uridine uptake, *Eur. J. Biochem.* **19**:502-508.

Peters, J. H., and Hausen, P., 1971b, Effect of PHA on lymphocyte membrane transport. II. Stimulation of "facilitated diffusion" of 3-O-methyl-glucose, *Eur. J. Biochem.* **19**:509-513.

Peterson, O. H., and Maruiyama, Y., 1984, Calcium-activated potassium channels and their role in secretion, *Nature (Lond.)* **307**:693–696.

Phillips, C. A., Girit, E. Z., and Kay, J. E., 1978, Changes in intracellular prostaglandin content during activation of lymphocytes by phytohemagglutinin, *FEBS Lett.* **94**:115–119.

Phillips, J. L., 1976, Specific binding of zinc transferrin to human lymphocytes, *Biochem. Biophys. Res. Commun.* **72**:634–639.

Phillips, J. L., and Azair, P., 1974, Zinc transferrin enhancement of nucleic acid synthesis in phytohemagglutinin-stimulated human lymphocytes, *Cell Immunol.* **10**:31–37.

Pike, M. C., and Snyderman, R., 1981, Requirement of transmethylation reactions for immune effector function, *Lymphokines* **3**:432–444.

Pogo, B. G. T., 1972, Early events in lymphocyte transformation by phytohemagglutinin, *J. Cell. Biol.* **53**:635–641.

Pogo, B. G. T., Allfrey, V. G., and Mirsky, A. E., 1966, RNA synthesis and histone acetylation during the course of gene activation in lymphocytes, *Proc. Natl. Acad. Sci. USA* **55**:805–812.

Polgar, P., Vera, J., Kelley, P., and Rutenburg, A,. 1973, Adenylate cyclase activity in normal and leukemic human leukocytes as determined by a radioimmunoassay for cyclic AMP, *Biochim. Biophys. Acta* **197**:378–383.

Polgar, P., Vera, J., and Rutenburg, A., 1977, An altered response to cyclic AMP stimulating hormones in intact human leukemic lymphocytes (39701), *Proc. Soc. Exp. Biol. Med.* **154**:493–495.

Pommier, G., Ripert, G., Azoulay, E., and Depieds, R., 1975, Effects of concanavalin A on membrane-bound enzymes from mouse lymphocytes, *Biochim. Biophys. Acta* **389**:483–494.

Pompidou, A., Mace, B., Esnous, D., Michel, P., and Cochin, C. H. U., 1980, The nuclear refringence test: A new method for the evaluation of blood lymphocytes nuclei response *in vitro* to lectins and immunomodulators in man, in: *International Symposium on New Trends in Human Immunology and Cancer Immunotherapy* (B. Serrou and C. Rosenfold, eds.), pp. 696–703, Doin Editeurs, Paris.

Pompidou, A., Rousset, S., Mace, B., Michel, P., Esnous, D., and Renard, N., 1984, Chromatin structure and nucleic acid synthesis in human lymphocyte activation by phytohemagglutinin, *Exp. Cell. Res.* **150**:213–225.

Pompidou, A., Michel, P., Esnous, D., Rouquet, F., and Coral, M., 1986, Early nuclear events during human T lymphocytes activation, in: *Sixth International Congress of Immunology Abstracts,* #43.

Purtell, M. J., and Anthony, D. D., 1975, Changes in ribosomal RNA processing paths in resting and phytohemagglutinin-stimulated guinea pig lymphocytes, *Proc. Natl. Acad. Sci. USA* **72**:3315–3319.

Quastel, M. R., and Kaplan, J. G., 1968, Inhibition by ouabain of human lymphocyte transformation induced by phytohemagglutinin *in vitro, Nature (Lond.)* **219**:198–200.

Quastel, M. R., and Kaplan, J. G., 1970, Early stimulation of potassium uptake in lymphocytes treated with PHA, *Exp. Cell. Res.* **63**:230–233.

Quastel, M. R., and Kaplan, J. G., 1975, Ouabain binding to intact lymphocytes: Enhancement by phytohemagglutinin and leucoagglutinin, *Exp. Cell. Res.* **94**:351–362.

Quastel, M. R., Milthorpe, P., Kaplan, J. G., and Vogelfanger, I. J., 1974, Further studies on M-ATPase in lymphocytes and plaque-forming cells: Possible species and functional differences between lymphocyte subclasses, in: *Lymphocyte Recognition and Effector Mechanisms* (K. Lindahl-Kiessling and D. Osoba, eds.), pp. 493–500, Academic, New York.

Rabinovitch, P. S., June, C. H., Grossman, A., and Ledbetter, J. A., 1986, Heterogeneity among T cells in intracellular free calcium responses after mitogen stimulation with PHA or anti-CD3, *J. Immunol.* **137**:952–961.

Rasmussen, S. A., and Davis, R. P., 1977, Effect of microtubular antagonists on lymphocyte mitogenesis, *Nature (Lond.)* **269**:249–251.

Reed, J. C., Alpers, J. D., Nowell, P. C., and Hoover, R. G., 1987, Sequential expression of proto-oncogenes during normal human lymphocyte mitogenesis, *Proc. Natl. Acad. Sci. USA* **83:** 3982–3986.

Reeves, J. P., 1975, Calcium-dependent stimulation of 3-O-methyglucose uptake in rat thymocytes by the divalent cation ionophore A23187, *J. Biol. Chem.* **250:**9428–9430.

Reilly, C. E., and Ferber, E., 1976, Concanavalin A induced changes of membrane-bound lysolecithin acyltransferase of thymocytes, in: *Surface Membrane Receptors* (R. A. Bradshaw, W. A. Frazier, R. C. Merrell, D. I. Gottlieb, and R. A. Hogue-Angeletti, eds.), pp. 199–213, Plenum, New York.

Resch, K., 1976, Membrane associated events in lymphocyte activation, in: *Receptors and Recognition.* 1. Series A (P. Cuatrecasas and M. F. Greaves, eds.), pp. 61–117, Chapman and Hall, Ltd., London.

Resch, K., and Ferber, E., 1972, Phospholipid metabolism of stimulated lymphocytes. Effects of phytohemagglutinin, concanavalin A and antiimmunoglobulin serum, *Eur. J. Biochem.* **27:** 153–161.

Resch, K., Ferber, E., Odenthal, J., and Fischer, H., 1971, Early changes in the phospholipid metabolism of lymphocytes following stimulation with phytohemagglutinin and with lysolecithin, *Eur. J. Immunol.* **1:**162–165.

Resch, K., Gelfand, E. W., Hansen, K., and Ferber, E., 1972, Lymphocyte activation: Rapid changes in the phospholipid metabolism of plasma membranes during stimulation, *Eur. J. Immunol.* **2:**598–601.

Resch, K., Prester, M., Ferber, E., and Gelfand, E. W., 1976, The inhibition of initial steps of lymphocyte transformation by cytochalasin B, *J. Immunol.* **117:**1705–1710.

Resch, K., Bovillon, D., Gemsa, D., and Averdunk, R., 1977, Drugs which disrupt microtubules do not inhibit the initiation of lymphocyte activation, *Nature (Lond.)* **265:**349–351.

Resch, K., Bovillon, D., and Gemsa, D., 1978, The activation of lymphocytes by the ionophore A23187, *J. Immunol.* **120:**1514–1520.

Resch, K., Wood, T., Northoff, H., and Cooper, H. L., 1981, Microtubules: Are they involved in the initiation of lymphocyte activation?, *Eur. J. Biochem.* **115:**659–664.

Resch, K., Schneider, S., and Szamel, M., 1983, Characterization of functional domains of the lymphocyte plasma membrane, *Biochim. Biophys. Acta* **733:**142–153.

Resch, K., Brennecke, M., Goppelt, M., Kaever, V., Szamel, M., 1984, The role of phospholipids in the signal transmission of activated lymphocytes-T, *Prog. Immunol.* **5:**349–360.

Rink, T. J., and Deutsch, C., 1983, Calcium-activated potassium channels in lymphocytes, *Cell Calcium* **4:**463–474.

Riordan, J. R., Slavik, M., and Kartner, N., 1977, Nature of the lectin-induced activation of plasma membrane Mg^{2+} ATPase, *J. Biol. Chem.* **252:**5449–5455.

Rittenhouse-Simmons, S., 1980, Indomethacin-induced accumulation of diglyceride in activated human platelets, *J. Biol. Chem.* **255:**2259–2262.

Robins, R. K., 1982, Purine nucleoside 3',5'-cyclic monophosphates as hormonal modulators of cellular proliferation, metastases and lymphocyte response, *Nucleosides and Nucleotides* **1:** 205–231.

Rochette-Egly, C., and Kempf, J., 1981, Cyclic nucleotides and calcium in human lymphocytes induced to divide, *J. Physiol. Paris* **77:**721–725.

Rocklin, R. E., 1976, Modulation of cellular immune responses *in vivo* and *in vitro* by histamine receptor-bearing lymphocytes, *J. Clin. Invest.* **57:**1051–1058.

Rode, H. N., Szamel, M., Schneider, S., and Resch, K., 1982, Phospholipid metabolism of stimulated lymphocytes. Preferential incorporation of polyunsaturated fatty acids into plasma membrane phospholipid upon stimulation with concanavalin A, *Biochim. Biophys. Acta* **688:** 66–74.

Rogers, J., Hesketh, T. R., Smith, G. A., Beaven, M. A., Melcalfe, J. C., Johnson, P., and

Garland, P. B., 1983a, Intracellular pH and free calcium changes in single cells using Quin 1 and Quin 2 probes and fluorescence microscopy, *FEBS Lett.* **161**:21–27.

Rogers, J., Hesketh, T. R., Smith, G. A., and Melcalfe, J. C., 1983b, Intracellular pH of stimulated thymocytes measured with a new fluorescent indicator, *J. Biol. Chem.* **258**:5994–5997.

Rola-Pleszczynski, M., 1985, Differential effects of leukotriene B_4 on $T_4{}^+$ and $T_8{}^+$ lymphocyte phenotype and immunoregulation functions, *J. Immunol.* **135**:1357–1360.

Rola-Pleszczynski, M. P., Borgeat, P., and Sirois, P., 1982, Leukotriene B_4 induces human suppressor lymphocytes, *Biochem, Biophys. Res. Commun.* **198**:1531–1536.

Roos, D., Loos, J. A., Bloom, A. J., and Scholte, B. M., 1970, Changes in the carbohydrate metabolism of mitogenically stimulated human peripheral lymphocytes. I. Stimulation by phytohemagglutinin, *Biochim. Biophys. Acta* **222**:565–582.

Roos, D., DeRoer, J., Huismans, L., and Boom, A., 1972, Dose-response of lymphocyte carbohydrate metabolism to phytohaemagglutinin, *Exp. Cell. Res.* **75**:185–190.

Rosenberg, S. A., and Levy, R., 1972, Communications: Synthesis of nuclear-associated proteins by lymphocytes within minutes after contact with phytohemagglutinin, *J. Immunol.* **108**:1105–1109.

Rosenberg, E. M., Conway, J. G., Tucci, M., and Doucet, E. W., 1980, Immunohistochemical studies of cyclic guanosine monophosphate and nuclear function, *J. Clin. Invest.* **66**:832–842.

Rosenfeld, M. G., Abrass, I. B., Mendelsohn, J., Roos, B. A., Boone, R. F., and Garren, L. D., 1972, Control of transcription of RNA rich in polyadenylic acid in human lymphocytes, *Proc. Natl. Acad. Sci. USA* **69**:2306–2311.

Rudd, C. E., Rogers, K. A., Brown, D. L., and Kaplan, J. G., 1979, Microtubules, colchicine, and lymphocyte blastogenesis, *Can. J. Biochem.* **57**:673–683.

Ruhl, H., and Kirchner, H., 1978, Monocyte-dependent stimulation of human T cells by zinc, *Clin. Exp. Immunol.* **32**:484–488.

Russell, D. H., 1973, *Polyamines in Normal and Neoplastic Growth*, Raven, New York.

Salari, H., Braquet, P., and Borgeat, P., 1984, Comparative effects of indomethacin, acetylenic acids, 15-HETE, nordihydroguaiaretic acid and BW-755 on the metabolism of arachidonic acid in human leukocytes and platelets, *Prostaglandins Leukotrienes Med.* **13**:53–60.

Samuelsson, B., 1982, The leukotrienes: An introduction, in: *Leukotrienes and Other Lipoxygenase Products. Advances in Prostaglandin, Thromboxane, and Leukotriene Research*, Vol. 9 (B. Samuelsson and R. Pauletti, eds.), pp. 1–18, Raven, New York.

Samuelsson, B., Goldyne, M., Granstrom, E., Hamberg, M., Hammarstrom, S., and Malmsten, C., 1978, Prostaglandins and thromboxanes, *Annu. Rev. Biochem.* **47**:997–1029.

Sasaki, T., and Hasagewa-Sasaki, H., 1981, Effects of anchorage-modulating doses of concanavalin A, microtubule-disrupting drugs and microfilament perturbants, cytochalasins, in the phosphatidylinositol response of rat lymph node cells, *Biochim. Biophys. Acta* **649**:449–454.

Sawyer, W. H., Hammarstrom, S., Moller, G., and Goldstein, I. J., 1975, Precipitin and mitogenic behavior of dimeric and tetrameric concanavalin A, *Eur. J. Immunol.* **5**:507–510.

Scavennec, J., Carcassonne, Y., Gastaut, J-A., Blanc, A., and Cailla, H., 1981, Relationship between the levels of cyclic cytidine 3′:5′-monophosphate and cyclic guanosine 3′:5′-monophosphate in urines and leukocytes and the type of human leukemias, *Cancer Res.* **41**:3222–3227.

Schellenberg, R. R., and Gillespie, E., 1977, Colchicine inhibits phosphatidylinositol turnover induced in lymphocytes by concanavalin A, *Nature (Lond.)* **265**:741–742.

Schellenberg, R. R., and Gillespie, E., 1980, Effects of colchicine, vinblastine, griseofulvin and deuterium oxide upon phospholipid metabolism in concanavalin A-stimulated lymphocytes, *Biochim. Biophys. Acta* **619**:522–532.

Scher, N. S., Quagliata, F., Malathi, V., Faig, D., Melton, R. A., and Silber, R., 1976, Cyclic adenosine 3′:5′-monophosphate phosphodiesterase activity in normal and chronic lymphocytic leukemia lymphocytes, *Cancer Res.* **36**:3958–3962.

Schreiner, G. F., and Unanue, E. R., 1975, The modulation of spontaneous and anti-Ig-stimulated motility of lymphocytes by cyclic nucleotides and adrenergic and cholinergic agents, *J. Immunol* **114**:802–809.

Schumm, D. E., and Webb, T. E., 1978, Effect of adenosine 3':5'-monophosphate and guanosine 3':5'-monophosphate on RNA release from isolated nuclei, *J. Biol. Chem.* **253**:8513–8517.

Schumm, D. E., Morris, H. P., and Webb, T. E., 1974, Early biochemical changes in PHA-stimulated peripheral blood lymphocytes from normal and tumor bearing rats, *Eur. J. Cancer* **10**:107–113.

Segel, G. B., and Lichtman, M. A., 1976, Potassium transport in human blood lymphocytes treated with phytohemagglutinin, *J. Clin. Invest.* **58**:1358–1369.

Segel, G. B., and Lichtman, M. A., 1981, Amino acid transport in human lymphocytes: Distinctions in the enhanced uptake with PHA treatment or amino acid deprivation, *J. Cell. Physiol.* **106**: 303–308.

Segel, G. B., Hollander, M. M., Gordon, B. R., Klemperer, M. R., and Lichtman, M. A., 1975, A rapid phytohemagglutinin induced alteration in lymphocyte potassium permeability, *J. Cell. Physiol.* **86**:327–335.

Segel, G. B., Lichtman, M. A., Hollander, M. M., Gordon, B. R., and Klemperer, M. R., 1976, Human lymphocyte potassium content during the initiation of phytohemagglutinin induced mitogenesis, *J. Cell. Physiol.* **88**:43–48.

Segel, G. B., Simon, W., and Lichtman, M. A., 1979a, Regulation of sodium and potassium transport in phytohemagglutinin-stimulated human blood lymphocytes, *J. Clin. Invest.* **64**:834–841.

Segel, G. B., Kovach, G., and Lichtman, M. A., 1979b, Sodium-potassium adenosine triphosphatase activity of human lymphocyte membrane vesicles: Kinetic parameters, substrate specificity, and effects of phytohemagglutinin, *J. Cell. Physiol.* **100**:109–118.

Segel, G. B., Simon, W., Lichtman, A. H., and Lichtman, M. A., 1981, The activation of lymphocyte plasma membrane (Na,K)-ATPase by EGTA is explained better by zinc than by calcium chelation, *J. Biol. Chem.* **256**:6629–6632.

Sell, S., and Linthicum, D. S., 1975, Distribution of surface Ig during lymphocyte transformation, in: *Lymphocytes and Their Interaction: Recent Observations* (R. C. Williams, ed.), Kroc Foundation Symposia Series, Vol. 4, pp. 57–75. Raven, New York.

Serhan, C. N., Fridovich, J., Goetzl, E. J., Dunham, P. B., and Weissmann, G., 1982, Leukotriene B$_4$ and phosphatidic acid are calcium ionophores, *J. Biol. Chem.* **257**:4746–4752.

Shapiro, H. M., Natale, P. J., and Kamentsky, L. A., 1979, Estimation of membrane potentials of individual lymphocytes by flow cytometry, *Proc. Natl. Acad. Sci. USA* **76**:5728–5730.

Sherline, P., and Mundy, G. R., 1977, Role of the tubulin–microtubular system in lymphocyte activation, *J. Cell. Biol.* **74**:371–376.

Shipp, M. A., and Reinherz, E. L., 1987, Differential expression of nuclear proto-oncogenes in T cells triggered with mitogenic and nonmitogenic T3 and T11 activation signals, *J. Immunol.* **139**:2143–2148.

Singer, S. J., and Nicolson, G. L., 1972, The fluid mosaic model of the structure of cell membranes, *Science* **175**:720–731.

Smit, J. W., Bloom, N. R., VanLuyn, M. J. A., and Halie, M. R., 1983, Lymphocytes with parallel tubular structures: Morphologically a distinctive subpopulation, *Blut* **46**:311–320.

Smith, J. W., Steiner, A. L., Newberry, W. M., and Parker, C. W., 1971, Cyclic adenosine 3',5'-monophosphate in human lymphocytes. Alterations after phytohemagglutinin stimulation, *J. Clin. Invest.* **50**:432–441.

Smith, K. A., 1982, Interleukin-2, *Immunobiology* **161**:157–173.

Soren, L., 1973, Variability of the time at which PHA-stimulated lymphocytes initiate DNA synthesis, *Exp. Cell Res.* **78**:201–208.

Spach, C., and Aschkenasy, A., 1979, Effects of a protein-free diet on the changes in cyclic AMP and cyclic GMP levels induced by immunization in splenic T and B lymphocytes in rat, *J. Nutr.* **109:**1265–1273.

Spiegel, R. J., Magrath, I. T., and Shutta, J. A., 1981, Role of cytoplasmic lipids in altering diphenylhexatriene fluorescence polarization in malignant cells, *Cancer Res.* **41:**452–458.

Stark, R., Liebes, L. F., Nevrla, D., and Silber, R., 1982, The quantitation of actin in human lymphocytes by isoelectric focusing, *Biochem. Med.* **27:**200–206.

Stenzel, K. M., Schwartz, R., Rubin, A. L., and Novogrodsky, A., 1978, Potentiation of lymphocyte activation by colchicine, *J. Immunol.* **121:**863–871.

Sternholm, R. L., and Falor, W. H., 1970, Early biochemical changes in phytohemagglutinin-stimulated human lymphocytes of blood and lymphocytes, *J. Reticuloendothel. Soc.* **7:**471–483.

Stoeck, M., Northoff, H., and Resch, K., 1983, Inhibition of mitogen-induced lymphocyte proliferation by ouabain, *J. Immunol.* **131:**1433–1437.

Stolc, V., 1980, Stimulatory effect of ionophores on adenosine 3′,5′-monophosphate content in human mononuclear leukocytes, *Biochem. Pharmacol.* **29:**1991–1994.

Strom, T. B., Lundin, A. P., and Carpenter, C. B., 1977, The role of cyclic nucleotides in lymphocyte activation and function, *Prog. Clin. Immunol.* **3:**115–153.

Sugiura, T., and Waku, K., 1984, Enhanced turnover of arachidonic acid-containing species of phosphatidylinositol and phosphatidic acid of concanavalin A-stimulated lymphocytes, *Biochim. Biophys. Acta* **796:**190–198.

Sundquist, K. G., Otteskog, P., Wanger, L. Thorstensson, R., and Utter, G., 1980, The morphology and microfilament organization in human blood lymphocytes: Effects of substratum and mitogen exposure, *Exp. Cell. Res.* **130:**327–337.

Suzuki T., Sadasivan, R., Saito-Taki, T., Stechschulte, D. J., and Balentine, L., 1980, Studies of Fc gamma-receptors of human B lymphocytes: Phospholipase A$_2$ activation of Fc gamma-receptors, *Biochemistry* **19:**6037–6043.

Szamel, M., and Resch, K., 1981a, Modulation of enzyme activities is isolated lymphocyte plasma membranes by enzymatic modification of phospholipid fatty acids, *J. Biol. Chem.* **256:**11618–11623.

Szamel, M., and Resch, K., 1981b, Inhibition of lymphocyte activation by ouabain. Interference with the early activation of membrane phospholipid metabolism, *Biochim. Biophys. Acta* **647:**297–301.

Szamel, M., Schneider, S., and Resch, K., 1981, Functional interrelationship between (Na$^+$ and K$^+$)-ATPase and lysolecithin acyltransferase in plasma membranes of mitogen-stimulated rabbit thymocytes, *J. Biol. Chem.* **256:**9198–9204.

Takemoto, D. J., Kaplan, S. A., and Appleman, M. M., 1979, Cyclic guanosine 3′,5′-monophosphate and phosphodiesterase activity in mitogen-stimulated human lymphocyte, *Biochem. Biophysica Res. Commun.* **90:**491–497.

Takemoto, D. J., Dunford, C., Vaughn, D., Kramer, K. J., Smith, A., and Powell, R. G., 1982, Guanylate cyclase activity in human leukemic and normal lymphocytes, *Enzyme* **27:**179–188.

Takigawa, M., and Waksman, B., 1980, Mechanisms of lymphocyte "deletion" by high concentrations of ligand. I. Cyclic AMP levels and cell death in T-lymphocytes exposed to high concentration of concanavalin A, *Cell. Immunol.* **58:**29–38.

Tam, C. F., and Walford, R. L., 1978, Cyclic nucleotide levels in resting and mitogen-stimulated spleen cell suspensions from young and old mice, *Mech. Aging Dev.* **7:**309–320.

Tam, C. F., and Walford, R. L., 1980, Alterations in cyclic nucleotides and cyclase-specific activities in T lymphocytes of aging normal humans and patients with Down's Syndrome, *J. Immunol.* **125:**1665–1670.

Tam, C., Smith, G., and Walford, R., 1979, Resting and concanavalin-A stimulated levels of cyclic nucleotides in splenic cells of aging mice with spontaneous cancers, *Life Sci.* **24:**311–322.

Tandon, N. N., Davidson, L. A., and Titus, E. O., 1983, Changes in (Na$^+$ and K$^+$) ATPase activity associated with stimulation of thymocytes by concanavalin A, *J. Biol. Chem.* **258:** 9850–9855.

Tatham, P. E. R., and Delves, P. J., 1984, Flow cytometric detection of membrane potential changes in murine lymphocytes induced by concanavalin A, *Biochem. J.* **221:**137–146.

Taylor, M. J., Metcalfe, J. C., Hesketh, T. R., Smith, G. A., and Moore, J. P., 1984, Mitogens increase phosphorylation of phosphoinositides in thymocytes, *Nature (Lond.)* **312:**462–463.

Toh, B. H., and Hard, G. C., 1977, Actin co-caps with concanavalin A receptors, *Nature (Lond.)* **269:**695–697.

Tomar, R. H., Darrow, T. L., and John, P. A., 1981, Response to and production of prostaglandins by murine thymus, spleen, bone marrow and lymph node cells, *Cell. Immunol.* **60:**335–346.

Touraine, J. L., Hadden, J. W., Touraine, F., Hadden, E. M., Estensen, R., and Good, R. A., 1977, Phorbol myristate acetate: A mitogen selective for a T-lymphocyte subpopulation, *J. Exp. Med.* **145:**460–465.

Toyoshima, S., and Osawa, T., 1975, Lectins from *Wistaria floribunda* seeds and their effect on membrane fluidity of human peripheral lymphocytes, *J. Biol. Chem.* **250:**1655–1660.

Toyoshima, S., Iwata, M., and Osawa, T., 1976, Kinetics of lymphocyte stimulation by concanavalin A, *Nature (Lond.)* **264:**447–449.

Toyoshima, S., Hirata, F., Axelrod, J., Beppu, M., Osawa, T., and Waxdal, M. J., 1982a, The relationship between phospholipid methylation and calcium influx in murine lymphocytes stimulated with native and modified Con A, *Mol. Immunol.* **19:**229–234.

Toyoshima, S., Hirata, F., Iwata, M., Axelrod, J., Osawa, T., and Waxdal, M. J., 1982b, Lectin-induced mitosis and phospholipid methylation, *Mol. Immunol.* **19:**467–476.

Trotter, J., and Ferber, E., 1981, CoA-dependent cleavage of arachidonic acid from phosphatidylcholine and transfer to phosphatidylethanolamine in homogenates of murine thymocytes, *FEBS Lett.* **128:**237–241.

Trotter, J., Fleisch, I., Schmidt, B., and Ferber, E., 1982, Acyltransferase-catalyzed cleavage of arachidonic acid from phospholipids and transfer to lysophosphatides in lymphocytes and macrophages, *J. Biol. Chem.* **257:**1816–1823.

Tsien, R. Y., Pozzan, T., and Rink, T. J., 1982, T-cell mitogens cause early changes in cytoplasmic free Ca^{2+} and membrane potential in lymphocytes, *Nature (Lond.)* **295:**68–70.

Tsuda, H., Maeda, H., and Kishimoto, S., 1981, Fluorescence polarization with FDA in leukemic cells: A clear difference between myelogenous and lymphocytic organs, *Br. J. Cancer* **43:**793–803.

Udey, M. C., and Parker, C. W., 1982, Effects of inhibitors of arachidonic acid metabolism on alpha-aminoisobutyric acid transport in human lymphocytes, *Biochem. Pharmacol.* **31:**337–345.

Udey, M. C., Chaplin, D. D., Wedner, M. J., and Parker, C. W., 1980, Early activation events in lectin-stimulated human lymphocytes, *J. Immunol.* **125:**1544–1550.

Van Blitterswijk, W. J., DeVeer, G., Krol, J. H., and Emmelot, P., 1982, Comparative lipid analysis of purified plasma membranes and shed extracellular membrane vesicles from normal murine thymocytes and leukemic GRSL cells, *Biochim. Biophys. Acta* **688:**495–504.

Van den Berg, K. J., and Betel, I., 1971, Early increase of amino acid transport in stimulated lymphocytes, *Exp. Cell. Res.* **66:**257–259.

Van den Berg, K. J., and Betel, I., 1973a, Increased transport of 2-aminoisobutyric acid in rat lymphocytes stimulated with concanavalin A, *Exp. Cell. Res.* **76:**63–72.

Van den Berg, K. J., and Betel, I., 1973b, Selective early activation of a sodium dependent amino acid transport system in stimulated rat lymphocyte, *FEBS Lett.* **29:**149–152.

Van den Berg, K. J., and Betel, I., 1974a, Correlation of early changes in amino acid transport and DNA synthesis in stimulated lymphocytes, *Cell. Immunol.* **10:**319–323.

Van den Berg, K. J., and Betel, I., 1974b, Regulation of amino acid uptake in lymphocytes stimulated by mitogens, *Exp. Cell. Res.* **84:**412–418.

Varesio, L., and Holden, J. T., 1980, Mechanisms of lymphocyte activation: Linkage between early protein synthesis and late lymphocyte proliferation, *J. Immunol.* **124:**2288–2294.

Varesio, L., Holden, H. T., Taramelli, D., 1980, Mechanism of lymphocyte activation, *J. Immunol.* **125:**2810–2816.

Wagshal, A., and Waksman, B., 1978, Regulatory substances produced by lymphocytes. VIII. Cell cycle specificity of inhibitory of DNA synthesis (IDS) action in lymphocytes, *J. Immunol.* **121:** 966–972.

Wagshal, A., Jegasothy, B., and Waksman, B., 1978, Regulatory substances produced by lymphocytes. VI. Cell cycle specificity of inhibitor of DNA synthesis action in L cells, *J. Exp. Med.* **147:**171–181.

Waksman, B. H., Dessaint, J-P., and Katz, S. P., 1980, Proteolysis, calcium and cyclic nucleotides in macrophage T-lymphocyte interaction, in: *Biochemical Characterization of Lymphokines* (A. L. deWeck, F. Kristensen, and M. Landz, eds.), pp. 435–443, Academic, New York.

Walls, E. V., Borghetti, A. F., Benzie, C. R., and Kay, J. E., 1984, Early events during the activation of human lymphocytes by the mitogenic monoclonal antibody OKT3. *Cell. Immunol.* **89:**30–38.

Walsh, J. V., and Singer, J. J., 1983, Ca^{2+}-activated K^+ channels in vertebrate smooth muscle cells, *Cell. Calcium* **4:**321–330.

Wands, J. R., Podolsky, D. K., and Isselbacher, K. J., 1976, Mechanism of human lymphocyte stimulation by concanavalin A: Role of valence and surface binding sites, *Proc. Natl. Acad. Sci. USA* **73:**2118–2122.

Wang, J. L., McClain, D. A., and Edelman, G. M., 1975a, Modulation of lymphocyte mitogenesis, *Proc. Natl. Acad. Sci. USA* **72:**1917–1921.

Wang, J. L., Gunther, G. R., and Edelman, G. M., 1975b, Inhibition by colchicine of the mitogenic stimulation of lymphocytes prior to the S phase, *J. Cell Biol.* **66:**128–144.

Wang, T., Sheppard, J. R., and Foker, J. E., 1978, Rise and fall of cyclic AMP required for onset of lymphocyte DNA synthesis, *Science* **201:**155–157.

Wang, T., Foker, J. E., and Malkinson, A. M., 1981, Protein phosphorylation in intact lymphocytes stimulated by concanavalin A, in *Exp. Cell. Res.* **134:**409–416.

Waterhouse, P. D., Anderson, P. L., and Brown, D. L., 1983, Increases in microtubule assembly and in tubulin content on mitogenically stimulated mouse splenic T lymphocytes, *Exp. Cell. Res.* **144:**367–376.

Watson, J., 1976, The involvement of cyclic nucleotide metabolism in the initiation of lymphocyte proliferation induced by mitogens, *J. Immunol.* **117:**1656–1663.

Watson, J., Epstein, R., and Cohn, M., 1973, Cyclic nucleotides as intracellular mediators of the expression of antigen-sensitive cells, *Nature (Lond.)* **246:**405–409.

Waxdal, M. J., 1980, Discussions, *Fourth International Congress on Immunology, Paris.*

Webb, D. R., and Jamieson, A. T., 1976, Control of mitogen-induced transformation: Characterization of a splenic suppressor cell and its mode of action, *Cell. Immunol.* **24:**45–57.

Webb, D. R., and Nowowiejski, I., 1981, Control of suppressor cell activation via endogenous prostaglandin synthesis: The role of T cells and macrophages, *Cell. Immunol.* **63:**321–328.

Webb, D. R., Stites, D. P., Perlman, J. D., Luong, D., and Fudenberg, H. H., 1973, Lymphocyte activation: The dualistic effect of cAMP, *Biochem. Biophys. Res. Commun.* **53:**1002–1008.

Webb, D. R., Belobradsky, B., Hanes, D., Stites, D. P., Perlman, J. D., and Fudenberg, H. H., 1975, Control of mitogen-induced lymphocyte activation, *Clin. Immunol. Immunopathol.* **4:** 226–240.

Weber, W. T., 1977, T-cell activation induced by cross-linking of anti-T cell directed antibodies with anti-immunoglobulin, in: *Regulatory Mechanisms in Lymphocyte Activation* (D. E. Lucas, ed.), p. 31, Academic, New York.

Weber, T. H., and Goldberg, M. L., 1975, Effects of leukoagglutinating phytohemagglutinin on cAMP and cGMP levels in lymphocytes, *Exp. Cell. Res.* **97:**432–435.

Weber, W., Schwock, G., Wielckens, K., Gartemann, A., and Hilz, H., 1981, cAMP receptor proteins and protein kinases in human lymphocytes: Fundamental alterations in chronic lymphocytic leukemaic cells, *Eur. J. Biochem.* **120**:585–592.

Wedner, H. J., and Parker, C. W., 1975, Protein phosphorylation in human peripheral lymphocytes-stimulation by phytohemagglutinin and N^6-monobutyryl cyclic AMP, *Biochem. Biophys. Res. Commun.* **62**:808–815.

Wedner, H. J., and Parker, C. W., 1976, Lymphocyte Activation, *Prog. Allergy* **20**:195–300.

Wedner, H. J., Dankner, R., and Parker, C. W., 1975, Cyclic GMP and lectin-induced lymphocyte activation, *J. Immunol.* **115**:1682–1687.

Weidemann, M. J., and Kolbuck-Braddon, M. E., 1982, The effect of trifluoperazine on concanavalin A-induced chemiluminescence, respiration and glycolysis in rat thymocytes, *Biochem. Internatl.* **4**:575–583.

Weiel, J. E., and Hamilton, T. A., 1984, Quiescent lymphocytes express intracellular transferrin receptors, *Biochem. Biophys. Res. Commun.* **119**:598–602.

Weinstein, Y., Chambers, D. A., Bourne, H. R., and Melmon, K. L., 1974, Cyclic GMP stimulates lymphocyte nucleic acid synthesis, *Nature (Lond.)* **251**:352–353.

Weinstein, Y., Segal, S., and Melmon, K. L., 1975, Specific mitogenic activity of 8-Br-guanosine 3′,5′-monophosphate (Br-cyclic GMP) on B lymphocytes, *J. Immunol.* **115**:112–117.

Weiss, A., Imboden, J., Hardy, K., Manger, B., Terhorst, C., and Stobi, J., 1986, The role of the T3/antigen receptor complex in T-cell activation, *Annu. Rev. Immunol.* **4**:593–619.

Weiss, B., and Winchurch, R. A., 1978, Analyses of cyclic nucleotide phosphodiesterases in lymphocytes from normal and aged leukemic mice, *Cancer Res.* **38**:1274–1280.

Wertz, P. W., and Mueller, G. C., 1978, Rapid stimulation of phospholipid metabolism in bovine lymphocytes by tumor-promoting phorbolesters, *Cancer Res.* **38**:2900–2904.

Wertz, P. W., and Mueller, G. C., 1980, Inhibition of 12-O-tetradecanoylphorbol-13-acetate accelerated phospholipid metabolism by 5,8,11,14-eicosatetraynoic acid, *Cancer Res.* **40**:776–781.

Wess, J. A., and Archer, D. L., 1981, Restoration by cyclic guanosine monophosphate and extracellular calcium of butylated hydroxyanisole-suppressed primary murine thymus-dependent antibody response, *Immunopharmacology* **3**:361–366.

Wess, J. A., and Archer, D. L., 1982, Evidence from *in vitro* murine immunologic assays that some phenolic food additives may function as antipromoters by lowering intracellular cyclic GMP levels, *Proc. Soc. Exp. Biol. Med.* **170**:427–430.

Whitesell, R. R., Johnson, R. A., Tarpley, H. L., and Regen, D. M., 1977, Mitogen-stimulated glucose transport in thymocytes. Possible role of Ca^{2+} and antagonism by adenosine 3′:5′-monophosphate, *J. Cell. Biol.* **72**:456–469.

Whitfield, J. F., and MacManus, J. P., 1972, Calcium-mediated effects of cyclic GMP on the stimulation of thymocyte proliferation by prostaglandin E_1, *Proc. Exp. Biol. Med.* **193**:818–824.

Whitfield, J. F., Rixon, R. H., Perris, A. D., and Youdale, T., 1969, Stimulation by calcium of the entry of thymic lymphocytes into the deoxyribonucleic acid-synthetic(S) phase of the cell cycle, *Exp. Cell. Res.* **57**:8–12.

Whitfield, J. F., MacManus, J. P., Boynton, A. L., Gillan, D. J., and Isaacs, R. J., 1974, Concanavalin A and the initiation of thymic lymphoblast DNA synthesis and proliferation by a calcium-dependent increase in cyclic GMP level, *J. Cell. Physiol.* **84**:445–458.

Whitfield, J. F., MacManus, J. P., Rixon, A. H., Boynton, A. L., Youdale, T., and Swierenga, S., 1976, The positive control of cell proliferation by the interplay of calcium and cyclic nucleotides: A review, *In Vitro* **12**:1–18.

Whitney, R. B., and Sutherland, R. M., 1972a, The influence of calcium, magnesium and cyclic adenosine 3′,5′-monophosphate on the mixed lymphocyte reaction, *J. Immunol.* **108**:1179–1183.

Whitney, R. B., and Sutherland, R. M., 1972b, Requirement for calcium ions in lymphocyte transformation stimulated by phytohemagglutinin, *J. Cell. Physiol.* **80:**329–338.

Whitney, R. B., and Sutherland, R. M., 1972c, Enhanced uptake of calcium by transforming lymphocytes, *Cell. Immunol.* **5:**137–147.

Whitney, R. B., and Sutherland, R. M., 1973a, Effects of chelating agents on the initial interaction of phytohemagglutinin with lymphocytes and the subsequent stimulation of amino acid uptake, *Biochim. Biophys. Acta* **298:**790–797.

Whitney, R. B., and Sutherland, R. M., 1973b, Characteristics of calcium accumulation by lymphocytes and alteration in the process induced by phytohemagglutinin, *J. Cell. Physiol.* **82:**9–20.

Williams, D. B., Perera, M. A., Facca, L. A., Heng, Y. M., Simon, G. T., Dorrington, K. J., and Klein, M. H., 1986, Role of calcium remobilization in antigen specific T-cell activation, in: *Sixth International Congress of Immunology Toronto, Canada* (abst. #26), p. 234.

Williams, J. M., Ransil, B. J., Shapiro, H. M., and Strom, T. B., 1984, Accessory cell requirement for activation antigen expression and cell cycle progression by human T-lymphocytes, *J. Immunol.* **133:**2986–2994.

Williams, R. O., and Loeb, L. A., 1973, Zinc requirement for DNA replication in stimulated human lymphocytes, *J. Cell. Biol.* **58:**594–601.

Wood, P. J., Pao, G., and Cooper, A., 1984, Changes in guinea pig plasma cyclic nucleotide levels during the development of transplantable leukemia, *Cancer* **53:**79–82.

Wright, P., Quastel, M. R., and Kaplan, J. G., 1973, Differential sensitivity of antigen- and mitogen-stimulated human leukocytes to prolonged inhibition of potassium transport, *Exp. Cell. Res.* **79:**87–94.

Yahara, I., and Edelman, G. M., 1972, Restriction of the mobility of lymphocyte immunoglobulin receptors by concanavalin A, *Proc. Natl. Acad. Sci. USA* **69:**608–612.

Yahara, I., and Edelman, G. M., 1973, The effects of concanavalin A on the mobility of lymphocyte surface receptors, *Exp. Cell. Res.* **81:**143–155.

Yahara, I., and Edelman, G. M., 1975, Modulation of lymphocyte receptor mobility by locally bound concanavalin A, *Proc. Nat. Acad. Sci.* **72:**1579–1583.

Yang, S. V., Chouaib, S., and Dupont, B., 1986, A common pathway for T lymphocyte activation involving both the CD3–Ti complex and CD2 sheep erythrocyte receptor determinants, *J. Immunol.* **137:**1097–1100.

Yasmeen, D., Laird, A. J., Hume, D. A., and Weidemann, M. J., 1977, Activation of 3-O-methyl-glucose transport in rat thymus lymphocytes by concanavalin A, *Biochim. Biophys. Acta* **500:** 89–102.

Yoshinaga, M., Waksman, B., and Malawista, S. E., 1972, Inhibition of lymphocyte triggering by cytochalasin B, *Transplant. Proc.* **4:**325–327.

Yunis, A. A., Arimura, G. K., and Kipnis, D. M., 1963, Amino acid transport in blood cells. I. Effect of cations and amino acid transport in human leukocytes, *J. Lab. Clin. Med.* **62:**465–476.

Zachowski, A., Lelievre, L., Aubry, J., Charlemagne, D., and Paraf, A., 1977, Roles of proteins from inner face of plasma membranes in susceptibility of adenosinetriphosphatase to ouabain, *Proc. Natl. Acad. Sci. USA* **74:**633–637.

Zimmerman, T. P., Schmitges, C. J., Wolberg, G., Deeprose, R. D., Duncan, G. S., Cuatrecasass, P., and Elion, G. B., 1980, Modulation of cyclic AMP metabolism by S-adenosylhomocysteine and S-3-deazadenosylhomocysteine in mouse lymphocytes, *Proc. Natl. Acad. Sci. USA* **77:** 5639–5643.

Zwiller, J., Revel, M.-O., and Malviya, A. N., 1985, Protein kinase C catalyzes phosphorylation of guanylate cyclase *in vitro, J. Biol. Chem.* **260:**1350–1356.

CHAPTER 6

TOXICITY TO THE IMMUNE SYSTEM: A REVIEW

JACK H. DEAN, JOEL B. CORNACOFF, and MICHAEL I. LUSTER

1. INTRODUCTION

Immunotoxicology is defined as the study of events that lead to undesired effects as a result of interaction of foreign substances (e.g., xenobiotics) with the immune system. Toxic responses might arise when the immune system either (1) acts as a passive target of chemical insult, leading to a relatively broad-spectrum loss or potentiation of function; or (2) responds to the antigenic specificity of the chemical as part of a specific immune response. In the latter instance, a more limited population of antigen-specific immune cells is the initial target of the chemical interaction, with the potential for toxic responses to occur (e.g., in the skin or lungs), subsequent to the specific interaction between the chemical antigen (hapten) and host antibody or sensitized cells.

Chemically induced toxicity involving the immune system as the target may result in an increased incidence of infectious disease, the development of neo-

Abbreviations used in this chapter: AB, antibody; CMI, cell-mediated immunity; Con A, concanavalin A; CSA, cyclosporin A; CTL, cytotoxic T lymphocyte; CY, cyclophosphamide; DBCT, di-*n*-butyltin dichloride; DES, diethylstilbestrol; DOTC, di-*n*-octyltin dichloride; DTH, delayed-type hypersensitivity; ELISA, enzyme-linked immunosorbent assay; GVH, graft versus host; HMI, humoral mediated immunity; Ig, immunoglobulin; IL-1, interleukin 1; IL-2, interleukin 2; Mφ, macrophage; MLR, mixed leukocyte response; MTD, maximum tolerated dose; NK, natural killer (cell); PBB, polybrominated biphenyls; PC, plasma cell; PCB, polychorinated biphenyls; PFC, plaque-forming cell; PG, prostaglandin; PGE₂, prostaglandin E₂; SRBC, sheep red blood cells; TCDD, 2,3,7,8-tetrachlorodibenzo-*p*-dioxin.

JACK H. DEAN and JOEL B. CORNACOFF • Sterling Research Group, Rensselaer, New York 12144.   MICHAEL I. LUSTER • National Toxicology Programs, National Institute of Environmental Health Science, Research Triangle Park, North Carolina 27709.

plasia, or autoimmune effects associated with immune dysregulation. The health consequences of exposure to chemicals that the immune system responds to as "nonself" (i.e., hypersensitivity) may be, *inter alia,* respiratory tract allergies to the specific substance (e.g., asthma, rhinitis) or allergic contact dermatitis to that substance, or autoimmune diseases in which the foreign substance modifies the host's tissue. Immunotoxicology is concerned with the identification and quantification of the components described above and with assessment of their importance in terms of human or animal health. In recent years, the science of toxicology has expanded along organ- or system-specific lines, to which are added studies on particular hazards.

    The immune system is a highly regulated network of lymphoid cells requiring continued renewal, activation, and differentiation for full immunocompetence. The functions of the immune system include discrimination of self from nonself and defense against infectious micro-organisms and spontaneously arising neoplasia. Cell depletion, dysregulation, and functional deficits within this cellular network can result in a pathological process marked by altered responses to self- and nonself-antigens or increased susceptibility to infectious agents and tumor cells. It can therefore be easily appreciated that the immune system may be a frequent target organ for cytotoxic drug and nondrug chemicals. A large number of diverse compounds or their metabolites possess the capacity to induce autoimmunity or allergic responses in susceptible individuals (e.g., diisocyantes, penicillamine) (Table I). Conversely, immunosuppression has been well documented to occur following exposure of humans or animals to a wide range of chemicals (Table II), including inorganic pollutants, halogenated and nonhalogenated aromatic hydrocarbons, and therapeutic agents. Although several chemicals of occupational or environmental concern have produced immune modification in rodents and are suspected of producing similar effects in humans, in most cases rigorous clinical confirmation of altered immunological responsiveness is incomplete. Immunomodulatory activity (i.e., immunosuppression or immune enhancement) has been beneficially exploited in the development of antineoplastic agents and so-called biological response modifiers (BRMs) proposed for immunotherapy of immune deficiency and certain types of neoplasia.

    The distribution of mononuclear phagocytes and lymphocytes throughout the body requires that they cope with the many xenobiotics (e.g., physical agents, chemicals, and drugs) that enter through the skin, blood, digestive tract, or pulmonary system. During the past decade, numerous studies have shown that exposure of rodents to chemicals or drugs by dosing protocols that did not cause overt toxicity often produced immune alterations sufficient to result in altered host resistance to challenge with infectious agents or neoplastic cells (Dean *et al.,* 1982, 1986b; Faith *et al.,* 1980; Vos, 1977). For certain environmental agents, the relevance of many of these rodent exposure studies to human health effects awaits further investigation. In the case of such drugs as cyclophosphamide, methotrexate, or cyclosporin A, the immune effects seen in rodents were comparable to immune alterations observed in the clinic (Dean *et al.,* 1987).

TABLE I

Xenobiotics Known or Presumed to Produce Autoimmune or Allergic Syndromes in Experimental Animals or Humans[a]

Autoimmune syndromes	Hypersensitivity/allergy
Acetazolamide	Antioxidants
Anticonvulsants	Antibiotics
Chloropromazine	Ampicillin
Chlorothiazides	Spiramycin
Gold salts	Penicillin
Hydralazine	Sulfathiazole
Isoniazid	Neomycin sulfate
Methyldopa	Castor beans
Penicillamine	Chloramine
Procainamide	Dusts
Propranolol	House
Quinidine	Organic
Rifampin	Cotton
Salicylates	Antibiotic
Sulfa	Wood
Sulfonamides	Diisocyanates
Vinyl chloride	TDI
	HDI
	MDI
	Dichlorphene
	Enzymes
	Hog trypsin
	Pancreatic papain
	Subtilin
	Ethylenediamine
	Formaldehyde
	Green coffee beans
	Grain and flour
	Insecticides
	Hexachlorophene
	Metals
	Pt
	Ni
	BE
	Hg
	Natural resins
	Phenylglycine acid
	Phosphorus (organic)
	Pyrolysis products of PVC
	Phthalic anhydride
	Resorcinal
	Trimellitic anhydride
	Vegetable gums

[a]From Dean et al. (1986a).

TABLE II
Xenobiotics Known to Produce Immunosuppression or Immunomodulation in Rodents[a]

Aflatoxin
Airborne pollutants
  O_3
  NO_2
  SO_2
  Asbestos
Benzene
Benzidine
Diethylstilbestrol
Drugs
  Therapeutic (partial listing)
    Cyclophosphamide
    Busulfan
    BCNU
    DTIC
    Prednisone
    6-Mercaptopurine
    5-FU
    Methotrexate
    Cyclosporin A
    Estradiol
  Abused
    Ethanol
    Cannabinoids
Halogenated aromatic hydrocarbons
  PCB
  PBB
  TCDD
  TCDF
Insecticides
  DDT
  Mirex
  Aldrin
  Lindane
  Carbaryl
Metals
  Pb
  Cd
  Hg
Organometals
  Dioctyltindichloride
  Dibutyltindichloride
  Methyl mercury
Phorbol esters
Polycyclic aromatic hydrocarbons
B[a]P
  1,2,5,6-DBA
  BA
  3-MCA
  7,12-DMBA
Urethane

[a]From Dean *et al.* (1986a).

2. HUMAN HEALTH EFFECTS

Intentional or accidental exposure of humans to certain of these immunotoxic xenobiotics has produced immunomodulation and an increased incidence of infectious disease or neoplasia (Kammüller et al., 1984; Penn, 1985). Several incidences of accidental exposure have been reported to result in immunological abnormalities (Table III): (1) Michigan farm residents exposed to PBB contaminating dairy products and meat showed impaired lymphocyte blastogenesis to mitogens and E rosette formation (Bekesi et al., 1978, 1987); (2) an increased frequency of infectious disease followed exposure of Taiwanese and Japanese to rice oil contaminated with PCB (Chang et al., 1982b; Wu et al., 1984); (3) pneumonitis and Sjögren-like syndrome resulted from the ingestion of isothiocyanate-derived imidazolidinethione compounds in adulterated rapeseed oil sold as olive oil in Spain (CDC, 1981; Gomez-Reino, 1987; Kammüller et al., 1984; Kammüller et al., 1986); and (4) altered skin-test reactivity to recall antigens and lymphocyte subset numbers occurred among Missouri residents exposed to TCDD (Hoffman et al., 1986). An increased evidence of pulmonary infections

TABLE III

Xenobiotics Reported to Produce Immunological Dysfunction in Both Rodents and Humans[a]

Chemical class	Agent	Immune disturbance		Reference
		Rodent	Human	
Aromatic amines	Benzidine	+	+	Gorodilova and Mandrik (1978)
Aromatic hydro-carbons	Benzene and other solvents	+	+	Lange et al. (1973); Denkhaus et al. (1986)
Polyhalogenated aromatic hydrocarbons	TCDD	+	+	Hoffman et al. (1986)
	PCB	+	+	Chang et al. (1982b)
	PBB	+	+	Bekesi et al. (1978)
Oxidant gases (air pollutants)	NO_2	+	+	Lunn et al. (1967); French et al. (1973)
	O_3	+	+	Lunn et al. (1967); French et al. (1973)
	SO_3	+	+	Lunn et al. (1967); French et al. (1973)
Others	Asbestos	+	+	Lew et al. (1986)
	DES	+	+	Kalland and Haukass (1981)

[a]Modified from Berlin et al. (1986).

has also been observed in humans following exposure to noxious gases (e.g., ozone, nitrogen dioxide, sulfur dioxide) and airborne particulates (French et al., 1973; Lunn et al., 1967; NRC, 1978, 1979). Although clinical studies of these accidental exposures have provided some data regarding human health effects, they do not define mechanisms of toxicity or clarify dose–response relationships. Rodent models continue to provide the only means for such determinations and are crucial to the safety evaluation of chemicals.

3. PREDICTABILITY OF ANIMAL STUDIES FOR IMMUNOTOXICITY

A large body of data has developed over the past 10 years demonstrating that xenobiotic exposure can produce immune dysfunction and altered host resistance in experimental animals following acute and chronic exposure (reviewed by Vos, 1977; Dean et al., 1982, 1986a; Luster et al., 1987), although only a limited number of reports indicate immune dysfunction following human exposure to xenobiotics (reviewed by Dean et al., 1982, 1986b; Berlin et al., 1987).

Among the issues of comparative toxicology among species are the selection of appropriate animal models and the design of experimental protocols that accurately correspond to xenobiotic or metabolite exposure in the species of predominant interest, most frequently humans, for risk assessment. It is crucial to weigh species variations in the design of toxicological studies for application to humans, since biological diversity may confound efforts for accurate predictions of toxicity. A well-designed toxicological study (e.g., the preclinical toxicology of CSA) provides reassurance that at least basic similarities exist in the toxicity between rodents and humans and that these similarities also extend to the immunotoxicology and immunopharmacology of immunologically active agents (Ryffiel et al., 1983; Thomas et al., 1984). During the premarket development of a drug or chemical, the compound is screened to determine its toxicity profile in one or more rodent species. Table IV summarizes the comparative immunosuppressive profile for the immunosuppressive drug CSA in several species. The immunological effects produced, as well as the doses producing these end points, were similar in all species. The rat was slightly more susceptible to the immunosuppressive effects of CSA than the mouse (2- to 10-fold higher dose required). This slight species difference was further reflected in the LD_{50} to CSA in these two rodent species (mouse: 2329 mg/kg p.o.; rat: 1480 mg/kg p.o.).

Despite the close correlation of toxicity profiles among species examined with CSA, toxic responses to a chemical are potentially variable among different species. Ideally, toxicity testing should be performed with a species that will elicit chemical-related pharmacology and toxicities similar to those anticipated in humans (i.e, the test animals and humans will metabolize the chemical similarly and will have identical target organ responses and toxicity). Toxicological stud-

TABLE IV
Species Comparison of Immune Responses Suppressed by Cyclosporin A[a,b]

Species	Response	Antigen/model	CSA dose
Mouse	AB production	SRBC, DNP–(Ficoll, Dextran)	50–300
	CMI (DTH)	Marrow graft	100–300
	GVH reaction	SRBC,BCG, oxazalone	50–250
Rat	AB production	SRBC, DNP–KLH, MHC	20–50
	GVH reaction	Marrow graft, lymph node assay	10–60
Guinea pig	CMI (DTH)	BCG, OVA, DNCB, DNFB	10–100
Dog	CMI (DTH)	Marrow graft	15–30
Rhesus monkey	AB production	SRBC	50–250

[a]From Dean and Thurmond (1987).
[b]Abbreviations used: AB, antibody; BCG, bacillus Calmette-Guérin; CMI, cell-mediated immunity; CSA, cyclosporin A dosage range (in mg/kg); DNCB, dinitrochlorobenzene; DNFB, dinitrofluorobenzene; DNP, dinitrophenol; DNP–KLH, DNP–keyhole limpet hemocyanin; MHC, histocompatability antigens; OVA, ovalbumin; SRBC, sheep red blood cells.

ies are conducted in a variety of animal species, since the ideal animal for extrapolation may not exist. Priority should be given to animal species that demonstrate metabolism, pharmacokinetics, pharmacological effects, and suspected target organ specificity as similar to humans as possible.

Rodent data on target organ toxicities and comparability of immunosuppressive doses have generally been predictive of what was later to be observed in the clinic with most immunosuppressive drugs. Exceptions to the predictive value of rodent toxicological data are infrequently seen but have occurred in studies of glucocorticoids, which are lympholytic in rodents, but not in primates (Haynes and Murad, 1985). Although certain compounds may exhibit different pharmacokinetics (absorption, disposition, metabolism, and pharmacological effect) in rodents than in humans, rodents still appear to be the most appropriate animal model for examining the immunotoxicity of non-species-specific compounds, based on established similarities of toxicological profiles as well as the ease of generating host susceptibility challenge and immune function data. Comparative toxicological studies must be continued and expanded as novel recombinant biological compounds enter safety testing, since host interactions and species specificity may present new toxicological profiles for consideration.

4. IMMUNOTOXICOLOGICAL ASSESSMENT IN RODENTS

The potential of the immune system as a target organ for xenobiotic toxicity stems from three characteristics of the system. First, functional immunocompetent cells are required for host resistance to infectious agents and neoplastic cells. Second, immunocompetent cells must undergo continual renewal via proliferation and differentiation to remain functional, and both processes are known to be quite sensitive to chemical perturbation. Third, a regulatory network of soluble factors and cell–cell contact is necessary for immunocompetence. Detrimental alterations in the balance of the immune regulatory network affecting critical interactions between lymphoid cells may cause detectable changes in discrete components of immune function. However, such alterations may still be within the functional or physiological reserve of the immune system and not produce significant impairment in the whole animal.

Immunotoxicity assessments require validation of the end points to be measured (quality control and biological relevance) as well as knowledgeable selection of animal models, exposure parameters, and other general toxicological parameters. The evaluation of functional immune capacity in rodents involves testing of specific immunologic functions *in vitro* and measurements of host resistance to disease. Correlations between *in vitro* functions and host resistance to disease have been demonstrated (Dean *et al.*, 1987). These may be combined with toxicological data to provide the most efficiently generated comparative data base for estimation of human risk.

Immune dysfunction produced by chemical or drug exposure is dependent on the type of immunological injury characteristic of the xenobiotic, the chemical threshold and toxicokinetics of the compound, and the functional reserve of the immune function affected. Dose selection is critical to the validity of immunologic assessment, since severe stress and malnutrition are known to impair immune responsiveness. The general toxicological data base (including LD_{50}, LD_{10}, and MTD data) should be used when available to establish preliminary exposure protocols. Three exposure levels are recommended to establish the dose effect relationships; the lowest dose should cause no alteration in immune function. The highest dose used should be considerably lower than the LD_{10} and should have no associated mortality—especially important in the design of host resistance studies. Selection of the exposure route should parallel the probable natural route of exposure in humans, which is frequently oral, carried out by feeding dosed laboratory animal chow or water, or by gavage. A requirement for an accurate delivered dose may require the use of the parenteral, subcutaneous, or intraperitoneal exposure routes. Because xenobiotic exposure of humans frequently occurs via the respiratory tract, a reasonable exposure protocol for laboratory animals would be by inhalation or intratracheal instillation. All *in vitro* assays described herein are performed *ex vivo* following *in vivo* exposure of the animal to the test compound.

Two hallmarks of the complexity of the immune system are the diversity of immunomodulatory mechanisms and the variety of adverse effects that may be induced by immunotoxicants or immunomodulatory drugs. Therefore, preclinical or prerelease testing of xenobiotics suspected of immunotoxicity represents a process of extreme importance. A flexible tiered approach to the safety assessment of potential immunotoxic chemicals or immunomodulatory drugs has been recommended as a logical and efficient testing protocol (Berlin et al., 1987). It was concluded that the immunological evaluation encompassing a battery of validated and refined methods must maintain a suitable degree of flexibility because of the varied nature and characteristics of xenobiotic-induced alterations of the immune system. Assessment tiers would be expected to improve in sensitivity, predictive value, and cost effectiveness as they are applied. Most of the methods previously proposed (Dean et al., 1979; Vos, 1977) have recently undergone scientific validation through a limited interlaboratory comparison in the United States and have been used extensively in several laboratories (Luster et al., 1988a; Vos and Dean, 1987). A preliminary correlation has been demonstrated between depression of certain immune functions and increased susceptibility to challenge with certain defined infectious agents and transplantable tumor cells (Dean et al., 1987). Recently, a preclinical rodent screen was proposed for determining the appropriate dosing schedule and underlying mechanisms of action of biological response-modifying drugs or biologicals newly proposed as therapeutic modalities (Talmadge et al., 1984) and for assessing their efficacy.

The structure of an immune-function assay tier may vary somewhat among the various groups working in immunotoxicology and immunopharmacology, partly because of the use of different animal species. This is particularly true regarding the application of bacterial, viral, and tumor challenge models. A flexible approach to immunotoxicity assessment (Moore et al., 1982) was adopted by the National Toxicology Program (NTP) as part of its Special Studies Panel for Immunotoxicology Assessment and has undergone extensive validation (Luster et al., 1988a). The phase 1 panel currently used for immunotoxicity evaluation at the Chemical Industry Institute of Toxicology (CIIT) and in the NTP is divided into two levels (Table V) and encompasses both in vivo and in vitro measures of quantitative and functional changes in immune status. Level 1 testing can be performed in the mouse or the rat as well as in several other species.

The recent evaluation of a wide range of chemicals has demonstrated that significant toxic effects manifested in the immune system of rodents include changes in lymphoid organ weights and histology, alterations in the humoral immune response (e.g., depressed ability to generate specific antibody plaque-forming cells), and depression of lymphocyte proliferation in response to foreign cell-associated antigens (Dean et al., 1986a; Luster et al., 1987). Routine toxicity assessments that fail to include the most basic indicators of immune dysfunction (i.e., alterations in lymphoid organ weights, cellularity, or histopathology) run a significant risk of overlooking a potentially immunotoxic chemical. Possible indicators (''flags'') of selective toxicity for the immune system that might be observed during the routine toxicological evaluation of a chemical are listed in Table VI.

TABLE V
Approach for Detecting Immunotoxic Alterations[a]

Parameters	Procedures
Level 1 (mouse or rat)	
Immunopathology	Routine hematology;[b] lymphoid organ weights (spleen, thymus), histology (spleen, thymus, lymph nodes),[b] cellularity (spleen and bone marrow)[b]
Cell-mediated immunity	
Proliferation	Mixed leukocyte response[b]
Tumoricidal	NK cell activity
Antibody-mediated immunity	Antibody PFC[b] or specific immunoglobulin level
Level 2 (mouse only)	
Immunopathology	Quantification of lymphocyte subpopulations using surface markers (monoclonal antibody reagents)
Host-resistance challenge models	PYB6 sarcoma;[b] B16F10 melanoma;[b] Listeria monocytogenes,[b] Streptococcus, or influenza virus[b]
Cell-mediated immunity	
Proliferation	Mitogen (Con A, LPS) response[b]
Tumoricidal	Cytotoxic T-cell cytolysis
Macrophage function	Phagocytosis, ectoenzymes

[a]From Dean et al. (1984a).
[b]Included in the National Toxicology Program Panel.

5. IMMUNOTOXIC XENOBIOTICS: BACKGROUND AND MECHANISM OF ACTION

A substantial data base exists demonstrating that a broad spectrum of environmental pollutants and drugs can alter immune function in laboratory animals. This identification of the immune system as a sensitive target organ for chemicals has prompted additional research into the subcellular and molecular events responsible for the immunotoxicological manifestation of certain xenobiotics. The following is a broad representation of compounds shown to modulate immune function and is representative of those xenobiotics that have been exam-

TABLE VI
Possible Indicators of Immunotoxic Effect Observed during
Toxicological Evaluation of Chemicals

Increased mortality due to infectious agent
Rapid onset of neoplasia
Altered hematology parameter
Changes in lymphoid organ:body weight ratio (thymus, spleen)
Changes in lymphoid organ cellularity (bone marrow, spleen)
Changes in histology of lymphoid organs (thymus, lymph nodes, spleen, bone marrow)

ined in depth. Each example provides a general overview and discusses the mechanism of injury in those cases in which it is known.

5.1. Polycyclic Aromatic Hydrocarbons

Polycyclic aromatic hydrocarbons (PAH) are a class of widely disseminated compounds consisting of three or more fused benzene rings. These compounds are formed as products of incomplete combustion of fossil fuels and can be found as environmental contaminants in automobile exhaust, soot, and tobacco smoke (Zedeck, 1980). Human exposures occur primarily through breathing polluted air, eating and drinking contaminated food and water, and tobacco smoke. Human health risks associated with PAH have centered primarily around their carcinogenic potential. A correlation that has emerged following examination of their immunotoxicity indicates that those PAH that are carcinogenic possess potent immunosuppressive properties, while those that are not carcinogenic lack substantial immunosuppressive effects (Ward et al., 1985). This has led to the suggestion that the potential of a chemical to cause immunosuppression may serve as a cofactor for carcinogenicity either by altering immunocompetence and allowing tumor neoantigens to bypass normal host-immune surveillance, or, once established, by preventing normal immune mechanisms from inhibiting tumor growth and metastasis, or both.

Suppression of humoral immunity has been frequently observed following exposure to a number of PAH, including benzo(a)pyrene (B[a]P), 7,12-dimethylbenzanthracene (DMBA), and 3-methylcholanthrene (3-MC) (reviewed by Ward et al., 1985; Dean et al., 1986a; Luster et al., 1987). These xenobiotics have been shown to suppress the antibody response to T-dependent (SRBC) and T-independent antigens (TNP-carrier) (Stjernsward, 1966; Dean et al., 1983; White et al., 1985; Ward et al., 1984). In the case of DMBA, the suppression in antibody-forming cell responses persisted for more than 8 weeks after exposure (Ward et al., 1986). While humoral immunosuppression following DMBA exposure may reside at the level of T-cell regulation, the finding of reduced progenitor B cells (CFU-BL) in exposed animals suggests that B cells may be directly targeted early in their maturational process (Ward et al., 1984). B(a)P has also been shown to impair production of IL1, implicating chemical-induced defects in accessory cell function as a contributing factor in decreased antibody-forming cell production (Lyte and Bick, 1986).

Cell-mediated immunity is also inhibited by PAH. Cytotoxic T-cell activity is suppressed by DMBA or 3-MC following in vitro as well as in vivo exposure in mice (Wojdani and Alfred, 1984; Dean et al., 1985, 1986a; Lill and Gangami, 1986). Additional measures of CMI suppressed following DMBA, B(a)P, and 3-MC exposure include mixed lymphocyte responsiveness and NK cell activity (Dean et al., 1985, 1986b; Ward et al., 1984; Urso et al., 1986; Lill and Gangami, 1986). Apparently, because of more pronounced CMI effects, DMBA, but not B(a)P, demonstrated a marked increase in host susceptibility to *Listeria monocytogenes* and PYB6 sarcoma challenges (Ward et al., 1984). The addition of IL-2 or T-helper cells, but not IL-1, to cultures of DMBA-exposed lymphocytes, restored CTL function, suggesting that T-helper cells may be a sensitive target following *in vitro* and *in vivo* exposure (House *et al.*, 1987).

The mechanism(s) by which PAH produce immunosuppression is not completely understood. The carcinogenic members of this class are believed to require metabolic activation to reactive species capable of forming nucleic acid and/or protein adducts. This is true in the case of methylated compounds, which form methylene carbonium ions. Hepatic PAH metabolism is not a prerequisite for immunosuppression, as the addition of B(a)P or DMBA to lymphocyte cultures results in suppression. Lymphocytes and monocytes are known to possess inducible cytochrome P-450 activity. Although not demonstrated in lymphocytes, B(a)P and DMBA can be oxidized to reactive species by prostaglandin synthetase.

5.2. Halogenated Aromatic Hydrocarbons

Halogenated aromatic hydrocarbons (HAH) represent a family of compounds with widespread environmental distribution. Primary sources of HAH result from commercial production as industrial chemicals, pesticides, flame retardants, and heat conductors, as well as by-products in the manufacture of halogenated biphenyls or phenols or at commercial incinerators. Laboratory studies have demonstrated that a number of HAH possess immunomodulatory potential, including specific chlorinated dibenzo-*p*-dioxins, dibenzofurans, hexachlorobenzene, polychlorinated biphenyl, and polybrominated biphenyls (reviewed by Thomas and Faith, 1985; Silkworth and Vecchi, 1985). In addition, selected isomers of this class of compounds have been associated with teratogenic, carcinogenic, neurotoxic, and hepatotoxic effects (reviewed by Kimbrough, 1980).

The first indication that PCBs affects the immune system stemmed from observations of altered weight and histology of lymphoid organs in experimental animal studies (Vos *et al.*, 1980). Functionally, PCB-mediated immunotoxicity in laboratory animals is characterized by suppressed humoral immunity. Administration of highly chlorinated biphenyls to guinea pigs (Vos *et al.*, 1980), rabbits (Koller and Thigpan, 1973), rhesus monkeys (Thomas and Hinsdill, 1978), or mice (Silkworth and Grabstein, 1982; Wierda *et al.*, 1981) inhibits antibody production. The effects on CMI are less clear. PCBs have been reported to suppress DTH reactions in guinea pigs (Vos and van Driel Grootenhuis, 1972) but not mitogenic responses, MLR, graft-versus-host reactions, or cytotoxic T-lymphocyte activity of spleen cells in mice (Silkworth and Loose, 1981). PCBs also alter host resistance to a number of infectious agents, including *Plasmodium berghei* (Loose *et al.*, 1978), *Listeria monocytogenes* (Smith *et al.*, 1978), *Salmonella typhimurium* (Thomas and Hinsdill, 1978), and herpes simplex (Imaniski *et al.*, 1980). Increased tumor growth following inoculation with Walkers 256 carcinoma cells (Kerkvliet and Kimeldorf, 1977) and Ehrlich's ascites tumor

(Keck, 1982), but not Moloney leukemia virus (Koller, 1977) or MKSA or L1210 tumor cell implants (Loose *et al.*, 1981), occurs in PCB-exposed animals. Immunological changes consistent with those seen in animal studies have been reported in persons accidentally exposed in Japan and Taiwan to PCBs and PCDFs through consumption of contaminated rice oil (Lee and Chang, 1985; Wu *et al.*, 1984).

The most widely studied HAH is 2,3,7,8-tetrachlorodebenzo-*p*-dioxin (TCDD). Predominant features of TCDD toxicity include myelosuppression, immunodysregulation, and thymic atrophy, which occur in most all species examined thus far and at concentrations that preclude overt toxicity (reviewed by Vos *et al.*, 1980; Dean and Lauer, 1983; Thomas and Faith, 1985; Luster *et al.*, 1987). TCDD administered to mice has been associated with thymic atrophy, myelotoxicity, inhibition of complement system components, suppression of lymphocyte function, as well as impaired host resistance to challenge with *Salmonella bern* and *Plasmodium yoelii*, but not *Listeria monocytogenes* (Luster *et al.*, 1980, 1985a). It appears that macrophage and NK function are spared from any measurable effect (Mantovani *et al.*, 1980; Lauer *et al.*, 1987). As probably occurs with a number of immunosuppressive HAH, the specific effects of TCDD on the immune system can vary depending on the age of the animal relative to chemical exposure. For example, the primary effect following perinatal TCDD exposure is persistent suppression of cellular immunity, a condition mimicking neonatal thymectomy (Vos and Moore, 1974). In contrast to perinatal exposure, TCDD exposure in adult mice, while still inducing deterioration of thymic tissue (predominantly cortical lymphoid depletion), causes a transient antiproliferative response in rapidly dividing cell populations including progenitor hematopoietic cells and B lymphocytes (Faith and Luster, 1979; Tucker *et al.*, 1986). The marked and persistent suppression of T-cell function seen in neonates is not manifested following adult exposure, although suppression of cytotoxic T-lymphocyte response are reported to occur (Clark *et al.*, 1981).

Regardless of the status of maturity at the time of exposure, immunosuppression by TCDD, as well as PCBs, is believed mediated throughout stereospecific and irreversible binding to an intracellular receptor protein found in the cellular targets for TCDD, including lymphoid tissue, bone marrow cells, and thymic epithelium (Thomas and Faith, 1985). This receptor is termed the *Ah* receptor and is controlled by the *Ah* locus, which is also responsible for microsomal enzyme production. Evidence for the association of TCDD immunotoxicity with *Ah* genotype was derived from immune studies comparing inbred strains of *Ah*-responsive and -nonresponsive mice in which the ability of TCDD to cause immunotoxicity coordinated with the presence of the *Ah* locus (Vecchi *et al.*, 1983; Tucker *et al.*, 1986). In addition, a good correlation exists between the binding affinities of various HAH and their abilities to induce immunotoxicity (Silkworth *et al.*, 1984; Tucker *et al.*, 1986).

The role, if any, of microsomal enzyme induction in the cellular mechanism(s) responsible for inducing immunotoxicity following the binding of TCDD to its receptor are unknown. The observation that thymic epithelium contains relatively high concentrations of receptor suggests that TCDD may be inducing maturational defects in developing thymocytes (Greenlee et al., 1985). Studies performed using thymic epithelial cell cultures have shown that binding of TCDD to the Ah receptor results in the terminal differentiation of these cells and the loss of supportive microenvironment required for thymocyte maturation (Greenlee et al., 1985). Data suggest that cellular targets other than T cells (e.g., bone marrow cells and B cells) may be susceptible to similar patterns of altered cell proliferation and maturation following TCDD binding to Ah receptor found in these cells (reviewed by Luster et al., 1987). Recent studies examining the effects of TCDD on B-cell maturation have shown that TCDD selectively inhibited late stages of the cell cycle and the development of B cells into plasma cells. TCDD was required at the time of initial lymphoid cell activation to be effective, suggesting that TCDD may interfere with early activation events of these cells (Luster et al., 1988b).

5.3. Pesticides

A number of pesticides have been examined for immunotoxic potential in laboratory animals, including organochlorines and organophosphates (for review, see Vos and Kranjc, 1983). The literature to date suggests that organochlorine compounds, including DDT, captan, and chlordane, can modulate immune function (Glick, 1974; Street and Sharma, 1975; Beggs et al., 1985; Spyker-Cranmer et al., 1982; Barnett et al., 1980; Kaminsky et al., 1986). Methylparathion has also been shown to suppress immune function (Street and Sharma, 1975) and host resistance (Fan et al., 1978). While the toxicity of most organophosphate pesticides is relatively low because of their rapid detoxification by carboxyesterases, certain contaminants formed during their manufacture and storage have the capacity to inhibit carboxyesterase activity; these have been shown to be immunotoxic (Rodgers et al., 1985a,b; Devans et al., 1985). O,O,S-Trimethylphosphorothioate (OOS-TMP), a contaminant found in malathion, fenitrothion, and acephate, is immunotoxic at concentrations lower than those observed for other manifestations of its toxicity. Rodgers et al. (1985a,b) demonstrated that murine exposure to OOS-TMP, but not malathion, caused lymphocytopenia, thymic atrophy, suppression of antibody synthesis and decreased CTL activity. Interestingly, neither IL-2 production nor lymphoproliferative responses were affected. Macrophages treated with OOS-TMP have shown evidence of chemically induced activation (e.g., inflammatory macrophages), suggesting that the immunosuppressive profile demonstrated with OOS-TMP in vivo may relate to alterations in tissue macrophages. While the molecular mechanisms involved in OOS-TMP immunosuppression have not been elucidated, alterations in cholinesterase activity do not seem to play a role since O,O,S-trimethylphosphorodithioate, a structural analogue of OOS-TMP, modulates cholinesterase activity without affecting immunocompetence (Rodgers *et al.*, 1985b; Devans *et al.*, 1985).

5.4. Aromatic Amines

Benzidine (4,4-diaminobiphenyl), employed industrially in the synthesis of dyes as well as analytical reagents in various laboratory tests, is a urinary bladder carcinogen in humans (Haley, 1975). In rodents, benzidine causes hepatomas, mammary tumors, and, to a lesser extent, lymphoreticular neoplasms, primarily lymphomas (Vesselinovitch *et al.*, 1975). Because considerable evidence indicates that the immune response to chemically induced tumors may modulate either tumor growth or progression, or both, it follows that an increased incidence of neoplastic disease may occur by chemical carcinogens that also suppress immune functions. In mice, suppression of CMI occurs at dose levels of benzidine that are tumorigenic (Luster *et al.*, 1985b). In addition, benzidine exposure decreases host resistance to challenge by transplantable tumor cells or *Listeria* (Luster *et al.*, 1985b). Relevant to these observations in mice, an unconfirmed study showed a relationship between immunosuppression and neoplasia in workers engaged in the manufacture of benzidine (Gorodilova and Mandrik, 1978). In this 4-year study, only workers identified as having suppressed CMI (based on skin tests) demonstrated precancerous conditions and subsequent neoplasms.

The mechanisms responsible for immunosuppression by benzidine may not be the same as those responsible for its carcinogenicity. The addition of benzidine *in vitro* to mitogen-activated lymphocytes mimics the suppression of lymphocyte responsiveness observed following *in vivo* exposure. *In vitro* studies suggest that alterations in metabolites of the arachidonic acid–lipoxygenase pathway by benzidine (benzidine can serve as a co-oxidative substrate for hydroperoxidase) are responsible for inhibiting lymphocyte activation (Luster *et al.*, 1985b).

5.5. Metals

5.5.1. Inorganic Metals

Heavy metals, including lead, cadmium, and mercury, have been shown by a number of investigators to be capable of altering immune responsiveness in laboratory animals; while immunosuppression is a frequent manifestation of exposure, immunopotentiation may also result (see reviews by Koller, 1980; Lawrence, 1985). This apparent divergence may stem from differences in animal species used, the dose and route of administration, and the type of assay system employed. Alterations in B-lymphocyte function have been the most frequent observation following exposure to lead and cadmium, although T-cell and macrophage dysfunctions have also been described (Faith et al., 1979; Blakely and Archer, 1981; Kerkvliet and Baecher-Steppan, 1982). Studies examining the effects of heavy metals on host resistance have shown a strong correlation between metal exposure and impaired ability to resist bacterial or viral challenges, an observation that does not always correlate with alterations in B- or T-cell activities. Along these lines, heavy metals have been shown to synergize with injected bacterial endotoxin in mice and to increase dramatically the likelihood of endotoxin shock (Cook et al., 1975; Cook and Karns, 1978). Lead acetate exposure in mice altered endotoxin-induced reticuloendothelial cell activities (Sakaguchi et al., 1982), including lipid peroxidation, reactive oxygen intermediates, as well as glutathione-associated enzymes—findings that may account for increased susceptibility following bacterial and viral challenge.

The divergent data reported on inorganic metal interactions with the immune system suggest that more than one mechanism may be operable in the immunotoxicity and impaired host resistance associated with this class of compounds. While defects in B-cell function have been suggested to reside at the level of plasma cell development (Koller, 1979), impaired accessory cell function and/or deficient complement system components have also been implicated (Ewers et al., 1982; Ito et al., 1982). The subcellular mechanism involved in metal-induced immunotoxicity is complex. Lead as well as cadmium are sulfhydryl alkylating agents with high binding affinity for cellular sulfhydryl groups, and it has been suggested that these metals alter lymphocyte function by modulating membrane bound thiols (Blakely and Archer, 1981). This observation is strengthened by the fact that suppressive effects of lead, at least in vitro, can be reversed by the addition of exogenous thiol reagents (Blakely and Archer, 1981).

The augmentation of B- or T-cell responsiveness discussed above could precipitate autoimmunity, and metals have been implicated in influencing autoimmune disorders, although the precise cellular mechanisms for this is poorly understood (Lawrence, 1985). Glomerulonephritis, arthritis, and interstitial nephritis have been suggested to have an immunological pathogenesis and have been associated with exposure to mercury, silver, and lead, respectively (for review, see Lawrence, 1985). Experimentally, administration of mercury has been shown to induce polyclonal activation of B cells resulting in increased antibody synthesis to self-antigens (Hirsch et al., 1982). Thus, metal-induced tissue damage resulting in altered self-antigens and loss of tolerance and/or stimulation of immune system components may be partially responsible for metal induced autoimmune diseases.

5.5.2. Organotins

Organotin compounds are used primarily as heat stabilizers, industrial and agricultural biocides, and industrial catalysts in the production of foams and rubbers. Immunotoxic properties have been attributed to a number of organic tin compounds (for review, see Seinen and Penninks, 1979; Vos et al., 1985). Rats fed dibutyltin exhibited a dose-related decrease in thymus, spleen, and lymph node weights histologically associated with depletion of lymphocytes (Krajnc et al., 1984) in the perarteriolar lymphocyte sheath (spleen and thymus) and para-cortical areas (lymph nodes). Depletion of lymphocytes from the thymic cortex occurs without causing cytolysis, myelotoxicity, or nonlymphoid toxicity (Miller and Scott, 1985). Immune function of rats exposed to dialkyltins demonstrated suppression of CMI parameters, including increased skin-graft rejection time, suppressed DTH, and decreased T-cell mitogenesis (Seinen, 1981). These im-munological defects appear to be species specific, since neither immune function nor lymphoid atrophy is impaired in mice or guinea pigs fed dialkyltins.

A cellular depletion mechanism may be partly responsible for observed decreases in CMI, since decreased T-cell mitogen responsiveness correlated with decreased numbers of circulating lymphocytes with T-cell surface markers. In addition, suppression of T-helper cells resulting in altered regulation may ac-count for the decreases observed in the T-dependent humoral immunity in these studies (Seinen et al., 1977; Seinen, 1981). More recently, another class of organotin compounds, triorganotins (e.g., tri-n-butylin; TBT) have been shown to induce thymic atrophy and to suppress CMI (Vos et al., 1984; Snoeij et al., 1986). Following oral administration in the rat, however, these compounds are rapidly dealkylated, and thymus atrophy is actually mediated by the dealkylated metabolite of tributylin, dibutyltin (Snoeij et al., 1987).

Studies examining the mechanisms involved in organotin-induced thymic atrophy demonstrated a significant increase in the consumption of glucose and accumulated pyruvate and lactate in thymocytes incubated with a number of dialkyltins (Penninks and Seinen, 1980). This class of compounds has been shown indirectly to inhibit α-keto acid-oxidizing enzyme complexes in mito-chondria, pyruvate dehydrogenase, and α-ketoglutarate dehydrogenase (Pen-ninks and Seinen, 1980; Penninks et al., 1983). Thus, organotins may interfere directly with lymphocyte function or thymocyte maturation by inhibiting glucose metabolism via disturbances in mitochondrial respiration. Apart from inhibiting cellular energetics, alterations found in DNA, RNA, and protein synthesis in isolated rat thymocytes may also account for the particular sensitivity of this primary lymphoid organ (Penninks et al., 1985; R. P. Miller et al., 1980).

5.6. Inhaled Pollutants

The respiratory tract is a major route of exposure for many industrial and environmental xenobiotics. Consequently, the lungs and associated pulmonary defense mechanisms are often targets of airborne chemicals. Because of their strategic location within the lung, alveolar macrophages provide a first-line defense mechanism against inhaled pollutants. An extensive data base exists on xenobiotic-induced alterations in alveolar macrophage function (reviewed by Brain, 1986). Additional immunological defense mechanisms also operative in the respiratory tract include HMI and CMI responses of lung bronchial-associated lymphoid tissue (Bice, 1985) as well as NK activity in interstitial lung tissue (Stein-Streilein et al., 1983). However, much less information is available on the mechanism by which inhaled pollutants modulate these immunological processes. Of the multitude of pollutants that exist in the ambient or industrial atmosphere, only a few have been examined for their immunotoxic potential. The following discussion represents some of these xenobiotics that have been studied in depth.

5.6.1. Benzene

The toxicity of benzene has been the subject of considerable research for more than a century, with particular emphasis on its hematologic and leukemogenic potential (for review, see Snyder and Kocsis, 1975). In humans, the predominant hemopathy associated with benzene exposure is pancytopenia, with associated bone marrow hypoplasia (Goldstein, 1977). While hematopoietic progenitor cells are particularly susceptible to benzene, the mature circulating lymphocyte also responds to benzene via an antiproliferative response (Snyder et al., 1980). For example, suppression of B- and T-cell mitogenesis and mixed leukocyte responsiveness has been reported following benzene inhalation in rodents (Rosen et al., 1984; Rosenthal and Snyder, 1987). In addition, Wierda and Irons (1982) demonstrated that administration of benzene or the hydroquinone and catechol metabolites to mice resulted in suppression of mitogenesis and antibody production. Host-resistance studies have demonstrated impaired resistance to Listeria monocytogenes in mice exposed to concentrations as low as 30 ppm benzene (Rosenthal and Snyder, 1985). Studies employing PYB6 tumor cell challenge similarly demonstrated increased susceptibility at concentrations of benzene that also impaired CTL-mediated tumor cell cytolysis (Rosenthal and Snyder, 1987). Additional evidence of increased host susceptibility was supported by early studies demonstrating increased susceptibility to tuberculosis (White and Gammon, 1914) and pneumonia (Winternitz and Hirschfelder, 1913) in benzene-exposed rabbits. These studies are consistent with reports of severe benzene toxicity in humans characterized by acute overwhelming infections (IARC, 1982). Additional evidence for the immunotoxic potential of benzene in humans includes reports of depressed levels of serum complement and IgG and IgA circulating immunoglobulins in chronically exposed workers (Smolik et al., 1973; Lange et al., 1973), although these populations were exposed to other vapors as well.

The mechanism of the toxic effects of benzene on immune system components remains unknown, partly because the precise toxic metabolite(s) responsible for immunotoxicity remain unidentified. A cellular depletion mechanism may be at least partially responsible for observed immunotoxicity, although evidence for defective B- and T-cell function also exists. The antiproliferative effects of benzene may relate to its ability to alter cytoskeletal development through the inhibition of microtubule assembly. Polyhydroxy metabolites of benzene (p-benzoquinone and hydroquinone) have been shown to bind to sulfhydryl groups on proteins necessary for the integrity and polymerization of microtubules (Pfeifer and Irons, 1981). This may alter cell membrane fluidity and may explain the sublethal effect of benzene on lymphocyte function.

5.6.2. Pollutant Gases

Ozone (O_3) is a photochemical oxidant resulting from atmospheric reactions of hydrocarbons and nitrogen oxides catalyzed by sunlight. The immunotoxicologic data on O_3 demonstrate a marked impairment in pulmonary host-defense mechanisms (reviewed by Graham and Gardner, 1985). Laboratory mice exposed to concentrations as low as 0.1 ppm show decreased host resistance to bacterial challenge (Coffin and Gardner, 1972). Ozone has also been shown to increase the incidence of pulmonary infections induced by a number of other pathogenic organisms, including *Streptococcus* sp., *Pasturella haemolytica,* and *Mycobacterium tuberculosis* (for review, see Graham and Gardner, 1985). The increased susceptibility may relate to O_3-induced impairment in alveolar macrophage function. Studies supporting this supposition have demonstrated that exposure to O_3 can significantly decrease the number of alveolar macrophages (Gardner and Graham, 1976), impair the phagocytic ability of alveolar macrophages (Gardner and Graham, 1976), and decrease the ability of macrophages to secrete reactive oxygen intermediates (Amoruso *et al.,* 1981) as well as interferon (Shingu *et al.,* 1980). Ozone-induced systemic immune dysfunction has also been demonstrated (Aranyi *et al.,* 1983) and cannot be ruled out as an additional factor in impaired host defense. Alterations in rabbit alveolar macrophage production of arachidonic acid metabolites (increased PGE_2) following *in vitro* and *in vivo* O_3 exposure has also been reported (Driscoll, 1986; Schleshinger and Driscoll, 1987). These investigators suggest that increased PGE_2 production may represent a potential mechanism for the impaired alveolar macrophage function consistently observed in O_3-exposed animals, i.e., a nonimmunological mechanism that may contribute to decreased host resistance. Ozone-induced impairment in mucociliary clearance and increased mucus secretions could result in an accumulation of pathogenic organisms in a controlled study (Kenoyer *et al.,* 1981; Last *et al.,* 1977).

Nitrogen dioxide (NO_2) exposure appears to result in patterns of altered host responses similar to those seen with O_3 exposure. Animals exposed to NO_2 responded to experimentally induced pulmonary infections in a concentration-dependent manner (for review, see Graham and Gardner, 1985). Many parameters of alveolar macrophage function are impaired by NO_2 exposure, including phagocytosis (Sone *et al.*, 1983), interferon production (Gardner *et al.*, 1979), recognition of tumorigenic cells (Sone *et al.*, 1983), as well as bactericidal capacity (Environmental Criteria and Assessment Office, 1982). Morphological alterations observed in alveolar macrophages following NO_2 exposure most likely underlie the functional deficits observed in these cells (Brummer *et al.*, 1977). Systemically, NO_2 has been shown to suppress splenic T- and B-cell mitogenic responses (Maigetter *et al.*, 1978) as well as the primary antibody response to SRBC (Fujimaki *et al.*, 1981). However, the role of systemic immunity in pulmonary infectivity models is not fully understood.

5.6.3. Asbestos

Asbestos exposure in humans has long been associated with respiratory diseases, including fibrosis, asbestosis, and mesothelioma. Often associated with these conditions are alterations in cellular and humoral immune responses (for review, see Miller and Brown, 1985). Asbestos-associated impairments in CMI in humans are characterized by decreases in DTH responses, numbers of circulating T cells, and T-cell mitogen proliferation (Gaumer *et al.*, 1981; Haslam *et al.*, 1978; Kagan *et al.*, 1977a; Lew *et al.*, 1986). In contrast to the T-cell suppression often observed in asbestosis patients, hyperactive B-cell functions are observed, manifested by increased levels of serum immunoglobulins IgA, IgM, and IgG, as well as increased secretory IgA production (Huuskonen *et al.*, 1978; Kagan *et al.*, 1977b; Lange *et al.*, 1974). Kagan *et al.* (1979) described a number of cases demonstrating an association between asbestos exposure and B-cell lymphoproliferative disorders, including neoplasia. In addition, NK cell reactivity has been reported to be altered in persons exposed to asbestos (Kubota *et al.*, 1985; Ginns *et al.*, 1985). Experimental studies have confirmed the immunomodulatory potential of asbestos, particularly at the level of the alveolar macrophage (K. Miller and Brown, 1985). Asbestos fibers reaching the distal airways are readily phagocytized by alveolar macrophages, eventually resulting in cell lysis and release of inflammatory products and lysosomal enzymes (K. Miller *et al.*, 1979). In this regard, fiber size (length) has been shown to be an important factor in inducing macrophage toxicity, with decreased toxicity associated with reduced fiber length (Brown *et al.*, 1978; Wade *et al.*, 1980). Direct T cell–fiber interactions have been reported to result in altered immunoregulations (Bozelka *et al.*, 1983). Suppression of *in vitro* T-dependent antibody responses following the addition of chrysotile asbestos to spleen cell cultures has also been shown (White and Munson, 1986), a finding associated with dysfunction of an adherent cell population.

The data concerning modulation of immune function in humans exposed to asbestos are consistent with the loss of immunoregulatory control of alveolar macrophages. Macrophages are generally thought to down-regulate immune function in the respiratory tract under normal physiological circumstances (Holt,

1986). In a situation analogous to that described for silica, asbestos may exert an adjuvant-like response resulting in augmentation of immune system reactivity (K. Miller and Brown, 1985). However, the reported increased release of PG by macrophage cell lines and primary alveolar macrophage cultures (Sirois *et al.*, 1980; Brown and Poole, 1980) would be more consistent with asbestos-induced immunosuppression. Experimental studies examining the interactions of murine alveolar macrophages have shown that asbestos-exposed alveolar macrophages lose the capacity to suppress or down-regulate both T-cell mitogenesis (Bozelka *et al.*, 1986) as well as B-cell mitogenesis and production of antibody to SRBC (Rosenthal and Luster, 1987). A more thorough understanding of the role of asbestos in immunotoxicity will result as the immunoregulatory function of alveolar macrophages becomes better defined.

5.6.4. Beryllium

Beryllium is an industrial pollutant used in the manufacture of copper, nonsparking tools, light-weight alloys, and nuclear reactor components. Environmental beryllium contamination arises from coal combustion and, to a lesser extent, from its use as a rocket propellant. In humans, beryllium is associated with a number of diseases that clearly have an immunological pathogenesis, namely beryllium dermatitis, acute beryllium pneumonitis, and chronic pulmonary granulomatosis (berylliosis) (for review, see Reeves and Preuss, 1985). While beryllium-induced neoplasia in humans is controversial (Science, 1977, 1981), osteocarcinoma and adenocarcinoma have been reported in experimental studies following administrations of beryllium oxide and beryllium sulfate, respectively (Gardner and Heslington, 1946; Vorwald *et al.*, 1955).

Immune system abnormalities associated with beryllium are believed to result from the antigenicity of various chemical forms of beryllium. Current dogma states that beryllium, a poorly soluble particle, is essentially a hapten that associates with tissue protein(s) resulting in a complete antigen (Reeves and Preuss, 1985). Evidence for this can be found in studies showing that in $BeSO_4$-sensitized guinea pigs, beryllium complexed with serum albumin resulted in a more intense cutaneous reaction than did $BeSO_4$ itself (Krivanek and Reeves, 1972). Clinical evidence of beryllium exposure is often associated with blastlike transformation of T lymphocytes obtained from bronchoalveolar lavage as well as peripheral blood (Hanifin *et al.*, 1970; Jones and Amos, 1975). The correlation of T-lymphocyte blast transformation and beryllium hypersensitivity is so strong that, for practical purposes, the test has been used as a surveillance tool for berylliosis (Deodhar *et al.*, 1973; Williams and Jones-Wiliams, 1982). Lymphocytes from beryllium workers restimulated with beryllium demonstrated increased production of macrophage migration inhibitory factors (Henderson *et al.*, 1972); this test has also been used diagnostically for beryllium hypersensitivity. Cutaneous hypersensitivity demonstrated by positive patch-test results have often been reported in beryllium-exposed workers (Curtis, 1959). In light of the recognition of beryllium as a tissue antigen, increased levels of circulating immunoglobulins have been detected in beryllium workers and berylliosis patients; however, these antibodies were not shown to be specific for beryllium (Resnick et al., 1970).

The precise mechanisms involved in beryllium-induced hypersensitivity remain poorly understood. The granulomatous hypersensitivity associated with beryllium is associated with a specific immune response to tissue contact and is mediated and perpetuated by the accumulation and proliferation of reticuloendothelial cells. It has been hypothesized that the pulmonary granuloma may represent a state of hypersensitivity induced by macrophage migration inhibitory factor, impeding the mobility of these cells in the presence of antigen (Reeves and Preuss, 1985). The presence of increased numbers of T cells in bronchoalveolar lavage fluid of patients suffering from beryllium disease strengthens this theory (Epstein et al., 1982). In fact, evidence of free activated pulmonary T cells is so frequent that berylliosis is often confused with sarcoidosis. While the human data demonstrating the immunotoxic capacity of this compound are overwhelming, more experimental work is needed to increase our understanding of the molecular mechanisms involved in beryllium diseases.

6. CONCLUSIONS AND FUTURE DIRECTION

The immune system is composed of several cell populations the maturation of which are subject to orderly control by endogenous hormones and exogenous bacterial product. These mediators possess activation, growth promotion, or differentiation properties and are under the influence of potent but not well understood regulators. From observations in rodents and limited studies in inadvertently exposed humans, it is apparent that a number of xenobiotics adversely affect the immune system through disruption of cell maturation, regulation, or cytotoxic processes. These examples and our current knowledge about the pathogenesis of disease support the possibility that chemical-induced damage to the immune system may be associated with a wide spectrum of diverse pathological conditions, some of which may become detectable only after a long latency. Likewise, exposure to immunoalterative xenobiotics might represent additional risk to persons with already fragile immune systems caused by malnutrition, infancy, old age, and other factors. However, caution must be exercised when attempting to extrapolate meaningful conclusions from experimental data or isolated epidemiological studies to risk assessment for low-level human exposure.

Because of the functional heterogeneity of the immune system, efforts to assess chemical-induced immunotoxicity in laboratory animals have historically been performed using a tiered approach with multiple assays (Dean et al., 1982;

Koller and Exon, 1985; Vos, 1980). The testing configuration described in this chapter (i.e., level I screening assays) is derived from a more comprehensive panel taken from the NTP guidelines for immunotoxicity evaluation in mice (Luster *et al.*, 1988a). A similar configuration has been included in the Environmental Protection Agency's FIFRA regulations for immunotoxicity testing of biochemical pesticides. Each of the assays in level I has undergone extensive scrutiny in order to determine intra- and interlaboratory reproducibility, accuracy, sensitivity, and predictability (Luster *et al.*, 1988a). The configuration (level 1) represents a limited screening effort that includes immunopathology as well as functional assays for CMI, HMI, and NK cell function. Although the probability of detecting potent immunotoxicants in level I is high, the likelihood of detecting weaker immunotoxicants, such as those that may affect only a specific cell population or subpopulation, is presumably less. Nonetheless, on the basis of the data on compounds that can be considered immunotoxic alter at least one parameter in level I. Thus although level I provides little information on the specific cell type responsible for the immune defect or its relevance to the host, it can readily discern immune alterations resulting from chemical exposure.

The value of incorporating immunological rodent data for the toxicological assessment of drugs, chemicals, and biologicals for human risk assessment has been increasingly accepted. The receding decade of research has provided a data base of immunotoxic and nonimmunotoxic compounds, studies correlating immune dysfunction and altered host resistance, and a better standardized panel of methods for detecting immunomodulatory chemicals. In the near future, research related to methodology is needed to (1) further refine and validate immune function tests and host resistance assays, particularly in the rat; (2) develop, refine, and validate better testing methods to evaluate the effects of chemical inhalation on lung immunity; (3) determine the need and relevance of methods for assessing hematopoietic and polymorphonuclear leukocyte function; (4) develop and evaluate *in vitro* methodology as screens for detecting chemical-induced immunotoxicity using rodent and human immune cells; (5) develop improved methods for evaluating chemical-induced hypersensitivity and autoimmunity; and (6) develop a testing battery to examine dysfunction in humans occupationally or environmentally exposed to chemicals shown to be immunotoxic in laboratory animals.

REFERENCES

Alfred, L. J., and Wojdani, A., 1983, Effects of methylcholanthrene and benzanthracene on blastogenesis and aryl hydrocarbon hydroxylase induction in splenic lymphocytes from three inbred strains of mice, *Int. J. Immunopharmacol.* **5:**123–129.

Amoruso, M. A., Witz, G., and Goldstein, B. D., 1981, Decreased superoxide anion radical production by rat alveolar macrophages following inhalation of ozone or nitrogen dioxide, *Life Sci.* **28:**2215–2221.

Aranyi, C., Vana, S. C., Thomas, P. T., Bradof, J. N., Fenters, J. D., Graham, J. A., and Miller, F. J., 1983, Effects of subchronic exposure to a mixture of O_3, SO_2, $(NH_4)_2SO_4$, on host defenses in mice, *Environ. Res.* **12**:55–71.

Barnett, J. B., Spyker-Cranmer, J. M., Avery, P. C., and Hoberman, A. M., 1980, Immunocompetence over the lifespan of mice exposed to *in vitro* to Carbofuran or Diazinon, *J. Environ. Pathol. Toxicol.* **4**:53–63.

Beggs, M., Menna, J. H., and Barnett, J. B., 1985, Effects of Chlordane on influenza type A virus and herpes simplex type 1 virus replication *in vitro*, *J. Toxicol. Environ. Health* **16**:173–188.

Bekesi, J. G., Holland, J. F., Anderson, H. A., Fischbein, A. S., Rom, W., Wolff, M. S., and Selikoff, I. J., 1978, Lymphocyte function of Michigan dairy farmers exposed to polybrominated biphenyls, *Science* **199**:1207–1209.

Bekesi, J. G., Roboz, J. P., Fischbein, A., and Selikoff, I. J., 1987, Clinical immunology studies in individuals exposed to environmental chemicals, in: *Immunotoxicology: Proceedings of an International Seminar on the Immunological System as a Target for Toxic Damage* (A. Berlin, J. Dean, M. H. Draper, E. M. B. Smith, and F. Spreafico, eds.), pp. 347–361, Martinus Nijhoff, Dordrecht.

Berlin, A., Dean, J., Draper, M., Smith, E. M. B., and Spreafico, F., 1987, Synopsis, conclusions, and recommendations, in: *Immunotoxicology* (A. Berlin, J. Dean, M. Draper, E. M. B. Smith, and F. Spreafico, eds.), pp. xi–xxvii, Martinus Nijhoff, Dordrecht.

Bice, D. E., 1985, Methods and approaches for assessing immunotoxicology of the lower respiratory tract, in: *Immunotoxicology and Immunopharmacology* (J. H. Dean, M. I. Luster, A. E. Munson, and H. Amos, eds.), pp. 1–10, Raven, New York.

Blakely, B. R., and Archer, D. L., 1981, The effects of lead acetate on the immune response of mice, *Toxicol. Appl. Pharmacol.* **61**:18–26.

Bozelka, B. E., Gaumer, H. R., Nordberg, J., and Salvaggio, J. E., 1983, Asbestos-induced alterations of human lymphoid cell mitogenic responses, *Environ. Res.* **30**:281–290.

Bozelka, B. E., Sestini, P., Hammad, Y., and Salvaggio, J. E., 1986, Effects of asbestos fibers on alveolar macrophage-mediated lymphocyte cytostasis, *Environ. Res.* **40**:172–180.

Brain, J. D., 1986, Toxicological aspects of alterations of pulmonary macrophage function, *Annu. Rev. Pharmacol. Toxicol.* **26**:547–565.

Brown, R. C., and Poole, A., 1980, Arachidonic acid release and prostaglandin synthesis in a macrophage-like cell line exposed to asbestos, *Agents Actions* **15**:336–340.

Brown, R. C., Chamberlain, M., Griffiths, M., and Timbrell, V., 1978, The effect of fiber size on the *in vitro* biological activity of three types of amphibole asbestos, *Int. J. Cancer* **22**:721–727.

Brummer, M. E. G., Schwartz, L. W., and McQuillen, N. K., 1977, A quantitative study of lung damage by scanning electron microscopy. Inflammatory cell responses to high ambient levels of ozone, *Scanning Electron Microsc.* **2**:513–518.

Centers for Disease Control, 1981, Follow-up on toxic pneumonia—Spain, *M. M. W. R.* **30**:436–438.

Chang, K. J., Hsieh, K. H., Lee, T. P., and Tung, T. C., 1982a, Immunologic evaluation of patients with polychlorinated biphenyl poisoning: Determination of phagocytic Fc and complement receptors, *Environ. Res.* **28**:329–334.

Chang, K. J., Hsieh, K. H., Tang, S. Y., Tung, T. C., and Lee, T. P., 1982b, Immunologic evaluation of patients with polychlorinated biphenyl poisoning: Evaluation of delayed-type skin hypersensitive response and its relation to clinical studies, *J. Toxicol. Environ. Health* **9**:217–223.

Clark, D. A., Gauldie, J., Szewcyk, M. R., and Sweeney, G., 1981, Enhanced suppressor cell activity as a mechanism of immunosuppression by TCDD, *Proc. Soc. Exp. Biol. Med.* **168**:290–299.

Coffin, D. L., and Gardner, D. E., 1972, Interactions of biological agents and chemical air pollutants, *Ann. Occup. Hyg.* **15**:219–235.

Cook, J. A., and Karns, L., 1978, Effects of RES stimulation and suppression on lead sensitization to endotoxin shock, *J. Reticuloendothelial Soc.* **24**:1A.

Cook, J. A., Hoffman, E. D., and DiLuzio, N. R., 1975, Influence of lead and cadmium on the susceptibility of rats to bacterial challenge, *Proc. Soc. Exp. Biol. Med.* **150**:741–747.

Curtis, G. H., 1959, The diagnosis of beryllium disease with special reference to the patch test, *Arch. Indust. Health* **19**:150–153.

Dean, J. H., and Lauer, L. D., 1983, Immunological effects following exposure to 2,3,7,8-tetrachlorodibenzo-*p*-dioxin: A review, in: *Public Health Risks of the Dioxins* (W. W. Lowrance, ed.), pp. 275–294, Rockefeller University, New York.

Dean, J. H., Padarathsingh, M. L., and Jerrells, T. R., 1979, Assessment of immunobiological effects induced by chemicals, drugs or food additives. I. Tier testing and screening approach, *Drug Chem. Toxicol.* **2**:5–17.

Dean, J. H., and Thurmond, L. M., 1987, Immunotoxicology: An overview, *Toxicol. Pathol.* **15**: 265–271.

Dean, J. H., Luster, M. I., and Boorman, G. A., 1982, Immunotoxicology, in: *Immunopharmacology* (P. Sirios and M. RolaPleszczynski, eds.), pp. 349–397, Elsevier, Amsterdam.

Dean, J. H., Luster, M. I., Boorman, G. A., Lauer, L. D., Luebke, R. W., and Lawson, L., 1983, Selective immunosuppression resulting from exposure to the carcinogenic congener of benzopyrene in B6C3F1 mice, *Clin. Exp. Immunol.* **52**:199–206.

Dean, J. H., Ward, E. C., Murray, M. J., Lauer, L. D., and House, R. V., 1985, Mechanisms of dimethylbenzanthracene-induced immunotoxicity, *Clin. Physiol. Biochem.* **3**:98–110.

Dean, J. H., Murray, M. J., and Ward, E. D., 1986a, Toxic responses of the immune system, in: *Casarett and Doull's Toxicology: The Basic Science of Poisons*, 3rd ed. (C. D. Klaassen, M. O. Amdur, and J. Doull, eds.), pp. 245–285, Macmillan, New York.

Dean, J. H., Ward, E. C., Murray, M. J., Lauer, L. D., House, R. V., Stillman, W. S., Hamilton, T. A., and Adams, D. O., 1986b, Immunosuppression following 7,12-dimethyl-benz(a)anthracene exposure in $B_6C_3F_1$ mice. II. Altered cell-mediated immunity and tumor resistance, *Int. J. Immunopharmacol.* **8**:189–198.

Dean, J. H., Thurmond, L. D., Lauer, L. D., and House, R. V., 1987, Comparative toxicology and correlative immunotoxicology in rodents, in: *Environmental Chemical Exposure and Immune System Integrity, Advances in Modern Environmental Toxicology* (E. J. Burger, R. G. Tardiff, and J. A. Bellanti, eds.), Vol. 13, pp. 85–100, Princeton Scientific Publishing Company, Princeton, New Jersey.

Denkhaus, W., Steldern, D. V. Botzenhardt, U., and Konietzko, H., 1986, Lymphocyte subpopulations in solvent-exposed workers, *Int. Arch. Occup. Environ. Health* **57**:109–115.

Deodhar, S. D., Barna, B., and VanOrdstrand, H. S., 1973, A study of the immunologic aspects of chronic berylliosis, *Chest* **63**:309–313.

Devans, B. H., Grayson, M. H., Imamura, T., and Rodgers, K. E., 1985, O,O,S-Trimethyl phosphorothioate effects on immunocompetence, *Pesticide Biochem. Physiol.* **24**:251–259.

Driscoll, K., 1986, Doctoral dissertation, New York University Medical Center, Department of Environmental Health, University microfilms.

Environmental Criteria and Assessment Office, 1982, Air quality for nitrogen oxides, EPA-600/8-82-026, pp. 22–39, U.S. Environmental Protection Agency, Research Triangle Park, North Carolina.

Epstein, P. E., Dauber, J. H., Rossman, M. D., and Daniele, R. P., 1982, Bronchoalveolar lavage in a patient with chronic berylliosis: Evidence for hypersensitivity pneumonitis, *Ann. Intern. Med.* **97**:213–216.

Ewers, U., Stiller-Winkler, R., and Idel, H., 1982, Serum immunoglobulin complement C3 and salivary IgA levels in lead workers, *Environ. Res.* **29**:351–357.

Faith, R. E., and Luster, M. I., 1979, Investigations on the effects of 2,3,7,8-tetrachlorodibenzo-*p*-dioxin on parameters of various immune functions, *Ann. N.Y. Acad. Sci.* **320**:564–571.

Faith, R. E., Luster, M. I., and Kimmel, C. A., 1979, Effect of chronic developmental lead exposure on cell mediated immune functions, *Clin. Exp. Immunol.* **35**:413–420.

Faith, R. E., Luster, M. I., and Vos, J. G., 1980, Effects on immunocompetence by chemicals of environmental concern, in: *Reviews in Biochemical Toxicology*, Vol. 2 (E. Hodgson, J. R. Bend, and R. M. Philpot, eds.), pp. 173–211, Elsevier/North-Holland, New York.

Fan, A., Street, J. C., and Nelson, R. M., 1978, Immune suppression in mice administered methyl parathion and carbofuran by diet, *Toxicol. Appl. Pharmacol.* **45**:235–242.

French, J. G., Lowrimore, G., Nelson, W. C., Finklea, J. F., English, T., and Hertz, M., 1973, The effect of sulfur dioxide and suspended sulfates on acute respiratory disease, *Arch. Environ. Health* **27**:129–133.

Fujimaki, H., Shimizu, F., and Kubota, K., 1981, Suppression of antibody response in mice by acute exposure to nitrogen dioxide. *In Vitro* study, *Environ. Res.* **26**:490–496.

Gardner, D. E., and Graham, J. A., 1976, Increased pulmonary disease mediated through altered bacterial defenses, in: *Pulmonary Macrophage and Epithelial Cells* (C. L. Sanders, R. P. Schneider, G. E. Doyle, and H. A. Ragan, eds.), pp. 1–21, *Proceedings of the Sixteenth Annual Hanford Biology Symposium*. ERDA Symposium Series, Richland, Washington.

Gardner, D. E., Graham, J. A., Illing, J. W., Blommer, E. J., and Miller, F. J., 1979, Impact of exposure patterns on the toxicological response to NO_2 and modifications by added stressors, in: *Proceedings of the U.S.–USSR Third Joint Symposium on Problems in Environmental Health*, pp. 17–40, National Institute of Environmental Health Sciences, Research Triangle Park, North Carolina.

Gardner, L. U., and Heslington, H. F., 1946, Osteo-sarcoma from intravenous beryllium compounds in rabbits, *Fed. Proc.* **5**:221.

Gaumer, H. R., Doll, N. Y., Kaimmal, Y., Schuyer, M., and Salvaggio, Y. E., 1981, Diminished suppressor cell function in patients with asbestosis, *Clin. Exp. Immunol.* **44**:108–116.

Ginns, L. C., Ryo, J. H., Rogol, P. R., Sprince, N. L., Oliver, L. C., and Larsson, C. L., 1985, Natural killer cell activity in cigarette smokers and asbestos workers, *Annu. Rev. Respir. Dis.* **131**:831–834.

Glick, B., 1974, Antibody-mediated immunity in the presence of Mirex and DDT, *Poultry Sci.* **53**:1476–1485.

Goldstein, B. D., 1977, Hematotoxicity in humans, *J. Toxicol. Environ. Health* **2**(suppl.):69–106.

Gomez-Reino, J., 1987, Immune system disorders associated with adulterated cooking oil, in: *Immunotoxicology. Proceedings of an International Seminar on the Immunological System as a Target for Toxic Damage* (A. Berlin, J. Dean, M. H. Draper, E. M. B. Smith, and F. Spreafico, eds.), pp. 376–388, Martinus Nijhoff, Dordrecht.

Gorodilova, V. V., and Mandrik, E. V., 1978, The use of some immunological reaction for studying the immune response in persons presenting a high oncological risk, *Soviet Med.* **8**:50–53.

Graham, J. A., and Gardner, D. E., 1985, Immunotoxicity of air pollutants, in: *Immunotoxicology and Immunopharmacology* (J. H. Dean, M. I. Luster, and A. E. Munson, eds.), pp. 367–380, Raven, New York.

Greenlee, W. F., Dold, K. M., Irons, R. D., and Osborne, R., 1985, Evidence for direct action of 2,3,7,8-tetrachlorodibenzo(*p*)dioxin on thymic epithelium, *Toxicol. Appl. Pharmacol.* **19**:112–120.

Haley, T. J., 1975, Benzidine revisited: A review of the literature and problems associated with the use of benzidine and its congeners, *Clin. Toxicol.* **8**:13–42.

Hanifin, J. M., Epstein, W. L., and Cline, M. J., 1970, *In vitro* studies of granulomatous hypersensitivity to beryllium, *J. Invest. Dermatol.* **55**:284–288.

Haslam, P. L., Lukoszek, A., Merchant, J. A., and Turner-Warwick, M., 1978, Lymphocyte responses to phytohemagglutinin in patients with asbestosis and pleural mesothelioma, *Clin. Exp. Immunol.* **31**:178–188.

Haynes, R. C., and Murad, F., 1985, Adrenocortical steroids and their synthetic analogs; inhibitors of adrenocortical steroid biosynthesis, in: *Goodman and Gilman's Pharmacological Basis of*

Therapeutics (A. G. Gilman, L. S. Goodman, T. W. Rall, and F. Murad, eds.), pp. 1459–1489, Macmillan, New York.

Henderson, W. R., Fukuyama, K., Epstein, W. L., and Spitler, L. F., 1972, In vitro demonstration of delayed hypersensitivity in patients with berylliosis, *J. Invest. Dermatol.* **58:**5–8.

Hirsch, F., Couderc, J., Sapin, C., Fournie, G., and Druet, P., 1982, Polyclonal effect of $HgCl_2$ in the rat, its possible role in an experimental autoimmune disease, *Eur. J. Immunol.* **12:**620–625.

Hoffman, R. E., Stehr-Green, P. A., Webb, K. B., Evans, G., Knutsen, A. P., Schramm, W. F., Staake, J. L., Gibson, B. A., and Steinberg, K. K., 1986, Health effects of long-term exposure to 2,3,7,8-tetrachlorodibenzo-*p*-dioxin, *J.A.M.A.* **255:**2031–2038.

Holt, P. A., 1986, Down regulation of immune responses in the lower respiratory tract: The role of alveolar macrophages, *Clin. Exp. Immunol.* **63:**261–270.

House, R. V., Lauer, L. D., Murray, M. J., and Dean, J. H., 1987, Suppression of T-helper cell function in mice following exposure to the carcinogen 7,12-dimethylbenz(a)anthracene and its restoration by interleukin 2, *Int. J. Immunopharmacol.* **9:**85–87.

Huuskonen, M. S., Rasanen, Y. A., Hankonen, H., and Asp, S., 1978, Asbestos exposure as a cause of immunologic stimulation, *Scand. J. Respir. Dis.* **59:**326–332.

Imaniski, J., Nomura, H., Matsubara, M., Kita, M., Won, S. J., Muzutani, T., and Kishida, T., 1980, Effect of polychlorinated biphenyl on viral infections in mice, *Infect. Immun.* **29:**275–277.

International Agency for Research on Cancer, 1982, Evaluation of the carcinogenic risk of chemical to humans: Some industrial chemicals and dye stuffs, *IARC Monogr.* **29:**93–148.

Ito, Y., Kurita, H., Yoshida, T., Shima, S., Niiya, Y., Tariumi, H., Nakayasu, T., Kamori, Y., and Sarai, S., 1982, Studies on serum specific protein levels in lead exposed workers, *Jpn. J. Indust. Health* **24:**390–391.

Jones, J. M., and Amos, H. E., 1975, Contract sensitivity in vitro: The effect of beryllium preparations on the proliferative response of specifically allergized lymphocytes and normal lymphocytes stimulated with PHA, *Int. Arch. Allergy* **48:**22–29.

Kagan, E., Solomon, A., Cochrane, J. C., Beissmer, E. K., Gluckman, J., Rocks, P. H., and Webster, I., 1977a, Immunological studies of patients with asbestosis. I. Studies of cell mediated immunity, *Clin. Exp. Immunol.* **28:**261–267.

Kagan, E., Solomon, A., Cochrane, J. C., Kuba, P., Rocks, P. H., and Webster, I., 1977b, Immunological studies of patients with asbestosis. II. Studies of circulating lymphoid numbers and humoral immunity, *Clin. Exp. Immunol.* **28:**268–275.

Kagan, E., Jacobson, R. J., Yeung, K. Y., Haildale, D. J., and Machnani, G. H., 1979, Asbestos-associated neoplasms of B-cell lineage, *Am. J. Med.* **67:**325–331.

Kalland, T., and Haukass, S. A., 1981, Effect of treatment with diethylstilbestrol–polyestradiol phosphate or estramustine phosphate (Estracyt) on natural killer cell activity in patients with prostatic cancer, *Invest. Urol.* **18:**437–441.

Kaminsky, N. E., Wells, D. S., Dauterman, W. C., Roberts, J. F., and Guthrie, F., 1986, Macrophage uptake of lipoprotein sequestered toxicant: A potential route of immunotoxicity, *Toxicol. Appl. Pharmacol.* **82:**474–480.

Kammüller, M. E., Penninks, A. H., and Seinen, W., 1984, Spanish toxic oil syndrome is a chemically induced GVHD-like epidemic, *Lancet* **1:**1174–1175.

Kammüller, M. E., Penninks, A. H., and Seinen, W., 1986, Cyclization products of phenylthiourea compounds in adulterated rapeseed oil as possible aetiologic factor in Spanish toxic oil syndrome, *Adv. Immunopharmacol.* **3:**439–442.

Keck, G., 1982, Effets de la contamination par les polychlorobiphenyles sur le developpement de la tumeur d'Ehrlich chez la souris suisse, *Toxicol. Eur. Res.* **3:**229–236.

Kenoyer, J. L., Phalen, R. F., and Davis, J. R., 1981, Particle clearance from the respiratory tract as a test of toxicity. Effect of ozone exposure on short and long term clearance, *Exp. Lung Res.* **2:**111–120.

Kerkvliet, N. I., and Baecher-Steppan, L., 1982, Immunotoxicology studies on lead: Effect of exposure on tumor growth and cell-mediated immunity after syngeneic or allogeneic stimulator, *Immunopharmacology* **4**:213–224.

Kerkvliet, N. I., and Kimeldorf, D. J., 1977, Antitumor activity of a polychlorinated biphenyl mixture, Aroclor 1254, in rats inoculated with Walker 256 carcinoma cells, *J. Natl. Cancer Inst.* **59**:951–955.

Kimbrough, R. D., 1980, *Halogenated Biphenyls, Terphenyls, Naphthalenes, Dibenzodioxins, and Related Products*, Elsevier/North-Holland, New York.

Koller, L. D., 1977, Enhanced polychlorinated biphenyl lesions in Moloney leukemia virus infected mice, *Clin. Toxicol.* **11**:107–116.

Koller, L. D., 1979, Effects of environmental contaminants on the immune system, *Adv. Vet. Sci. Comp. Med.* **23**:267–295.

Koller, L. D., 1980, Immunotoxicology of heavy metals, *Int. J. Immunopharmacol.* **2**:269–279.

Koller, L. D., and Exon, J. H., 1985, The rat as a model for immunotoxicity assessment, in: *Immunotoxicity and Immunopharmacology* (J. H. Dean, M. I. Luster, A. E. Munson, and H. Amos,eds.), pp. 99–112, Raven, New York.

Koller, L. D., and Thigpen, J. E., 1973, Reduction of antibody to pseudorabies virus in polychlorinated biphenyl-exposed rabbits, *Am. J. Vet. Res.* **34**:1605–1606.

Krajnc, E. I., Wester, P. W., Loeber, J. G., van Leeuwen, F. X. R., Vos, J. G., Vaessen, H. A. M. G., and van der Heijden, G. A., 1984, Toxicity of bis(tri-*n*-butyltin) oxide in the rat. I. Short-term effects on general parameters and on the endocrine and lymphoid systems, *Toxicol. Appl. Pharmacol.* **75**:363–386.

Krivanek, N. D., and Reeves, A. L., 1972, The effect of chemical forms of beryllium on the production of the immunologic response. *Am. Indust. Hyg. Assoc. J.* **33**:45–52.

Kubota, M., Kagamimori, S., Yokoyama, K., and Okada, A., 1985, Reduced natural killer activity of lymphocytes from patients with asbestosis, *Br. J. Indust. Med.* **42**:276–280.

Lange, A., Smolik, R., Zatonski, W., and Szymanska, J., 1973, Serum immunoglobulin levels in workers exposed to benzene, toluene and xylene, *Int. Arch. Arbeitsmed.* **31**:37–44.

Lange, A., Smolik, R., Zatonski, W., and Szymanska, Y., 1974, Autoantibodies and serum immunoglobulin levels in asbestos workers, *Int. Arch. Arbeitsmed.* **32**:313–325.

Last, J. A., Jennings, M., Schwartz, L. E., and Cross, C. E., 1977, Glycoprotein secretion by tracheal explants cultured from rats exposed to ozone, *Am. Rev. Respir. Dis.* **116**:695–703.

Lauer, L. D., Tucker, A. N., House, R. V., Barbera, P. W., Fenters, J. D., Ehrlich, J. P., Burleson, G. R., and Dean, J. H., 1987, Altered B cell function is a predominant feature of TCDD exposure in adult mice, submitted.

Lawrence, D. A., 1985, Immunotoxicity of heavy metals, in: *Immunotoxicology and Immunopharmacology* (J. H. Dean, M. I. Luster, A. E. Munson, and H. Amos, eds.), pp. 341–353, Raven, New York.

Lee, T. P., and Chang, K. J., 1985, Health effects of polychlorinated biphenyls, in: *Immunotoxicology and Immunopharmacology* (J. H. Dean, M. I. Luster, A. E. Munson, and H. Amos, eds.), pp. 415–422, Raven, New York.

Lew, F., Tsang, P., Holland, J. F., Warner, N., Selikoff, I. J., and Bekesi, J. G., 1986, High frequency of immune dysfunctions in asbestos workers and in patients with malignant mesothelioma, *J. Clin. Immunol.* **6**:225–233.

Lill, P. H., and Gangemi, J. D., 1986, Suppressive effects of 3-methylcholanthrene on the *in vitro* antitumor activity of naturally cytotoxic cells, *J. Toxicol. Environ. Health* **17**:347–356.

Loose, L. D., Silkworth, J. B., Pittman, K. A., Benitz, K. F., and Mueller, W., 1978, Impaired host resistance to endotoxin and malaria in polychlorinated biphenyl- and hexachlorobenzene-treated mice, *Infect. Immun.* **20**:30–35.

Loose, L. D., Silkworth, J. B., Charbonneau, T., and Blumenstock, F., 1981, Environmental chemical-induced macrophage dysfunction, *Environ. Health Perspect.* **39**:79–91.

Lunn, J. E., Knowelden, J., and Handyside, A. J., 1967, Patterns of respiratory illness in Sheffield school children, *Br. J. Prev. Soc. Med.* **21**:7–16.

Luster, M. I., Boorman, G. A., Dean, J. H., Harris, M. W., and Luebke, R. W., 1980, Examination of bone marrow immunologic parameters and host susceptibility following pre- and postnatal exposure to 2,3,7,8-tetrachlorodibenzo(p)dioxin, *Int. J. Immunopharmacol.* **2**:301–310.

Luster, M. I., Hong, L. H., Tucker, A. N., Clark, G., Greenlee, W. F., and Boorman, G. A., 1985a, Acute myelotoxic responses in mice induced *in vivo* and *in vitro* by 2,3,7,8-tetrachlorodibenzo-p-dioxin, *Toxicol. Appl. Pharmacol.* **81**:156–165.

Luster, M. I., Tucker, A. N., Hayes, H. T., Pung, O. J., Burka, T., McMillan, R., and Eling, T., 1985b, Immunosuppressive effects of benzidine in mice: Evidence of alterations in arachidonic acid metabolism, *J. Immunol.* **135**:2754–2761.

Luster, M. I., Blank, J. A., and Dean, J. H., 1987, Molecular and cellular basis of chemically induced immunotoxicity, *Annu. Rev. Pharmacol. Toxicol.* **27**:23–49.

Luster, M. I., Munson, A. E., Thomas, P. T., Holsapple, M. P., Fenters, J. D., White, K. L., Lauer, L. D. D., Germolec, D. R., Rosenthal, G. J., and Dean, J. H., 1988a, Development of a testing battery to assess chemical-induced immunotoxicity: National Toxicology Program's guidelines for immunotoxicity evaluation in mice, *Fundam. Appl. Toxicol.* **10**:2–19.

Luster, M. I., Germolec, D. R., Clark, G., Wiegand, G., and Rosenthal, G. J., 1988b, Selective effects of 2,3,7,8-tetrachlorodibenzo-p-dioxin and corticosteroid on *in vitro* activation, proliferation and differentiation of murine B-lymphocytes, *J. Immunol.* **140**:928–935.

Lyte, M., and Bick, P. H., 1986, Modulation of interleukin 1 production by macrophages following benzo(a)pyrene exposure, *Int. J. Immunopharmacol.* **8**:377–381.

Maigetter, R. Z., Fenters, J. D., Findlay, J. C., Ehrlich, R., and Gardner, D. E., 1978, Effects of exposure to nitrogen dioxide on T and B cells in mouse spleen, *Toxicol. Lett.* **2**:157–161.

Mantovani, A., Vecchi, A., Luini, W., Sironi, M., Candiani, G., Spreafico, F., and Garattini, S., 1980, Effect of 2,3,7,8-tetrachlorodibenzo-p-dioxin on macrophage and NK cell mediated cytotoxicity in mice, *Biomedicine* **32**:200–204.

Miller, K., and Brown, R. C., 1985, The immune system and asbestos associated disease, in: *Immunotoxicology and Immunopharmacology* (J. H. Dean, M. I. Luster, A. E. Munson, and H. Amos, eds.), pp. 429–440, Raven, New York.

Miller, K., and Scott, M. P., 1985, Immunologic consequences of dioctyltin dichloride (DOTC)-induced thymic injury, *Toxicol. Appl. Pharmacol.* **78**:395–403.

Miller, K., Weintraub, Z., and Kagan, E., 1979, Manifestations of cellular immunity in the rat after prolonged asbestos inhalation. I. Physical interactions between alveolar macrophages and splenic lymphocytes, *J. Immunol.* **123**:1029–1038.

Miller, R. P., Hartung, R., and Cornish, H. H., 1980, Effects of diethyltindichlorides on amino acids and nucleoside transport in suspended rat thymocytes, *Toxicol. Appl. Pharmacol.* **55**:564–571.

Moore, J. A., Huff, J. E., and Dean, J. H., 1982, The National Toxicology Program and immunological toxicology, *Pharmacol. Rev.* **43**:13–16.

National Research Council, 1978, *Sulfur Oxides*, National Academy of Sciences, Washington, D. C.

National Research Council, 1979, *Airborne Particles*, National Academy of Sciences, Washington, D. C.

Penn, I., 1985, Neoplastic consequences of immunosuppression, in: *Immunotoxicology and Immunopharmacology* (J. H. Dean, M. I. Luster, A. E. Munson, and H. Amos, eds.), pp. 79–89, Raven, New York.

Penninks, A. H., and Seinen, W., 1980, Toxicity of organotin compounds. IV. Impairment of energy metabolism of rat thymocytes by various dialkyltin compounds, *Toxicol. Appl. Pharmacol.* **56**:221–231.

Penninks, A. H., Verschuren, P. M., and Seinen, W., 1983, Di-n-butyltindichloride uncouples oxidative phosphorylation in rat liver mitochondria, *Toxicol. Appl. Pharmacol.* **70**:115–120.

Penninks, A. H., Kuper, F., Spit, B. J., and Seinen, W., 1985, On the mechanism of dialkyltin induced thymus involution, *Immunopharmacology* **10**:1–10.

Pfeifer, R., and Irons, R. D., 1981, Inhibition of lectin-stimulated lymphocyte agglutination and mitogenesis by hydroquinone: Reactivity with intracellular sulfhydryl groups, *Exp. Mol. Pathol.* **35**:189–198.

Reeves, A. L., and Preuss, O. P., 1985, The immunotoxicity of beryllium, in: *Immunotoxicology and Immunopharmacology* (J. H. Dean, M. I. Luster, A. E. Munson, and H. Amos, eds.), pp. 441–455, Raven, New York.

Resnick, H., Roche, M., and Morgan, W. K. C., 1970, Immunoglobulin concentrations in berylliosis, *Am. Rev. Respir. Dis.* **101**:504–510.

Rodgers, K. E., Imamura, T., and Devans, B. H., 1985a, Effects of subchronic treatment with *O,O,S*-trimethyl phosphorothioate on cellular and humoral immune response systems, *Toxicol. Appl. Pharmacol.* **81**:310–318.

Rodgers, K. E., Imamura, T., and Devans, B. H., 1985b, Investigations into the mechanism of immunosuppression caused by acute treatment with *O,O,S*-trimethyl phosphorothioate. I. Characterization of the immune cell population affected, *Immunopharmacology* **10**:171–180.

Rosenthal, G. J., and Luster, M. I., 1987, Asbestos-induced reversal of the normal down regulatory function of alveolar macrophages, *Fed. Proc.* **46**:539.

Rosenthal, G. J., and Snyder, C. A., 1985, Modulation of the immune response to *Listeria monocytogenes* by benzene inhalation, *Toxicol. Appl. Pharmacol.* **80**:502–510.

Rosenthal, G. J., and Snyder, C. A., 1987, Inhaled benzene reduces aspects of cell-mediated tumor surveillance in mice, *Toxicol. Appl. Pharmacol.* **88**:35–43.

Rozen, M. G., Snyder, C. A., and Albert, R. E., 1984, Depressions in B- and T-lymphocyte mitogen-induced blastogenesis in mice exposed to low concentrations of benzene, *Toxicol. Lett.* **20**:343–349.

Ryffel, B., Donatsch, P., Madorin, M., Matter, B. E., Ruttimann, G., Schon, H., Stoo, R., and Wilson, J., 1983, Toxicological evaluation of cyclosporin A, *Arch. Toxicol.* **53**:107–141.

Sakaguchi, O., Abe, H., Sakaguchi, S., and Hsu, C. C., 1982, Effect of lead acetate on superoxide anion generation and its scavengers in mice given endotoxin, *Microbiol. Immunol.* **26**:767–778.

Schleshinger, R. B., and Driscoll, K. E., 1987, Respiratory tract defense mechanisms and their interaction with air pollutants, in: *Current Topics in Pharmacology and Toxicology* (in press).

Science, 1977, Occupational cancer: Government challenged in beryllium proceeding, **198**:898–901.

Science, 1981, Beryllium report disputed by listed author, **211**:556–557.

Seinen, W., 1981, Immunotoxicity of alkyltin compounds, in: *Immunologic Considerations in Toxicology* (R. P. Sharma, ed.), Vol. 1, pp. 103–119, CRC Press, Boca Raton, Florida.

Seinen, W., and Penninks, A., 1979, Immune suppression as a consequence of a selective cytotoxic activity of certain organometallic compounds on thymus dependent lymphocytes, *Ann. N.Y. Acad. Sci.* **320**:499–517.

Seinen, W., Vos, J. G., Van Krieken, R., Penninks, A. H., Brands, R., and Hooykaas, H., 1977, Toxicity of organotin compounds. III. Suppression of thymus-dependent immunity in rats by di-*n*-butyltin dichloride, *Toxicol. Appl. Pharmacol.* **42**:213–224.

Shingu, H., Sugiyama, M., Watanabe, M., and Nakajima, T., 1980, Effects of ozone and photochemical oxidants on interferon production by rabbit alveolar macrophages, *Bull. Environ. Contam. Toxicol.* **24**:433–438.

Silkworth, J. B., and Grabstein, E. M., 1982, Polychlorinated biphenyl immunotoxicity: Dependence on isomer planarity and the Ah gene complex, *Toxicol. Appl. Pharmacol.* **65**:109–115.

Silkworth, J. B., and Loose, L. D., 1981, Assessment of environmental contaminant-induced lymphocyte dysfunction, *Environ. Health Perspect.* **39**:105–128.

Silkworth, J. B., and Vecchi, A., 1985, The role of the Ah receptor in halogenated aromatic hydrocarbon immunotoxicity, in: *Immunotoxicology and Immunopharmacology* (J. H. Dean, M. I. Luster, A. E. Munson, and H. A. Amos, eds.), pp. 263–275, Raven, New York.

Silkworth, J. B., Antrim, L., and Grabstein, E. M., 1984, Correlations between polychlorinated biphenyl immunotoxicity. The aromatic hydrocarbon locus, and liver microsomal enzyme induction in C57BL/6 and DBA/2 mice, *Toxicol. Appl. Pharmacol.* **75**:156–165.

Sirois, P., Rola-Pleszczynski, M., and Begin, R., 1980, Phospholipase A activity and prostaglandin synthesis from alveolar macrophages exposed to asbestos, *Prostaglandins Med.* **5**:31–37.

Smith, S. H., Sanders, V. M., Barrett, B. A., Borzelleca, J. F., and Munson, A. E., 1978, Immunotoxicological evaluation on mice exposed to polychlorinated biphenyls, *Toxicol. Appl. Pharmacol.* **45**:336 (abst.).

Smolik, R., Grzybek-Hryncewicz, K., Lange, A., and Zatonski, W., 1973, Serum complement level in workers exposed to benzene, toluene and xylene, *Int. Arch. Arbeitsmed.* **31:**243–247.

Snoeij, N. J., Van Iersel, A. A. J., Penninks, A. H., and Seinen, W., 1986, Triorganotin-induced cytotoxicity to rat thymus, bone marrow, and red blood cells as determined by several *in vitro* assays, *Toxicology* **39:**71–83.

Snoeij, N. J., Penninks, A. H., and Seinen, W., 1987, Toxicity of triorganotin compounds. Species-dependency, dose–effect relationships and kinetics of the thymus atrophy induced by tri- and diorganotin compounds, in press.

Snyder, C. A., Goldstein, B. D., Sellakumar, A. R., Bromberg, I., Laskin, S., and Albert, R. E., 1980, The inhalation toxicology of benzene. Incidence of hematopoietic neoplasms and hematotoxicity in AKR/J and C57BL/6 mice, *Toxicol. Appl. Pharmacol.* **54:**323–331.

Snyder, R., and Kocsis, J. J., 1975, Current concepts of chronic benzene toxicity, *CRC Crit. Rev. Toxicol.* **3:**265–288.

Sone, S., Brennan, L. M., and Creasia, W. A., 1983, *In vivo* and *in vitro* NO_2 exposure enhances phagocytic and tumoricidal activities of rat alveolar macrophages, *J. Toxicol. Environ. Health* **11:**151–163.

Spyker-Cranmer, J. M., Barnett, J., Avery, D. L., and Cranmer, M. F., 1982, Immunoteratology of Chlordane: Cell mediated and humoral immune responses in adult mice exposed in utero, *Toxicol. Appl. Pharmacol.* **62:**402–408.

Stjernsward, J., 1966, Effect of noncarcinogenic and carcinogenic hydrocarbons on antibody forming cells measured at the cellular level, *J. Natl. Cancer Inst.* **36:**1189–1195.

Street, J. C., and Sharma, R. P., 1975, Alteration of induced cellular and humoral immune responses by pesticides and chemicals of environmental concern. Qualitative studies of immunosuppression by DDT, Arochlor 1254, Carbaryl, Carbofuran, and methylparathion, *Toxicol. Appl. Pharmacol.* **32:**587–602.

Talmadge, J. E., Oldham, R. K., and Fidler, I. J., 1984, Practical considerations for the establishment of a screening procedure for the assessment of biological response modifiers, *J. Biol. Response Mod.* **3:**88–109.

Thomas, A. W., Whitting, P. H., and Simpson, J. G., 1984, Cyclosporin: Immunology, toxicity and pharmacology in experimental animals, *Agents Actions* **15:**306–327.

Thomas, P., and Faith, R., 1985, Adult and perinatal immunotoxicity by halogenated aromatic hydrocarbons, in: *Immunotoxicology and Immunopharmacology* (J. H. Dean, M. I. Luster, A. E. Munson, and H. Amos, eds.), pp. 305–313, Raven, New York.

Thomas, P. T., and Hinsdill, R. D., 1978, Effect of polychlorinated biphenyls on the immune responses of Rhesus monkeys and mice, *Toxicol. Appl. Pharmacol.* **44:**41–51.

Tucker, A. N., Vore, S. J., and Luster, M. I., 1986, Suppression of B cell differentiation by 2,3,7,8-tetrachlorodibenzo-*p*-dioxin, *Mol. Pharmacol.* **29:**372–377.

Urso, P., Gengozian, N., Rossi, R. M., and Johnson, R. A., 1986, Suppression of humoral and cell mediated immune responses *in vitro* by benzo(a)pyrene, *J. Immunopharmacol.* **8:**223–241.

Vecchi, A., Sironi, M., Canegrati, M. A., Recchia, M., and Garattini, S., 1983, Immunosuppressive effects of 2,3,7,8-tetrachlorodibenzo-*p*-dioxin in strains of mice with different susceptibility to induction of aryl hydrocarbon hydroxylase, *Toxicol. Appl. Pharmacol.* **68:**434–441.

Vesselinovitch, S. D., Rao, K. V. N., and Mihailovich, N., 1975, Factors modulating benzidine carcinogenicity bioassay, *Cancer Res.* **35:**2814–2819.

Vorwald, A. J., Pratt, P. C., and Urban, E. J., 1955, The production of pulmonary cancer in albino rats exposed by inhalation to an aerosol to beryllium sulfate, *Acta Unio Int. Contra Cancrum* **11:** 735.

Vos, J. G., 1977, Immune suppression as related to toxicology, *CRC Crit. Rev. Toxicol.* **5:**67–101.

Vos, J. G., 1980, Immunotoxicology assessment: Screening and function studies, *Arch. Toxicol.* **4** (suppl.):95–108.

Vos, J. G., and Dean, J. H., 1987, The immune system: Evaluation of methods for immunotoxicity assessment, in: *Proceedings of the SGOMEC Meeting, Health and Welfare, Ottawa, Canada* (in press).

Vos, J. G., and Krajnc, E. I., 1983, Immunotoxicology of pesticides, in: *Developments in the Science and Practice of Toxicology* (A. W. Hayers, R. C. Schnell, and T. S. Miya, eds.), pp. 229–239, Elsevier, New York.

Vos, J. G., and Moore, J. A., 1974, Suppression of cellular immunity in rats and mice by natural treatment with 2,3,7,8-tetrachlorobibenzo-*p*-dioxin, *Int. Arch. Allergy Appl. Immunol.* **47:**777–789.

Vos, J. G., and van Driel Grootenhuis, L., 1972, PCB-induced suppression of the humoral and cell-mediated immunity in guinea pigs, *Sci. Total Environ.* **1:**289–302.

Vos, J. G., Faith, R. E., and Luster, M. I., 1980, Immune alterations, in: *Halogenated Biphenyls, Terphenyls, Napthalenes, Dibenzodioxins, and Related Products* (R. D. Kimbrough, ed.), pp. 241–266, Elsevier, Amsterdam.

Vos, J. G., de Klerk, A., Krajnc, E. I., Kruizinga, W., van Ommen, B., and Rozing, J., 1984, Toxicity of bis(tri-*n*-butyltin) oxide in the rat. II. Suppression of thymus dependent immune responses and of parameters of nonspecific resistance after short term exposure, *Toxicol. Appl. Pharmacol.* **75:**387–408.

Vos, J. G., Krajnc, E. I., and Wester, P. W., 1985, Immunotoxicity of bis(tri-*n*-butyltin) oxide, in: *Immunotoxicology and immunopharmacology* (J. H. Dean, M. I. Luster, A. E. Munson, and H. Amos, eds.), pp. 327–340, Raven, New York.

Wade, M. J., Lipkin, L. E., Stanton, M. F., and Frank, A. L., 1980, P338D1 *in vitro* cytotoxicity assay as applied to asbestos and other minerals. Its possible relevance to carcinogenesis, in: *The In Vitro Effects of Mineral Dusts* (R. C. Brown, I. P., Gormly, M. Chamberlain, and R. Davis, eds.), pp. 351–357, Academic, London.

Ward, E. C., Murray, M. J., Lauer, L. D., House, R. V., Irons, R., and Dean, J. H., 1984, Immunosuppression following 7,12-dimethylbenzanthracene exposure in B6C3F1 mice. I. Effects on humoral immunity and host resistance, *Toxicol. Appl. Pharmacol.* **75:**299–308.

Ward, E. C., Murray, M. J., and Dean, J. H., 1985, Immunotoxicity of nonhalogenated polycyclic aromatic hydrocarbons, in: *Immunotoxicology and immunopharmacology* (J. H. Dean, M. I. Luster, A. E. Munson, and H. Amos, eds.), pp. 291–304, Raven, New York.

Ward, E. C., Murray, M. J., Lauer, L. D., House, R. V., and Dean, J. H., 1986, Persistent suppression of humoral and cell mediated immunity in mice following exposure to the polycyclic aromatic hydrocarbon 7,12-dimethylbenzanthracene, *Int. J. Immunopharmacol.* **8:**13–22.

White, K. L., and Munson, A. E., 1986, Suppression of the *in vitro* humoral immune response by chrysotile asbestos, *Toxicol. Appl. Pharmacol.* **82:**493–504.

White, K. L., Lysy, H. H., and Holsapple, M. P., 1985, Immunosuppression by polycyclic aromatic hydrocarbons: A structure–activity relationship in B6C3F1 and DBA/2 mice, *Immunopharmacology* **9:**155–164.

White, W. C., and Gammon, A. M., 1914, The influence of benzol inhalations on experimental pulmonary tuberculosis in rabbits, *Trans. Assoc. Am. Physicians* **29:**332–337.

Wierda, D., and Irons, R. D., 1982, Hydroquinone and catechol reduce the frequency of progenitor B lymphocytes in mouse spleen and bone marrow, *Immunopharmacology* **4:**41–54.

Wierda, D., Irons, R. D., and Greenlee, W. F., 1981, Immunotoxicity in C57Bl/6 mice exposed to benzene and Aroclor 1254, *Toxicol. Appl. Pharmacol.* **60:**410–417.

Williams, W. R., and Jones-Williams, W., 1982, Development of beryllium lymphocyte transformation tests in chronic beryllium disease, *Int. Arch. Allergy* **67:**175–180.

Winternitz, M. C., and Hirschfelder, A. D., 1913, Studies upon experimental pneumonia in rabbits, I–III. *J. Exp. Med.* **17:**657–665.

Wojdani, A., and Alfred, L. J., 1984, Alterations in cell mediated immune functions induced in mouse splenic lymphocytes by polycyclic aromatic hydrocarbons, *Cancer Res.* **44:**942–945.

Wu, J. C., Lu, Y. C., Kao, H. Y., Pan, C. C., and Lin, R. Y., 1984, Cell-mediated immunity in patients with polychlorinated biphenyl poisoning, *J. Formosa Med. Assoc.* **83:**419–429.

Zedeck, M. S., 1980, Polycyclic aromatic hydrocarbons: A review, *J. Environ. Pathol. Toxicol.* **3:**537–567.

INDEX